Resilience and Mental Health: Challenges Across the Lifespan

Resilience and Mental Health

Challenges Across the Lifespan

Edited by

Steven M. Southwick
Yale University School of Medicine, New Haven

Brett T. Litz
Boston University School of Medicine, Boston

Dennis Charney
The Mount Sinai School of Medicine, New York

Matthew J. Friedman
Dartmouth University School of Medicine, White River Junction

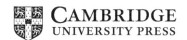
CAMBRIDGE
UNIVERSITY PRESS

CAMBRIDGE
UNIVERSITY PRESS

University Printing House, Cambridge CB2 8BS, United Kingdom

One Liberty Plaza, 20th Floor, New York, NY 10006, USA

477 Williamstown Road, Port Melbourne, VIC 3207, Australia

4843/24, 2nd Floor, Ansari Road, Daryaganj, Delhi - 110002, India

79 Anson Road, #06-04/06, Singapore 079906

Cambridge University Press is part of the University of Cambridge.

It furthers the University's mission by disseminating knowledge in the pursuit of education, learning and research at the highest international levels of excellence.

www.cambridge.org
Information on this title: www.cambridge.org/9780521898393

© Cambridge University Press 2011

First published 2011
3rd printing 2014

A catalogue record for this publication is available from the British Library

Library of Congress Cataloging in Publication data
Resilience and mental health: challenges across the lifespan / [edited by]
    Steven M. Southwick ... [et al.].
        p. ; cm.
    Includes bibliographical references and index.
    ISBN 978-0-521-89839-3 (hardback)
    1. Mental health.   2. Stress (Psychology)   3. Adaptability (Psychology)
    I. Southwick, Steven M.   II. Title. [DNLM: 1. Mental Health.   2. Resilience,
    Psychological.   3. Adaptation, Psychological.   4. Stress Disorders,
    Traumatic–prevention & control.   5. Stress, Psychological–psychology. WM 105]
    RA790.R447 2011
    616.89–dc23   2011016713

ISBN 978-0-521-89839-3 Hardback

....

Every effort has been made in preparing this book to provide accurate and up-to-date information which is in accord with accepted standards and practice at the time of publication. Although case histories are drawn from actual cases, every effort has been made to disguise the identities of the individuals involved. Nevertheless, the authors, editors and publishers can make no warranties that the information contained herein is totally free from error, not least because clinical standards are constantly changing through research and regulation. The authors, editors and publishers therefore disclaim all liability for direct or consequential damages resulting from the use of material contained in this book. Readers are strongly advised to pay careful attention to information provided by the manufacturer of any drugs or equipment that they plan to use.

Contents

List of contributors   *page* vii
Preface   xi

Section 1   Pathways to resilience   1
Section editor: Brett T. Litz

1   **Neurobiology of resilience**   1
Adriana Feder, Dennis Charney, and Kate Collins

2   **Resilience in the face of stress: emotion regulation as a protective factor**   30
Allison S. Troy and Iris B. Mauss

3   **Cognitive factors and resilience: how self-efficacy contributes to coping with adversities**   45
Charles C. Benight and Roman Cieslak

4   **Personality factors in resilience to traumatic stress**   56
Mark W. Miller and Kelly M. Harrington

5   **Social ties and resilience in chronic disease**   76
Denise Janicki-Deverts and Sheldon Cohen

6   **Religious and spiritual factors in resilience**   90
David W. Foy, Kent D. Drescher, and Patricia J. Watson

Section 2   Resilience across the lifespan   103
Section editor: Dennis Charney

7   **Resilience in children and adolescents**   103
Ann S. Masten, Amy R. Monn, and Laura M. Supkoff

8   **Toward a lifespan approach to resilience and potential trauma**   120
George A. Bonanno and Anthony D. Mancini

9   **Resilience in older adults**   135
Diane L. Elmore, Lisa M. Brown, and Joan M. Cook

Section 3   Resilience in families, communities, and societies   149
Section editor: Fran H. Norris

10   **Family resilience: a collaborative approach in response to stressful life challenges**   149
Froma Walsh

11   **Community resilience: concepts, assessment, and implications for intervention**   162
Fran H. Norris, Kathleen Sherrieb, and Betty Pfefferbaum

12   **Trauma, culture, and resiliency**   176
Carl C. Bell

Section 4   Specific challenges   189
Section editor: Matthew J. Friedman

13   **Loss and grief: the role of individual differences**   189
Anthony D. Mancini and George A. Bonanno

14   **Reorienting resilience: adapting resilience for post-disaster research**   200
Jennifer Johnson and Sandro Galea

15   **Rape and other sexual assault**   218
Heidi S. Resnick, Constance Guille, Jenna L. McCauley, and Dean G. Kilpatrick

16   **The stress continuum model: a military organizational approach to resilience and recovery**   238
William P. Nash, Maria Steenkamp, Lauren Conoscenti, and Brett T. Litz

17   **Resilience in the face of terrorism: linking resource investment with engagement**   253
Stevan E. Hobfoll, Brian Hall, Katie J. Horsey, and Brittain E. Lamoureux

18 **Resilience in the context of poverty** 264
John C. Buckner and Jessica S. Waters

19 **Resiliency in individuals with serious mental illness** 276
Piper S. Meyer and Kim T. Mueser

Section 5 Training for resilience 289
Section editor: Steven M. Southwick

20 **Interventions to enhance resilience and resilience-related constructs in adults** 289
Steven M. Southwick, Robert H. Pietrzak, and Gerald White

21 **Childhood resilience: adaptation, mastery, and attachment** 307
Angie Torres, Steven M. Southwick, and Linda C. Mayes

22 **Military mental health training: building resilience** 323
Carl Andrew Castro and Amy B. Adler

23 **Public health practice and disaster resilience: a framework integrating resilience as a worker protection strategy** 340
Dori B. Reissman, Kathleen M. Kowalski-Trakofler, and Craig L. Katz

Index 359

Contributors

Amy B. Adler
Clinical Research Psychologist and Chief of Science, US Army Medical Research Unit, Europe, Walter Reed Army Institute of Research, Heidelberg, Germany

Carl C. Bell
President/CEO, Community Mental Health Council, Inc. and Clinical Professor of Psychiatry and Public Health, University of Illinois, Chicago, IL, USA

Charles C. Benight
Department of Psychology and Trauma, Health, and Hazards Center, University of Colorado, Colorado Springs, CO, USA

George A. Bonanno
Professor of Education and Psychology, Teachers College, Columbia University, New York, USA

Lisa M. Brown
Associate Professor, Department of Aging and Mental Health, University of South Florida, Tampa, FL, USA

John C. Buckner
Staff Scientist, Department of Psychiatry, Children's Hospital Boston, Boston, MA, USA

Carl Andrew Castro
Director, Military Operational Medicine Research Program, US Army Medical Research and Material Command, Fort Detrick, MD, USA

Dennis Charney
Dean and Professor of Psychiatry, Neuroscience and Pharmacology and Systems Therapeutics, Mount Sinai School of Medicine, New York, USA

Roman Cieslak
Department of Psychology, Warsaw School of Social Psychology and Trauma, Health, and Hazards Center, University of Colorado, Colorado Springs, CO, USA

Sheldon Cohen
Director of the Laboratory for the Study of Stress, Immunity and Disease, Carnegie Mellon University, Pittsburgh, PA, USA

Kate Collins
Graduate Assistant, Mount Sinai School of Medicine, New York, USA

Lauren Conoscenti
National Center for PTSD, VA Boston Healthcare System and Boston University, Boston, MA

Joan M. Cook
Assistant Professor, Psychiatry, Yale School of Medicine and National Center for PTSD, West Haven, CT, USA

Kent D. Drescher
Health Science Specialist, Palo Alto VA Healthcare System and National Center for PTSD, Menlo Park, CA, USA

Diane L. Elmore
Associate Executive Director, Public Interest Government Relations Office, American Psychological Association, Washington, DC, USA

Adriana Feder
Assistant Professor, Psychiatry, Mount Sinai School of Medicine, New York, USA

David W. Foy
Professor, Department of Psychology, GSEP-Pepperdine University, Encino, CA, USA

Matthew J. Friedman
Professor of Psychiatry and of Pharmacology and Toxicology and Executive Director of the National Center for Posttraumatic Stress Disorder, US Department of Veterans Affairs, Dartmouth Medical School, White River Junction, VT, USA

Sandro Galea
Gelman Professor, Department of Epidemiology, Mailman School of Public Health, Columbia University, New York, USA

Constance Guille
Clinical Instructor of Psychiatry, National Crime Victims Research and Treatment Center, Medical University of South Carolina, Charleston, SC, USA

Brian Hall
Research Study Coordinator, Rush Medical College and Kent State University, Kent, OH, USA

Kelly M. Harrington
VA Boston Healthcare System, National Center for PTSD and Division of Psychiatry, Boston University School of Medicine, Boston, MA, USA

Stevan E. Hobfoll
Professor and Chairperson, Department of Behavioral Sciences, Rush Medical College, Chicago, IL, USA

Katie J. Horsey
Kent State University, Kent, OH, USA

Denise Janicki-Deverts
Research Fellow, Carnegie Mellon University, Pittsburgh, PA, USA

Jennifer Johnson
Research Assistant, Center for Global Health, University of Michigan, Ann Arbor, MI, USA

Craig L. Katz
Disaster Psychiatry Outreach and Department of Psychiatry, Mount Sinai School of Medicine, New York, USA

Dean G. Kilpatrick
Director, National Crime Victims Research and Treatment Center and Vice Chair for Education, Psychiatry, Medical University of South Carolina, Charleston, SC, USA

Kathleen M. Kowalski-Trakofler
Pittsburgh Research Laboratory, Office of Mining Safety and Health Research, National Institute for Occupational Safety and Health, US Centers for Disease Control and Prevention, Pittsburgh, PA, USA

Brittain E. Lamoureux
Kent State University, Kent, OH, USA

Brett T. Litz
Massachusetts Veterans Epidemiological Research and Information Center, National Center for PTSD, VA Boston Healthcare System and Boston University, Boston, MA, USA

Anthony D. Mancini
Teachers College, Columbia University, New York, USA

Ann S. Masten
Distinguished McKnight University Professor, University of Minnesota, Minneapolis, MN, USA

Iris B. Mauss
Assistant Professor, Department of Psychology, University of Denver, Denver, CO, USA

Linda C. Mayes
Chair of the Directorial Team at the Anna Freud Centre, London and Arnold Gesell Professor of Child Psychiatry and Psychology, Yale Child Study Center, New Haven, CT, USA

Jenna L. McCauley
Instructor, Psychiatry and Behavioral Sciences, National Crime Victims Research and Treatment Center, Medical University of South Carolina, Charleston, SC, USA

Piper S. Meyer
Department of Psychology, University of North Carolina at Chapel Hill, Chapel Hill, NC, USA

Mark W. Miller
VA Boston Healthcare System, National Center for PTSD and Division of Psychiatry, Boston University School of Medicine, Boston, MA, USA

Amy R. Monn
Researcher, University of Minnesota, Minneapolis, MN, USA

Kim T. Mueser
Departments of Psychiatry and of Community and Family Medicine, Dartmouth Psychiatric Research Center, Concord, NH, USA

William P. Nash

Captain, Medical Corps, US Navy (Retired), VA San Diego Healthcare System, and University of California, San Diego, CA, USA

Fran H. Norris

Research Professor of Psychiatry and of Community and Family Medicine, Department of Veterans Affairs National Center for PTSD and National Consortium for the Study of Terrorism and Responses to Terrorism, Dartmouth Medical School, White River Junction, VT, USA

Betty Pfefferbaum

National Consortium for the Study of Terrorism and Responses to Terrorism, National Child Traumatic Stress Network of the Terrorism and Disaster Center, University of Oklahoma Health Sciences Center, Oklahoma City, OK, USA

Robert H. Pietrzak

Assistant Professor of Psychiatry, Yale University School of Medicine, New Haven, CT, USA

Dori B. Reissman

Office of the Director, National Institute for Occupational Safety and Health, US Centers for Disease Control and Prevention and Commissioned Medical Corps of the US Public Health Service, Washington DC, USA

Heidi S. Resnick

Professor, National Crime Victims Research and Treatment Center, Charleston, SC, USA

Kathleen Sherrieb

Department of Veterans Affairs National Center for PTSD and National Consortium for the Study of Terrorism and Responses to Terrorism, Dartmouth Medical School, White River Junction, VT, USA

Steven M. Southwick

Professor, Yale University School of Medicine National Center for Posttraumatic Stress Disorder, and VA Connecticut Healthcare System, New Haven, CT, USA

Maria Steenkamp

Clinical Psychology, Boston University, Boston, MA, USA

Laura M. Supkoff

Researcher, University of Minnesota, Minneapolis, MN, USA

Angie Torres

Postdoctoral Fellow, Yale Child Study Center, New Haven, CT, USA

Allison S. Troy

Department of Psychology, University of Denver, Denver, CO, USA

Froma Walsh

Firestone Professor Emerita and Co-Director of the Chicago Center for Family Health, University of Chicago, Chicago, IL, USA

Jessica S. Waters

Research Assistant, Department of Psychiatry, Children's Hospital Boston, Boston, MA, USA

Patricia J. Watson

National Center for PTSD and VA Medical and Regional Office Center, White River Junction, VT, USA

Gerald White

Co-founder, Survivor Corps, Washington, DC, USA

Preface

Humans are remarkably resilient in the face of crises, traumas, disabilities, attachment losses, and ongoing adversities. In fact, resilience to stress and trauma may be the norm rather than the exception. However, to date, most research in the field of traumatic stress has focused on neurobiological, psychological, and social factors associated with trauma-related psychopathology and deficits in psychosocial functioning. While much has been learned in these areas of research, particularly about post-traumatic stress disorder (PTSD), far less is known about resilience to stress and healthy adaptation to stress and trauma.

The study of resilience is enormously challenging. The first hurdle involves definition. Currently, there is no single agreed-upon definition of resilience in the clinical or scientific literature. In a review of the published literature on risk, vulnerability, resistance, and resilience, Layne and colleagues (2007) described the lack of precision and numerous terminological inconsistencies in the meanings of these concepts, and identified at least eight distinct meanings for the term "resilience." For example, definitions of resilience have ranged from symptom-free functioning following trauma exposure (Bonanno *et al.*, 2006) to positive adaptation despite adversity (Garmezy, 1993), and even to enhanced psychobiological regulation of stress/fear-related brain circuitry, neurotransmitters, and hormones (Charney, 2004). The American Psychological Association (2010) has defined resilience as "the process of adapting well in the face of adversity, trauma, tragedy, threats or even significant sources of threat."

Further complicating the study of resilience is the notion that resilience can be conceptualized as an *outcome* in the face of stress and trauma or as a *process* that mediates the response to stress and trauma. Examples of resilience as an outcome include symptom-free functioning (defined as "resistance" by some researchers); not meeting criteria for PTSD following traumatic exposure; developing symptoms of trauma-related psychopathology, but recovering from those symptoms (often called "recovery"); and functioning well in spite of trauma-related psychopathology (functional resilience). Clearly these outcome-related definitions of resilience differ markedly from one another.

Process-oriented definitions of resilience include cognitions, emotional reactions, and behaviors that are adaptive in response to stress and trauma. For example, active coping and seeking social support have been described as resilient processes that facilitate resistance to, or recovery from, traumatic stressors. Other processes shown to be adaptive in relation to stress and trauma include the capacity to generate positive emotions, to accept that which cannot be changed, and to reframe the negative into positive.

Resilience is multidimensional in nature. Consequently, people who are faced with adversity can exhibit competence in some domains but not others. For example, traumatized adults may demonstrate resilience in areas such as work but falter in other areas such as family relationships. Typically at-risk or resilient individuals display an unevenness of functioning across domains. As noted by Masten and colleagues (Chapter 7), it is unrealistic to expect that anyone, no matter how resilient, will consistently perform at a uniformly high or low level across all areas of their life. Consequently, some researchers define resilience as excellence in one salient domain with at least average adjustment in other domains.

In some cases resilience and related constructs have been viewed as enduring because they are believed to be present even when the individual is not challenged by stress. In other cases, factors associated with resilience have been referred to as risk-activated moderating factors because they only become fully activated when the individual is challenged. Masten offers the analogy of an automobile airbag that inflates during a collision but not during everyday driving. For example, some forms of social support, such as assistance by emergency personnel and social services, may only become activated in the immediate aftermath of a traumatic event.

In addition to being multidimensional, resilience is dynamic rather than static. Resilience trajectories may be uneven, with some people demonstrating resilience at one age but not another, or in one circumstance but not another. Some researchers have conceptualized resilience as one of a set of possible trajectories following severe stress or trauma. For example, Norris and colleagues (2009) analyzed two population-based longitudinal datasets that were collected after the terror attacks of September 11, 2001 and the 1999 floods in Mexico and found five different symptom trajectories among study participants. They specifically differentiated what they called resilience (i.e., initial moderate or severe symptoms followed by a sharp decrease) from resistance (i.e., no symptoms or mild and stable symptoms) and recovery (i.e., initially moderate or severe symptoms followed by a gradual decrease).

Resilient processes are not strictly intrapsychic and biological; rather they reflect the transaction or interaction between the person and his or her environment. For example, stressful events are processed through perception and subjective appraisal, which, in turn, moderates impact. The subsequent response (e.g., a coping behavior) to the stressor is shaped and constrained by environmental (e.g., social supports) as well as personal (e.g., biological) factors and resources. The individual who adapts to stress does not do so in isolation but rather in the context of available resources, other human beings, families, specific cultures and religions, organizations, and communities and societies, all of which adapt to challenges as well.

Stresses and losses can hamper or reduce resources that would otherwise be employed to manage and recover from stressors. For example, death of a loved one can greatly constrain social and relational resources when those providing solace and support to others must also cope with his/her own grief and loss. Stress can also adversely affect sleep and wellness behaviors that are needed to restore biological, psychological, and functional capacities.

Readers should bear in mind that the type and degree of stress and trauma typically have a marked impact on resilience processes and outcomes. At the extreme end of stress and trauma, even the best trained elite athletes, professionals, and warriors have a limit beyond which they can no longer function adequately, at least for a period of time.

This edited textbook on resilience has brought together experts from a broad array of scientific fields whose research has focused on adaptive responses to stress. The chapters, which are organized into five sections, summarize the current literature on the adaptive responses to stress from various relevant fields and domains.

Section 1 introduces the reader to state of the art advances in theory and empirical research on pathways to resilience, approaching this discussion from multiple perspectives. Decades of research on mental disorders, psychosomatic disease, and abnormalities in social behavior have led to advances in our understanding of the biological, psychological, and social processes and mechanisms that are associated with enduring distress and malfunction in the face of stress and trauma. The ultimate value of the study of pathways to resilience is to develop universal, selective, and targeted programs to prevent damaging responses to stress and adversity in at-risk groups.

The pathways to resilience and positive outcomes after exposure to stress are multidimensional and multisystemic and typically require complex multivariate modeling. The study of human resilience also requires an interdisciplinary approach, which has been rare in this relatively young field. Nevertheless, the chapters in this section will help the reader to appreciate the state of the art advances in theory and empirical research pertaining to different perspectives of pathways to resilience, which is a good starting place toward the goal of developing a more paradigmatic and interdisciplinary approach. The chapters review the full range of salutogenic factors that moderate and mediate the relationship between exposure to acute stress, trauma, and chronic adversity and the multidimensional outcomes (biological, spiritual, social, behavioral, and cognitive). These include neurobehavioral and neurohormonal factors, social and interpersonal variables, spiritual practices, social cognition, emotion regulation strategies, and personality variables.

Section 2 examines developmental determinants of resilience across the lifespan, from infancy to old age. Although there are both conceptual differences and similarities in the concept of resilience across the lifespan, there is little research comparing responses to traumatic stress as a function of development. What information that does exist suggests that children cope as well as, if not better than, adults. Furthermore, factors such as attachment relationships, social support, religion, intelligence and problem-solving ability, and cognitive flexibility promote resilience in both children and adults.

Scientists interested in human resilience are beginning to study much larger systems, at the level of society, culture, and government to enhance adaptive responses to traumas, such as natural disasters or pandemics, where many systems are involved that impact resilience in individuals, families, and communities. However, a great deal of work remains to fully understand how resilience can be facilitated throughout life. Further investigation is needed to determine the best methods for fostering resilience in children, adults, and the elderly. Resilience is multifaceted and the interplay needs to be better understood among a number of variables including type and severity of trauma, genetic predisposition, psychosocial context, personality, social support and relationships, family, community, and culture. Ultimately, the goal is to identify a personalized roadmap to help people of all ages to maintain and enhance resilience and experience personal growth in the face of the challenges of daily life, stressful life events, and major traumas.

Section 3 describes the impact of social context, in the form of family, community and society, on adaptation to adversity. Since the earliest days of research on human resilience, it has been understood that individuals are embedded in social networks that can augment or undermine their capacity to thrive in the face of adversity. The resilience of children, for example, depends highly on the strength of their bonds with parents and others who nurture their development. Ecologies of human behavior are often portrayed as nested systems that exert increasingly complex layers of influence (Bronfenbrenner, 1977). *Microsystems* are the primary settings, such as families, schools, and places of work; *mesosystems* are intersecting microsystems; and *macrosystems* are the matrices of rules, laws, and cultural norms that shape the nature of society's political, economic, legal, and educational systems.

Together capturing such an ecological perspective on resilience, the three chapters in Section 3 summarize current knowledge about the influences of family, community, and culture on individual well-being. Beyond this, these chapters explore the resilience of families and societies themselves. The family, for example, is more than just a resource for individual resilience but is itself a functional unit that may exhibit resilience as a whole. Varied and evolving family structures and life courses create challenges and opportunities for resilience.

In the face of collective stressors, such as disasters, survivors are connected and dependent upon one another's coping strategies, and individual resilience, as well as family resilience, is inextricably linked to the community's ability to prepare for, respond to, and adapt to adverse conditions. Furthermore, just as individuals and families are embedded in communities, so too are communities embedded in larger systems of influence. Among the most important of these is culture. Recovery from trauma involves the reconstruction of meaning, and constructs of meaning are inseparable from culture. Culture exerts a strong influence on the multitude of protective factors discussed throughout this text, including personality, optimism, cognitive styles and attributions, worldview, social support, beliefs about illness and health, and healing practices.

The chapters in Section 4 focus on challenges to resilience when dealing with specific adversities, including loss and grief, disasters, rape and assault, combat, terrorism, poverty, and chronic mental illness. Previous sections of this book have addressed general cross-cutting attributes of resilience that would be applicable to almost any situation. In addition, however, there are specific skill sets that may be useful in some contexts, but not in others. In this section, the reader learns how different challenges demand more specific manifestations of resilience. In short, the different challenges posed by bereavement, disasters, rape, combat, terrorism, poverty, and chronic mental illness appear to require different, and more context-specific, expressions of resilience. For example, as with service men and women returning from Iraq and Afghanistan, what constitutes adaptive and resilient behavior in a war zone may be dysfunctional or disruptive in a post-deployment, marital, or domestic context. Resilience following bereavement or rape may also be different, in some respects, than resilience in coping with poverty or chronic mental illness.

In Section 4 the reader learns that even in the context of painful loss, the bereaved retain a capacity for generative experiences, positive emotions, and the capacity to derive comfort from others while overcoming loss. Section 4 also considers that resilience, in the face of disasters, is expressed at the individual, family, and community level, and that resilience evaluations need to accommodate these various contexts, ideally synergistically and comprehensively.

The challenges associated with coming to terms with sexual assault are enormous. Section 4 describes the advantages of using approach-oriented coping strategies for this group of survivors, and points out that these strategies are at the core of early interventions designed to promote recovery and resilience.

Terrorism presents yet another special challenge to the modern world. Resilient responses or variables that indicate successful navigation of these challenges are discussed in the context of *conservation of resources and engagement theory*, where resilience is characterized by "engagement" (i.e., a persistent, pervasive, and positive affect-motivational state), "dedication" (i.e., a commitment to key life tasks), "absorption" (i.e., the sense of full involvement and excitement over life tasks), and "vigor" (i.e., high levels of energy and mental resilience when meeting life challenge). Resilience in the face of combat and operational experiences during war also requires a unique vantage point and conceptual framework, where operational resilience (e.g., successful performance, mission readiness) needs to be distinguished from psychological resilience.

Resilience in the context of poverty, which is an enduring source of adversity, powerlessness, stress, and limited opportunities for personal and social advancement is both complex and understudied. In Section 4, the reader learns that poverty should be studied at the individual and community level. For individuals, resilience is understood as self-regulation and adaptive flexibility in the service of goal-directed behavior. At the community level, this translates into social cohesion and collective efficacy.

Finally, Section 4 discusses methods that may be used to mobilize resilience and optimize functional capacity among individuals with chronic mental illness. Using a recovery model, which eschews the traditional psychopathology model, the focus of these methods is on improving well-being through empowerment and enhancement of autonomous function.

As these chapters attest, although resilience consists of general attributes that serve individuals well in almost any context, there are also very specific expressions of resilience that are context dependent and that may require different sets of adaptive capacity. Mental toughening and combat readiness for a marine may require different biopsychosocial capabilities than the coping strategies needed by a recently raped individual, than acquisition of social capital by an impoverished inner city youth, or than the capacity to generate positive emotions by a homeless individual with chronic schizophrenia.

The final section brings together what is currently known about enhancing resilience and includes chapters specifically devoted to children, military members, and disaster workers. While much is known about cognitive styles, emotions, and behaviors of children and adults who adapt well in the face of adversity, to date, there have been relatively few methodologically rigorous investigations of actual strategies and techniques designed to enhance resilience.

Some resilience-enhancing interventions have been developed to strengthen coping skills in stress- and trauma-exposed individuals, both with and without psychiatric disorders. Others focus on preventing the development of stress- and trauma-related morbidity. While most resilience-enhancing programs have been designed for specific at-risk populations (e.g., firefighters, police, military personnel), some are more general in nature. Other relevant interventions include those that have not specifically been designed to enhance resilience but that enhance aspects of functioning, such as optimism and social support, which are known to be associated with resilience.

Children, in general, are remarkably resilient. Their resilience develops as a set of abilities and processes including positive attachment, the capacity to attract social support, self-motivating rewards critical for mastery and self-efficacy, effective modulation of the stress response, and successful monitoring and regulation of emotions. These abilities and processes form the foundation for resilience in adulthood. As with adults, stress tends to enhance resilience so long as the stress is manageable and not overwhelming. Interventions designed to enhance resilience must address capacities and skills that are appropriate to the physical, emotional, and cognitive maturity of the child.

The specific approach to resilience training often depends on anticipated stressors. Consequently, resilience training for a prospective fireman will differ from training for a prospective humanitarian worker. For example, the US Army Battlemind Training System, a mental health resilience-building program, is specifically designed to prepare service members for the mental challenges of training, operations, combat, and transitioning home. It addresses military-specific concerns about relevance, practicality, utility, user acceptability, and stigma.

When evaluating public health practices to enhance disaster resilience, it is important to adopt an ecological framework that addresses interdependencies between people and the contexts in which they respond. Therefore, it is useful to consider a wide range of interventions including engineering design; safety codes and standards; legislation; land use management; interagency planning and coordination; public education; leadership training; worker training; medical, emotional, and cognitive readiness; regulation of operational tempo and degree of worker exposure; as well as close monitoring of medical and psychological status of those who have been exposed to the disaster.

In future efforts to develop effective interventions to enhance resilience, it will be important to address a number of critical questions. Is the intervention designed to be administered prior to stress and trauma exposure as a means to prevent trauma-related morbidity or is it designed to enhance resilience in survivors of trauma? Is the intervention designed for a specific population and a specific type of stressor? What skills and strengths will be targeted for development by the intervention? Is there sufficient scientific evidence to support the association between these skills and resilience, and how will mastery of these skills be assessed? Will the intervention be most effective using a classroom-based model or a scenario-based model? What are the most appropriate control groups? What are the most relevant outcome measures for the intervention? These are just some of the critical issues that will need to be addressed in order to further advance interventions designed to enhance resilience.

In summary, each of the five sections in this edited textbook examine adaptive responses to trauma, spanning from factors that contribute to and promote resilience, to populations and societal systems in which resilience is employed, to specific applications and contexts of resilience, and interventions designed to better enhance resilience. The reader is reminded that this textbook aims to review relevant concepts pertaining to adaptive responses to trauma, but that just as resilience continually changes and adapts for each individual and context, the study of resilience is continually changing and improving as scientists and researchers learn more.

References

American Psychological Association (2010). *The road to resilience*. Washington, DC: American Psychological Association, http://www.apa.org/helpcenter/road-resilience.aspx (accessed June 25, 2010).

Bonanno, G. A., Galea, S., Bucciarelli, A., & Vlahov, D. (2006). Psychological resilience after disaster: New York City in the aftermath of the September 11th terrorist attack. *Psychological Science*, **17**, 181–186.

Bronfenbrenner, U. (1977). Toward an experimental ecology of human development. *American Psychologist*, **32**, 513–531.

Charney, D. S. (2004). Psychobiological mechanisms of resilience and vulnerability: implications for successful adaptation to extreme stress. *American Journal of Psychiatry*, **161**, 195–216.

Garmezy, N. (1993). Children in poverty: resilience despite risk. *Psychiatry: Interpersonal and Biological Processes*, **56**, 127–136.

Layne, C. M., Warren, J. S., Watson, P. J., & Shalev, A. Y. (2007). Risk, vulnerability, resistance, and resilience: toward an integrative conceptualization of posttraumatic adaptation. In T. K. M. Friedman & P. Resick (eds.), *Handbook of PTSD: Science and practice* (pp. 497–520). New York: Guilford Press.

Norris, F. H., Tracy, M., & Galea, S. (2009). Looking for resilience: understanding the longitudinal trajectories of responses to stress. *Social Science and Medicine*, **68**, 2190–2198.

Neurobiology of resilience

Adriana Feder, Dennis Charney, and Kate Collins

Introduction

Resilience is commonly conceptualized as the ability to adapt and thrive despite experiencing adversity (Masten *et al.*, 1995; Elder, 1998; Masten & Coatsworth, 1998). A resilient individual has been tested (Rutter, 2006) and continues to demonstrate healthy psychological and physiological stress responses (McEwen, 2003; Charney, 2004). For most, it is possible to conjure an image of such a person: a woman who chooses to work with sexual assault survivors after she herself is raped; a child growing up in poverty who earns a scholarship to college; a hurricane survivor who rebuilds her own home and helps to revitalize her community.

For over three decades, scientists have worked to identify the states and traits characteristic of resilience, with the aim of developing more effective and more diverse evidence-based prophylactic and treatment interventions to combat the deleterious impact of stress on human body and brain. While the value of understanding the neurobiological substrates of resilience has always been appreciated, the lack of tools available to assess the integrity of neural structure and function has impeded progress. Hence, early research on resilience focused on illuminating the psychological and social determinants of stress resistance (Rutter, 1985; Masten & Coatsworth, 1998; Masten, 2001; Bonanno, 2004).

While recent advances in scientific technology have made the exploration of biological processes associated with resilient phenotypes more feasible, it remains constrained by reliance on behavioral observations and self-report to identify resilient individuals. Because we have very few direct measures of neural health, a person's descriptions of his or her internal experience and the degree of functional impairment observed must serve as its proxy. Hence, it is not surprising that researchers have had difficulty operationalizing resilience on a neurobiological level. Some neuroscientists have focused on the capacity to experience stress without developing mental illness (Conrad & Hammen, 1989; Tiet *et al.*, 1998; New *et al.*, 2009); others have placed less emphasis on the development of psychiatric symptoms and, instead, focus on the ability to recover from a mental illness with (or without) treatment (Nitschke *et al.*, 2009).

We believe that a different archetype will be necessary as neuroscience progresses and scientists come to define neural health with increasingly accurate biological assays, and become less dependent on behavioral measures. In order to articulate the formulation of resilience employed in this chapter, we return to its original meaning as defined by physicists: the capability of an object to resume its original size and shape after deformation. While maintaining a clear parallel with the definition of resilience utilized in psychosocial investigation, this signification is more easily translated into a neurobiological model: acute adaptations in neural systems in response to stress constitute deformation, and the ability of those systems to resume optimal or pre-stress operations is resilience.

Allostasis and resilience

Homeostasis is the maintenance of the small set of physiological states that must be rigidly preserved to ensure survival. Even minute changes in variables such as temperature, osmolarity, pH, or oxygen tension will result in death. In contrast, a multitude of other parameters can be, and often are, altered. Such modifications constitute the body's efforts to respond to and counteract stressors that could disturb homeostasis. Sterling and Eyer (1988) introduced the term allostasis to describe this dynamic regulation of secondary

Table 1.1 Key terminology.

Term	Definition
Homeostasis	Maintenance of those states essential to survival (pH, osmolarity, temperature, oxygen tension, etc.)
Stress	Stimulus or stimuli that threaten homeostasis
Allostasis	Dynamic regulation of non-essential set-points in response to stress in order to preserve critical variables
Allostatic load	The damage the body incurs as a result of allostasis
Resilience	The degree to which the body is able to minimize allostatic load

set-points in defense of homeostasis. Subsequently, McEwen and Stellar (1993) observed that, while essential to survival, any allostatic deviation from the optimal internal milieu takes a toll on the body. They coined the phrase "allostatic load" to refer to the physiological cost of adaptation to stressors. In this context, the severity of the allostatic load, as a measure of the brain's *in*ability to resume its pre-allostatic state, is inversely proportional to the degree of resilience. That is, resilience is the capacity to minimize allostatic load. Table 1.1 summarizes these definitions.

In this chapter, we begin by reviewing the systems most directly involved in the acute stress response, highlighting both their contribution to allostasis and their allostatic load. The genetic, physiological, psychological, and environmental factors that appear to contain allostatic load and, therefore, promote resilience are also delineated. Subsequently, we describe other variables whose allostatic role is less clear but are known to modulate the intensity and efficacy of the acute processes and, therefore, to influence resilience. We conclude with a discussion of emerging integrated models of resilience and the potential applications of this work.

Acute stress-response systems

The hypothalamic–pituitary–adrenal axis

The hypothalamic–pituitary–adrenal (HPA) axis, composed of the hypothalamus, pituitary, and adrenal glands, is the primary mechanism responsible for coordinating the body's response to stress. When a stimulus is perceived as threatening, the paraventricular nucleus of the hypothalamus releases corticotropin-releasing hormone (CRH) and arginine-vasopressin into the portal vessels. These subsequently trigger the production and secretion of adrenocorticotropic hormone (ACTH) from the anterior lobe of the pituitary.

This, in turn, stimulates increases in the production and release of the glucocorticoids cortisol and dehydroepiandrosterone (DHEA) from the adrenal gland (Rosenfeld *et al.*, 1971). The glucocorticoids travel throughout the body inciting the physiological changes required to cope with the stressor.

Allostatic contribution

Cortisol promotes arousal, attention, and memory formation and increases blood glucose and blood pressure, while suppressing growth, reproductive, and immune processes. By comparison, DHEA, its sulfated derivative (DHEA-S), and its metabolites have antiglucocorticoid and antiglutamatergic properties in several tissues, including the brain (Browne *et al.*, 1992), and appear to support memory and cognition (Rose *et al.*, 1997). They deter corticosteroid-induced hippocampal neurotoxicity by interfering with the glucocorticoid receptor (GR) uptake in the hippocampus (Kimonides *et al.*, 1998; Bastianetto *et al.*, 1999; Morfin & Starka, 2001), and they amplify long-term potentiation of hippocampal neurons, likely by modulating transmission at the *N*-methyl-D-aspartate (NMDA) receptor (Chen *et al.*, 2006).

Allostatic load

Chronic excessive cortisol exposure is thought to increase vulnerability to hypertension, immunosuppression, osteoporosis, insulin resistance, truncal obesity, dyslipidemia, dyscoagulation, atherosclerosis, cardiovascular disease (Whitworth *et al.*, 2005), anxiety, and depressive disorders (Carroll *et al.*, 2007). A substantial body of literature exploring cortisol dysregulation in major depressive disorder (MDD) and post-traumatic stress disorder (PTSD) has emerged in the past few decades (reviewed by Handwerger, 2009). Handwerger concluded that the available literature links the development of PTSD after single-trauma exposure to chronic (if not acute) reductions in basal cortisol levels, relative suppression of the cortisol response in the low-dose dexamethasone suppression test, and heightened cortisol responses in anticipation of, and in response to, stress. These findings support a hypothesis that the GRs of the HPA axis are hypersensitive in single-trauma PTSD. However, as Handwerger (2009), notes, patients with PTSD and histories of chronic or multiple traumas such as child abuse often display different patterns of cortisol dysregulation than either healthy volunteers or individuals with PTSD precipitated by a single adulthood trauma. She posits that this mediator may account for conflicting findings in the literature (e.g., Baker *et al.*, 2005; Inslicht *et al.*, 2006; Wheler *et al.*, 2006).

In addition to the exact impact of trauma history, what remains unclear is the timeline of the onset of cortisol dysregulation observed in patients with PTSD. Is it a pre-existing risk factor or does it emerge only in the aftermath of the trauma? Studies showing that glucocorticoid administration inhibits traumatic memory formation (Bierer *et al.*, 2006) support a vulnerability model. For example, patients undergoing surgery and/or hospitalization in the intensive care unit who are pre-treated with stress doses of glucocorticoids are less likely to have traumatic memories of their hospital stay after discharge than patients treated with placebo (Brunner *et al.*, 2006; Schelling *et al.*, 2006; Weis *et al.*, 2006). In contrast, studies showing that individuals with elevated cortisol at the time of trauma are more likely to be subsequently diagnosed with PTSD could be cited as evidence of a post-hoc model (Baker *et al.*, 2005; Inslicht *et al.*, 2006).

Handwerger's (2009) review also concluded that 40–60% of adults with MDD display hypercortisolemia and non-suppression in the dexamethasone suppression test. This pattern may be even more common in psychotic than non-psychotic depression. In contrast, when changes in cortisol levels following exposure to acute stressors are assessed, no clear pattern distinguishes patients with MDD from controls. A recent study with a very large sample (1588) also documented statistically significant morning basal cortisol elevation in patients with present or a history of MDD but failed to differentiate between those with MDD and healthy volunteers in cortisol response to the dexamethasone suppression test (Vreeburg *et al.*, 2009).

Factors promoting resilience

Several animal models and some investigations in humans suggest that the relative efficiency of the HPA axis is predictive of the degree of resilience (de Kloet *et al.*, 2005). That is, its successful acute activation when triggered by a threat, and subsequent and timely deactivation when danger has passed, are adaptive and promote physical and mental health. Conversely, both hypo- and hyperactive HPA axis activity are associated with psychological and physical illness. Hence, factors that enhance the functioning of the feedback mechanisms that regulate the axis are likely to promote resilient phenotypes.

Single nucleotide polymorphisms

Single nucleotide polymorphisms (SNPs) that influence HPA reactivity have been identified in the genes coding for the mineralocorticoid receptor (MR), GR, gamma-aminobutyric acid (GABA) A receptor, α-adrenoceptor (Masten *et al.*, 1995), μ-opioid receptor, as well as the serotonin transporter, catechol-O-methyltransferase (COMT), monoamine oxidase A, brain-derived neurotrophic factor (BDNF), and angiotensin-converting enzyme. Comprehensive reviews are available elsewhere (Derijk & de Kloet, 2008; Derijk, 2009) but many SNPs will be briefly discussed in this chapter.

Ratio of dehydroepiandrosterone to cortisol

The ratio of DHEA and its derivatives to cortisol has proved to be predictive of adaptive responses to stress in multiple populations (Morgan *et al.*, 2004). The ratio of DHEA-S to cortisol was positively correlated with performance during rigorous survival training (Morgan *et al.*, 2004) and negatively correlated with dissociative symptoms (Korte *et al.*, 2005). This ratio is also negatively correlated with the severity of negative mood symptoms in women with PTSD (Rasmusson *et al.*, 2004). Secretion of DHEA in response to ACTH injections in these same women was highest in those reporting the mildest symptoms (Rasmusson *et al.*, 2004). Higher DHEA plasma levels have been positively correlated with improvement and effective coping in an investigation of veterans being treated for PTSD (Morgan *et al.*, 2004; Yehuda *et al.*, 2006a) and negatively correlated with depressive symptoms (Goodyer *et al.*, 1998; Gallagher & Young, 2002; Young *et al.*, 2002).

The inverse relationships observed between DHEA levels and psychopathology prompted researchers to test its viability as a treatment. Use of DHEA outperformed placebo in 145 patients with human immunodeficiency/acquired immunodeficiency syndrome

(HIV/AIDS) being treated for MDD (Rabkin *et al.*, 2006): 51% of patients randomized to DHEA reported symptom relief in comparison to only 31% of those assigned to the placebo group when assessed with the Hamilton Depression Rating Scale and the Clinical Global Impression Scale.

Integrity of feedback mediated by glucocorticoid and mineralocorticoid receptors

Functional variants have been identified in humans of the genes for brain MRs and GRs, which are involved, respectively, in setting the threshold and in regulating the termination of the HPA axis response to stress (de Kloet *et al.*, 2007). For example, carriers of the N363S variant of GR were shown to exhibit higher cortisol responses to the Trier Social Stress Test, a stress-inducing public speaking and mental arithmetic task (Krishnan *et al.*, 2007). Interestingly, four SNPs of *FKBP5* (rs9296158, rs3800373, rs1360780, and rs9470080), a gene coding for a "chaperone" protein that regulates GR sensitivity, were found to interact with severity of childhood abuse in the prediction of PTSD symptoms in adults (Bradley *et al.*, 2008). Another study demonstrated an association between genetic variation in *FKBP5* and inefficient recovery of HPA axis activity after the Trier Social Stress Test in healthy participants, identifying a potential risk factor for chronically elevated cortisol levels and, ultimately, stress-related psychopathology (Derijk & de Kloet, 2008).

Extrahypothalamic corticotropin-releasing hormone

Allostatic contribution

In addition to its role in the HPA pathway, CRH also contributes to the inhibition of a variety of neurovegetative functions, such as food intake, sexual activity, growth, and reproduction. Increased activity of extrahypothalamic CRH-containing neurons in the amygdala appears to activate fear-related behaviors, while those in the cortex may reduce reward expectation.

Two G-protein-coupled CRH receptors have been characterized, CRH-1 and CRH-2. Both are expressed in the pituitary, the hippocampus, the amygdala, and throughout the neocortex (with greater density in the prefrontal, cingulate, striate, and insular cortices). Only CRH-1 has been detected in the locus coeruleus, the nucleus of the solitary tract, the thalamus, and the

striatum, and only CRH-2 in the choroid plexus, certain hypothalamic nuclei, the nucleus prepositus, and the bed nucleus of the stria terminalis (Sanchez *et al.*, 1999). Mice bred to be deficient in either CRH-1 or CRH-2 display contradictory behavioral profiles when exposed to stress. The CRH-1-deficient mice demonstrate less anxiety-like behavior and fail to mount an adequate stress response in comparison with controls, while CRH-2-deficient mice evince more anxiety-like behavior and are hypersensitive to stress (Bale *et al.*, 2000; Coste *et al.*, 2000). Trials of CRH-1 antagonists indicate that this receptor activates the behavioral, endocrine, and visceral responses to stress; in contrast, CRH-2 generally serves to dampen these effects (Tache & Bonaz, 2007). However, CRH-2 does have some anxiogenic effects; it appears to enhance the CRH-1-mediated suppression of feeding behavior, for example, and to augment stress-induced behaviors via action in the lateral septum of the amygdala (Bakshi *et al.*, 2002). What is more, stress appears to modify CRH receptor expression in the rodent dorsal raphe nucleus, increasing the CRH-2 and decreasing the CRH-1 availability (Waselus *et al.*, 2009). Therefore, additional research will be required to illuminate the complex interactions between these receptors.

Allostatic load

As described above, CRH-1 signaling appears to be primarily anxiogenic. Exposure to excessive CRH during development appears to have a lasting and deleterious impact on mental and social health. In adults, increased levels of CRH in cerebrospinal fluid have been linked to PTSD and major depression (Bremner *et al.*, 1997; Baker *et al.*, 1999; Nemeroff, 2002). The data from studies measuring plasma CRH levels in patients with PTSD are mixed (Voisey *et al.*, 2009).

Factors promoting resilience

Early life stress has been linked to chronically high levels of CRH in human and animal studies (Heim & Nemeroff, 2001), providing yet more evidence that environmental stability during childhood equips a body to resist damage when stressed. Yet genetic factors appear to mediate the impact of childhood trauma on CRH system integrity. A recent study in two independent populations found that polymorphisms and haplotypes of the gene for CRH (e.g., a haplotype formed by three SNPs in intron 1) affected the influence of child abuse on depressive symptoms in adulthood, with certain alleles (rs7209436, rs242940) and haplotypes exerting a protective effect (Berton *et al.*,

2006). In addition, scientists were able to reverse social impairments associated with developmental exposure to high levels of CRH by administering a CRH antagonist to the dorsal raphe of rodents (Lukkes *et al.*, 2009), suggesting that these compounds may be effective treatments for people suffering from social anxiety stemming from early adverse experiences.

Monoamines

Monoamines (norepinephrine [NE], serotonin [5-HT], and dopamine) were the original neuromodulators implicated in emotion regulation. Hence, it is hardly surprising that they have been identified as players in allostasis.

Norepinephrine

The locus coeruleus is co-activated with the HPA axis in response to stress. This is a nucleus located within the dorsal wall of the rostral pons in the lateral floor of the fourth ventricle, and the primary site of NE genesis in the brain. Having the hypothalamus, amygdala, and prefrontal cortex as both afferents and efferents, the locus coeruleus plays a key role in regulating emotional and physiological reactions to stimuli.

Allostatic contribution

When provoked by stress, the locus coeruleus contributes to the excitation of the HPA axis and the sympathetic nervous system, while inhibiting the parasympathetic nervous system, resulting in a state of arousal. Further inhibition of the prefrontal cortex allows instinctual "fight or flight" behaviors to dominate, unchecked by the more nuanced cognitions of the forebrain (Charney & Bremner, 1999). Researchers recently demonstrated that NE levels in the prefrontal cortex also, in part, determine the dopaminergic response to stress. Higher levels of NE appear to favor dominance of mesolimbic dopamine signaling and active coping, lower levels of NE leading to mesocortical dopamine signaling and passive coping.

The activation of the HPA and locus coeruleus–NE systems under acute stress also facilitates the encoding and relay of aversively charged emotional memories, beginning at the amygdala. Animal studies have shown that injections of NE into the amygdala enhance memory consolidation; in contrast, blocking NE activity during stress impedes the encoding of fearful memories. In rats, blocking the lateral nucleus of the amygdala to the effects of NE during reactivation of a fearful

memory prevents the process of memory reconsolidation and appears to permanently impair that memory (Debiec & LeDoux, 2006).

Allostatic load

Although locus coeruleus activity is important for mounting an effective stress response, hyperactivity or sustained activity of the locus coeruleus is likely deleterious and is associated with depression, anxiety disorders, fear, intrusive memories, and an increased risk of hypertension and cardiovascular disease (Charney *et al.*, 1987, 1992; Southwick *et al.*, 1997; Wong *et al.*, 2000; Geracioti *et al.*, 2001). For example, both plasma and cerebrospinal fluid levels of NE were found to be elevated in patients with PTSD (Yehuda *et al.*, 1995; Baker *et al.*, 1997).

The neuron response in the locus coeruleus to stress-related stimuli is mediated in part by α_2-adrenoceptors, which are inhibitory autoreceptors localized to the cell bodies of locus coeruleus neurons. These α_2-adrenoceptors serve an important role in providing negative feedback and containment of the NE response to stress. Antagonism of α_2-adrenoceptors with idazoxan or yohimbine increases the response of locus coeruleus neurons to excitatory stimuli without altering their baseline firing rate (Simson & Weiss, 1988). Neumeister and colleagues (2005) found that humans homozygous for a polymorphism that compromises the integrity of α_2-adrenoceptor function had higher levels of NE at rest and more sustained increases in NE, heart rate, and anxiety in response to a yohimbine challenge compared with non-carriers.

Exposure to stressors from which the animal cannot escape results in behavioral deficits termed *learned helplessness*. The learned helplessness state is regarded as an animal model of MDD and is associated with depletion of NE (Bremner *et al.*, 1996). The depletion of NE during exposure to an inescapable stressor may function as a blockade of α_2-adrenoceptors and precipitate hypersensitization of locus coeruleus neurons to stimuli (Simson & Weiss, 1988).

Factors promoting resilience

Variables that promote efficiency and/or prevent hypersensitivity or chronic activation of the NE system would likely result in resilience. For example, the levels of COMT, which degrades NE and dopamine, would influence the quality and duration of NE activation. Polymorphisms in the gene that codes for COMT have been identified and found to affect cognition and anxiety levels. Individuals with low functioning COMT variants (hence, higher levels of circulating NE) tend to have better attention and working memory, but higher anxiety (Heinz & Smolka, 2006). Individuals with low functioning COMT also exhibit higher neural responsiveness in the limbic system and visuospatial attention system when presented with unpleasant stimuli, suggesting that they have heightened reactivity to potential threats (Smolka et al., 2005).

There is also evidence linking severe stress in early life to hyperfunctioning of the locus coeruleus–NE system in adulthood. In one study of police recruits, participants watched aversive videos and subsequently gave saliva samples. Those recruits with a history of childhood trauma had significantly higher levels of a salivary metabolite of NE than did control peers (Otte et al., 2005).

Beta-blockers (e.g., propranolol), agents that prevent stimulation of β-adrenoceptors by both NE and epinephrine, inhibit some aspects of memory consolidation when administered to animals immediately before or after a learning task. These findings suggested that treatment with beta-blockers in the acute aftermath of trauma exposure might prevent PTSD. Propranolol, in comparison with placebo treatment, was associated with greater reductions in physiological reactivity when recalling memories of trauma three months later (Pitman et al., 2002). Unfortunately, subsequent similar investigations have failed to replicate the promising results (Orr et al., 2006).

Serotonin

Serotonin has been implicated in the regulation of a number of complex processes including anxiety, fear, mood, aggression, and impulse control. However, because 5-HT has at least 17 unique receptors and additional enzymes and proteins that influence its metabolism and release, it remains exceedingly difficult to understand exactly how it exerts its influence (Cools et al., 2008; Dayan & Huys, 2009). Researchers have approached the study of 5-HT by exposing humans or animals believed to have compromised 5-HT signaling (5-HT-impaired subjects) to stressors and observing the results. In humans, genetic testing can identify individuals with specific polymorphisms known to impair the function of their 5-HT system for participation in experiments. Alternatively, the quantity of 5-HT available can be reduced via nutritional manipulation (tryptophan depletion). Animals can be genetically or physically modified.

Allostatic contribution

Such investigations of 5-HT-impaired subjects have demonstrated that 5-HT tempers physiological responsivity to threats in part via modulation of amygdala and prefrontal activation (Inoue et al., 1993; Cools et al., 2005; Heinz et al., 2005; Pezawas et al., 2005). Stress exposure triggers more activity in those regions in 5-HT-impaired individuals than in controls (Cools et al., 2008). Furthermore, multiple studies in humans and animals have revealed a negative association between tonic 5-HT levels and negative bias (reviewed by Cools et al., 2008). That is, 5-HT-impaired individuals have more difficulty perceiving and processing positive and rewarding stimuli than aversive stimuli. This 5-HT impairment has also been linked to impulsivity. In animals, 5-HT impairment results in an inability to refuse or ignore rewarding stimuli. In humans, it renders individuals less likely to refuse or ignore a stimulus that was once rewarding, even if it is no longer rewarding. These 5-HT-impaired subjects also make more commission errors on go–no-go cognitive tests. These tests ask participants to act ("go") in some situations and to refrain from acting ("no-go") in others. The 5-HT-impaired subjects are as likely as controls to act when acting is appropriate. However, they are more likely to act even when acting is not appropriate, demonstrating a failure of inhibitory mechanisms (reviewed by Cools et al., 2008). This 5-HT impairment is also thought to contribute to the pathophysiology of MDD, PTSD, and other anxiety disorders. Although this was originally inferred from the serendipitous discovery that agents that increased 5-HT transmission were often effective antidepressants, decades of additional research have documented more direct evidence to support this hypothesis. For example, the density of 5-HT$_{1A}$ receptors is reduced in depressed patients when they are depressed as well as in remission (Belda & Armario, 2009), and density is also decreased in patients with panic disorder (Bogdan & Pizzagalli, 2006).

Given that 5-HT impairment is associated with increased physiological responsivity to stress, increased attention to negative stimuli, and impulsivity, as well as with MDD and PTSD, it is possible to deduce that effective 5-HT neurotransmission would contribute to allostasis in situations where tranquility, optimism, and/or behavioral control are adaptive.

Allostatic load

There is no evidence that physiologically appropriate levels of 5-HT are harmful. However, agents that facilitate its neurotransmission have a clear allostatic load. Common side-effects of selective serotonin reuptake inhibitors such as fluoxetine and citalopram include sexual dysfunction, such as reduced desire, deficits in the ability to achieve orgasm, or quality of orgasm; nausea; dry mouth; headache; diarrhea; rash; nervousness, agitation, and restlessness; increased sweating; and weight gain. Serotonin syndrome, one of the most severe of the possible adverse effects, is characterized by the presence of symptoms in three domains: cognitive (mental confusion, hypomania, hallucinations, agitation, headache, coma); autonomic (shivering, sweating, hyperthermia, hypertension, tachycardia, nausea, diarrhea); and somatic (myoclonus [muscle twitching], hyperreflexia [manifested by clonus], tremor). As indicated by the range of risk imposed by the symptoms listed in each domain, cases can range from mild to severe (Boyer & Shannon, 2005).

Factors contributing to resilience

Given the wealth of data implicating suboptimal 5-HT signaling in the pathophysiology of mood and anxiety disorders, any factors that promote the health of this system would likely support resilience. Numerous studies have explored the role of genetics, and specifically a well-known polymorphism in the gene for the serotonin transporter (5HTTLPR) in conferring vulnerability to depression. Three genotypes are possible: two copies of the long allele (LL), two copies the short allele (SS), or one of each (SL). A handful of studies found that that the short allele renders individuals more likely to develop MDD after stressful life experiences (Caspi et al., 2003; Gillespie et al., 2005). However, two recent meta-analyses concluded that the relationship between these variables is not significant (Munafo et al., 2009; Risch et al., 2009). Verhagen and colleagues (2009) suggest that the effect of the 5HTTLPR polymorphism on MDD is co-dependent on the presence of co-morbid disorders and sex. In their work, the S-allele of the 5-HTTLPR polymorphism has been associated with significantly lower rates of particular lifetime co-morbid disorders. Therefore, they argue that the presence of co-morbid psychiatric disorders should be taken into account to clarify the association of the 5HTTLPR polymorphism with MDD phenotypes.

In animal models, embryonic and early postnatal shutdown of expression of a type of 5-HT receptor (5-HT$_1$), via either genetic (e.g., knockout mice) or environmental (e.g., high levels of juvenile CRH) means, produces an anxiety phenotype that endures, even following the restoration of the receptors (Heisler et al., 1998; Parks et al., 1998; Gross et al., 2002). Reductions in these same 5-HT$_1$ receptors in adulthood create only a state-dependent anxious phenotype, reinstating the receptors restores original behavior. These results suggest that altered function of 5-HT receptors early in life can produce long-term abnormalities in the regulation of anxiety behaviors (Gross et al., 2002) and underscores the importance of early childhood environment in inclining an individual to resilience or vulnerability to mood and anxiety disorders.

Interactions between the 5-HT and other neuromodulating systems also appear to be relevant to the efficacy of its signaling. For example, increases in adrenal steroid release, characteristic of an active HPA axis, result in a corresponding decrease in 5-HT$_1$ receptor density and mRNA levels by activating MRs (Lopez et al., 1998). There may also be important functional interactions between 5-HT$_{1A}$ and benzodiazepine receptors. One study of 5-HT$_{1A}$ knockout mice reported a downregulation of benzodiazepine GABA α_1- and α_2-receptor subunits as well as benzodiazepine-resistant anxiety in the elevated-plus maze (Sibille et al., 2000). However, a subsequent study did not replicate these results using mice with a different genetic background (Pattij et al., 2002), raising the possibility that genetic background can affect functional interplay between 5-HT$_{1A}$ and benzodiazepine systems.

Dopamine

With five known receptors, dopamine is another multitasking neuromodulator, involved in numerous psychological and physiological processes (psychosis and movement among the most well known). Its function in the experience of reward and pleasure has been most thoroughly investigated in mood and anxiety disorders. The "mesocorticolimbic" dopamine pathway, composed of neurons in the ventral tegmental area, ventral striatum (nucleus accumbens), amygdala, medial prefrontal cortex, ventral pallidum and mediodorsal thalamus, is thought to be most relevant to reward. This circuit is linked to brain regions involved in attention, goal-directed behavior, motivation, reinforcement, emotion regulation, cognitive function, and social interactions. Dopamine neuron activity in the ventral tegmental area is dependent upon expectation of and receipt of reward: the neurons are activated in response to a reward (e.g., food, sex, social interaction), or even the expectation of a reward, and are inhibited by an aversive stimulus or the absence of an expected reward (Carter *et al.*, 2009). (However, certain dopaminergic neurons are also activated by aversive stimuli, suggesting their involvement in mood regulation more generally [Carter *et al.*, 2009].) Hence animal models suggest that the response of the dopaminergic system changes as a function of the nature and duration of the stress experienced by an animal.

Allostatic contribution

Exposure to brief, novel stressors appears to result in an immediate increase in mesolimbic dopamine release (Puglisi-Allegra *et al.*, 1991; Pascucci *et al.*, 2007). These changes in signaling serve to arouse the animal and catalyze coping behaviors. If the animal determines that it is possible to behaviorally modulate the dose or intensity of the stressor, increased mesolimbic dopamine release can be maintained regardless of the severity or duration of exposure (Puglisi-Allegra *et al.*, 1991). The animal continues to struggle as long as the behavior is rewarded.

However, if coping tactics are ineffective (and the stress is uncontrollable), the animal does not receive the reward it originally expected. Mesolimbic dopamine transmission will drop off to lower than normal levels, contributing to the inhibition of behavioral responses to stress (Puglisi-Allegra *et al.*, 1991; Pascucci *et al.*, 2007). This may serve as a survival mechanism in situations where conservation of energy better serves the animal than continuing a futile struggle.

In addition, Belda and Armario (2009) explored the impact of dopamine antagonists on HPA axis activity with immobilization stress in rats. Both D_1 and D_2 receptor antagonists reduced HPA axis activity and the duration of activation, indicating that dopamine stimulates HPA axis activity during and after stress via these receptors.

Allostatic load

Stress reduces sensitivity to reward in humans (Bogdan & Pizzagalli, 2006), and altered reward circuitry appears to characterize both MDD (Nestler & Carlezon, 2006) and PTSD. Indeed, an increasing number of studies implicate the mesocorticolimbic circuit in both resilience and vulnerability to developing mood and anxiety symptoms. Special forces soldiers, considered highly resilient because of their ability to perform well even under extreme stress, showed increased reactivity of reward-processing regions compared with healthy civilian controls (Vythilingam *et al.*, 2009). Conversely,

dissatisfaction with social rewards in healthy males was associated with increased activation in prefrontal (top-down control) areas during performance of a monetary task (Siegrist *et al.*, 2005).

Patients with PTSD are both less likely to expect a reward and experience less satisfaction upon receipt of a reward than controls (Hopper *et al.*, 2008). Further, functional magnetic resonance imaging (fMRI) investigations suggest that they demonstrate less activation in the nucleus accumbens and medial prefrontal cortex in response to reward (Sailer *et al.*, 2008). However, their activation does not differ from controls in response to a loss or disappointment. In rodents, exposure to a social defeat paradigm (time in a cage with a larger aggressive animal) increased activity of dopamine neurons in the ventral tegmental area via increased activity-dependent release of BDNF onto nucleus accumbens neurons. Animals that recovered normal functioning after the exposure upregulated potassium channels in the ventral tegmental area, minimizing the increase in neuronal excitability and in BDNF release (Eisch *et al.*, 2003; Meaney & Szyf, 2005). Those that continued to demonstrate anxious behaviors did not (Eisch *et al.*, 2003, Krishnan *et al.*, 2008).

In a study conducted by Pizzagalli and colleagues (2009), subjects with MDD, in contrast to controls, showed attenuated responses to reward in the left nucleus accumbens and the caudate bilaterally. However, there were no group differences in these regions in response to neutral or negative outcomes. In this same sample, self-reported severity of anhedonia and depressed mood group were associated with reduced caudate volume bilaterally. In imaging investigations, individuals with a history of MDD, but no present clinically significant depressive symptoms, were less responsive to pleasant visual stimuli in the ventral striatum than were controls. In contrast, they were more responsive to aversive visual stimuli in the caudate nucleus. When the visual stimuli were paired with corresponding olfactory stimuli, subjects with MDD evinced relatively less activity in the prefrontal cortex (McCabe *et al.*, 2009). Adolescents with MDD have also been shown to mount a weaker striatal response but a more robust dorsolateral and medial prefrontal cortex response than controls during reward anticipation and reward outcome (Forbes *et al.*, 2009). Altered activation of reward circuits in depressed compared with healthy adolescents was associated with self-reports of reduced positive affect in naturalistic settings (Forbes *et al.*, 2009). Differential reward system function has also been demonstrated in children of depressed versus never-depressed parents (Monk *et al.*, 2008).

Factors contributing to resilience

States and traits that facilitate effective functioning of mesolimbic dopamine signaling and buttress the circuitry of reward might promote active coping and decrease vulnerability to MDD and anxiety. For example, the persistence of the state of reduced mesolimbic dopaminergic transmission that results from uncontrollable stress appears to be, in part, genetically determined; some strains of mice become sensitized to the reduction in mesolimbic dopamine and re-initiate coping behaviors, while others will evince progressively fewer and fewer coping behaviors (Puglisi-Allegra *et al.*, 1990). In humans, genes affecting the integrity of dopamine signaling influence severity of PTSD. An SNP (C957T) in the gene for the D_2 receptor (*DRD2*) has been linked to PTSD risk. Individuals with PTSD are more likely to carry the C allele compared with the controls (Voisey *et al.*, 2009). In a study of combat veterans with PTSD, the A1+ allele of *DRD2* was associated with increased PTSD symptoms and higher co-morbid anxiety and depression (Lawford *et al.*, 2006). The A1+ allele has previously been linked to social dysfunction in children, compromised visuospatial functioning in adolescents, and increased family stress (Lawford *et al.*, 2006).

The A2 allele of *DRD2* appears to confer MDD risk. Occurrence of stressful life events was associated with increased risk of subsequent depressive symptoms in individuals with the A2/A2 genotype. No such association was detected in participants with A1/A1 or A1/A2 genotypes (Elovainio *et al.*, 2007).

Exposure to stress during development also appears to alter functioning of dopaminergic circuitry. Adult rats exposed to social defeat as adolescents had lower levels of medial prefrontal cortex dopamine, increased NE in the dentate gyrus, and decreased NE in the dorsal raphe (Watt *et al.*, 2009).

The Val158Met COMT polymorphism also appears to contribute to variability between individuals in neural responses to reward anticipation, even in healthy individuals.

Neuropeptides

Neuropeptide Y

Neuropeptide Y (NPY), composed of 36 amino acid residues and one of the most abundant neuropeptides, is involved in regulation of feeding and sexual behavior, circadian rhythms, cardiovascular symptoms, and the immune and stress responses (Hökfelt *et al.*, 1998). There are at least four metabotropic, G-protein-coupled NPY receptors expressed in the human brain (Y_1, Y_2, Y_3, Y_5) (Blomqvist & Herzog, 1997) whose activation precipitates inhibitory responses such as the inhibition of cyclic AMP accumulation (Lin *et al.*, 2004).

Allostatic contribution

There are important interactions between NPY and CRH (Heilig *et al.*, 1994; Britton *et al.*, 2000): NPY counteracts the anxiogenic effects of CRH at various locations within the stress–anxiety circuit, including the amygdala, hippocampus, hypothalamus, and locus coeruleus. Activation of the Y_1 receptor inhibits several metabolic and behavioral stress responses, including gastrointestinal effects, anxious behavior, and decreased sleep (Eva *et al.*, 2006).

Allostatic load

No known health risks are associated with excess exposure to NPY. However, knockout models have revealed that each of the NPY receptors have unique purposes. For example, while mice without any NPY display increased levels of anxious behavior (spending less time in the open field on the open field test) and increased startle amplitude (Bannon *et al.*, 2000), Y_2 receptor knockout mice display less anxious behavior than controls, suggesting that Y_2 receptors may be anxiogenic.

Mice bred to overexpress NPY are more vulnerable to developing obesity when maintained on a high-sucrose diet, and as their age advances (Kaga *et al.*, 2001). They are also relatively hypersensitive to ethanol (Thiele *et al.*, 1998).

Factors promoting resilience

In general, increased levels of NPY seem to promote resilience and reduce anxiety in both animal models and humans. In a study of special forces soldiers, who are considered to be highly stress resilient, higher NPY levels during rigorous military training were associated with better performance (McGaugh, 2004). Other studies found higher plasma and cerebrospinal fluid NPY in combat-exposed veterans without PTSD than in those with PTSD (Sah *et al.*, 2009). These findings in humans are consistent with recent studies in rats: central administration of NPY in rats inhibits the development, and promotes the extinction, of fear conditioning, with NPY antagonists exerting the opposite actions. These effects are mediated at least in part via the amygdala (Morgan et al., 2000). Moreover, intra-amygdala NPY administration promotes resilient responses to stress, in the form of reduced anxiety-like behaviors in response to acute restraint (Yehuda et al., 2006b).

Elevated NPY is negatively correlated with depression and anxiety in human and animal models (Heilig et al., 1993, 2004; Karlsson et al., 2005). A variety of antidepressant drugs increase NPY levels in humans and animals (Nikisch et al., 2005; Goyal et al., 2009; Bjornebekk et al., 2010). Electroconvulsive therapy has produced similar elevations in animal studies (Mikkelsen & Woldbye, 2006; Nikisch & Mathe, 2008).

Galanin

Galanin is a neuropeptide composed of 30 amino acid residues and with three known receptors (GAL-1, GAL-2, GAL-3). All are thought to be involved in allostasis (Walton et al., 2006). A dense galanin fiber system originates in the locus coeruleus and innervates the hippocampus, hypothalamus, amygdala, and prefrontal cortex among other areas (Perez et al., 2001). Galanin-releasing neurons are thought to be located immediately adjacent to the central amygdala and appear to be activated by non-noradrenergic afferents that themselves are activated by NE (Barrera et al., 2006).

Allostatic contribution

Both GAL-1, an autoreceptor (Sevcik et al., 1993; Xu et al., 2001), and GAL-2 appear to be anxiolytic. Knockout mice for GAL-1 and GAL-2 evince increased anxiety-like behavior (Holmes et al., 2003; Rajarao et al., 2007; Lu et al., 2008a). Galnon, a non-specific galanin agonist, has been shown to elevate GABA levels in the rat amygdala and results in anxiolytic effects in some (open-maze and hyperthermia), but not all (mouse tail suspension, rat forced swim) animal models (Unschuld et al., 2008). Galanin reduces NE, 5-HT, and dopamine levels in the prefrontal cortex via inhibition (Holmes & Picciotto, 2006). Hence, scientists have proposed that galanin recruitment during stress may serve as a buffer, minimizing the intensity of the anxiety experienced as a result of NE over-activation (Karlsson & Holmes, 2006). Galanin-overexpressing transgenic mice are unresponsive to the anxiogenic effects of the α_2-adrenoceptor antagonist yohimbine. Consistent with this observation, galanin injected directly into the central nucleus of the amygdala blocked the anxiogenic effects of stress, which is associated with increased NE release in the central nucleus of the amygdala (Khoshbouei et al., 2002).

Allostatic load

The GAL-3 receptor has anxiogenic effects. Galanin acting at the GAL-3 receptor may precipitate decreases in 5-HT signaling by hyperpolarizing 5-HT neurons in the dorsal raphe nucleus and reducing levels of 5-HT in the hippocampus and prefrontal cortex, leading to increased vulnerability to anxiety and isolation. In animal models, GAL-3 antagonists have increased prosocial behaviors and decreased anxiety and depression-like behaviors (Swanson et al., 2006; Kozlovsky et al., 2009).

Factors promoting resilience

In humans, certain polymorphisms of the gene for the GAL-3 receptor have been linked with anxiety and alcoholism (Belfer et al., 2006). In a recent study exploring an animal model of galanin functioning in PTSD, rats were exposed to a predator. Those rats who exhibited minimal anxiety-like symptoms after the exposure were observed to have a lasting upregulation of galanin mRNA in the C area of the hippocampus in the prefrontal cortex, while those who became symptomatic evinced galanin mRNA downregulation in the same areas (Kozlovsky et al., 2009). In addition, those symptomatic animals treated with galnon displayed fewer anxiety-like behaviors and upregulated their galanin mRNA. Immediate post-exposure treatment with galnon significantly reduced prevalence rates of extreme responders, reduced trauma-cue freezing responses, corrected the corticosterone response, and increased CA1 expression of 5-HT$_{1A}$ and BDNF mRNA compared with controls treated with saline.

Agents modulating the efficacy and intensity of the acute stress response

Sex hormones (gonadal steroids)

Epidemiological studies have repeatedly demonstrated that women are twice as likely to suffer from depressive and anxiety disorder. It appears that this gender disparity in risk and resilience is mediated in part by the impact of sex hormones on HPA axis activity.

Testosterone

Testosterone, a steroid hormone from the androgen group derived from cholesterol, induces protein synthesis and growth of tissues with androgen receptors. It can also act, after conversion to estradiol, via the estrogen receptors. In men, who have much higher levels of testosterone than women, it is produced primarily in the Leydig cells in the testes; in women, it is produced in the thecal cells of the ovaries, and in the placenta during pregnancy. Testosterone increases muscle mass and bone density, facilitates maturation of the sex organs and development of secondary sex characteristics in men, and promotes libido.

Testosterone administration in women reliably reduces physiological reactivity to stress, as evinced by decreases in skin conductance, heart rate, and startle (Hermans et al., 2006, 2007), as well as attention bias toward and conscious recognition of angry faces (van Honk et al., 1999, 2005; van Honk & Schutter, 2007; Wirth & Schultheiss, 2007). It also increases activity of brain areas associated with aggression and impulse control (amygdala, hypothalamus, brainstem, and Brodmann area 47 of the orbitofrontal cortex) (Hermans et al., 2008). A profile of high testosterone and low cortisol in the absence of testosterone administration is also associated with increased activity in these regions compared with controls. In addition, testosterone levels are known to correlate positively with aggression (Zitzmann & Nieschlag, 2001; Bender et al., 2006; Yu & Shi, 2009), social status (Flugge et al., 2001; Anestis, 2006; Setchell et al., 2008; Czoty et al., 2009), athletic success (Edwards et al., 2006; Edwards & O'Neal, 2009; Oliveira et al., 2009), and the subjective feelings of success, dominance, and social connectedness, all experiences that are known to be associated with resilience (as discussed above).

However, stress is associated with reductions in testosterone levels, which is observed both in soldiers after a psychologically and physically stressful training exercise and in marathon runners following a difficult race (Morgan et al., 2004; Franca et al., 2006). Hypogonadism is associated with depressive symptoms, while testosterone replacement is associated with improvement in mood and relief from other depressive symptoms, and decreases in CRH-stimulated release of cortisol and the cortisol-to-ACTH ratio (Daly et al., 2001). Some men with a polymorphism within the gene encoding the androgen receptor that makes them less susceptible to androgen effects are at a higher risk for developing MDD (Zitzmann, 2006; Colangelo et al., 2007). While the results of studies testing the antidepressant potential of testosterone have been inconsistent, a recent meta-analysis concluded that testosterone administration was more likely to result in reduced depression severity than placebo and noted that the effect was particularly strong in patients with hypogonadism or HIV/AIDS (Zarrouf et al., 2009). Hence, one reasonable hypothesis is that adequate supplies of testosterone, by reducing physiological and psychological stress reactivity, serve as a buffer. Those with lower basal levels (including women) would be more vulnerable because the stress-induced decrease in testosterone would make them prone to more severe, and therefore more costly, stress responses.

However, as with most agents that impact allostatic load, there can be too much of a good thing. High levels of testosterone are associated not only with productive feelings of competence but also with mood lability and increased propensity for violence. Studies of the neuropsychiatric effects of androgen administration in healthy men are few but informative. Some have observed statistically significant, if not always clinically significant, increases in mood lability and distractibility (Su et al., 1993); others have not (O'Connor, 2002). Emergence of hypomania and mania has also been noted (Su et al., 1993; Pope et al., 2000). Increased levels of testosterone have been found in male prison inmates with frequent episodes of violent behavior (Forbes et al., 2009; McCabe et al., 2009). While testosterone's ability to reduce conscious recognition of emotions such as anger might serve to control fear and facilitate active responses to threat (van Honk & Schutter, 2007), this same effect might also predispose individuals to antisocial behavior. There is also some evidence to suggest that pairing reduced levels of cortisol with increased levels of testosterone may augment its effect and contribute to criminal and aggressive tendencies (Terburg et al., 2009).

Estrogens

Estrogens, steroid hormones produced through enzymatic modulation of androgens, act primarily via estrogen receptors. In women, who have much higher levels than men, estrogens are produced primarily in the ovarian follicles, the corpus luteum and the placenta during pregnancy; in men, testosterone is converted into estradiol to act in the skeletal and central nervous systems. Estrogens promote the development of female secondary sex characteristics and regulate the menstrual cycle in women, and they contribute to sperm maturation in men. In addition, they support the health and functioning of many other body systems.

Estrogens can either potentiate or inhibit the body's stress response. Normally menstrual cycling female rodents have higher basal and stress-induced levels of ACTH and corticosterone than males, as do proestrous compared with diestrous females (Young *et al.*, 2001; Solomon & Herman 2009). Administration of superphysiological doses of estrogens to gonadally intact female rats or estradiol to ovariectomized rats raises ACTH and corticosterone levels (Carey *et al.*, 1995). However, physiological doses of estradiol have been shown to reduce the ACTH response to acute stress in female rats, while estrogen antagonists had the opposite effect (Young *et al.*, 2001). Proestrous compared with diestrous females evince less anxious behavior.

In women, physiological doses of estrogens constrain stress-induced activation of neurons in the frontal cortex, hippocampal, and paraventricular nucleus. Estrogens have been shown to blunt HPA axis responses to psychological stress in postmenopausal women (Komesaroff *et al.*, 1999; Cucinelli *et al.*, 2002) and to blunt the ACTH response to CRH in postmenopausal women with high levels of body fat. In addition, eight weeks of estrogen supplementation in perimenopausal women blunted increases in systolic and diastolic blood pressure, cortisol, ACTH, plasma epinephrine and NE, and in NE responses of the entire body to stress (Young, 1996). Pregnancy and lactation, states associated with high levels of estrogens, also result in decreased ACTH and cortisol signaling. Conversely, premenstrual, postpartum, and premenopausal states are associated with an increased prevalence of MDD and anxiety disorders (reviewed by Douma *et al.*, 2005).

It is clear that estrogens are able to modulate the degree of stress response and, consequently, the degree of allostatic load. Whether or not estrogens enhance or suppress stress responsivity appears to depend, in part, on the targeted receptor. Two unique estrogen receptors have been identified: ERα and ERβ (Green *et al.*, 1986; Kuiper *et al.*, 1996). Systemic or paraventricular nucleus administration of agents that selectively target ERα, in concert with a stressor, precipitated increases in ACTH, corticosterone, and paraventricular nucleus *fos* RNA; agents that selectively target ERβ have the opposite impact. Hence, ERβ are thought to underlie estrogen's protective benefits, and vice versa (Weiser *et al.*, 2008; Solomon & Herman 2009).

Estrogens are also known to interact with the monoaminergic (McEwen, 2002), GABA, and neuro-peptide systems (Table 1.2). These interactions also play a role in determining the allostatic load. Further research is needed to specifically determine the mechanisms, and ultimate importance, of these relationships.

What is understood about the very complex role of estrogens in the central nervous system was recently reviewed by Solomon & Herman (2009). They concluded that stable, physiological doses of estrogens in gonadally intact females appear to be largely protective, while fluctuation and instability in estrogen levels confer vulnerability.

Brain-derived neurotrophic factor

Neurotrophins are proteins that promote survival, development, and function of neurons by regulating growth, and associated metabolic functions such as protein synthesis, and neurotransmitter production. Hence, they play a role in determining the brain's response to stressors. Brain-derived neurotrophic factor is highly produced in the brain and is known for its support of adult hippocampal function in rodent models.

Studies have demonstrated that stress leads to a reduction of BDNF in the rodent hippocampus. Further, chronic antidepressant treatment can reverse this effect (Gutman *et al.*, 2008). Postmortem studies suggest that a parallel process occurs in the human hippocampus. In contrast, in the rodent nucleus accumbens, chronic stress increases BDNF levels (Duman & Monteggia, 2006; Sajdyk *et al.*, 2008). This change in BDNF concentrations results in a proportional increase in depressive-like behaviors such as passive coping, social avoidance, and anhedonia. That is, the more symptomatic an animal, the larger the increase in BDNF concentration in the nucleus accumbens, while "resilient" animals show no parallel increase. Humans with depression also show increased BDNF levels in the nucleus accumbens (Eisch *et al.*, 2003).

It is unclear what role exactly BDNF plays in resilience. As with other factors, its impact is different in different contexts. In mice, an SNP (G196A, Val66Met) in the gene encoding BDNF is associated with reduced hippocampal volume and significantly impairs BDNF's intracellular trafficking and activity-dependent release (Heinz & Smolka, 2006). Mice expressing the A allele evince more anxiety-like behavior and impaired hippocampal-dependent learning. Yet, they are more resilient to chronic stress (Eisch *et al.*, 2003; Heinz &

Table 1.2 Estrogen's influence on other stress-responsive systems.

System	Interaction	Reference
5-HT	Increased expression of the gene for tryptophan hydroxylase and protein production	Bethea *et al.*, 2002
	Increased 5-HT$_{2A}$ receptor binding	Moses *et al.*, 2000
	Decreased serotonin transporter expression	Pecins-Thompson *et al.*, 1998
	Decreased 5-HT$_{1A}$ mRNA and 5-HT$_{1A}$ binding in both presynaptic (dorsal raphe) and postsynaptic sites	Bethea *et al.*, 2002
	Decreased levels of inhibitory G proteins involved in intracellular signal transduction mediated by the 5-HT$_{1A}$ receptor	Raap *et al.*, 2000; Mize *et al.*, 2001
Norepinephrine and dopamine	Modulated α$_1$-adrenoceptor expression	Colucci *et al.*, 1982
	Modulated β-adrenoceptor receptor expression	Klangkalya & Chan, 1988
	Modulated norepinephrine and dopamine release	Alfinito *et al.*, 2009
GABA	Increased GABA$_A$ benzodiazepine receptor expression	Maggi & Perez, 1986
Neuropeptides	Increased neuropeptide Y release and gene expression	Hilke *et al.*, 2009
	Increased galanin release and gene expression	Hilke *et al.*, 2005

5-HT, serotonin; GABA, gamma-aminobutyric acid.

Smolka, 2006). These data underscore the complex effects of BDNF on the brain, which are highly specific to the brain region.

Epigenetic mechanisms

Chromosomes are constructed from chromatin, which consists of DNA, RNA, and proteins. The most abundant of these proteins are histones, which serve as the framework around which DNA is wound. When chromatin structure is modified, stable changes in gene expression result, which can be passed on to subsequent generations when they occur in germ cells. These "epigenetic" events impact gene expression by altering DNA transcription rather than sequence, and often involve chemical modification of histones via acetylation or methylation, or of DNA via methylation (Kim *et al.*, 2007). The often durable up- and downregulation of the stress-response systems following trauma appear to be mediated by epigenetic change.

For example, rats raised with low levels of maternal nurturing evince increased methylation of the promoter region for GR at the binding site for nerve growth factor-inducible factor in the hippocampus, an epigenetic change associated with reduced GR expression (Weaver *et al.*, 2004; Meaney & Szyf, 2005). This epigenetic change emerges in the first week of life and persists into adulthood. The rats, both as pups and adults, have a more robust corticosterone response to stress and express lower levels of GR in the hippocampus compared with genetically identical controls raised with more nurturing mothers. They are also more anxious and are less nurturing to their own offspring.

Perhaps even more dramatic evidence of epigenetic influences on resilience comes from comparisons of genetically identical rats raised not in purposefully different environments but in very controlled and nearly identical environments. These animals do not always demonstrate the same response (behaviorally or epigenetically) to the same stressors. For example, when a population of inbred mice is exposed to a social defeat paradigm (Pezawas *et al.*, 2005; Munafo *et al.*, 2008), some demonstrate behavioral changes indicative of anxiety and depression, while others do not (Eisch *et al.*, 2003; Krishnan *et al.*, 2007). In one study, the resilient animals not only failed to demonstrate many of the changes in gene expression seen in the ventral tegmental area–nucleus accumbens of vulnerable mice but also evinced distinct changes in gene expression absent in their vulnerable counterparts (Eisch *et al.*, 2003). For example, resilient mice induced several potassium channel subunits in dopamine neurons in the ventral tegmental area. This change served as prophylaxis against a stress-triggered increase in ventral tegmental area excitability and subsequent release of BDNF into the nucleus accumbens (Eisch *et al.*, 2003; Meaney & Szyf, 2005). Resilience has also been associated with the induction of ΔFosB in neurons in the ventrolateral region of the periaqueductal gray in the midbrain. The ΔFosB suppressed the production of the neuropeptide substance P in these cells, which, in turn, reduced substance P transmission to target regions such as the nucleus accumbens (Berton *et al.*, 2007). Interestingly, in some of the vulnerable animals, chronic, but not acute, treatment with imipramine reversed the effect (Wilkinson *et al.*, 2009).

These findings buttress the view that resilience is not simply the absence of maladaptive changes that occur in vulnerable individuals but also is mediated by a unique set of adaptive changes. In addition, the absence of any obvious external variables that determined which of the identical animals were resilient and which were not suggests that some epigenetic changes that influence an organism's resilience and vulnerability to stress are unpredictable. It is important to note that the maladaptive or adaptive nature of any epigenetic changes, or even genetic polymorphisms, is likely context dependent. Belsky and colleagues (2009) proposed that, "putative 'vulnerability genes' or 'risk alleles' might, at times, be more appropriately conceptualized as 'plasticity genes', because they seem to make individuals more susceptible to environmental influences – for better and for worse."

Neural circuitry of fear

The ability to distinguish between threatening and non-threatening stimuli is essential to ensure optimal HPA axis efficiency. A neural circuit of coordinated signaling between the amygdala, hippocampus and ventromedial prefrontal cortex) is thought to be associated with fear and fear-related learning (Dedovic *et al.*, 2005; Ulrich-Lai & Herman, 2009). Animal and human studies suggest that the amygdala is the primary site of fear-conditioning acquisition (Rauch *et al.*, 2006). That is, the amygdala facilitates the learning that allows cues associated with a fearful stimulus (e.g., footshock, predator odor) to become aversive themselves (Felmingham *et al.*, 2007; Liberzon & Sripada, 2008). Contextual and temporal aspects of fear conditioning are processed by the hippocampus (Davis & Whalen, 2001). Both amygdala- and hippocampus-dependent fear conditioning in animals has been related to long-term potentiation and other forms of synaptic plasticity. Accordingly, blockade of NMDA glutamate receptors in the amygdala blocks cue-associated fear conditioning. In the hippocampus, it blocks context-dependent fear conditioning (Bast, 2007). Reactivation of memories (i.e., re-exposure to the cue or context) can lead to either reconsolidation (further strengthening of the memory) or to extinction, with extinction generally requiring more intensive training. Extinction of fear conditioning involves not only the amygdala but also the ventromedial prefrontal cortex; activation in these structures, as well as thickness of the ventromedial prefrontal cortex, has been associated with extinction success (Rauch *et al.*, 2006; Yehuda & LeDoux, 2007). In addition, emerging evidence suggests that this area of the brain is the site of the neural processing required to adapt to context when assessing the degree of threat associated with a particular stimuli. In a recent fMRI study, participants were repeatedly exposed to stimuli that changed from threatening to safe, and vice versa. Activity in the ventromedial prefrontal cortex was correlated with success in modifying neural and physiological responses accordingly (Delgado *et al.*, 2006).

The experience of fear, and more specifically the ability to learn to associate stimuli with danger, is essential to ensuring that the stress response is timely, adequate, and facilitates survival. However, in order to prevent hyperactivity of the HPA axis, it is also important that an individual be able to extinguish fear-related memories, so that stimuli that are only dangerous in some contexts do not continue to be interpreted physiologically as valid threats. Therefore, the integrity of the neural circuitry of fear and fear learning would promote resilience. While the genetic and environmental

Trigger: A woman passes her friend on the street. She waves and says hello. Her friend doesn't make eye contact		
Interpretation A My friend ignored me purposefully. He must be angry with me	**Interpretation B** My friend ignored me purposefully. He is such a self-centered jerk!	**Interpretation C** My friend didn't see me. He would have responded if he had seen me
Physiological response/awareness Guilt, depression I must have done something wrong. I am a bad person	**Physiological response/ awareness** Anger, hopelessness My friend is trying to hurt me. No one can be trusted. I will always be alone	**Physiological response/ awareness** Resignation, disappointment I wish he had seen me. It would be nice to talk to him
Behavior Avoid friend, other social contact	**Behavior** Call friend and berate him	**Behavior** Call friend to arrange a meeting
Outcome Vulnerable	**Outcome** Vulnerable	**Outcome** Resilient

Figure 1.1 Elements of emotion and the impact of cognitive interpretation trigger.

variables that determine the functional capacity of this circuit have yet to be identified, several treatments for PTSD attempt to inhibit fear-conditioning learning and enhance extinction learning. For example, because long-term potentiation is known to be involved in extinction learning, a partial agonist of the NMDA receptor (D-cycloserine) that facilitates long-term potentiation is administered during prolonged exposure therapy (Goldstein *et al.*, 1996). Blockade of β-adrenoceptors in the amygdala can also block cue-dependent fear conditioning, and beta-blockers have been tested in patients exposed to trauma, with mixed results (Baker *et al.*, 1999; Morrow *et al.*, 1999). In addition, fear conditioning and its extinction are regulated by activation of GRs in the hippocampus and perhaps in the amygdala, which suggests the possible use of glucocorticoids in the treatment of trauma (Lemieux & Coe, 1995). However, whether β-adrenoceptor and GR levels or functioning differs in resilient versus non-resilient individuals has not yet been studied.

Psychological processes

A number of psychosocial states and traits have been repeatedly associated with resilience, including positive emotions, optimism, active coping, social support, and prosocial behavior. All of these can be understood as strategies that support the efficacy and reduce the intensity and duration of stress responsivity.

Positive and negative emotions

Theorists conceptualize emotion as a multifaceted entity with the following components: an internal or external trigger, an interpretation of the trigger, an appraisal of the interpretation, a physiological reaction, and (possibly) conscious awareness and overt behavior (Power & Dalgleish, 1997). Consider the following sequence: a woman passes an old friend on the street and waves hello. The friend does not make eye contact or respond in any way and continues walking (trigger). A number of possible interpretations, and the resulting consequences, that provide an apt illustration of how emotions can influence stress response are outlined in Figure 1.1.

The transient and/or context-dependent experience of negative emotion serves a purpose and promotes successful adaptation. An attentional bias toward stimuli that signal danger and mobilization of physiological resources support the arousal necessary for life-saving responses to threat such as "fight and flight" (Isen *et al.*, 1987; Lazarus, 1991; Folkman & Moskowitz, 2000). However, chronic negativity is taxing to the body. A recent meta-analysis of 729 studies found that hostility, aggression, and type A behavior are associated with increased cardiovascular activity in response to stress, while anxiety, neuroticism, and generalized negative affect are associated with poorer cardiovascular recovery following stress (Chida & Hamer, 2008).

In contrast, positive states and traits are associated with reduced HPA axis reactivity (Chida & Hamer, 2008), as well as faster cardiovascular recovery from negativity-induced stressors (Levenson, 2003), and have been associated with physical and psychological risk only when very unrealistic (e.g., manic delusions of grandeur and invincibility leading to poor decision making). The broaden and build theory of Fredrikson (2001) posits that the impact of positive emotions is cumulative; repeated positive emotional experiences over time prime the system for optimal response to negative stimuli by expanding physical, psychological, intellectual, and social resources. The experience of positive emotions can also tune the degree of stress response by supporting interpretations of events that are associated with safety (Figure 1.1).

Given the protective capacity of positivity and the necessary but taxing nature of negative emotions, it also follows that resources that promote positive emotions and/or quick recovery and general affective flexibility (emotion regulation) would promote resilience (Masten & Coatsworth, 1998; Siegrist et al., 2005). A neural model of emotion regulation consisting of ventral and dorsal systems has been described, with various patterns of abnormalities associated with a range of psychiatric disorders (Hyman et al., 2006; Nestler & Carlezon, 2006). Studies in mood and anxiety disorders have most consistently identified abnormalities in amygdala, hippocampus, subgenual anterior cingulated cortex, and prefrontal cortex function (Johnstone et al., 2007).

In healthy individuals, differential amygdala reactivity to negative stimuli could represent an intermediate phenotype associated with differential vulnerability to anxiety and depressive disorders (Jabbi et al., 2007). Indeed, several studies have linked the short allele of 5HTTLPR and the A allele of COMT with higher anxiety levels, vulnerability to negative mood, increased amygdala reactivity to negative stimuli, and differential amygdala–cortical functional coupling (Phillips et al., 2003a, 2003b; Gillespie et al., 2005; Munafo et al., 2008). Furthermore, differences in corticolimbic connectivity suggest a possible genetic predisposition toward inflexible emotion processing (Phillips et al., 2003a). As mentioned above, recent imaging studies have shown evidence of multiple gene interactions on limbic reactivity to unpleasant stimuli (Jabbi et al., 2007). In addition, studies of healthy children and young adults at high familial risk for depression and controls at low familial risk for depression have yielded evidence of volumetric differences and diverging neural responses to emotional stimuli between the groups (Munn et al., 2007; Monk et al., 2008; Wolfensberger et al., 2008).

The specific strategies of emotion regulation that have been linked to resilience include the active coping internal mechanisms of reframing/reappraisal, humor, optimism, and meaning-making, and the nature of social interactions (competence and prosocial behavior). These are now discussed in more detail.

Reframing/reappraisal

In general, the ability to use one's cognitive facilities to frame an event in a relatively positive light promotes a quick recovery from distress. Neurobiological mechanisms that underlie some of these processes include memory suppression, memory consolidation, and cognitive control of emotion (Ochsner et al., 2004; Goldin et al., 2008). One mechanism of emotion regulation – cognitive reappraisal – has received particular attention. Functional MRI studies have shown increased activation in lateral and medial prefrontal cortex regions and decreased amygdala activation during reappraisal, with increased activation in lateral prefrontal cortex associated with reappraisal success (Ochsner et al., 2004; Goldin et al., 2008). It has, therefore, been hypothesized that the prefrontal cortex regulates the intensity of emotional response by modulating activation of the amygdala. An fMRI study using mediation analysis demonstrated that the ventrolateral prefrontal cortex acts on both the amygdala and the nucleus accumbens, resulting in opposite behavioral responses: the pathways through the amygdala and the nucleus accumbens were associated with reduced and increased reappraisal success, respectively (Wager et al., 2008). These findings are consistent with animal studies, which have established that the amygdala and nucleus accumbens work in concert to regulate an individual's responses to both negative and positive emotional stimuli. Consequently, variability in the function of these two pathways might underlie individual differences in emotional response and regulation in stressful contexts. Greater use of reappraisal in everyday life has also been linked to greater prefrontal cortex activation and lower amygdala activation to negative stimuli, suggesting a possible central mechanism through which reappraisal could promote successful coping and reduce the risk of mood disorder onset (Drabant et al., 2006). A further fMRI study found that resilient women with a history of sexual trauma were more successful at cognitively enhancing emotional responses to aversive pictures compared with women with PTSD after sexual trauma and healthy, non-traumatized controls. This increased capacity to enhance emotional responses was associated with increased prefrontal cortex activation (New et al., 2009).

Humor

Humor is a second strategy known to contain the threatening nature of stressful situations through cognitive reappraisal. Identified as one of the most mature defense mechanisms, humor may lessen the likelihood of developing stress-induced depression (Deaner & McConatha, 1993; Thorson & Powell, 1994; Manne et al., 2003). Humor, it has been suggested, may reduce depressive symptoms by reducing tension and discomfort (Vaillant, 1992), and by attracting social support (Silver et al., 1990). A network of subcortical regions that constitute core elements of the dopaminergic reward system are activated during humor-related tasks (Mobbs et al., 2003; Moran et al., 2004). In an event-related fMRI study of healthy volunteers, Mobbs et al. (2003) found that funny cartoons, in comparison with non-funny cartoons, elicited activation of the amygdala, ventral striatum/nucleus accumbens, ventral tegmental area, anterior thalamus, and subadjacent hypothalamus. A time-series analysis showed that activity in the nucleus accumbens increased with degree of humor intensity. The nucleus accumbens has been repeatedly linked to psychologically and pharmacologically mediated rewards, and the amygdala has been associated with processing of positive emotions, laughter, and reward magnitude, in addition to its well-known role in fear and fear-related behaviors (Mobbs et al., 2003; Moran et al., 2004).

Optimism

Optimism, the inclination to adopt the most hopeful interpretation of any event, is a trait that influences emotion regulation and is associated not only with resilience (Block & Kremen, 1996; Klohnen, 1996) but also with greater life satisfaction (Chang et al., 1997) and increased psychological and physical health (Affleck & Tennen, 1996; Goldman et al., 1996). Interestingly, brain imaging studies have linked the cognitive and emotional experiences of optimism to increased activity in the amygdala and anterior cingulated cortex (Sharot et al., 2007) This pattern contrasts with evidence of reduced anterior cingulated cortex activity in MDD. This is hardly surprising given that hopelessness and helplessness, polar opposites of optimism, are characteristic symptoms of depression.

Meaning-making

The ability to find meaning in even the most distressing events is another cognitive strategy that can effectively buffer against negative feelings and their consequences, and which is associated with resilience. A sense of purpose and an internal framework of beliefs about right and wrong are characteristic of resilient individuals (Southwick et al., 2005; Alim et al., 2008). Religious and spiritual beliefs and practices might also facilitate recovery and finding meaning after trauma (Southwick et al., 2005). Brain imaging studies are beginning to identify the neural correlates of human morality (Raine & Yang, 2006).

Active coping

Reframing/reappraisal, humor, optimism, and meaning-making are all active coping strategies, in that an individual expends cognitive effort to shape his or her own emotional response. Active coping, including fight and flight (rather than freeze) responses are associated with a more transient activation of the HPA axis (Korte et al., 2005), although the relationship between HPA axis activity and active or passive coping might not be straightforward, as positive associations have also been found (Lu et al., 2008b). Physical exercise, which can be viewed as a form of active coping, has positive effects on mood, attenuates stress responses, and is thought to promote neurogenesis (reviewed by aan het Rot et al., 2009).

Social competence and prosocial behavior

In addition to these internal mechanisms, the nature of one's social interactions can also promote or constrain positive emotionality. For instance, an fMRI study of married women demonstrated that holding hands with their husband attenuated neural responses to the threat of receiving a shock, a response that was proportional to the quality of their relationship (Coan et al., 2006).

Resilient individuals are often altruistic and are able to attract and make use of social support (Masten & Coatsworth, 1998; Southwick et al., 2005; Maier et al., 2006; Lyons & Parker, 2007). It seems likely that empathic capacity would facilitate social competence and prosocial behavior. Signaling by oxytocin, a neuropeptide, has been linked with empathic skill (Domes et al., 2007). In animal models, central release of oxytocin and vasopressin regulates anxiety and social behavior (Storm & Tecott, 2005). In rodent species, oxytocin and vasopressin increase social recognition, pair bonding, and affiliation (Insel, 1997). In humans, administration of intranasal oxytocin to healthy men was associated with increased trust. This change may be mediated by the amygdala (Kosfeld *et al.*, 2005). In a separate investigation, oxytocin reduced amygdala activation in response to fear-inducing visual stimuli, and reduced connectivity between the amygdala and brainstem areas mediating autonomic and behavioral fear responses (Kirsch *et al.*, 2005). It has been proposed that oxytocin and vasopressin may enhance the reward value of social stimuli and reduce potential fear responses (Skuse & Gallagher, 2009).

"Mirror neurons," cortical neurons that fire similarly both when an animal performs a task themselves and when the animal observes another animal of the same species performing that task, are also potentially relevant to the experience of empathy (Rizzolatti & Craighero, 2004). This system, in conjunction with limbic brain regions, may play a role in understanding others' emotions and intentions (Schulte-Ruther *et al.*, 2007). In a recent study, children rated as more empathic and socially skilled than their peers evinced greater activation in presumed mirror neuron and associated limbic areas during imitation of emotional faces (Pfeifer *et al.*, 2008). Adults engaged in tasks that require thinking about the mental states of both self and other activate the ventromedial prefrontal cortex. Patients with lesions in this area have deficits in social emotions such as shame, guilt, and empathy.

Conclusions

This chapter has used an allostatic framework to define resilience and to explore its neurobiological substrates. Given the preponderance and complexity of questions still unanswered, it is clear that years of further study will be needed to fully understand the dynamic mechanisms that support resilient phenotypes. However, a model of resilience has begun to emerge from the knowledge acquired so far. Throughout life, genetic and environmental agents (and perhaps some stochastic epigenetic events) interact with and reshape the circuitry responsible for and influenced by the stress response. Because the integrity of these dynamic neural systems involved in fear, reward, emotion regulation, and social behavior determines the degree of resilience, resilience can also be understood as a fluid state, rather than a static trait. Consequently, it seems likely that individuals could become more resilient with exposure to enhancing protective factors.

Indeed, clinicians have begun to design, implement, and evaluate translational strategies to improve resilience. Already, group-based interventions have proven effective in eliciting durable increases in resilience to work-related and terrorism-related stress (Butler *et al.*, 2009; Willert *et al.*, 2009). Certain forms of psychotherapy appear to enhance psychological attributes associated with resilience (Lee *et al.*, 2004). In addition, the US military has identified minimization of the psychiatric burden of war as a high priority and is just beginning the largest-scale study to date of psychosocial resilience-enhancing tactics (Reed & Love, 2009).

It is likely that new interventions will emerge with further improvements in technology. For example, new pharmacological agents that influence the function of the HPA axis, as well as the monoamine, neuropeptide, and other neurochemical stress-response systems, could be developed. It is even possible that individuals could be trained to modulate their own brain activity using real-time fMRI-based neurofeedback (Weiskopf *et al.*, 2004; Caria *et al.*, 2007). As the body of resilience scholarship and its impact on the academic and clinical communities continues to grow, there appears to be much cause for hope.

References

aan het Rot, M., Collins, K. A., & Fitterling, H. L. (2009). Physical exercise and depression. *Mount Sinai Journal of Medicine*, **76**, 204–214.

Affleck, G. & Tennen, H. (1996). Construing benefits from adversity: Adaptational significance and dispositional underpinnings. *Journal of Personality*, **64**, 899–922.

Alfinito, P. D., Chen, X., Mastroeni, R., Pawlyk, A. C., & Deecher, D. C. (2009). Estradiol increases catecholamine levels in the hypothalamus of ovariectomized rats during the dark-phase. *European Journal of Pharmacology*, **616**, 334–339.

Alim, T. N., Feder, A., Graves, R. E., *et al.* (2008). Trauma, resilience, and recovery in a high-risk African-American population. *American Journal of Psychiatry*, **165**, 1566–1575.

Anestis, S. F. (2006). Testosterone in juvenile and adolescent male chimpanzees (*Pan troglodytes*): effects of dominance rank, aggression, and behavioral style. *American Journal of Physical Anthropology*, **130**, 536–545.

Baker, D. G., West, S. A., Orth, D. N., *et al.* (1997). Cerebrospinal fluid and plasma beta-endorphin in combat veterans with post-traumatic stress disorder. *Psychoneuroendocrinology*, **22**, 517–529.

Baker, D. G., West, S. A., Nicholson, W. E., *et al.* (1999). Serial CSF corticotropin-releasing hormone levels and adrenocortical activity in combat veterans with posttraumatic stress disorder. *American Journal of Psychiatry*, **156**, 585–588.

Baker, D. G., Ekhator, N. N., Kasckow, J. W., *et al.* (2005). Higher levels of basal serial CSF cortisol in combat veterans with posttraumatic stress disorder. *American Journal of Psychiatry*, **162**, 992–994.

Bakshi, V. P., Smith-Roe, S., Newman, S. M., Grigoriadis, D. E., & Kalin, N. H. (2002). Reduction of stress-induced behavior by antagonism of corticotropin-releasing hormone (CRH2) receptors in lateral septum or CRH1 receptors in amygdala. *Journal of Neuroscience*, **22**, 2926–2935.

Bale, T. L., Contarino A., Smith, G. W., *et al.* (2000). Mice deficient for corticotropin-releasing hormone receptor-2 display anxiety-like behaviour and are hypersensitive to stress. *Nature Genetics*, **24**, 410–414.

Bannon, A. W., Seda, J., Carmouche, M., *et al.* (2000). Behavioral characterization of neuropeptide Y knockout mice. *Brain Research*, **868**, 79–87.

Barrera, G., Hernandez, A., Poulin, J. F., *et al.* (2006). Galanin-mediated anxiolytic effect in rat central amygdala is not a result of corelease from noradrenergic terminals. *Synapse*, **59**, 27–40.

Bast, T. (2007). Toward an integrative perspective on hippocampal function: From the rapid encoding of experience to adaptive behavior. *Reviews in the Neurosciences*, **18**, 253–281.

Bastianetto, S., Ramassamy, C., Poirier, J., & Quirion, R. (1999). Dehydroepiandrosterone (DHEA) protects hippocampal cells from oxidative stress-induced damage. *Brain Research, MolecularBrain Research*, **66**, 35–41.

Belda, X. & Armario, A. (2009). Dopamine D_1 and D_2 dopamine receptors regulate immobilization stress-induced activation of the hypothalamus–pituitary–adrenal axis. *Psychopharmacology (Berl)*, **206**, 355–365.

Belfer, I., Hipp, H., McKnight, C., *et al.* (2006). Association of galanin haplotypes with alcoholism and anxiety in two ethnically distinct populations. *Molecular Psychiatry*, **11**, 301–311.

Belsky, J., Jonassaint, C., Pluess, M., *et al.* (2009). Vulnerability genes or plasticity genes? *Molecular Psychiatry*, **14**, 746–754.

Bender, N., Heg, D., Hamilton, I. M., *et al.* (2006). The relationship between social status, behaviour, growth and steroids in male helpers and breeders of a cooperatively breeding cichlid. *Hormones and Behavior*, **50**, 173–182.

Berton, O., McClung, C. A., Dileone, R. J., *et al.* (2006). Essential role of BDNF in the mesolimbic dopamine pathway in social defeat stress. *Science*, **311**, 864–868.

Berton, O., Covington, H. E. 3rd, Ebner, K., *et al.* (2007). Induction of deltaFosB in the periaqueductal gray by stress promotes active coping responses. *Neuron*, **55**, 289–300.

Bethea, C. L., Mirkes, S. J., Shively, C. A., & Adams, M. R. (2002). Steroid regulation of tryptophan hydroxylase protein in the dorsal raphe of macaques. *Biological Psychiatry*, **47**, 562–576.

Bierer, L. M., Tischler, L., Labinsky, E., *et al.* (2006). Clinical correlates of 24-h cortisol and norepinephrine excretion among subjects seeking treatment following the World Trade Center attacks on 9/11. *Annals of the New York Academy of Sciences*, **1071**, 514–520.

Bjornebekk, A., Mathe, A. A., & Brene, S. (2010). The antidepressant effects of running and escitalopram are associated with levels of hippocampal NPY and Y_1 receptor but not cell proliferation in a rat model of depression. *Hippocampus*, **20**, 820–828.

Block, J. & Kremen, A. M. (1996). IQ and ego-resiliency: Conceptual and empirical connections and separateness. *Journal of Personality and Social Psychology*, **70**, 349–361.

Blomqvist, A. G. & Herzog, H. (1997). Y-receptor subtypes – how many more? *Trends in Neuroscience*, **20**, 294–298.

Bogdan, R. & Pizzagalli, D. A. (2006). Acute stress reduces reward responsiveness: Implications for depression. *Biological Psychiatry*, **60**, 1147–1154.

Bonanno, G. A. (2004). Loss, trauma, and human resilience: Have we underestimated the human capacity to thrive after extremely aversive events? *American Psychologist*, **59**, 20–28.

Boyer, E. W. & Shannon, M. (2005). The serotonin syndrome. *New England Journal of Medicine*, **352**, 1112–1120.

Bradley, R. G., Binder, E. B., Epstein, M. P., *et al.* (2008). Influence of child abuse on adult depression: Moderation by the corticotropin-releasing hormone receptor gene. *Archives of General Psychiatry*, **65**, 190–200.

Bremner, J. D., Krystal, J. H., Southwick, S. M., & Charney, D. S. (1996). Noradrenergic mechanisms in stress and anxiety: I. preclinical studies. *Synapse*, **23**, 28–38.

Bremner, J. D., Licinio, J., Darnell, A., *et al.* (1997). Elevated CSF corticotropin-releasing factor concentrations in posttraumatic stress disorder. *American Journal of Psychiatry*, **154**, 624–629.

Britton, K. T., Akwa, Y., Spina, M. G., & Koob, G. F. (2000). Neuropeptide Y blocks anxiogenic-like behavioral action of corticotropin-releasing factor in an operant conflict test and elevated plus maze. *Peptides*, **21**, 37–44.

Browne, E. S., Wright, B. E., Porter, J. R., & Svec, F. (1992). Dehydroepiandrosterone: Antiglucocorticoid action in mice. *American Journal of Medical Science*, **303**, 366–371.

Brunner, R., Schaefer, D., Hess, K., *et al.* (2006). Effect of high-dose cortisol on memory functions. *Annals of the New York Academy of Sciences*, **1071**, 434–437.

Butler, L. D., Koopman, C., Azarow, J., *et al.* (2009). Psychosocial predictors of resilience after the September 11, 2001 terrorist attacks. *Journal of Nervous and Mental Disorders*, **197**, 266–273.

Carey, M. P., Deterd, C. H., de Koning, J., Helmerhorst, F., & de Kloet, E. R. (1995). The influence of ovarian steroids on hypothalamic–pituitary–adrenal regulation in the female rat. *Journal of Endocrinology*, **144**, 311–321.

Caria, A., Veit, R., Sitaram, R., *et al.* (2007). Regulation of anterior insular cortex activity using real-time fMRI. *Neuroimage* **35**, 1238–1246.

Carroll, B. J., Cassidy, F., Naftolowitz, D., *et al.* (2007). Pathophysiology of hypercortisolism in depression. *Acta Psychiatric Scandinavica Supplement,* **433**, 90–103.

Carter, R. M., Macinnes, J. J., Huettel, S. A., & Adcock, R. A. (2009). Activation in the VTA and nucleus accumbens increases in anticipation of both gains and losses. *Frontiers in Behavioral Neuroscience*, **3**, 21.

Caspi, A., Sugden, K., Moffitt, T. E., *et al.* (2003). Influence of life stress on depression: Moderation by a polymorphism in the 5-*HTT* gene. *Science*, **301**, 386–389.

Chang, E., Maydeu-Olivares, A., & D'Zurilla, T. J. (1997). Optimism and pessimism as partially independent constructs: Relationship to positive and negative affectivity and psychological well-being. *Personality and Individual Differences*, **23**, 433–440.

Charney, D. S. (2004). Psychobiological mechanisms of resilience and vulnerability: Implications for successful adaptation to extreme stress. *American Journal of Psychiatry*, **161**, 195–216.

Charney, D. S. & Bremner, J. D. (1999). The neurobiology of anxiety disorders. In D. S. Charney, E. J. Nestler, & B. S. Bunney (eds.), *Neurobiology of mental illness* (pp. 494–517). New York: Oxford University Press.

Charney, D. S., Woods, S. W., Goodman, W. K., & Heninger, G. R. (1987). Neurobiological mechanisms of panic anxiety: Biochemical and behavioral correlates of yohimbine-induced panic attacks. *American Journal of Psychiatry*, **144**, 1030–1036.

Charney, D. S., Woods, S. W., Krystal, J. H., Nagy, L. M., & Heninger, G. R. (1992). Noradrenergic neuronal dysregulation in panic disorder: The effects of intravenous yohimbine and clonidine in panic disorder patients. *Acta Psychiatric Scandinavica*, **86**, 273–282.

Chen, L., Dai, X. N., & Sokabe, M. (2006). Chronic administration of dehydroepiandrosterone sulfate (DHEAS) primes for facilitated induction of long-term potentiation via sigma 1 (sigma1) receptor: Optical imaging study in rat hippocampal slices. *Neuropharmacology*, **50**, 380–392.

Chida, Y. & Hamer, M. (2008). Chronic psychosocial factors and acute physiological responses to laboratory-induced stress in healthy populations: A quantitative review of 30 years of investigations. *Psychological Bulletin*, **134**, 829–885.

Coan, J. A., Schaefer, H. S., & Davidson, R. J. (2006). Lending a hand: Social regulation of the neural response to threat. *Psychological Science*, **17**, 1032–1039.

Colangelo, L. A., Sharp, L., Kopp, P., *et al.* (2007). Total testosterone, androgen receptor polymorphism, and depressive symptoms in young black and white men: The CARDIA male hormone study. *Psychoneuroendocrinology*, **32**, 951–958.

Colucci, W. S., Gimbrone, M. A. Jr., McLaughlin, M. K., Halpern, W., & Alexander, R. W. (1982). Increased vascular catecholamine sensitivity and alpha-adrenergic receptor affinity in female and estrogen-treated male rats. *Circulation Research*, **50**, 805–811.

Conrad, M. & Hammen, C. (1989). Role of maternal depression in perceptions of child maladjustment. *Journal of Consulting and Clinical Psychology*, **57**, 663–667.

Cools, R., Calder, A. J., Lawrence, A. D., *et al.* (2005). Individual differences in threat sensitivity predict serotonergic modulation of amygdala response to fearful faces. *Psychopharmacology (Berl)*, **180**, 670–679.

Cools, R., Roberts, A. C., & Robbins, T. W. (2008). Serotoninergic regulation of emotional and behavioural control processes. *Trends in Cognitive Science*, **12**, 31–40.

Coste, S. C., Kesterson, R. A., Heldwein, K. A., *et al.* (2000). Abnormal adaptations to stress and impaired cardiovascular function in mice lacking corticotropin-releasing hormone receptor-2. *Nature Genetics*, **24**, 403–409.

Cucinelli, F., Soranna, L., Barini, A., *et al.* (2002). Estrogen treatment and body fat distribution are involved in corticotropin and cortisol response to corticotropin-releasing hormone in postmenopausal women. *Metabolism, Clinical and Experimental*, **51**, 137–143.

Czoty, P. W., Gould, R. W., & Nader, M. A. (2009). Relationship between social rank and cortisol and testosterone concentrations in male cynomolgus monkeys (*Macaca fascicularis*). *Journal of Neuroendocrinology*, **21**, 68–76.

Daly, R. C., Su, T. P., Schmidt, P. J., *et al.* (2001). Cerebrospinal fluid and behavioral changes after methyltestosterone administration: Preliminary findings. *Archives of General Psychiatry*, **58**, 172–177.

Davis, M. & Whalen, P. J. (2001). The amygdala: Vigilance and emotion. *Molecular Psychiatry*, **6**, 13–34.

Dayan, P. & Huys, Q. J. (2009). Serotonin in affective control. *Annual Reviews in the Neurosciences*, **32**, 95–126.

de Kloet, E. R., Joels, M., & Holsboer, F. (2005). Stress and the brain: From adaptation to disease. *Nature Reviews in the Neurosciences*, **6**, 463–475.

de Kloet, E. R., Derijk, R. H., & Meijer, O. C. (2007). Therapy insight: Is there an imbalanced response of mineralocorticoid and glucocorticoid receptors in depression? *Nature Clinical and Practical Endocrinology and Metabolism*, **3**, 168–179.

Deaner, S. L. & McConatha, J. T. (1993). The relation of humor to depression and personality. *Psychological Reports*, **72**, 755–763.

Debiec, J. & LeDoux, J. E. (2006). Noradrenergic signaling in the amygdala contributes to the reconsolidation of fear memory: Treatment implications for PTSD. *Annals of the New York Academy of Sciences*, **1071**, 521–524.

Dedovic, K., Renwick, R., Mahani, N. K., *et al.* (2005). The Montreal Imaging Stress Task: Using functional imaging to investigate the effects of perceiving and processing psychosocial stress in the human brain. *Journal of Psychiatry and Neuroscience*, **30**, 319–325.

Delgado, M. R., Olsson, A., & Phelps, E. A. (2006). Extending animal models of fear conditioning to humans. *Biological Psychology*, **73**, 39–48.

Derijk, R. H. (2009). Single nucleotide polymorphisms related to HPA axis reactivity. *Neuroimmunomodulation*, **16**, 340–352.

Derijk, R. H. & de Kloet, E. R. (2008). Corticosteroid receptor polymorphisms: Determinants of vulnerability and resilience. *European Journal of Pharmacology*, **583**, 303–311.

Domes, G., Heinrichs, M., Michel, A., Berger, C., & Herpertz, S. C. (2007). Oxytocin improves "mind-reading" in humans. *Biological Psychiatry*, **61**, 731–733.

Douma, S. L., Husban D. C., O'Donnell, M. E., Barwin, B. N., & Woodend, A. K. (2005). Estrogen-related mood disorders: Reproductive life cycle factors. *Advances in Nursing Science*, **28**, 364–375.

Drabant, E. M., Hariri, A. R., Meyer-Lindenberg, A., *et al.* (2006). Catechol *O*-methyltransferase val158met genotype and neural mechanisms related to affective arousal and regulation. *Archives of General Psychiatry*, **63**, 1396–1406.

Duman, R. S. & Monteggia, L. M. (2006). A neurotrophic model for stress-related mood disorders. *Biological Psychiatry*, **59**, 1116–1127.

Edwards, D. A., Wetzel, K., & Wyner, D. R. (2006). Intercollegiate soccer: Saliva cortisol and testosterone are elevated during competition, and testosterone is related to status and social connectedness with teammates. *Physiology and Behavior*, **87**, 135–143.

Edwards, D. A. & O'Neal, J. (2009). Oral contraceptives decrease saliva testosterone but do not affect the rise in testosterone associated with athletic competition. *Hormones and Behavior*, **56**, 195–198.

Eisch, A. J., Bolanos, C. A., de Wit, J., *et al.* (2003). Brain-derived neurotrophic factor in the ventral midbrain-nucleus accumbens pathway: A role in depression. *Biological Psychiatry*, **54**, 994–1005.

Elder, G. H. Jr. (1998). The life course as developmental theory. *Child Development*, **69**, 1–12.

Elovainio, M., Jokela, M., Kivimaki, M., *et al.* (2007). Genetic variants in the *DRD2* gene moderate the relationship between stressful life events and depressive symptoms in adults: Cardiovascular risk in Young Finns study. *Psychosomatic Medicine*, **69**, 391–395.

Eva, C., Serra, M., Mele, P., Panzica, G., & Oberto, A. (2006). Physiology and gene regulation of the brain NPY Y1 receptor. *Frontiers in Neuroendocrinology*, **27**, 308–339.

Felmingham, K., Kemp, A., Williams, L., *et al.* (2007). Changes in anterior cingulate and amygdala after cognitive behavior therapy of posttraumatic stress disorder. *Psychological Science*, **18**, 127–129.

Flugge, G., Kramer, M., & Fuchs, E. (2001). Chronic subordination stress in male tree shrews: Replacement of testosterone affects behavior and central alpha(2)-adrenoceptors. *Physiology and Behavior*, **73**, 293–300.

Folkman, S. & Moskowitz, J. T. (2000). Positive affect and the other side of coping. *American Psychology*, **55**, 647–654.

Forbes, E. E., Hariri, A. R., Martin, S. L., *et al.* (2009). Altered striatal activation predicting real-world positive affect in adolescent major depressive disorder. *American Journal of Psychiatry*, **166**, 64–73.

Franca, S. C., Barros Neto, T. L., Aqresta, M. C., Lotufo, R. F., & Kater, C. E. (2006). Divergent responses of serum testosterone and cortisol in athlete men after a marathon race. *Arquivos Brasileiros de Endocrinologia e Metabologia*, **50**, 1082–1087.

Fredrickson, B. L. (2001). The role of positive emotions in positive psychology. The broaden-and-build theory of positive emotions. *American Psychologist*, **56**, 218–226.

Gallagher, P. & Young, A. (2002). Cortisol/DHEA ratios in depression. *Neuropsychopharmacology*, **26**, 410.

Geracioti, T. D. Jr., Baker, D. G., Ekhator, N. N., *et al.* (2001). CSF norepinephrine concentrations in posttraumatic stress disorder. *American Journal of Psychiatry*, **158**, 1227–1230.

Gillespie, N. A., Whitfield, J. B., Williams, B., Heath, A. C., & Martin, N. G. (2005). The relationship between stressful life events, the serotonin transporter (5-HTTLPR) genotype and major depression. *Psychological Medicine*, **35**, 101–111.

Goldin, P. R., McRae, K., Ramel, W., & Gross, J. J. (2008). The neural bases of emotion regulation: Reappraisal and suppression of negative emotion. *Biological Psychiatry*, **63**, 577–586.

Goldman, S. L., Kraemer, D. T., & Salovey, P. (1996). Beliefs about mood moderate the relationship of stress to illness and symptom reporting. *Journal of Psychosomatic Research*, **41**, 115–128.

Goldstein, L. E., Rasmusson, A. M., Bunney, B. S., & Roth, R. H. (1996). Role of the amygdala in the coordination of behavioral, neuroendocrine, and prefrontal cortical monoamine responses to psychological stress in the rat. *Journal of Neuroscience*, **16**, 4787–4798.

Goodyer, I. M., Herbert, J., & Altham, P. M. (1998). Adrenal steroid secretion and major depression in 8- to 16-year-olds, III. Influence of cortisol/DHEA ratio at presentation on subsequent rates of disappointing life events and persistent major depression. *Psychological Medicine*, **28**, 265–273.

Goyal, S. N., Upadhya, M. A., Kokare, D. M., Bhisikar, S. M., & Subhedar, N. K. (2009). Neuropeptide Y modulates the antidepressant activity of imipramine in olfactory bulbectomized rats: Involvement of NPY Y1 receptors. *Brain Research*, **1266**, 45–53.

Green, S., Walter, P., Kumar, V., et al. (1986). Human oestrogen receptor cDNA: Sequence, expression and homology to v-Erb-A. *Nature*, **320**, 134–139.

Gross, C., Zhuang, X., Stark, K., et al. (2002). Serotonin 1A receptor acts during development to establish normal anxiety-like behaviour in the adult. *Nature*, **416**, 396–400.

Gutman, A. R., Yang, Y., Ressler, K. J., & Davis, M. (2008). The role of neuropeptide Y in the expression and extinction of fear-potentiated startle. *Journal of Neuroscience*, **28**, 12682–12690.

Handwerger, K. (2009). Differential patterns of HPA activity and reactivity in adult posttraumatic stress disorder and major depressive disorder. *Harvard Reviews of Psychiatry*, **17**, 184–205.

Heilig, M., McLeod, S., Brot, M., et al. (1993). Anxiolytic-like action of neuropeptide Y: Mediation by Y1 receptors in amygdala, and dissociation from food intake effects. *Neuropsychopharmacology*, **8**, 357–363.

Heilig, M., Koob, G. F., Ekman, R., & Britton, K. T. (1994). Corticotropin-releasing factor and neuropeptide Y: Role in emotional integration. *Trends in Neuroscience*, **17**, 80–85.

Heilig, M., Zachrisson, O., Thorsell, A., et al. (2004). Decreased cerebrospinal fluid neuropeptide Y (NPY) in patients with treatment refractory unipolar major depression: Preliminary evidence for association with preproNPY gene polymorphism. *Journal of Psychiatric Research*, **38**, 113–121.

Heim, C. & Nemeroff, C. B. (2001). The role of childhood trauma in the neurobiology of mood and anxiety disorders: Preclinical and clinical studies. *Biological Psychiatry*, **49**, 1023–1039.

Heinz, A. & Smolka, M. N. (2006). The effects of catechol *O*-methyltransferase genotype on brain activation elicited by affective stimuli and cognitive tasks. *Reviews in the Neurosciences*, **17**, 359–367.

Heinz, A., Braus, D. F., Smolka, M. N., et al. (2005). Amygdala–prefrontal coupling depends on a genetic variation of the serotonin transporter. *Nature Neuroscience*, **8**, 20–21.

Heisler, L. K., Chu, H. M., Brennan, T. J., et al. (1998). Elevated anxiety and antidepressant-like responses in serotonin 5-HT1A receptor mutant mice. *Proceedings of the National Academy of Sciences of the USA*, **95**, 15049–15054.

Hermans, E. J., Putman P., Baas, J. M., Koppeschaar, H. P., & van Honk, J. (2006). A single administration of testosterone reduces fear-potentiated startle in humans. *Biological Psychiatry*, **59**, 872–874.

Hermans, E. J., Putman P., Baas, J. M., et al. (2007). Exogenous testosterone attenuates the integrated central stress response in healthy young women. *Psychoneuroendocrinology*, **32**, 1052–1061.

Hermans, E. J., Ramsey, N. F., & van Honk, J. (2008). Exogenous testosterone enhances responsiveness to social threat in the neural circuitry of social aggression in humans. *Biological Psychiatry*, **63**, 263–270.

Hilke, S., Theodorsson, A., Fetissov, S., et al. (2005). Estrogen induces a rapid increase in galanin levels in female rat hippocampal formation: Possibly a nongenomic/indirect effect. *European Journal of Neuroscience*, **21**, 2089–2099.

Hilke, S., Holm, L., Man, K., Hökfelt, T., & Theodorsson, E. (2009). Rapid change of neuropeptide Y levels and gene-expression in the brain of ovariectomized mice after administration of 17β-estradiol. *Neuropeptides*, **43**, 327–332.

Hökfelt, T., Broberger, C., Zhang, X., et al. (1998). Neuropeptide Y: Some viewpoints on a multifaceted peptide in the normal and diseased nervous system. *Brain Research Reviews*, **26**, 154–166.

Holmes, A. & Picciotto, M. R. (2006). Galanin: A novel therapeutic target for depression, anxiety disorders and drug addiction? *CNS Neurology Disorders and Drug Targets* 5, 225–232.

Holmes, A., Kinney, J. W., Wrenn, C. C., et al. (2003). Galanin GAL-R1 receptor null mutant mice display increased anxiety-like behavior specific to the elevated plus-maze. *Neuropsychopharmacology*, **28**, 1031–1044.

Hopper, J. W., Pitman, R. K., Su, Z., et al. (2008). Probing reward function in posttraumatic stress disorder: Expectancy and satisfaction with monetary gains and losses. *Journal of Psychiatric Research*, **42**, 802–807.

Hyman, S. E., Malenka, R. C., & Nestler, E. J. (2006). Neural mechanisms of addiction: The role of reward-related learning and memory. *Annual Reviews in the Neurosciences*, **29**, 565–598.

Inoue, T., Koyama, T., & Yamashita, I. (1993). Effect of conditioned fear stress on serotonin metabolism in the rat brain. *Pharmacology Biochemistry and Behavior*, **44**, 371–374.

Insel, T. R. (1997). A neurobiological basis of social attachment. *American Journal of Psychiatry*, **154**, 726–735.

Inslicht, S. S., Marmar, C. R., Neylan, T. C., *et al.* (2006). Increased cortisol in women with intimate partner violence-related posttraumatic stress disorder. *Annals of the New York Academy of Sciences*, **1071**, 428–429.

Isen, A. M., Daubman, K. A., & Nowicki, G. P. (1987). Positive affect facilitates creative problem solving. *Journal of Personality and Social Psychology*, **52**, 1122–1131.

Jabbi, M., Korf, J., Kema, I. P., *et al.* (2007). Convergent genetic modulation of the endocrine stress response involves polymorphic variations of 5-HTT, COMT and MAOA. *Molecular Psychiatry*, **12**, 483–490.

Johnstone, T., van Reekum, C. M., Urry, H. L., Kalin, N. H., & Davidson, R. J. (2007). Failure to regulate: Counterproductive recruitment of top-down prefrontal-subcortical circuitry in major depression. *Journal of Neuroscience*, **27**, 8877–8884.

Kaga, T., Inui, A., Okita, M., *et al.* (2001). Modest overexpression of neuropeptide Y in the brain leads to obesity after high-sucrose feeding. *Diabetes*, **50**, 1206–1210.

Karlsson, R. M. & Holmes, A. (2006). Galanin as a modulator of anxiety and depression and a therapeutic target for affective disease. *Amino Acids*, **31**, 231–239.

Karlsson, R. M., Holmes, A., Heilig, M., & Crawley, J. N. (2005). Anxiolytic-like actions of centrally-administered neuropeptide Y, but not galanin, in C57BL/6J mice. *Pharmacology, Biochemistry and Behavior*, **80**, 427–436.

Khoshbouei, H., Cecchi, M., Dove, S., Javors, M., & Morilak, D. A. (2002). Behavioral reactivity to stress: Amplification of stress-induced noradrenergic activation elicits a galanin-mediated anxiolytic effect in central amygdala. *Pharmacology, Biochemistry and Behavior*, **71**, 407–417.

Kim, J. M., Stewart, R., Kim, S. W., *et al.* (2007). Interactions between life stressors and susceptibility genes (5-*HTTLPR* and *BDNF*) on depression in Korean elders. *Biological Psychiatry*, **62**, 423–428.

Kimonides, V. G., Khatibi, N. H., Svendsen, C. N., Sofroniew, M. V., & Herbert, J. (1998). Dehydroepiandrosterone (DHEA) and DHEA-sulfate (DHEAS) protect hippocampal neurons against excitatory amino acid-induced neurotoxicity. *Proceedings of the National Academy of Sciences of the USA*, **95**, 1852–1857.

Kirsch, P., Esslinger, C., Chen, Q., *et al.* (2005). Oxytocin modulates neural circuitry for social cognition and fear in humans. *Journal of Neuroscience*, **25**, 11489–11493.

Klangkalya, B. & Chan, A. (1988). The effects of ovarian hormones on beta-adrenergic and muscarinic receptors in rat heart. *Life Science*, **42**, 2307–2314.

Klohnen, E. C. (1996). Conceptual analysis and measurement of the construct of ego-resiliency. *Journal of Personality and Social Psychology*, **70**, 1067–1079.

Komesaroff, P. A., Esler, M. D., & Sudhir, K. (1999). Estrogen supplementation attenuates glucocorticoid and catecholamine responses to mental stress in perimenopausal women. *Journal of Clinical Endocrinology and Metabolism*, **84**, 606–610.

Korte, S. M., Koolhaas, J. M., Wingfield, J. C., & McEwen, B. S. (2005). The Darwinian concept of stress: Benefits of allostasis and costs of allostatic load and the trade-offs in health and disease. *Neuroscience and BioBehavioral Reviews*, **29**, 3–38.

Kosfeld, M., Heinrichs, M., Zak, P. J., Fischbacher, U., & Fehr, E. (2005). Oxytocin increases trust in humans. *Nature*, **435**, 673–676.

Kozlovsky, N., Matar, M. A., Kaplan, Z., Zohar, J., & Cohen, H. (2009). The role of the galaninergic system in modulating stress-related responses in an animal model of posttraumatic stress disorder. *Biological Psychiatry*, **65**, 383–391.

Krishnan, V., Han, M. H., Graham, D. L., *et al.* (2007). Molecular adaptations underlying susceptibility and resistance to social defeat in brain reward regions. *Cell*, **131**, 391–404.

Krishnan, V., Han, M. H., Mazei-Robison, M., *et al.* (2008). AKT signaling within the ventral tegmental area regulates cellular and behavioral responses to stressful stimuli. *Biological Psychiatry*, **64**, 691–700.

Kuiper, G. G., Enmark, E., Pelto-Huikko, M., Nilsson, S., & Gustafsson, J. A. (1996). Cloning of a novel receptor expressed in rat prostate and ovary. *Proceedings of the National Academy of Sciences of the USA*, **93**, 5925–5930.

Lawford, B. R., Young, R., Noble, E. P., Kann, B., & Ritchie, T. (2006). The D_2 dopamine receptor (DRD2) gene is associated with co-morbid depression, anxiety and social dysfunction in untreated veterans with post-traumatic stress disorder. *European Psychiatry*, **21**, 180–185.

Lazarus, R. S. (1991). Progress on a cognitive-motivational-relational theory of emotion. *American Psychologist*, **46**, 819–834.

Lee, V., Cohen, S. R., Edgar, L., Laizner, A. M., & Gagnon, A. J. (2004). Clarifying "meaning" in the context of cancer research: A systematic literature review. *Palliative Support Care*, **2**, 291–303.

Lemieux, A. M. & Coe, C. L. (1995). Abuse-related posttraumatic stress disorder: Evidence for chronic neuroendocrine activation in women. *Psychosomatic Medicine*, **57**, 105–115.

Levenson, R. W. (2003). Blood, sweat, and fears: The autonomic architecture of emotion. *Annals of the New York Academy of Sciences*, **1000**, 348–366.

Liberzon, I. & Sripada, C. S. (2008). The functional neuroanatomy of PTSD: A critical review. *Progress in Brain Research*, **167**, 151–169.

Lin, S., Boey, D., & Herzog, H. (2004). NPY and Y receptors: Lessons from transgenic and knockout models. *Neuropeptides*, **38**, 189–200.

Lopez, J. F., Chalmers, D. T., Little, K. Y., & Watson, S. J. (1998). A.E. Bennett Research Award. Regulation of serotonin 1A, glucocorticoid, and mineralocorticoid receptor in rat and human hippocampus: Implications for the neurobiology of depression. *Biological Psychiatry*, **43**, 547–573.

Lu, X., Ross, B., Sanchez-Alavez, M., Zorrilla, E. P., & Bartfai, T. (2008a). Phenotypic analysis of *GalR2* knockout mice in anxiety- and depression-related behavioral tests. *Neuropeptides*, **42**, 387–397.

Lu, A., Steiner, M. A., Whittle, N., *et al.* (2008b). Conditional mouse mutants highlight mechanisms of corticotropin-releasing hormone effects on stress-coping behavior. *Molecular Psychiatry*, **13**, 1028–1042.

Lukkes, J., Vuong, S., Scholl, J., Oliver, H., & Forster, G. (2009). Corticotropin-releasing factor receptor antagonism within the dorsal raphe nucleus reduces social anxiety-like behavior after early-life social isolation. *Journal of Neuroscience*, **29**, 9955–9960.

Lyons, D. M. & Parker, K. J. (2007). Stress inoculation-induced indications of resilience in monkeys. *Journal of Trauma and Stress*, **20**, 423–433.

Maggi, A. & Perez, J. (1986). Estrogen-induced up-regulation of gamma-aminobutyric acid receptors in the CNS of rodents. *Journal of Neurochemistry*, **47**, 1793–1797.

Maier, S. F., Amat, J., Baratta, M. V., Paul, E., & Watkins, L. R. (2006). Behavioral control, the medial prefrontal cortex, and resilience. *Dialogues in Clinical Neuroscience*, **8**, 397–406.

Manne, S., Duhamel, K., Ostroff, J., *et al.* (2003). Coping and the course of mother's depressive symptoms during and after pediatric bone marrow transplantation. *Journal of the American Academy of Child and Adolescent Psychiatry*, **42**, 1055–1068.

Masten, A. S. (2001). Ordinary magic. Resilience processes in development. *American Psychologist*, **56**, 227–238.

Masten, A. S. & Coatsworth, J. D. (1998). The development of competence in favorable and unfavorable environments. Lessons from research on successful children. *American Psychologist*, **53**, 205–220.

Masten, A. S., Coatsworth, J. D., Neemann, J., *et al.* (1995). The structure and coherence of competence from childhood through adolescence. *Child Development*, **66**, 1635–1659.

McCabe, C., Cowen, P. J., & Harmer, C. J. (2009). Neural representation of reward in recovered depressed patients. *Psychopharmacology (Berl)*, **205**, 667–677.

McEwen, B. S. (2002). Estrogen actions throughout the brain. *Recent Progress in Hormonal Research*, **57**, 357–384.

McEwen, B. S. (2003). Mood disorders and allostatic load. *Biological Psychiatry*, **54**, 200–207.

McEwen, B. S. & Stellar, E. (1993). Stress and the individual: Mechanisms leading to disease. *Archives of Internal Medicine*, **153**, 2093–2101.

McGaugh, J. L. (2004). The amygdala modulates the consolidation of memories of emotionally arousing experiences. *Annual Reviews in the Neurosciences*, **27**, 1–28.

Meaney, M. J. & Szyf, M. (2005). Environmental programming of stress responses through DNA methylation: Life at the interface between a dynamic environment and a fixed genome. *Dialogues in Clinical Neuroscience*, **7**, 103–123.

Mikkelsen, J. D. & Woldbye, D. P. (2006). Association of the 5-HT2A receptor gene polymorphism 102T/C with ischemic stroke. *Journal of Psychiatric Research*, **40**, 153–159.

Mize, A. L., Poisner, A. M., & Alper, R. H. (2001). Estrogens act in rat hippocampus and frontal cortex to produce rapid, receptor-mediated decreases in serotonin 5-HT(1A) receptor function. *Neuroendocrinology*, **73**, 166–174.

Mobbs, D., Greicius, M. D., Abdel-Azim, E., Menon, V., & Reiss, A. L. (2003). Humor modulates the mesolimbic reward centers. *Neuron*, **40**, 1041–1048.

Monk, C. S., Klein, R. G., Telzer, E. H., *et al.* (2008). Amygdala and nucleus accumbens activation to emotional facial expressions in children and adolescents at risk for major depression. *American Journal of Psychiatry*, **165**, 90–98.

Moran, J. M., Wig, G. S., Adams, R. B. Jr., Janata, P., & Kelley, W. M. (2004). Neural correlates of humor detection and appreciation. *Neuroimage*, **21**, 1055–1060.

Morfin, R. & Starka, L. (2001). Neurosteroid 7-hydroxylation products in the brain. *International Reviews in Neurobiology*, **46**, 79–95.

Morgan, C. A. 3rd, Wang, S., Southwick, S. M., *et al.* (2000). Plasma neuropeptide-Y concentrations in humans exposed to military survival training. *Biological Psychiatry*, **47**, 902–909.

Morgan, C. A. 3rd, Southwick, S., Hazlett, G., *et al.* (2004). Relationships among plasma dehydroepiandrosterone sulfate and cortisol levels, symptoms of dissociation, and objective performance in humans exposed to acute stress. *Archives of General Psychiatry*, **61**, 819–825.

Morrow, B. A., Elsworth, J. D., Rasmusson, A. M., & Roth, R. H. (1999). The role of mesoprefrontal dopamine neurons in the acquisition and expression of conditioned fear in the rat. *Neuroscience*, **92**, 553–564.

Moses, E. L., Drevets, W. C., Smith, G., *et al.* (2000). Effects of estradiol and progesterone administration on human serotonin 2A receptor binding: A PET study. *Biological Psychiatry*, **48**, 854–860.

Munafo, M. R., Brown, S. M., & Hariri, A. R. (2008). Serotonin transporter (5-HTTLPR) genotype and amygdala activation: A meta-analysis. *Biological Psychiatry*, **63**, 852–857.

Munafo, M. R., Durrant, C., Lewis, G., & Flint, J. (2009). Gene X environment interactions at the serotonin transporter locus. *Biological Psychiatry*, **65**, 211–219.

Munn, M. A., Alexopoulos, J., Nishino, T., *et al.* (2007). Amygdala volume analysis in female twins with major depression. *Biological Psychiatry*, **62**, 415–422.

Nemeroff, C. B. (2002). Recent advances in the neurobiology of depression. *Psychopharmacological Bulletin*, **36**(Suppl 2), 6–23.

Nestler, E. J. & Carlezon, W. A. Jr. (2006). The mesolimbic dopamine reward circuit in depression. *Biological Psychiatry*, **59**, 1151–1159.

Neumeister, A., Charney, D. S., Belfer, I., *et al.* (2005). Sympathoneural and adrenomedullary functional effects of alpha2C-adrenoreceptor gene polymorphism in healthy humans. *Pharmacogenetics and Genomics*, **15**, 143–149.

New, A. S., Fan J., Murrough, J. W., *et al.* (2009). A functional magnetic resonance imaging study of deliberate emotion regulation in resilience and posttraumatic stress disorder. *Biological Psychiatry*, **66**, 656–664.

Nikisch, G. & Mathe, A. A. (2008). CSF monoamine metabolites and neuropeptides in depressed patients before and after electroconvulsive therapy. *European Psychiatry*, **23**, 356–359.

Nikisch, G., Agren, H., Eap, C. B., *et al.* (2005). Neuropeptide Y and corticotropin-releasing hormone in CSF mark response to antidepressive treatment with citalopram. *International Journal of Neuropsychopharmacology*, **8**, 403–410.

Nitschke, J. B., Sarinopoulos I., Oathes, D. J., *et al.* (2009). Anticipatory activation in the amygdala and anterior cingulate in generalized anxiety disorder and prediction of treatment response. *American Journal of Psychiatry*, **166**, 302–310.

Ochsner, K. N., Ray, R. D., Cooper, J. C., *et al.* (2004). For better or for worse: Neural systems supporting the cognitive down- and up-regulation of negative emotion. *Neuroimage*. **23**, 483–499.

O'Connor, D. B. (2002). Exogenous testosterone, aggression, and mood in eugonadal and hypogonadal men. *Physiology and Behavior*, **75**, 557–566.

Oliveira, T., Gouveia, M. J., & Oliveira, R. F. (2009). Testosterone responsiveness to winning and losing experiences in female soccer players. *Psychoneuroendocrinology*, **34**, 1056–1064.

Orr, S. P., Milad, M. R., Metzger, L. J., *et al.* (2006). Effects of beta blockade, PTSD diagnosis, and explicit threat on the extinction and retention of an aversively conditioned response. *Biological Psychology*, **73**, 262–271.

Otte, C., Neylan, T. C., Pole, N., *et al.* (2005). Association between childhood trauma and catecholamine response to psychological stress in police academy recruits. *Biological Psychiatry*, **57**, 27–32.

Parks, C. L., Robinson, P. S., Sibille, E., Shenk, T., & Toth, M. (1998). Increased anxiety of mice lacking the serotonin 1A receptor. *Proceedings of the National Academy of Sciences of the USA*, **95**, 10734–10739.

Pascucci, T., Ventura, R., Latagliata, E. C., Cabib, S., & Puglisi-Allegra, S. (2007). The medial prefrontal cortex determines the accumbens dopamine response to stress through the opposing influences of norepinephrine and dopamine. *Cerebral Cortex*, **17**, 2796–2804.

Pattij, T., Groenink, L., Hijzen, T. H., *et al.* (2002). Autonomic changes associated with enhanced anxiety in 5-HT(1A) receptor knockout mice. *Neuropsychopharmacology*, **27**, 380–390.

Pecins-Thompson, M., Brown, N. A., & Bethea, C. L. (1998). Regulation of serotonin re-uptake transporter mRNA expression by ovarian steroids in rhesus macaques. *Brain Research, Molecular Brain Research*, **53**, 120–129.

Perez, S. E., Wynick, D., Steiner, R. A., & Mufson, E. J. (2001). Distribution of galaninergic immunoreactivity in the brain of the mouse. *Journal of Comparative Neurology*, **434**, 158–185.

Pezawas, L., Meyer-Lindenberg, A., Drabant, E. M., *et al.* (2005). *5-HTTLPR* polymorphism impacts human cingulate-amygdala interactions: A genetic susceptibility mechanism for depression. *Nature Neuroscience*, **8**, 828–834.

Pfeifer, J. H., Iacoboni, M., Mazziotta, J. C., & Dapretto, M. (2008). Mirroring others' emotions relates to empathy and interpersonal competence in children. *Neuroimage*, **39**, 2076–2085.

Phillips, M. L., Drevets, W. C., Rauch, S. L., & Lane, R. (2003a). Neurobiology of emotion perception, I: The neural basis of normal emotion perception. *Biological Psychiatry*, **54**, 504–514.

Phillips, M. L., Drevets, W. C., Rauch, S. L., & Lane, R. (2003b). Neurobiology of emotion perception, II: Implications for major psychiatric disorders. *Biological Psychiatry*, **54**, 515–528.

Pitman, R. K., Sanders, K. M., Zusman, R. M., *et al.* (2002). Pilot study of secondary prevention of posttraumatic stress disorder with propranolol. *Biological Psychiatry*, **51**, 189–192.

Pizzagalli, D. A., Holmes, A. J., Dillon, D. G., *et al.* (2009). Reduced caudate and nucleus accumbens response to rewards in unmedicated individuals with major depressive disorder. *American Journal of Psychiatry*, **166**, 702–710.

Pope, H. G. Jr., Kouri, E. M., & Hudson, J. I. (2000). Effects of supraphysiologic doses of testosterone on mood and aggression in normal men: A randomized controlled trial. *Archives of General Psychiatry*, **57**, 133–140; discussion 155–156.

Power, M. & Dalgleish, T. (1997). *Cognition and emotion from order to disorder*. New York: Taylor and Francis.

Puglisi-Allegra, S., Kempf, E., & Cabib, S. (1990). Role of genotype in the adaptation of the brain dopamine system to stress. *Neuroscience, BioBehavioral Reviews*, **14**, 523–528.

Puglisi-Allegra, S., Imperato, A., Angelucci, L., & Cabib, S. (1991). Acute stress induces time-dependent responses in dopamine mesolimbic system. *Brain Research*, **554**, 217–222.

Raap, D. K., DonCarlos, L., Garcia, F., *et al.* (2000). Estrogen desensitizes 5-HT(1A) receptors and reduces levels of G(z), G(i1) and G(i3) proteins in the hypothalamus. *Neuropharmacology*, **39**, 1823–1832.

Rabkin, J. G., McElhiney, M. C., Rabkin, R., McGrath, P. J., & Ferrando, S. J. (2006). Placebo-controlled trial of dehydroepiandrosterone (DHEA) for treatment of nonmajor depression in patients with HIV/AIDS. *American Journal of Psychiatry*, **163**, 59–66.

Raine, A. & Yang, Y. (2006). Neural foundations to moral reasoning and antisocial behavior. *Social Cognitive and Affective Neuroscience*, **1**, 203–213.

Rajarao, SJR., Platt, B., Sukoff, S. J., *et al.* (2007). Anxiolytic-like activity of the non-selective galanin receptor agonist, galnon. *Neuropeptides*, **41**, 307–320.

Rasmusson, A. M., Vasek J., Lipschitz, D. S., *et al.* (2004). An increased capacity for adrenal DHEA release is associated with decreased avoidance and negative mood symptoms in women with PTSD. *Neuropsychopharmacology*, **29**, 1546–1557.

Rauch, S. L., Shin, L. M., & Phelps, E. A. (2006). Neurocircuitry models of posttraumatic stress disorder and extinction: Human neuroimaging research – past, present, and future. *Biological Psychiatry*, **60**, 376–382.

Reed, J. & Love, S. (2009). Army developing master resiliency training. *Military Health System News*, August 17. Washington, DC: Department of Defense, http://www.health.mil/News_And_Multimedia/News/detail/09-08-17/Army_Developing_Master_Resiliency_Training.aspx (accessed February 16, 2011).

Risch, N., Herrell, R., Lehner, T., *et al.* (2009). Interaction between the serotonin transporter gene (5-HTTLPR), stressful life events, and risk of depression: A meta-analysis. *Journal of the American Medical Association*, **301**, 2462–2471.

Rizzolatti, G. & Craighero, L. (2004). The mirror-neuron system. *Annual Reviews in the Neurosciences*, **27**, 169–192.

Rose, K. A., Stapleton, G., Dott, K., *et al.* (1997). Cyp7b, a novel brain cytochrome P450, catalyzes the synthesis of neurosteroids 7alpha-hydroxy dehydroepiandrosterone and 7alpha-hydroxy pregnenolone. *Proceedings of the National Academy of Sciences of the USA*, **94**, 4925–4930.

Rosenfeld, R. S., Hellman, L., Roffwarg, H., *et al.* (1971). Dehydroisoandrosterone is secreted episodically and synchronously with cortisol by normal man. *Journal of Clinical Endocrinology and Metabolism*, **33**, 87–92.

Rutter, M. (1985). Resilience in the face of adversity. protective factors and resistance to psychiatric disorder. *British Journal of Psychiatry*, **147**, 598–611.

Rutter, M. (2006). Implications of resilience concepts for scientific understanding. *Annals of the New York Academy of Sciences*, 1094, 1–12.

Sah, R., Ekhator, N. N., Strawn, J. R., *et al.* (2009). Low cerebrospinal fluid neuropeptide Y concentrations in posttraumatic stress disorder. *Biological Psychiatry*, **66**, 705–707.

Sailer, U., Robinson, S., Fischmeister, F. P., *et al.* (2008). Altered reward processing in the nucleus accumbens and mesial prefrontal cortex of patients with posttraumatic stress disorder. *Neuropsychologia*, **46**, 2836–2844.

Sajdyk, T. J., Johnson, P. L., Leitermann, R. J., *et al.* (2008). Neuropeptide Y in the amygdala induces long-term resilience to stress-induced reductions in social responses but not hypothalamic-adrenal-pituitary axis activity or hyperthermia. *Journal of Neuroscience*, **28**, 893–903.

Sanchez, M. M., Young, L. J., Plotsky, P. M., & Insel, T. R. (1999). Autoradiographic and in situ hybridization localization of corticotropin-releasing factor 1 and 2 receptors in nonhuman primate brain. *Journal of Comparative Neurology*, **408**, 365–377.

Schelling, G., Roozendaal, B., Krauseneck, T., *et al.* (2006). Efficacy of hydrocortisone in preventing posttraumatic stress disorder following critical illness and major surgery. *Annals of the New York Academy of Sciences*, **1071**, 46–53.

Schulte-Ruther, M., Markowitsch, H. J., Fink, G. R., & Piefke, M. (2007). Mirror neuron and theory of mind mechanisms involved in face-to-face interactions: A functional magnetic resonance imaging approach to empathy. *Journal of Cognitive Neuroscience*, **19**, 1354–1372.

Setchell, J. M., Smith, T., Wickings, E. J., & Knapp, L. A. (2008). Social correlates of testosterone and ornamentation in male mandrills. *Hormones and Behavior*, **54**, 365–372.

Sevcik, J., Finta, E. P., & Illes, P. (1993). Galanin receptors inhibit the spontaneous firing of locus coeruleus neurones and interact with μ-opioid receptors. *European Journal of Pharmacology*, **230**, 223–230.

Sharot, T., Riccardi, A. M., Raio, C. M., & Phelps, E. A. (2007). Neural mechanisms mediating optimism bias. *Nature*, **450**, 102–105.

Sibille, E., Pavlides, C., Benke, D., & Toth, M. (2000). Genetic inactivation of the serotonin(1A) receptor in mice results in downregulation of major GABA(A) receptor alpha subunits, reduction of GABA(A) receptor binding, and benzodiazepine-resistant anxiety. *Journal of Neuroscience*, **20**, 2758–2765.

Siegrist, J., Menrath, I., Stocker, T., *et al.* (2005). Differential brain activation according to chronic social reward frustration. *Neuroreport*, **16**, 1899–1903.

Silver, J. M., Sandberg, D. P., & Hales, R. E. (1990). New approaches in the pharmacotherapy of posttraumatic stress disorder. *Journal of Clinical Psychiatry*, **51**(Suppl), 33–38; discussion 44–46.

Simson, P. E. & Weiss, J. M. (1988). Altered activity of the locus coeruleus in an animal model of depression. *Neuropsychopharmacology*, **1**, 287–295.

Skuse, D. H. & Gallagher, L. (2009). Dopaminergic-neuropeptide interactions in the social brain. *Trends in Cognitive Science*, **13**, 27–35.

Smolka, M. N., Schumann, G., Wrase, J., *et al.* (2005). Catechol-*O*-methyltransferase VAL158MET genotype affects processing of emotional stimuli in the amygdala and prefrontal cortex. *Journal of Neuroscience*, **25**, 836–842.

Solomon, M. B. & Herman, J. P. (2009). Sex differences in psychopathology: Of gonads, adrenals and mental illness. *Physiology and Behavior*, **97**, 250–258.

Southwick, S. M., Krystal, J. H., Bremner, J. D., *et al.* (1997). Noradrenergic and serotonergic function in posttraumatic stress disorder. *Archives of General Psychiatry*, **54**, 749–758.

Southwick, S. M., Vythilingam, M., & Charney, D. S. (2005). The psychobiology of depression and resilience to stress: Implications for prevention and treatment. *Annual Reviews in Clinical Psychology*, **1**, 255–291.

Sterling, P. & Eyer, J. (1988). Allostasis: A new paradigm to explain arousal pathways. In S. R. Fisher (ed.), *Handbook of life stress, cognition, and health* (pp. 629–649). New York: Wiley.

Storm, E. E. & Tecott, L. H. (2005). Social circuits: Peptidergic regulation of mammalian social behavior. *Neuron*, **47**, 483–486.

Su, T. P., Pagliaro, M., Schmidt, P. J., *et al.* (1993). Neuropsychiatric effects of anabolic steroids in male normal volunteers. *Journal of the American Medical Association*, **269**, 2760–2764.

Swanson, C. J., Blackburn, T. P., Zhang, X., *et al.* (2006). Anxiolytic- and antidepressant-like profiles of the galanin-3 receptor (Gal3) antagonists SNAP 37889 and SNAP 398. *Proceedings of the National Academy of Sciences of the USA*, **102**, 17489–17494.

Tache, Y. & Bonaz, B. (2007). Corticotropin-releasing factor receptors and stress-related alterations of gut motor function. *Journal of Clinical Investigation*, **117**, 33–40.

Terburg, D., Morgan, B., & van Honk, J. (2009). The testosterone–cortisol ratio: A hormonal marker for proneness to social aggression. *International Journal of Law Psychiatry*, **32**, 216–223.

Thiele, T. E., Marsh, D. J., St. Marie, L., Bernstein, I. L., & Palmiter, R. D. (1998). Ethanol consumption and resistance are inversely related to neuropeptide Y levels. *Nature* **396**, 366–369.

Thorson, J. A. & Powell, F. C. (1994). Depression and sense of humor. *Psychological Reports*, **75**, 1473–1474.

Tiet, Q. Q., Bird, H. R., Davies, M., *et al.* (1998). Adverse life events and resilience. *Journal of American Academy of Child and Adolescent Psychiatry*, **37**, 1191–1200.

Ulrich-Lai, Y. M., & Herman, J. P. (2009). Neural regulation of endocrine and autonomic stress responses. *Nature Reviews in the Neurosciences*, **10**, 397–409.

Unschuld, P. G., Ising, M., Erhardt, A., *et al.* (2008). Polymorphisms in the galanin gene are associated with symptom severity in female patients suffering from panic disorder. *Journal of Affective Disorders*, **105**, 177–184.

Vaillant, G. E. (1992). *Ego mechanisms of defense: A guide for clinicians and researchers.* Washington, DC: American Psychiatric Press.

van Honk, J. & Schutter, D. J. (2007). Testosterone reduces conscious detection of signals serving social correction: Implications for antisocial behavior. *Psychological Science*, **18**, 663–667.

van Honk, J., Tuiten, A., Verbaten, R., *et al.* (1999). Correlations among salivary testosterone, mood, and selective attention to threat in humans. *Hormones and Behavior*, **36**, 17–24.

van Honk, J., Peper, J. S., & Schutter, DJLG. (2005). Testosterone reduces unconscious fear but not consciously experienced anxiety: Implications for the disorders of fear and anxiety. *Biological Psychiatry*, **58**, 218–225.

Verhagen, M., van der Meij, A., Janzing, J. G., *et al.* (2009). Effect of the 5-*HTTLPR* polymorphism in the serotonin transporter gene on major depressive disorder and related comorbid disorders. *Psychiatric Genetics*, **19**, 39–44.

Voisey, J., Swagell, C. D., Hughes, I. P., *et al.* (2009). The *DRD2* gene 957C>T polymorphism is associated with posttraumatic stress disorder in war veterans. *Depression and Anxiety*, **26**, 28–33.

Vreeburg, S. A., Hoogendijk, W. J., van Pelt, J., *et al.* (2009). Major depressive disorder and hypothalamic–pituitary–adrenal axis activity: Results from a large cohort study. *Archives of General Psychiatry*, **66**, 617–626.

Vythilingam, M., Nelson, E. E., Scaramozza, M., *et al.* (2009). Reward circuitry in resilience to severe trauma: An fMRI investigation of resilient special forces soldiers. *Psychiatry Research: Neuroimaging*, **172**, 75–77.

Wager, T. D., Davidson, M. L., Hughes, B. L., Lindquist, M. A., & Ochsner, K. N. (2008). Prefrontal-subcortical pathways mediating successful emotion regulation. *Neuron*, **59**, 1037–1050.

Walton, K. M., Chin, J. E., Duplantier, A. J., & Mather, R. J. (2006). Galanin function in the central nervous system. *Current Opinions in Drug Discovery and Development*, **9**, 560–570.

Waselus, M., Nazzaro, C., Valentino, R. J., & Van Bockstaele, E. J. (2009). Stress-induced redistribution of corticotropin-releasing factor receptor subtypes in the dorsal raphe nucleus. *Biological Psychiatry*, **66**, 76–83.

Watt, M. J., Burke, A. R., Renner, K. J., & Forster, G. L. (2009). Adolescent male rats exposed to social defeat exhibit altered anxiety behavior and limbic monoamines as adults. *Behavioral Neuroscience*, **123**, 564–576.

Weaver, I. C., Cervoni, N., Champagne, F. A., *et al.* (2004). Epigenetic programming by maternal behavior. *Nature Neuroscience*, **7**, 847–854.

Weis, F., Kilger, E., Roozendaal, B., *et al.* (2006). Stress doses of hydrocortisone reduce chronic stress symptoms and improve health-related quality of life in high-risk patients after cardiac surgery: A randomized study. *Journal of Thoracic and Cardiovascular Surgery*, **131**, 277–282.

Weiser, M. J., Foradori, C. D., & Handa, R. J. (2008). Estrogen receptor beta in the brain: From form to function. *Brain Research Reviews*, **57**, 309–320.

Weiskopf, N., Scharnowski, F., Veit, R., *et al.* (2004). Self-regulation of local brain activity using real-time functional magnetic resonance imaging (fMRI). *Journal of Physiology*, **98**, 357–373.

Wheler, G. H., Brandon, D., Clemons, A., *et al.* (2006). Cortisol production rate in posttraumatic stress disorder. *Journal of Clinical Endocrinology and Metabolism*, **91**, 3486–3489.

Whitworth, J. A., Williamson, P. M., Mangos, G., & Kelly, J. J. (2005). Cardiovascular consequences of cortisol excess. *Vascular Health and Risk Management*, **1**, 291–299.

Wilkinson, M. B., Xiao, G., Kumar, A., *et al.* (2009). Imipramine treatment and resiliency exhibit similar chromatin regulation in the mouse nucleus accumbens in depression models. *Journal of Neuroscience*, **29**, 7820–7832.

Willert, M. V., Thulstrup, A. M., & Hertz, J. (2009). Changes in stress and coping from a randomized controlled trial of a three-month stress management intervention. *Scandinavian Journal of Work and Environmental Health*, **35**, 145–152.

Wirth, M. M. & Schultheiss, O. C. (2007). Basal testosterone moderates responses to anger faces in humans. *Physiology and Behavior*, **90**, 496–505.

Wolfensberger, SPA., Veltman, D. J., Hoogendijk, WJG., Boomsma, D. I., & de Geus, EJC. (2008). Amygdala responses to emotional faces in twins discordant or concordant for the risk for anxiety and depression. *Neuroimage*, **41**, 544–552.

Wong, M. L., Kling, M. A., Munson, P. J., *et al.* (2000). Pronounced and sustained central hypernoradrenergic function in major depression with melancholic features: Relation to hypercortisolism and corticotropin-releasing hormone. *Proceedings of the National Academy of Sciences of the USA*, **97**, 325–330.

Xu, Z. Q., Tong, Y. G., & Hökfelt, T. (2001). Galanin enhances noradrenaline-induced outward current on locus coeruleus noradrenergic neurons. *Neuroreport*, **12**, 1779–1782.

Yehuda, R. & LeDoux, J. (2007). Response variation following trauma: A translational neuroscience approach to understanding PTSD. *Neuron*, **56**, 19–32.

Yehuda, R., Boisoneau, D., Lowy, M. T., & Giller, E. L. Jr. (1995). Dose–response changes in plasma cortisol and lymphocyte glucocorticoid receptors following dexamethasone administration in combat veterans with and without posttraumatic stress disorder. *Archives of General Psychiatry*, **52**, 583–593.

Yehuda, R., Brand, S. R., Golier, J. A., & Yang, R. K. (2006a). Clinical correlates of DHEA associated with post-traumatic stress disorder. *Acta Psychiatrica Scandinavica*, **114**, 187–193.

Yehuda, R., Brand, S., & Yang, R. K. (2006b). Plasma neuropeptide Y concentrations in combat exposed veterans: Relationship to trauma exposure, recovery from PTSD, and coping. *Biological Psychiatry*, **59**, 660–663.

Young, A. H., Gallagher, P., & Porter, R. J. (2002). Elevation of the cortisol–dehydroepiandrosterone ratio in drug-free depressed patients. *American Journal of Psychiatry*, **159**, 1237–1239.

Young, E. A. (1996). Sex differences in response to exogenous corticosterone: A rat model of hypercortisolemia. *MolecularPsychiatry*, **1**, 313–319.

Young, E. A., Altemus, M., Parkison, V., & Shastry, S. (2001). Effects of estrogen antagonists and agonists on the ACTH response to restraint stress in female rats. *Neuropsychopharmacology*, **25**, 881–891.

Yu, Y. Z. & Shi, J. X. (2009). Relationship between levels of testosterone and cortisol in saliva and aggressive behaviors of adolescents. *Biomedical and Environmental Science*, **22**, 44–49.

Zarrouf, F. A., Artz, S., Griffith, J., Sirbu, C., & Kommor, M. (2009). Testosterone and depression: Systematic review and meta-analysis. *Journal of Psychiatric Practice*, **15**, 289–305.

Zitzmann, M. (2006). Testosterone and the brain. *Aging Male*, **9**, 195–199.

Zitzmann, M. & Nieschlag, E. (2001). Testosterone levels in healthy men and the relation to behavioural and physical characteristics: Facts and constructs. *European Journal of Endocrinology*, **144**, 183–197.

Chapter

2

Resilience in the face of stress: emotion regulation as a protective factor

Allison S. Troy and Iris B. Mauss

Introduction

Everyone experiences stress at one time or another – from major events such as the death of a loved one, to more minor stressors such as financial difficulties. Not surprisingly, exposure to stress is generally associated with a wide range of negative outcomes, including decreased well-being, increased incidence of disease, post-traumatic stress disorder, generalized anxiety disorder, and major depressive disorder (Dohrenwend & Dohrenwend, 1974; Kendler *et al.*, 1999; Monat *et al.*, 2007). However, not all individuals who are exposed to even high levels of stress develop such negative outcomes. In fact, recent evidence suggests that a considerable number of individuals exhibit resilience, which is commonly defined as maintained or improved mental health in the face of stress, after short disruptions (if any) to normal functioning (Freitas & Downey, 1998; Rutter, 1999; Luthar *et al.*, 2000; Bonanno, 2005). Note that this definition, which we adapt here, conceptualizes resilience as a potential outcome after exposure to stress rather than a psychological trait that leads to positive outcomes (c.f. Norris *et al.*, 2008).

It, therefore, appears that, in the face of comparable stressors, some individuals exhibit significantly impaired functioning while others show impressive resilience. Understanding the factors that govern the great individual variance in outcomes after stress is important for understanding mental health and for developing interventions and prevention programs that foster resilience. What factors, then, might predict resilience? One key to this question might lie in the fact that stressful events are inherently highly emotional (Sarason *et al.*, 1978; Lazarus, 1999). For this reason, people's ability to *regulate* emotions may be a critically important factor in determining resilience

(Figure 2.1). The present chapter will review relevant literatures and suggest that there is indeed evidence to support this thesis. More specifically, we will propose that a specific type of emotion regulation, *cognitive* emotion regulation, holds particular promise for contributing to resilience.

Scope of the chapter

The concepts we examine here are complex: the topics of stress, mental health, and emotion regulation each have generated a vast body of research. To maintain conceptual clarity, the chapter will focus on specific types of stressor, specific types of emotion regulation, and specific types of relationship between these constructs and resilience. This is achieved as follows.

The first way in which the present review is narrowed is by focusing on stressful life events from among the various types of stressor that can affect people (Sarason *et al.*, 1978; Lu, 1994; Ensel & Lin, 1996; Mazure *et al.*, 2000; Tennant, 2002). Common stressful life events include relatively minor events, such as a disagreement with a spouse, to more major events, such as the unexpected loss of a job, a serious illness or injury of oneself, or the death of a friend or family member. Because this definition of stress exposure includes stressors that, arguably, everyone has experienced one time or another, the present model of resilience is fairly general in its implications. However, the stressors will not include traumatic events such as abuse, exposure to crime, or exposure to war, or events that could be considered "positive" stressors such as marriage or the birth of a child, because, based on the current literature, it is not clear whether the proposed model of resilience would generalize to these types of stressor. While it is possible that cognitive emotion regulation ability is also an important contributor

Resilience and Mental Health: Challenges Across the Lifespan, ed. Steven M. Southwick, Brett T. Litz, Dennis Charney, and Matthew J. Friedman. Published by Cambridge University Press. © Cambridge University Press 2011.

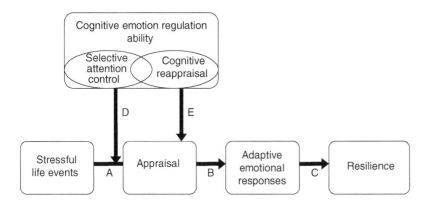

Figure 2.1 Proposed moderation of the relationship between stressful life events and resilience by cognitive emotion regulation ability. Each of the links in the model is indicated by a letter (A–E). Links D and E are positioned to imply that D usually occurs earlier in the emotion generative process than E, and that E operates by directly changing appraisals; however, this is not meant to imply a strict time course with regard to cognitive emotion regulation. The links are described in detail in the text.

to resilience with regard to trauma and positive events, more research is needed in order to test this hypothesis.

Second, the proposed framework will focus on emotion regulation ability as a *moderator*, such that people with high cognitive emotion regulation ability should exhibit increased likelihood of resilience after stress exposure compared with those low in cognitive emotion regulation ability (Figure 2.1). Emotion regulation has also been proposed as a *mediator* in the context of adjustment to stress (Schwartz & Proctor, 2000; McCarthy *et al.*, 2006; Silk *et al.*, 2007). According to such mediator models, stress exposure leads to emotion dysregulation, which, in turn, leads to negative outcomes. Both mediator and moderator models are useful in examining the relationship between stress and mental health. The present chapter focuses on emotion regulation as a moderating factor because a moderator model lends itself more clearly to understanding individual differences in resilience. One implication of this approach is that emotion regulation ability is conceptualized as a relatively independent variable that is not strongly affected by stress exposure. This is not to say, however, that this ability is set in stone. Rather, we believe that the ability to use cognitive emotion regulation is shaped and influenced by a number of situational and individual factors, and it can, in turn, be flexibly applied across a wide range of emotional contexts. According to this model of resilience, however, the ability to use cognitive emotion regulation is most important in the context of stress.

In order to provide evidence for the moderator model of resilience shown in Figure 2.1, empirical evidence that supports main effects of cognitive emotion regulation on positive outcomes will be reviewed,

as well as evidence that cognitive emotion regulation is a moderator of the relationship between stress and outcomes. Studies of the main effects of emotion regulation do not directly test resilience because they do not explicitly consider the context of stress. However, evidence of this type will be included for two reasons. First, the literature to date has simply focused more on the main effects of emotion regulation. Second, and more importantly, we believe that the relationship between cognitive emotion regulation and positive outcomes is likely to generalize to stressful contexts. In addition, where research has directly tested the interactions between emotion regulation and stress, it is described as evidence that directly supports the moderator model.

In order to lay the groundwork for the present review, appraisal theories of emotion and cognitive emotion regulation are discussed.

A framework for resilience: appraisal theory and cognitive emotion regulation

Appraisal theories are commonly used in the fields of emotion, emotion regulation, and coping to understand individuals' emotional reactions (Lazarus & Folkman, 1984). The central point of appraisal theories is that "the way we evaluate an event determines how we react emotionally" (Lazarus, 1999, p. 87). In other words, it is not a particular event that causes a particular emotion but, rather, it is a person's subjective appraisals of the event that lead to an emotional reaction (Lazarus & Folkman, 1984; Ortony *et al.*, 1988; Scherer, 1988; Lazarus, 1991). In this way, appraisals have generally been defined as the meaning and significance that a person assigns to an event or stimulus.

In support of appraisal theories, research has found that people exposed to comparable events, either in the laboratory or in a naturalistic setting, will display a wide variety of emotional reactions depending on their appraisal of the event (Folkman & Lazarus, 1985; Smith & Ellsworth, 1987; Scherer & Ceschi, 1997; Siemer *et al.*, 2007; Figure 2.1, links A and B). Because appraisals appear to play such an important role in the generation of an emotion, emotion regulation strategies that target appraisals should be particularly effective. Consequently, once an individual's appraisal of a situation has changed, so will the emotional reaction.

Given the centrality of appraisals in the generation of emotion, cognitive emotion regulation strategies that entail appraisal change may provide particularly effective ways to manage emotions. Cognitive emotion regulation has been broadly defined as changing one's attention to or one's appraisals of a situation in order to change an emotion's duration, intensity, or both (Ochsner & Gross, 2005). This definition is in contrast to non-cognitive types of emotion regulation such as expressive suppression, which consists of changing only the outward expression of an emotion (Gross & Thompson, 2007).

Two groups of cognitive emotion regulation strategies have shown particular promise as effective ways to manage emotions: attention control (AC) and cognitive reappraisal (CR) (Ochsner & Gross, 2005). Attention control consists of selectively attending toward or away from certain stimuli (either internal or external) in order to change their emotional impact (Ochsner & Gross, 2005). Note that internal stimuli are included in this definition, which refers to people's own thoughts and feelings. Selective attention to certain aspects of a situation changes individuals' appraisals, which, in turn, changes individuals' emotional states. For example, consider someone who is faced with giving a speech to a large crowd of people and chooses to focus on how friendly and engaged everyone in the first row looks. This person's appraisal of the situation will be less threat provoking than that of someone who instead focuses on the people who are asleep in the back row. Essentially, by filtering the affective information that enters one's awareness in a stressful situation, the appraisals one makes will be less threatening, in turn leading to fewer negative emotions (Figure 2.1, links A, B, and D). In this way, AC is conceptualized as a moderator of the relationship between stressful life events and appraisals.

Cognitive reappraisal involves reframing a situation in order to change its emotional impact. In the context of stress, this could involve changing one's appraisal to another less-threatening or more positive interpretation of the event (Gross & Thompson, 2007). Because CR most often occurs after an initial appraisal of an event has taken place, it is depicted as occurring slightly later in the emotion generation process than AC (Gross, 1998a; Figure 2.1, link E). We acknowledge that it is possible for CR to occur either earlier or later in the generation of emotion than described in this definition. In the proposed model, however, the temporal sequence of these strategies is not critical for determining their effectiveness. Instead, we believe that the ability to change appraisals is what ultimately determines the effectiveness of a given strategy. Going back to the public speaking example, one could initially look out at the huge audience and make the appraisal that this audience appears quite uninterested in the impending talk and is, therefore, threatening. Then, one could reappraise the situation by telling oneself that the few people who are paying such close attention could have great feedback that could really help to improve the speech in the future, thereby decreasing anxiety. By using CR to change appraisals of a threatening situation, individuals can effectively transform their ensuing emotions (Figure 2.1, links E and B).

Clearly, there is some overlap between AC and CR. Because attention and appraisals appear to be critically linked, it may be that the use of one of these strategies makes it more likely that the other strategy will also be used (Totterdell & Parkinson, 1999). For example, it may become much easier for someone to engage in a positive reappraisal of the public-speaking situation if he or she is selectively attending to the friendly people in the front row. Conversely, as he or she is busy reappraising the audience by considering how truly unthreatening everyone is, he or she may be more likely to notice the friendly people sitting in the front row and less likely to notice the people sleeping in the back. Although AC and CR are, therefore, by no means mutually exclusive, they will be described separately to maintain conceptual clarity. To acknowledge the fact that these two types of cognitive emotion regulation are not completely separable, they are pictured as overlapping circles in Figure 2.1.

In sum, as illustrated in Figure 2.1, the appraisal–theoretical framework suggests that AC and CR may be linchpin processes in contributing to resilience. Specifically, these types of strategy for cognitive emotion regulation should contribute to resilience (link C) by helping individuals to decrease negative emotional responses (links D and E). The following sections will review evidence to support this model.

Empirical findings: attention control and resilience

Theoretically, if a person does not attend to negative stimuli, this person will make appraisals of the environment that are less threatening. In turn, these changed appraisals will lead to fewer negative emotional reactions (Folkman & Lazarus, 1985; Gross & Thompson, 2007). For this reason, it has been widely hypothesized that the ability to distract oneself from negative stimuli, including one's own negative feelings, is an important protective factor against long-term negative outcomes. In the context of depression, for example, Nolen-Hoeksema (1991, p. 577) hypothesized that depressed individuals must "be distracted from their ruminative thoughts long enough for their depressed mood to be relieved substantially." Laboratory studies of distraction support this hypothesis. For example, in studies with depressed patients as well as normative samples, participants who distracted themselves from their sad moods by completing an emotionally neutral task were able to attenuate their negative feelings (Morrow & Nolen-Hoeksema, 1990; Erber & Tesser, 1992). Similarly, in a group of depressed adolescents, Park and colleagues (2004) found that participants induced to use distraction by reading about 45 neutral items (boats, kettle, etc.) decreased their depressed mood compared with participants who read about more emotional, self-focused items (feelings, body sensations, etc.).

While these laboratory studies suggest that distraction staves off depressed mood, the positive effects associated with distraction seem to wear off with time, giving those who use distraction only short-term benefits. For example, Kross and Ayduk (2008, study 2) found that after a laboratory sadness induction distraction decreased depressed mood immediately after the emotion induction. However, in follow-up sessions one day and seven days after the induction, the protective effects of distraction had disappeared and levels of self-reported depressed mood had significantly increased relative to other experimental groups that had not used distraction. The authors explained these results by pointing out that distraction does nothing to change how emotional experiences are dealt with in future situations; consequently, the utility of distraction appears to be limited to the short term (Kross & Ayduk,

2008). This is similar to the contention of Campbell-Sills and Barlow (2007, p. 556) that distraction is simply "a 'band-aid' approach rather than a long-term solution to excessive anxiety and/or depression." Indeed, there is evidence to suggest that distraction may be not just ineffective but even detrimental to long-term coping. For example, research has found that individuals who use avoidance coping strategies such as distraction when they are stressed are more likely to develop depression in the long run (Felsten, 2002; Powers et al., 2002; Holahan et al., 2005).

Given the negative long-term consequences associated with distraction, perhaps its opposite – focusing on what is wrong in a given situation – could lead to more positive outcomes. This negative focus is often referred to as rumination, which has been defined as repetitively focusing on oneself, one's negative emotions, and their anticipated negative consequences (Nolen-Hoeksema, 1991; Nolen-Hoeksema et al., 2008). Unfortunately, this ruminative response style in the face of stress decreases the likelihood of resilience. For example, among people who are already depressed, those who engage in rumination about their own depressed mood experience significantly longer depressive episodes, which suggests that rumination leads to a vicious cycle of negative emotions that are difficult to escape (Nolen-Hoeksema, 1991). The use of rumination has also been associated with higher levels of anxiety and symptoms of post-traumatic stress (Nolen-Hoeksema et al., 2008). This relationship between rumination and negative outcomes also seems to be present in the context of stress. In a study of caregivers for terminally ill patients, for example, results indicated that caregivers who used more rumination in response to their negative moods were more depressed than caregivers who used less rumination (Nolen-Hoeksema et al., 1994).

Such correlational studies, of course, do not allow for inferences about the causal role of rumination. Importantly, however, a prospective study by Nolen-Hoeksema and Morrow (1991) provided some support for the notion that rumination is a risk factor for depression. Their questionnaire study obtained participants' reports of ruminative response style and depressive symptoms. By chance, 14 days later, the Loma Prieta earthquake hit the area close to where these data had been collected. Participants who had previously reported using more of a ruminative response style were significantly more depressed at follow-up sessions 10 days and 50 days following the earthquake compared with individuals who reported using less of a ruminative response style. These results were significant even when controlling for depressed mood before the earthquake, suggesting that rumination indeed had a causal role in depressed mood. Several other prospective longitudinal studies using both adults and children have found a similar pattern: individuals who use rumination during periods of stress are more likely to develop depressive disorders and to experience more prolonged periods of depression in the long-run (reviewed by Nolen-Hoeksema *et al.*, 2008).

More recent laboratory studies that have manipulated the use of rumination have added further support to the contention that rumination plays a causal role in the occurrence of negative mood states. For example, Singer and Dobson (2007) found that remitted depressed patients who were instructed to ruminate after a negative emotion induction had higher levels of depressed mood compared with participants who were instructed to use distraction. Other studies using normative samples have also found that instructions to ruminate after negative mood inductions exacerbate negative mood states compared with those who were not instructed to ruminate (Broderick, 2005; Ray *et al.*, 2008). Overall, it seems that when people in stressful situations repetitively focus their attention on their own negative emotions, resilience becomes a less likely outcome.

In addition to the studies on rumination, research on attentional biases in depression suggest that a bias towards external negative affective stimuli (i.e., negative stimuli other than one's own emotional states) might also decrease the likelihood of resilience and lead to increased vulnerability to negative outcomes. In several studies using paradigms such as the dot-probe task, researchers have found that clinically depressed patients (Mogg *et al.*, 1995; Mathews *et al.*, 1996) as well as individuals with induced or naturally occurring dysphoria (Bradley *et al.*, 1997) displayed a negative attentional bias, attending relatively more to negatively valenced emotional stimuli than to neutral or positive stimuli. This negative attentional bias in depression has also been found using other tasks such as the dichotic listening task (Ingram *et al.*, 1994) and an affective interference task (Gotlib *et al.*, 2005).

In addition, using a negative affective priming task to measure selective attention to affective words, Joormann (2004) found an attentional bias towards irrelevant negative distractors in participants who were currently dysphoric, as well as in non-depressed individuals with a previous history of depression.

Furthermore, a sample of children at high risk for depression selectively attended to negative facial expressions after a negative mood induction, whereas children who were not at risk for depression selectively attended to positive facial expressions during an emotional faces dot-probe task (Joormann *et al.*, 2007). These findings suggest that negative attentional bias is not simply a side-effect of current depression, but may constitute a vulnerability to depression.

Taken together, these findings suggest that there is a main effect between AC and mental health outcomes. Specifically, distraction, rumination, and negative biases in attention are associated with vulnerabilities to negative outcomes over time. In addition, the findings reviewed above could have important implications in the context of stress and resilience – if an individual cannot effectively disengage attention away from negative aspects of themselves or the situation, the appraisals of a stressor could become much more threatening, the resulting negative emotions could become more intense and long lasting, and resilience will become more difficult to attain. At the other extreme, however, those who completely distract themselves away from negative information enjoy short-term benefits but appear ill-equipped to effectively cope with further exposure to stressors later on.

Indeed, research using the emotional Stroop task, which measures individuals' ability to ignore irrelevant emotional material, has provided evidence that pre-existing differences in AC can prospectively predict adjustment to stress. For example, MacLeod and Hagan (1992) found that women who displayed the most pronounced bias towards negative information later reported the greatest amount of distress upon learning that they had been diagnosed with cervical pathology. Similarly, MacLeod (1999) found that a Stroop measure predicted Singaporean students' emotional adjustment after migrating to Australia. Specifically, the students with the most pronounced negative attentional bias reported the greatest levels of anxiety after immigration.

These prospective studies support the hypothesis that individual differences in AC can exert a moderating effect on the relationship between stress and outcomes over time (Figure 2.1, link D). Specifically, maladaptive forms of AC such as negative attentional biases appear to result in heightened negative affective responses (Figure 2.1, link D) and are associated with more vulnerability to negative outcomes and less resilience (Figure 2.1, link C).

Conversely, then, individuals who use adaptive AC should respond to a stressor with an attenuated negative affective response, making resilience more likely. However, what constitutes "adaptive AC"? The findings reviewed so far suggest a dilemma: directing attention away from the negative aspects of a situation (as is done in distraction), on the one hand, is only adaptive in the short term but seems to have deleterious consequences in the longer term. On the other hand, focusing on the negative aspects of a situation (as is done in rumination) appears to lead to deleterious consequences in almost all contexts. One answer to this dilemma might lie in the degree and context rather than in the kind of AC strategies used. Perhaps it is just maladaptive to *completely* and *inflexibly* distract oneself from or *completely* and *inflexibly* focus on negative stimuli. In contrast, a more flexible employment of some of both strategies – *selectively* focusing attention – could lead to resilience in the face of stress. Additionally, the maladaptive types of AC described above are stimulus-driven strategies. Perhaps more goal-driven strategies based on an individual's present goals and needs would be more adaptive. In this way, selective AC could be employed flexibly across a wide range of contexts in order to suit an individual's current needs instead of according to particular stimulus contingencies.

Indeed, studies of selective attention support this hypothesis. For example, recent research using eye-gaze tracking has found that individuals who are high in trait optimism – that is, individuals who are generally characterized by high well-being – display an attentional bias away from negative material (Isaacowitz, 2005). At first glance, this looks like distraction. However, research from Aspinwall and Brunhart (1996) suggests that optimists are not using chronic pollyannaism to simply filter out all negative information; instead, optimists appear to attend only to what is relevant for their own well-being. For example, they found that when optimists who engage in habitual sun tanning were given health information about damage from ultraviolet radiation, they spent more time reading the threatening information, whereas optimists who did not habitually sun tan did not selectively attend to the same information. The optimists also displayed better recall for the relevant health risk information than for irrelevant information, adding to the contention that optimists do selectively attend to negative material if it is relevant (Aspinwall & Brunhart, 1996). More recent research on optimism has replicated these results (Abele & Gendolla, 2007).

These findings on optimists have led to the "pragmatic information-processing hypothesis," which posits that it is not the valence of information that drives selective attention in optimists but rather the level of personal relevance that will determine whether affective information is attended to or not (Abele & Gendolla, 2007).

With these findings in mind, it is not surprising that optimists tend to exhibit greater levels of well-being and lower rates of depression than pessimists (Scheier & Carver, 1993). By filtering out unneeded negative information, the optimists' appraisals of these stimuli may be less disturbing, leading, in turn, to fewer negative emotions. Although this phenomenon has not been examined in the context of high stress, it is plausible that optimists avoid the negative effects of distraction by attending to negative information when it is relevant. At the same time, when negative information becomes irrelevant, perhaps because it has been processed, optimists may effectively direct attention away from it. Hypothetically, by attending away from unneeded information in the environment, individuals with this type of selective attention would display less-threatening appraisals of the stressor in the first place, thus leading to an attenuated negative emotional response and resilience.

Does this mean that if someone does not naturally possess the ability to selectively focus attention away from negative stimuli, that person is doomed if stressors arise? Recent studies that have examined training paradigms for selective attentional biases suggest that the answer to this question is negative. These studies have shown that, with training, pre-existing attentional bias patterns can be changed (either acquired or attenuated). For example, in a laboratory study, participants were taught to acquire attentional biases either toward or away from affectively negative versus neutral stimuli using a computer task (MacLeod *et al.*, 2002, study 1). After completing the training procedure, participants in the negative attention condition exhibited greater bias towards negative stimuli while participants in the neutral attention condition exhibited greater bias towards neutral stimuli. A more recent study of attentional bias training extended the findings of MacLeod *et al.* by showing that positive attentional biases can also be taught (Wadlinger & Isaacowitz, 2008). These positive biases also have observable behavioral effects on subsequent tasks, such that the participants who had been trained to attend to positive stimuli subsequently looked less at negative images during a stress induction (Wadlinger & Isaacowitz, 2008).

These findings are important in suggesting that people's selective attention to emotional stimuli seem to be changeable. Such training procedures may have important therapeutic value for promoting resilience, particularly among individuals with pre-existing negative attentional biases. In a follow-up study, MacLeod and colleagues (2002, study 2) indeed found that participants who had learned to exhibit a negative attentional bias responded to a stress induction with a pronounced increase in negative emotions. Participants who had been trained to attend away from the negative stimuli and towards neutral stimuli did not exhibit this increase in negative emotion. The authors concluded that the acquired attentional biases contributed causally to these differences in negative emotions. These findings are very important in providing evidence that individual differences in selective AC might influence emotional adjustment to a stressor (Figure 2.1, link D).

It is promising to think that people who exhibit maladaptive patterns of AC can be led down a more resilient path by learning to attend to different kinds of stimulus in the environment. Indeed, recent work by Siegle and colleagues (2008) suggests that training in selective AC may be an effective treatment component for depression. They used an adjunctive intervention for depression called cognitive control training – importantly, the protocol included AC training, in which patients learnt to selectively attend to certain sounds coming out of speakers, while ignoring irrelevant sounds. After receiving two weeks of this AC training (in the context of cognitive control training), patients exhibited greater improvements in depressive symptoms than patients who received treatment as usual (Siegle *et al.*, 2008). Notably, the AC training consisted of short sessions (15 minutes) that used non-affective stimuli such as bird sounds. This suggests that this particular type of AC training may be tapping into a generic ability that is not simply limited to affective stimuli. In turn, this type of generic ability may make it more likely that people can use it in a flexible and context-dependent way.

Although these training paradigms have not been examined in the context of long-term adjustment to stress, the optimism literature discussed above suggests that the flexible use of these attentional biases across contexts would be most adaptive. For example, individuals who display biases away from irrelevant negative information but who attend to relevant negative information would be most likely to be resilient in the long term. Taken as a whole, these training studies suggest that selective AC is best conceptualized as an ability that can be improved with practice. Furthermore, they provide support for the hypothesis that selective AC plays an important role with regard to adaptive emotion regulation and resilience.

Clearly, more research is needed on the clinical utility of AC. As mentioned above, blind pollyannaism is not the answer to coping with stress. Rather, research suggests that selective AC is most adaptive, with attention paid to relevant but not irrelevant negative stimuli. It is unclear, however, how people coping with real-world stressors decide which negative information is "irrelevant" and could, therefore, be safely ignored. One promising idea is that "relevant" information, in the context of stress, can best be conceptualized as the aspects of the stressor that are changeable, and therefore subject to active problem solving and coping. Unchangeable aspects of a stressor could perhaps be considered "irrelevant" and filtered out using selective AC, thereby reducing the amount of negative information that enters awareness. This hypothesis has not yet been tested, however.

Taken together, the evidence reviewed in this section supports the moderating effect of AC on the relationship between stress and resilience. Specifically, strategies such as distraction and rumination appear to be maladaptive: by indiscriminately diverting attention away from negative stimuli (as in distraction), or indiscriminately focusing attention on negative stimuli (as in rumination), individuals who use these strategies are more vulnerable to outcomes such as depression in the context of stress. Although these two different strategies appear to be opposites, ironically, they both lead to negative outcomes over time, perhaps because of the cumulative aspect of ineffectively regulated negative emotions. The AC strategies that promote resilience, by comparison, appear to involve selectively attending away from irrelevant negative stimuli and towards more positive or neutral stimuli, suggesting that a more modulated attentional response (instead of the extreme approaches of distraction and rumination) is more adaptive in the context of stress. Therefore, by filtering out unnecessary negative information in a goal-directed way (Figure 2.1, moderation, link D), it becomes more likely that individuals will make less-threatening appraisals of stressful situations (Figure 2.1, link A) and, as a result, will experience fewer negative emotions (Figure 2.1, link B), in turn increasing the likelihood of resilience (Figure 2.1, link C). The next section will examine the main effects and the moderating effects of another type of cognitive emotion regulation strategy, CR, in the context of stress and resilience (Figure 2.1, link E).

Empirical findings: cognitive reappraisal and resilience

In contrast to AC, CR usually takes place after an initial appraisal has been made (Figure 2.1). Often, CR involves reframing an emotionally negative situation in a more positive way to decrease feelings of negative emotion (Gross, 1998a; Gross & Thompson, 2007). Notably, however, CR can also be used to increase the experience of positive emotions (Folkman & Moskowitz, 2000; Shiota, 2006; Krompinger et al., 2008). Because of its direct impact on appraisals, CR has been widely hypothesized to be an adaptive strategy, particularly in the context of stress – by reappraising a stressor in a less negative and/or more positive way, individuals can change their emotional reaction to the stressor for the better.

Neuroimaging studies of reappraisal have supported the hypotheses that this strategy is effective in changing the activation of brain regions associated with emotion, such as the amygdala and the insula. These areas of the brain can be either increased or decreased in activity in accordance with the goal of reappraisal (Ochsner & Gross, 2005, 2008; Urry et al., 2006; Eippert et al., 2007; Goldin et al., 2008). For example, when reappraisal was used to decrease negative emotions, results indicated that the experience of negative emotion was reduced, and activity in the amygdala and insula was decreased (Goldin et al., 2008). In addition, neuroimaging studies comparing distraction to reappraisal have found that these two strategies are supported by different areas of the brain, suggesting that people who claim to use reappraisal are not simply distracting themselves from negative stimuli (Kalisch et al., 2005, 2006).

Behavioral and autonomic-physiological studies lend further support to the hypothesis that CR can effectively change the experience of emotions without negative "side-effects." For example, Gross (1998b) showed emotional film clips to undergraduates and asked them to reappraise their emotions, suppress emotional behaviors, or simply watch the film. Results from this and similar laboratory studies indicate that individuals instructed to use CR report experiencing less negative emotion than the other experimental groups, but show no maladaptive physiological responding (Lazarus et al., 1965; Dandoy & Goldstein,

1990; Gross, 1998b; Jackson et al., 2000). Subsequent research using self-report trait measures of reappraisal have extended Gross' findings by examining the affective consequences of individual differences in CR use. For example, Mauss and colleagues (2007) found that individuals who reported frequently using CR as an emotion regulation strategy – relative to those who reported not using this strategy – experienced less anger and an adaptive pattern of physiological responding in a laboratory anger provocation.

Extending these findings beyond the laboratory, Gross and John (Gross & John, 2003; John & Gross, 2004) have examined the consequences of CR use for individuals' well-being in daily life. They found that individuals who report frequently using CR ("reappraisers") also report greater overall well-being. Together, these studies suggest that there are individual differences in CR use, and that those who report using CR are able to effectively downregulate their experience of negative emotion. In addition, reappraisers also seem to be rewarded with increases in positive outcomes over time, which supports the claim that CR has an important main effect on resilience. Specifically, those who use CR across a wide range of negative emotional contexts are more likely to experience positive outcomes and less likely to experience negative outcomes.

Studies that have examined the upregulation of positive emotions using CR have provided converging evidence. For example, the study of individual differences in CR and responding to an anger induction also showed that individuals who reported frequently using CR experienced more positive emotions during laboratory anger induction (Mauss et al., 2007). In the context of high stress, Folkman and Moskowitz (2000) noted that, among caregivers for people with AIDS, those who reported frequently using reappraisal consistently experienced more positive emotions both during caregiving and after the death of the patient. Specifically, these caregivers used positive reappraisal to change the meaning of the negative situations they were experiencing. For example, many thought about how their efforts were benefiting their patients. In another study on daily stressors among undergraduates, Shiota (2006) found that the self-reported trait use of positive reappraisal was positively associated with positive affect. These studies together support the notion that CR can be effectively used to increase one's experience of positive emotions even in highly stressful situations.

Although research on CR has focused considerably less on increases in positive emotion than on decreases in negative emotion, some studies suggest that experiencing positive emotions in the face of stress is an important facet of achieving resilience. In support of this point, resilient individuals are more likely to find positive meaning in the stressors they experience (Moskowitz, 2001; Tugade & Fredrickson, 2004). Fredrickson and colleagues (2003, p. 367) posited that this is because resilient people "use positive emotions strategically or intelligently to achieve their superior coping outcomes." This strategic use of positive emotional experience is likely based, in part, on adaptive emotion regulation strategies such as CR. For the remainder of the chapter, the term CR will be used to refer to both the upregulation of positive emotions and the downregulation of negative emotions, unless otherwise noted.

The studies reviewed so far suggest that CR is associated with positive outcomes in healthy populations. Additional research suggests that CR also explains variation in mental health. For example, across a series of studies, Garnefski and colleagues have found a consistent negative association between self-reported use of CR and depression (Garnefski et al., 2001, 2003; Garnefski & Kraaij, 2006). In addition, several longitudinal studies have found that this relationship remains robust over time. In one study using a sample of people aged 67 years and older, the negative relationship between CR and depression was replicated at a follow-up session two and a half years after the first session (Kraaij et al., 2002). In another longitudinal study that examined CR in the context of high stress, Pakenham (2005) investigated outcomes in a sample of people caring for patients with multiple sclerosis. Results indicated that self-reported use of CR had a buffering effect on the relationship between stress and negative outcomes, including depression.

In order to better understand the effects of CR in the context of high stress, Carrico and colleagues (2005) conducted a longitudinal, experimental intervention using cognitive-behavioral stress management with a sample of highly stressed males with HIV. Over the treatment period of 10 weeks, men who received the intervention showed significant decreases in depressive symptomatology relative to the control group, and this decrease was mediated by self-reported increases in the use of positive reframing, a strategy similar to CR, suggesting that CR was the mechanism of positive change after the intervention.

Taken together, it seems that CR confers advantages to those who use it, suggesting that this regulation strategy may be an important factor in resilience. Specifically, the use of CR appears to change appraisals of a stressor, thus leading to an attenuated negative emotional reaction (as depicted in Figure 2.1, links E and B). This adaptive emotional reaction, in turn, appears to increase the likelihood of resilience (Figure 2.1, link C). However, some open questions still remain. First, the efficacy of CR in the context of high life stress is not yet well understood. Although some studies have examined CR in stressed populations (c.f. Carrico et al., 2005; Pakenham, 2005), most of these studies included only one specific stressor, such as having HIV. This makes it difficult to know whether these findings would generalize to other types and intensities of stressor. Also, apart from a few notable exceptions (Garnefski et al., 2001, 2003; Garnefski & Kraaij, 2006), most research on CR has not examined its relationship to negative outcomes such as depression and anxiety symptoms, and even fewer studies have examined the potential moderating effects of CR on resilience versus negative outcomes. This makes it difficult to know whether CR can indeed buffer people from developing negative outcomes in the context of high life stress.

Additionally, nearly all of the existing research on CR has relied on self-report questionnaire measures of the frequency of CR use. Although these trait measures of CR have proven very useful, we argue that specifically the *ability* to effectively and flexibly manage emotions across different contexts serves as an important and strong moderator of the relationship between stress and depression. It is, therefore, important to measure CR ability in addition to frequency of CR use. One last limitation of research that has relied on self-report measures of CR is the the confounds inherent in self-reports, such as self-presentational biases. Going forward, it is important to use more objective laboratory measures of CR that are less influenced by self-report biases.

In our recent research, we sought to address these open questions (Troy et al., 2010). We tested the idea that CR ability could act as a moderator of the relationship between stress and depression – serving as a protective factor for those who are high in CR ability, and acting as a vulnerability factor for those who are low in CR ability. To test this hypothesis, a laboratory measure of CR ability was developed that measures changes in two affective domains: self-reported emotion, specifically sadness, and physiological responding. In order to measure CR ability in the laboratory, a sadness induction was conducted using short film clips. Ability in CR was quantified by calculating changes in sadness (using self-report and physiological changes) from a sad baseline film clip to a subsequent film clip in which the participants were instructed to reappraise. Specifically, participants were given instructions that asked them to think about the emotional situation depicted in the film in a more positive way. These instructions gave specific examples of how to reappraise, such as trying to imagine the unexpected good outcomes that the characters in the film clip could experience. Decreases in feelings of sadness and physiological indices of negative emotion when instructed to reappraise indexed the ability to use CR. This laboratory measure of CR ability was used with a community sample of 90 women who had experienced a stressful life event in the past three months. The women also filled out questionnaires that measure life stress and depressive symptoms.

The results indicated that CR ability moderated the relationship between intensity of life stress and depressive symptoms. Specifically, at high levels of stress, women who were high in CR ability exhibited significantly lower levels of depressive symptoms than women who were low in CR ability. Indeed, they were statistically indistinguishable from women who experienced low levels of life stress. At low levels of stress, CR ability did not have a moderating effect on depressive symptoms. This interaction was found using the self-reported as well as the physiological indices of CR ability. Additionally, nearly all participants reported that they tried very hard to use reappraisal when they were instructed to do so. This finding, combined with the significant interactions using both self-report and physiological changes, supports the conclusion that the observed results are not simply the product of demand characteristics or some other form of emotion regulation such as distraction.

Together, these results suggest that CR ability has important implications for resilience. First, CR only affected individuals' well-being in the context of high stress. Second, the fact that this sample contained a wide range of stressors and levels of stress suggests that CR may be an adaptive regulatory strategy across many types of stressful situation. In addition, by using a laboratory measure of CR ability, this study is one of the first to demonstrate that an ability specifically to downregulate negative emotions by using reappraisal

is an important factor contributing to adjustment to stress. Taken as a whole, the literature on stress, resilience, and CR supports a scientific model of resilience in which the ability to use CR serves as a moderator of the relationship between stress and resilience (Figure 2.1, link D) Specifically, CR can be used to change appraisals of a stressor, thus leading to an attenuated negative emotional response (Figure 2.1, link B). This downregulated emotional response is, in turn, associated with resilience (Figure 2.1, link C).

More work is needed in this area to improve understanding of the causal mechanisms, and further studies examining changes in emotions besides sadness, both positive and negative, are also warranted. The results of a recent study suggest that the ability to effectively regulate one's emotion, such as sadness, may also extend to the ability to effectively regulate other negative emotions, and even positive emotions such as joy, although this study did not look specifically at CR ability (Mikolajczak *et al.*, 2008). Additionally, the present review suggests that some *but not all* individuals are able to use CR to regulate emotions in the context of stress. This raises important questions. For example, why are some people quite good at using CR while others appear unable or unwilling to use this strategy? What processes support effective emotion regulation? While there is some preliminary evidence to suggest that specific aspects of cognitive control may support effective cognitive emotion regulation (Mikels *et al.*, 2008), this question remains to be fully explored. In addition, it remains unclear whether training paradigms (similar to those used in the selective attention literature) may allow those who are low in CR ability to increase their ability with practice. Future research on the plasticity of CR ability is needed in order to answer this open question.

An additional area for future research lies in the heterogeneity of processes involved in reappraisal. Reappraisal has been described, so far as the reframing of an emotional situation in a more positive way in order to change its emotional impact. However, there are several other ways in which reappraisal can be applied. For example, reappraisal has been used in other studies to reframe an emotional situation in a more objective, detached way (Gross, 1998b; Ochsner *et al.*, 2004), to imagine that an emotional event is being observed from a great distance (Ayduk & Kross, 2008), or to imagine that the situation is not real (Deveney & Pizzagalli, 2008). Research examining these other forms of reappraisal has found that they too appear to be adaptive ways to decrease negative emotions. Indeed, one study that compared the utility of different reappraisal strategies found that there are multiple ways in which CR can be used to effectively downregulate negative emotions (Ochsner *et al.*, 2004). In the context of stress and resilience, it remains unclear whether certain reappraisal strategies are more adaptive than others. It may be, for example, that distancing reappraisal is particularly adaptive for the downregulation of negative emotions in the context of uncontrollable stressors whereas positive reappraisal strategies may be more adaptive in the context of stressors that can be changed or controlled, in that this approach may facilitate appraisals that lead to more active coping and problem solving in the face of stress. Further work on optimal matching of specific reappraisal strategies to different emotional contexts will help to shed light on these hypotheses.

Lastly, the model outlined in Figure 2.1 has the potential to inform future clinical interventions. For example, several existing clinical interventions such as cognitive-behavioral stress management and cognitive-behavioral therapy target cognitive change as a mechanism for the prevention of psychological disorders as well as for growth. One important component of these therapies is to challenge distorted appraisals and replace them with more realistic, positive appraisals of a situation. This practice clearly overlaps with CR (Campbell-Sills & Barlow, 2007). The research reviewed above lends additional empirical support to these interventions. Based on this research, moreover, it seems that interventions could be particularly effective in highly stressed individuals before pathology develops. People who are highly stressed and low in emotion regulation ability may be particularly vulnerable, but also particularly responsive to treatments that are aimed at improving CR ability. Using the laboratory paradigm described above, such vulnerable people could be relatively easily identified. Clearly, more research on CR ability (both basic and applied) is warranted in order to answer these open empirical questions. Overall, however, as research in the area of CR, stress, and resilience progresses, it is our hope that more treatments might be informed by or improved upon using findings from this field. Moving forward, it is our hope that researchers and clinicians examining emotion regulation can work together to find the optimal way to promote resilient emotion regulation among at-risk populations.

Conclusions

Exposure to stress is an emotional experience for most people and, on average, stress exposure has been linked to impaired mental health outcomes such as depression. There is, however, wide variation in people's adjustment to stress – many people exhibit resilience after a stressor, while others experience negative long-term outcomes. This variance in adjustment to stress suggests that there must be some endogenous factors that serve a protective role: those who possess these factors are more likely to experience resilience, while those who do not are more vulnerable to negative outcomes. Because of the emotional nature of stressors, there has been an increasing focus on individual differences in emotion regulation as one such potential protective factor. Based on appraisal theories of emotion, which argue that it is one's appraisal of a stressor that leads to an emotional reaction (Figure 2.1, links A and B), we have put forth a framework for resilience (Figure 2.1). In this framework, the ability to use cognitive emotion regulation to adaptively change appraisals of a stressor moderates the relationship between stress and resilience. By changing one's appraisals of a stressor, the resulting emotions can be changed in adaptive ways, leading to increased chances of resilience even in highly stressful situations (Figure 2.1, link C).

To support the proposed framework, two different types of cognitive emotion regulation that appear to be particularly effective at changing appraisals in the context of stress have been explored. First, a review of studies of AC suggested that adaptive strategies in the context of stress consist of using AC selectively and flexibly according to an individual's current goals rather than in rigid, inflexible ways. For example, it appears to be maladaptive to attend to negative stimuli when they are irrelevant to one's well-being but it is adaptive to do so when they are relevant. People who are able to flexibly and effectively use this type of AC appear to be more resilient in the long term, while people who use maladaptive, stimulus-driven types of AC such as distraction and rumination are more vulnerable to long-term negative outcomes such as depression (Figure 2.1, link D).

Second, the role of CR, another form of cognitive emotion regulation, was examined. This consists of reframing emotional stimuli to decrease their negative emotional impact. The literature suggests that CR can be used to change the intensity of negative emotions in response to stressful situations. In the context of high life stress, individuals who report frequently using CR are less likely to exhibit depression. In addition, recent work suggests that CR ability moderates the relationship between stress and depression. In this way, CR ability may be playing an important protective role for those individuals who are able to effectively reappraise in the context of stress (Figure 2.1, link E).

In summary, it appears that the ability to use both types of cognitive emotion regulation serves as a protective factor against the development of negative outcomes in the context of stress. People who are able to use cognitive emotion regulation strategies in adaptive ways when experiencing stress are able to effectively manage the intensity of their negative emotions by changing the appraisals that they make. When these negative emotions are effectively and adaptively down-regulated, resilience becomes more likely.

Acknowledgements

The authors would like to thank Betsy App, Benjamin Hankin, Jutta Joormann, Jeremy Reynolds, Amanda Shallcross, and members of the Emotion Regulation Laboratory at the University of Denver for their feedback on a draft of this chapter.

References

Abele, A. E. & Gendolla, G. H. E. (2007). Individual differences in optimism predict the recall of personally relevant information. *Personality and Individual Differences*, **43**, 1125–1135.

Aspinwall, L. G. & Brunhart, S. M. (1996). Distinguishing optimism from denial: Optimistic beliefs predict attention to health threats. *Personality and Social Psychology Bulletin*, **22**, 993–1003.

Ayduk, O. & Kross, E. (2008). Enhancing the pace of recovery: Self-distanced analysis of negative experiences reduces blood pressure reactivity. *Psychological Science*, **19**, 229–231.

Bonanno, G. A. (2005). Resilience in the face of potential trauma. *Current Directions in Psychological Science*, **14**, 135–138.

Bradley, B. P., Mogg, K., & Lee, S. C. (1997). Attentional biases for negative information in induced and naturally occurring dysphoria. *Behaviour Research and Therapy*, **35**, 911–927.

Broderick, P. C. (2005). Mindfulness and coping with dysphoric mood: Contrasts with rumination and distraction. *Cognitive Therapy and Research*, **29**, 501–510.

Campbell-Sills, L. & Barlow, D. H. (2007). Incorporating emotion regulation into conceptualizations and treatments of anxiety and mood disorders. In J. J. Gross (ed.), *Handbook of emotion regulation* (pp. 542–560). New York: Guilford Press.

Carrico, A. W., Antoni, M. H., Weaver, K. E., Lechner, S. C., & Schneiderman, N. (2005). Cognitive–behavioural stress management with HIV-positive homosexual men: Mechanisms of sustained reductions in depressive symptoms. *Chronic Illness*, **1**, 207–215.

Dandoy, A. C. & Goldstein, A. C. (1990). The use of cognitive appraisal to reduce stress reactions: A replication. *Journal of Social Behavior and Personality*, **5**, 275–285.

Deveney, C. M. & Pizzagalli, D. A. (2008). The cognitive consequences of emotion regulation: An ERP investigation. *Psychophysiology*, **45**, 435–444.

Dohrenwend, B. S. & Dohrenwend, B. P. (eds.) (1974). *Stressful life events: Their nature and effects*. New York: Wiley.

Eippert, F., Veit, R., Weiskopf, N., *et al.* (2007). Regulation of emotional responses elicited by threat-related stimuli. *Human Brain Mapping*, **28**, 409–423.

Ensel, W. M. & Lin, N. (1996). Distal stressors and the life stress process. *Journal of Community Psychology*, **24**, 66–82.

Erber, R. & Tesser, A. (1992). Task effort and the regulation of mood: The absorption hypothesis. *Journal of Experimental Social Psychology*, **28**, 339–359.

Felsten, G. (2002). Minor stressors and depressed mood: Reactivity is more strongly correlated than total stress. *Stress and Health*, **18**, 75–81.

Folkman, S. & Lazarus, R. S. (1985). If it changes it must be a process: Study of emotion and coping during three stages of a college examination. *Journal of Personality and Social Psychology*, **48**, 150–170.

Folkman, S. & Moskowitz, J. T. (2000). Stress, positive emotion, and coping. *Current Directions in Psychological Science*, **9**, 115–118.

Freitas, A. L. & Downey, G. (1998). Resilience: A dynamic perspective. *International Journal of Behavioral Development*, **22**, 263–285.

Fredrickson, B. L., Tugade, M. M., Waugh, C. E., & Larkin, G. R. (2003). What good are positive emotions in crises? A prospective study of resilience and emotions following the terrorist attacks on the United States on September 11, 2001. *Journal of Personality and Social Psychology*, **84**, 365–376.

Garnefski, N. & Kraaij, V. (2006). Relationships between cognitive emotion regulation strategies and depressive symptoms: A comparative study of five specific samples. *Personality and Individual Differences*, **40**, 1659–1669.

Garnefski, N., Kraaij, V., & Spinhoven, P. (2001). Negative life events, cognitive emotion regulation and emotional problems. *Personality and Individual Differences*, **30**, 1311–1327.

Garnefski, N., Boon, S., & Kraaij, V. (2003). Relationships between cognitive strategies of adolescents and depressive symptomatology across different types of life event. *Journal of Youth and Adolescence*, **32**, 401–408.

Goldin, P. R., McRae, K., Ramel, W., & Gross, J. J. (2008). The neural bases of emotion regulation: Reappraisal and suppression of negative emotion. *Biological Psychiatry*, **63**, 577–586.

Gotlib, I. H., Yue, D. N., & Joormann, J. (2005). Selective attention in dysphoric individuals: The role of affective interference and inhibition. *Cognitive Therapy and Research*, **29**, 417–432.

Gross, J. J. (1998a). The emerging field of emotion regulation: An integrative review. *Review of General Psychology*, **2**, 271–299.

Gross, J. J. (1998b). Antecedent- and response-focused emotion regulation: Divergent consequences for experience, expression, and physiology. *Journal of Personality and Social Psychology*, **74**, 224–237.

Gross, J. J. & John, O. P. (2003). Individual differences in two emotion regulation processes: Implications for affect, relationships, and well-being. *Journal of Personality and Social Psychology*, **85**, 348–362.

Gross, J. J. & Thompson, R. A. (2007). Emotion regulation: Conceptual foundations. In J. J. Gross (ed.), *Handbook of emotion regulation* (pp. 3–24). New York: Guilford Press.

Holahan, C. J., Moos, R. H., Holahan, C. K., Brennan, P. L., & Schutte, K. K. (2005). Stress generation, avoidance coping, and depressive symptoms: A 10-year model. *Journal of Consulting and Clinical Psychology*, **73**, 658–666.

Ingram, R. E., Bernet, C. Z., & McLaughlin, S. C. (1994). Attentional allocation processes in individuals at risk for depression. *Cognitive Therapy and Research*, **18**, 317–332.

Isaacowitz, D. M. (2005). The gaze of the optimist. *Personality and Social Psychology Bulletin*, **31**, 407–415.

Jackson, D. C., Malmstadt, J. R., Larson, C. L., & Davidson, R. J. (2000). Suppression and enhancement of emotional responses to unpleasant pictures. *Psychophysiology*, **37**, 512–522.

John, O. P. & Gross, J. J. (2004). Healthy and unhealthy emotion regulation: Personality processes, individual differences, and life span development. *Journal of Personality*, **72**, 1301–1333.

Joormann, J. (2004). Attentional bias in dysphoria: The role of inhibitory processes. *Cognition and Emotion*, **18**, 125–147.

Joormann, J., Talbot, L., & Gotlib, I. H. (2007). Biased processing of emotional information in girls at risk for depression. *Journal of Abnormal Psychology*, **116**, 135–143.

Kalisch, R., Wiech, K., Critchley, H. D., *et al.* (2005). Anxiety reduction through detachment: Subjective, physiological, and neural effects. *Journal of Cognitive Neuroscience*, **17**, 874–883.

Kalisch, R., Wiech, K., Herrmann, K., & Dolan, R. J. (2006). Neural correlates of self-distraction from anxiety and a process model of cognitive emotion regulation. *Journal of Cognitive Neuroscience*, **18**, 1266–1276.

Kendler, K. S. Karkowski, L. M., & Prescott, C. A. (1999). Causal relationship between stressful life events and the onset of major depression. *American Journal of Psychiatry*, **156**, 837–841.

Kraaij, V., Pruymboom, E., & Garnefski, N. (2002). Cognitive coping and depressive symptoms in the elderly: A longitudinal study. *Aging and Mental Health*, **6**, 275–281.

Krompinger, J. W., Moser, J. S., & Simons, R. F. (2008). Modulations of the electrophysiological response to pleasant stimuli by cognitive reappraisal. *Emotion*, **8**, 132–137.

Kross, E. & Ayduk, O. (2008). Facilitating adaptive emotional analysis: Distinguishing distanced-analysis of depressive experiences from immersed-analysis and distraction. *Personality and Social Psychology Bulletin*, **34**, 924–938.

Lazarus, R. S. (1991). Cognition and motivation in emotion. *American Psychologist*, **46**, 352–367.

Lazarus, R. S. (1999). *Stress and emotion: A new synthesis.* New York: Springer.

Lazarus, R. S. & Folkman, S. (1984). *Stress, appraisal, and coping.* New York: Springer.

Lazarus, R. S., Opton, E. M. Jr., Nomikos, M. S., & Rankin, N. O. (1965). The principle of short-circuiting of threat: Further evidence. *Journal of Personality*, **33**, 622–635.

Lu, L. (1994). University transition: Major and minor life stressors, personality characteristics and mental health. *Psychological Medicine*, **24**, 81–87.

Luthar, S. S., Cicchetti, D., & Becker, B. (2000). The construct of resilience: A critical evaluation and guidelines for future work. *Child Development*, **71**, 543–562.

MacLeod, C. (1999). Anxiety and anxiety disorders. In T. Dalgleish & M. Powers (eds.), *The handbook of cognition and emotion* (pp. 447–477). Chichester, UK: Wiley.

MacLeod, C. & Hagan, R. (1992). Individual differences in the selective processing of threatening information, and emotional responses to a stressful life event. *Behaviour Research and Therapy*, **30**, 151–161.

MacLeod, C., Rutherford, E., Campbell, L., Ebsworthy, G., & Holker, L. (2002). Selective attention and emotional vulnerability: Assessing the causal basis of their association through the experimental manipulation of attentional bias. *Journal of Abnormal Psychology*, **111**, 107–123.

Mathews, A., Ridgeway, V., & Williamson, D. A. (1996). Evidence for attention to threatening stimuli in depression. *Behaviour Research and Therapy*, **34**, 695–705.

Mauss, I. B., Cook, C. L., Cheng, J. Y. J., & Gross, J. J. (2007). Individual differences in cognitive reappraisal: Experiential and physiological responses to an anger provocation. *International Journal of Psychophysiology*, **66**, 116–124.

Mazure, C. M., Bruce, M. L., Maciejewski, P. K., & Jacobs, S. C. (2000). Adverse life events and cognitive-personality characteristic in the prediction of major depression and anti-depressant response. *American Journal of Psychiatry*, **157**, 896–903.

McCarthy, C. J., Lambert, R. G., & Moller, N. P. (2006). Preventive resources and emotion regulation expectances as mediators between attachment and college students' stress outcomes. *International Journal of Stress Management*, **13**, 1–22.

Mikels, J. A., Reuter-Lorenz, P. A., Beyer, J. A., & Fredrickson, B. L. (2008). Emotion and working memory: Evidence for domain-specific processes for affective maintenance. *Emotion*, **8**, 256–266.

Mikolajczak, M., Nelis, D., Hansenne, M., & Quoidbach, J. (2008). If you can regulate sadness, you can probably regulate shame: Associations between trait emotional intelligence, emotion regulation and coping efficiency across discrete emotions. *Personality and Individual Differences*, **44**, 1356–1368.

Mogg, K., Bradley, B. P., & Williams, R. (1995). Attentional bias in anxiety and depression: The role of awareness. *British Journal of Clinical Psychology*, **34**, 17–36.

Monat, A., Lazarus, R. S., & Reevy, G. (eds.) (2007). *The Praeger handbook on stress and coping,* Vol. 1. Westport, CT: Praeger.

Morrow, J. & Nolen-Hoeksema, S. (1990). Effects of responses to depression on the remediation of depressive affect. *Journal of Personality and Social Psychology*, **58**, 519–527.

Moskowitz, J. T. (2001). Emotion and coping. In T. J. Mayne & G. A. Bonanno (eds.), *Emotions: Current issues and future directions* (pp. 311–336). New York: Guilford Press.

Nolen-Hoeksema, S. (1991). Responses to depression and their effects on the duration of depressive episodes. *Journal of Abnormal Psychology*, **100**, 569–582.

Nolen-Hoeksema, S. & Morrow, J. (1991). A prospective study of depression and posttraumatic stress symptoms after a natural disaster: The 1989 Loma Prieta earthquake. *Journal of Personality and Social Psychology*, **1**, 115–121.

Nolen-Hoeksema, S., Parker, L. E., & Larson, J. (1994). Ruminative coping with depressed mood following loss. *Journal of Personality and Social Psychology*, **67**, 92–104.

Nolen-Hoeksema, S., Wisco, B. E., & Lyubomirski, S. (2008). Rethinking rumination. *Perspectives on Psychological Science*, **3**, 400–424.

Norris, F. H., Stevens, S. P., Pfefferbaum, B., Wyche, K. F., & Pfefferbaum, R. L. (2008). Community resilience as a metaphor, theory, set of capacities, and strategy for disaster readiness. *American Journal of Community Psychology*, **41**, 127–150.

Ochsner, K. N. & Gross, J. J. (2005). The cognitive control of emotion. *Trends in Cognitive Sciences*, **9**, 242–249.

Ochsner, K. N. & Gross, J. J. (2008). Cognitive emotion regulation: Insights from social cognitive and affective neuroscience. *Current Directions in Psychological Science*, **17**, 153–158.

Ochsner, K. N., Ray, R. D., Cooper, J. C., *et al.* (2004). For better or for worse: Neural systems supporting the cognitive down and up-regulation of negative emotion. *Neuroimage*, **23**, 483–499.

Ortony, A., Clore, G. L., & Collins, A. (1988). *The cognitive structure of emotions.* New York: Cambridge University Press.

Pakenham, K. I. (2005). Relations between coping and positive and negative outcomes in carers of persons with multiple sclerosis (MS). *Journal of Clinical Psychology in Medical Settings*, **12**, 25–38.

Park, R. J., Goodyer, I. M., & Teasdale, J. D. (2004). Effects of induced rumination and distraction on mood and overgeneral autobiographical memory in adolescent major depressive disorder and controls. *Journal of Child Psychology and Psychiatry*, **45**, 996–1006.

Powers, D. V., Gallagher-Thompson, D., & Kraemer, H. C. (2002). Coping and depression in Alzheimer's caregivers: Longitudinal evidence of stability. *Journal of Gerontology*, **57B**, 205–211.

Ray, R. D., Wilhelm, F. H., & Gross, J. J. (2008). All in the mind's eye? Anger rumination and reappraisal. *Journal of Personality and Social Psychology*, **94**, 133–145.

Rutter, M. (1999). Resilience concepts and findings: Implications for family therapy. *Journal of Family Therapy*, **21**, 119–144.

Sarason, I. G., Johnson, J. H., & Siegel, J. M. (1978). Assessing the impact of life changes: Development of the life experiences survey. *Journal of Consulting and Clinical Psychology*, **46**, 932–946.

Scheier, M. F. & Carver, C. S. (1993). On the power of positive thinking: The benefits of being optimistic. *Current Directions in Psychological Science*, **2**, 26–30.

Scherer, K. R. (1988). Criteria for emotion-antecedent appraisal: A review. In V. Hamilton, G. H. Bower, & N. H. Frijda (eds.), *Cognitive perspectives on emotion and motivation* (pp. 89–126). New York: Kluwer Academic/Plenum Press.

Scherer, K. R. & Ceschi, G. (1997). Lost luggage: A field study of emotion antecedent appraisal. *Motivation and Emotion*, **21**, 211–235.

Schwartz, D. & Proctor, L. J. (2000). Community violence exposure and children's social adjustment in the school peer group: The mediating roles of emotion regulation and social cognition. *Journal of Consulting and Clinical Psychology*, **68**, 670–683.

Shiota, M. N. (2006). Silver linings and candles in the dark: Differences among positive coping strategies in predicting subjective well-being. *Emotion*, **6**, 335–339.

Siemer, M., Mauss, I., & Gross, J. J. (2007). Same situation – different emotions: How appraisals shape our emotions. *Emotion*, **7**, 592–600.

Siegle, G. J., Ghinassi, F., & Thase, M. E. (2008). Neurobehavioral therapies in the 21st century: Summary of an emerging field and an extended example of cognitive control training for depression. *Cognitive Therapy and Research*, **31**, 235–262.

Silk, J. S., Vanderbilt-Adriance, E., Shaw, D. S., *et al.* (2007). Resilience among children and adolescents at risk for depression: Mediation and moderation across social and neurobiological contexts. *Development and Psychopathology*, **19**, 841–865.

Singer, A. R. & Dobson, K. S. (2007). An experimental investigation of the cognitive vulnerability to depression. *Behaviour Research and Therapy*, **45**, 563–575.

Smith, C. A. & Ellsworth, P. C. (1987). Patterns of appraisal and emotion related to taking an exam. *Journal of Personality and Social Psychology*, **52**, 475–488.

Tennant, C. (2002). Life events, stress and depression: A review of recent findings. *Australian and New Zealand Journal of Psychiatry*, **36**, 173–182.

Totterdell, P. & Parkinson, B. (1999). Use and effectiveness of self-regulation strategies for improving mood in a group of trainee teachers. *Journal of Occupational Health Psychology*, **4**, 219–232.

Tugade, M. M. & Fredrickson, B. L. (2004). Resilient individuals use positive emotions to bounce back from negative emotional experiences. *Journal of Personality and Social Psychology*, **86**, 320–333.

Troy, A. S., Wilhelm, F. H., Shallcross, A. J., & Mauss, I. B. (2010). Seeing the silver lining: Cognitive reappraisal ability moderates the relationship between stress and depression. *Emotion*, **10**, 783–795.

Urry, H. L., van Reekum, C. M., Johnstone, T., *et al.* (2006). Amygdala and ventromedial prefrontal cortex are inversely coupled during regulation of negative affect and predict the diurnal pattern of cortisol secretion among older adults. *Journal of Neuroscience*, **26**, 4415–4425.

Wadlinger, H. A. & Isaacowitz, D. M. (2008). Looking happy: The experimental manipulation of a positive visual attention bias. *Emotion*, **8**, 121–126.

Chapter

3

Cognitive factors and resilience: how self-efficacy contributes to coping with adversities

Charles C. Benight and Roman Cieslak

We are disturbed not by events, but by the views which we take of them

(Epictetus, stoic philosopher, c. 55–135)

Introduction

Human ability to survive and to thrive in challenging or threatening situations has always fascinated people, inspiring artists and philosophers. People who proved their resilience, personal strengths, or moral virtues (as philosophers used to say) have been the focus of admiration and pride. They have been glorified as heroes in innumerate folktales and immortalized in countless works of art. The stoic philosophers, however, argued that ordinary people may face extraordinary circumstances and remain undisturbed by challenging situations. The quotation from Epictetus that opens this chapter introduces a major topic in this chapter: the role of cognitive processes in human resilience. Although there are many differences in cognitive approaches to understand resilience, all of them echo Epictetus' aphorism that perception of reality and processing of vital information are critical components of coping with adversities.

Many definitions and measures capturing the concept of resilience have been proposed and are discussed in other chapters in this book, including physiological resistance (Selye, 1936), temperamental or personality predispositions (Kobasa, 1979; Scheier & Carver, 1985; Antonovsky, 1987; Strelau, 1998), trajectories of psychological distress outcomes (Bonanno, 2004), coping flexibility (Cheng, 2003), and self-perceptions of ability to manage one's life (Davidson *et al.*, 1982). The focus in this chapter relates to the role of cognitive determinants of successful adaptation.

The first cognitive psychological conceptualization of factors relevant for surviving and adapting to changing stressful demands can be traced back to works of Sigmund Freud and his successors. These authors wrote in depth about how people manage extreme experiences using more or less adaptive cognitive defensive mechanisms. The later work of Victor Frankl poignantly describes the importance of perceptions in surviving the horror of his three-year imprisonment in a Nazi concentration camp (Frankl, 1962). Since these early approaches to stress and resilience, the cognitive revolution in psychology changed our understanding of the stress and coping process (Lazarus, 1966).

This chapter focuses on the contemporary cognitive factors deemed critical in understanding resilience. We agree with Luthar and colleagues (2000, p. 543), who stated that "resilience refers to a dynamic process encompassing positive adaptation within the context of significant adversity." We also argue that resilience is more a process than an outcome of individual coping efforts or a single factor (e.g., personality trait) contributing to effective coping with adversities. The risk in studies of resilience lies in the broad search for an agreed definition while the underlying processes remain unknown. Following an old logic principle ascribed to Ockham, this chapter will avoid multiplying entities beyond necessity. Instead, we will demonstrate how existing approaches focusing on cognitive factors vital to coping with adversities might be easily applied through theoretically available models to advance our knowledge of human resilience.

Among these approaches, Bandura's social cognitive theory (SCT) is a viable framework to understand resilience (Bandura, 1997). Other cognitive approaches that might be applied to the study of resilience will also be briefly introduced. The focus will then be on SCT, presenting its primary concepts and studies showing its usefulness in studies of resilience. Some possible

Resilience and Mental Health: Challenges Across the Lifespan, ed. Steven M. Southwick, Brett T. Litz, Dennis Charney, and Matthew J. Friedman. Published by Cambridge University Press. © Cambridge University Press 2011.

developments of this theory, which, in our opinion, could help in the understanding of the multidimensional and complex process of adaptation and coping with adversities, will also be discussed. This chapter focuses on adult adaptation to adversity and does not include how children might fit into these models.

Cognitive approaches to resilience

The process of regulating between environmental demands and available resources is seen as critical for human functioning in many theories of stress (Lazarus & Folkman, 1984; Hobfoll, 1989, 2001) and stress-related models (House, 1981; Karasek & Theorell 1990; Demerouti *et al.*, 2001; Siegrist *et al.*, 2004). Although the primary focus here is on cognitive factors derived from SCT (such as self-efficacy beliefs) and the dynamic process involved in managing environmental demands and resources, it is important to consider other theories that also acknowledge the crucial role of human cognitions in coping with adversities and adaptation processes.

The transactional theory of stress (Lazarus & Folkman, 1984) lists stress appraisals as key cognitive mediators and distinguishes between primary appraisal and secondary appraisal. In primary appraisal, individuals evaluate how important a specific demand is for their own well-being, judging if it is irrelevant (i.e., demands are not perceived as linked to a person), positive (i.e., the transaction may lead to positive consequences without taxing or exceeding resources), or stressful (i.e., the transaction may lead to positive or negative consequences, but resources need to be engaged). A stressful situation may be further appraised as harm/loss, threat, or challenge (Lazarus & Folkman, 1984). If the perception is that the consequences of a specific stress transaction may be positive, despite the amount of resources invested, the stressful situation is interpreted as a challenge. Harm/loss or threat appraisals, contrastingly, are made under situations where stress demands exceed available resources, leading to negative outcomes. Perceiving adversity as a challenge is a hallmark characteristic of resilience.

The perception of available resources is called secondary appraisal. These appraisals relate to an evaluation of available physical, social, psychological, and material resources and the ability to use them (self-efficacy) in dealing with environmental demands (Lazarus & Folkman, 1984). Specific coping strategies are undertaken as a result of both primary and secondary appraisals.

There are an overwhelming number of studies supporting the transactional model of stress (see Folkman & Moskowitz, 2004). Recently, research has demonstrated that appraisals made during stressful situations have an impact not only on psychological response but also on physiological response to stressors. For example, there is a strong effect of anticipatory cognitive appraisals on the cortisol stress response (Gaab *et al.*, 2005). Primary and secondary appraisals may explain up to 35% of the variance for cortisol reactivity among people who were exposed to a standard stressful situation (Gaab *et al.*, 2005). Importantly, Epel *et al.* (1998) suggested that cognitive appraisals that lead to a challenge approach to adversities may actually strengthen the physical and psychological resilience of the individual.

Other cognitive processes such as causal attributions about an adverse event may be important to consider when understanding resilience. Causal attributions may refer to the stability, controllability, and generalizability related to the stressor. For example, a stressor attributed to unstable, controllable, and specific causes can lead to a sense of challenge in dealing with the adversity (Abramson *et al.*, 1978).

Therefore, although not typically discussed as resilience, previous research utilizing cognitive processes such as appraisals and attributions conceptualizes successful coping as central to positive adaptation. Inherent in these models is an interactive process whereby an individual regulates his/her behavior through ongoing interactions with the adverse environment.

Carver and Scheier (1981) discussed an interactive control feedback system to understand this self-regulation. This system targets individualized appraisals of success or failure in reaching important self-goals, leading to cognitive and behavioral adjustments through a cybernetic feedback system. More recently, Carver (1998) developed a more complex model of different trajectories for understanding functional and dysfunctional responses to adverse events, including resilience. This model assumes four different possible trajectories following an adverse event. The trajectories include succumbing, survival with impairment, resilience, thriving. It is noteworthy that Carver (1998) introduced thriving as a possible outcome separate from resilience, and that environmental engagement and goal valence are also important to consider. Carver emphasized perceptions of personal confidence as critically important to consider. He stated (p. 256), "people with a sense of confidence and mastery move onward and upward and people with sufficient doubt suffer continued or repeated declines." As with secondary appraisal described by Lazarus and Folkman (1984), a sense of competence to meet adversity demands provides a sense of control that is critical for healthy adaptation (Epel *et al.*, 1998). Bandura (1997) and others have repeatedly shown this to be a central variable in understanding human behavior. Based on this, we argue that a sense of control to manage adversity is a necessary condition for resilience (or thriving) to occur. To understand this process more thoroughly, the SCT framework is utilized to examine the mechanisms that drive resilience.

Social cognitive theory approach to resilience

Social cognitive theory is a broad theory of human behavior (Bandura, 1997). It emphasizes the importance of interactions among three primary factors that predict future behavior: the environment, the person, and behavior (Figure 3.1). Through dynamic interactions with environmental conditions, human beings are able to be strategic in adapting to changing demands. Self-regulative behavior is accomplished through feedback systems both internally (cognitive appraisal processes) and externally (changes in environmental conditions). Self-evaluation is a critical component in the feedback process to ascertain successful or unsuccessful achievements of desired goals. By interpreting one's successes and failures, individuals alter their cognitions and behaviors in order to shape desired environmental conditions. We argue that self-appraisals play a central role in resilience.

A key construct within this self-regulatory dynamic interplay between the person, the environment, and

behaviors is *self-efficacy*. Self-efficacy is part of the self-evaluative cognitive process and is defined as the perceived capability to enact a certain behavior. Self-efficacy perceptions have been found to be highly predictive of behavior across a vast array of human functioning (e.g., athletics, education, health, work performance, stress [Bandura, 1997]). Within the context of stress and coping, self-efficacy perceptions have been labeled coping self-efficacy. Consequently, *coping self-efficacy* in the context of severe adversity is defined as the perceived capability for managing post-traumatic recovery or stressful demands (Benight & Bandura, 2004).

Self-efficacy perceptions are developed through interactive feedback, with success or failure as one strives toward valued goals. Self-efficacy perceptions are enhanced through mastery experiences, verbal persuasion of valued social connections, observations of relevant others' successes, and adequate self-management of physical arousal. Conversely, failure, negative social feedback, inadequate social models, and unmanageable anxiety lead to derailment of self-efficacy beliefs. These perceptions are highly predictive of motivational behaviors such as goal setting and behavioral perseverance following environmental impediments (Bandura, 1997). Clearly, it could be argued that such cognitive appraisals play an important role in positive trajectories following adversity (i.e., the resilience or thriving trajectories described by Carver [1998]). Other researchers have also cited the importance of perceptions of confidence in understanding resilience and optimal functioning (Ford & Smith, 2007).

Self-efficacy can be viewed as a more general construct or as a domain-specific construct. General self-efficacy is a trait-like factor that reflects one's beliefs about one's own capabilities in dealing with demands across different situations. Although general self-efficacy may be seen as a personality trait (e.g., Schyns & von Collani, 2002), it may be also argued that cross-situational coherence in self-efficacy appraisals might be explained without referring to a personality trait construct (Cervone, 1997, 2000). In contrast to general self-efficacy, task- or domain-specific self-efficacy is more proximally related to a target task, behavior, or goal. Individuals' beliefs about their ability to perform a particular task, execute a specific behavior, or achieve a goal predict health behavior change (Luszczynska & Schwarzer, 2003), teachers' performances (Skaalvik & Skaalvik, 2007), and managing computers (Compeau & Higgins, 1995), to name a few.

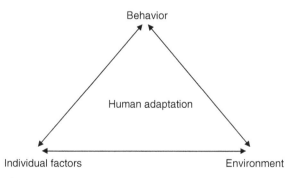

Figure 3.1 Interactions among environmental, individual, and behavioral factors predict human adaptation.

Self-efficacy perceptions are not the *only* cognitive factors influencing predictors of stress-response or post-traumatic outcomes. As discussed above, stress appraisals, attributions, perception of controllability, or general self-efficacy have all been shown to be predictive of behaviors. However, specific self-efficacy perceptions have been shown to be stronger predictors of outcomes than these other cognitive processes (Bandura, 1997).

As mentioned above, coping self-efficacy relates to beliefs about one's own abilities to manage demands specific to coping with trauma or stressful events (Benight & Bandura, 2004). A demand becomes stressful when there is a lack of adequate resources to deal with this demand (Lazarus & Folkman, 1984; Hobfoll, 1989). The process of regulation between demands and resources is seen as critical for human functioning in many theories of stress (Lazarus & Folkman, 1984; Hobfoll, 1989, 2001). We argue that the classical self-regulation mechanism described in SCT (Figure 3.1) might be extended by incorporating the regulating mechanisms between demands and resources (Figure 3.2). In other words, the self-regulation mechanisms among behavioral, personal, and environmental factors may be viewed as the dynamic interplay between demands and resources. This approach to self-regulation could be compared with a three-dimensional graph, in which multivectorial relationships represent the mechanisms discussed above. For example, for resilient individuals coping with environmental

demands from such adversities as a flood, terrorism, or a hurricane, all three types of resource (i.e., environmental, personal, and behavioral) will be used to offset the environmental demands to achieve positive functioning. Of course, internal demands (e.g., intrusive thoughts) must also be managed through available psychosocial resources.

In the context of this three-dimensional model of self-regulation, self-efficacy beliefs would remain a crucial mechanism predicting successful adaptation (i.e., resilience). In a study testing this expectation, both demands- and resources-related self-efficacy should be considered (e.g., "I am capable to work effectively even with time pressure" and "I am capable to get support from friends when needed," respectively). Our laboratory has recently shown that a measure assessing self-efficacy for specific job demands *and* for resource utilization mediates the effects of work stressors on job burnout (Lua, 2008).

Figure 3.3 depicts a model that might be used to test the effect of demands and resources on selected resilient adaptation outcomes. Rather than solely focusing on the specific measures of resilience or thriving outcomes, or on indices of resources or demands, the model highlights the mediational role of self-efficacy perceptions in understanding the dynamics of resilient coping with adversities. The dynamic nature of the model is represented by showing that changes in critical variable levels across time, both before and after exposure to traumatic or stressful events, are important to consider.

As SCT suggests, the ability to generate positive self-efficacy beliefs is not static but changes over time and as environmental conditions change (c.f. Mischel & Shoda, 1995). In other words, one can develop self-efficacy beliefs to cope with a particular demand, but demonstrate a lack of such beliefs about one's ability to cope with other demands as environmental conditions change. This approach toward understanding the adaptation after exposure to traumatic or stressful events focuses on the mechanisms underlying the process of resilient adaptation and requires monitoring the *levels* of critical components of the coping process and the *changes* in these factors (i.e., demands, resources, context-specific coping self-efficacy, and various aspects of functioning as indices of adaptation).

Rather than drawing possible trajectories of recovery resulting from coping with adversities, the model attempts to identify dynamic factors that *trigger, boost*, and *maintain* effective coping through the utilization and cultivation of internal and external resources. In

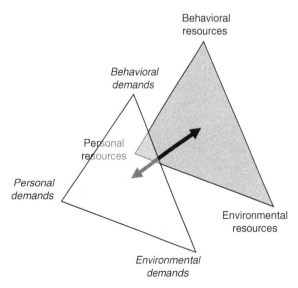

Figure 3.2 Three-dimensional model of self-regulation.

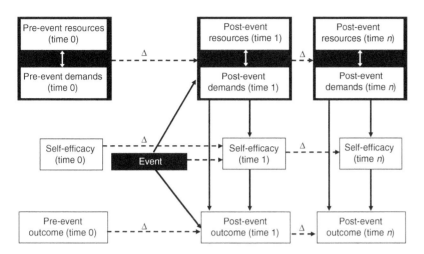

Figure 3.3 The mediating role of self-efficacy in coping with adversities.

our view, coping self-efficacy is an active, crucial cognitive component that can facilitate a sense of control to influence essential social and personal resources that are relevant to maintaining, regaining, or enhancing well-being. For example, the beneficial effect of social support on depressive symptoms can be more thoroughly explained when self-efficacy is considered as a mediating factor (Fiori *et al.*, 2006). Modern analytic techniques such as latent growth curve modeling and structural equation modeling allow us to test these more sophisticated theoretical approaches to understanding adaptation to adversity.

The importance of the environmental context

As discussed above, self-efficacy may modify the relationship between resources and demands as people confront adversities. These demands may vary, ranging from external demands caused by chronic stress at work or daily stressors to internal demands resulting from an exposure to a traumatic event. In our model (Figure 3.3), we argue that one should always control for the effects of specificity of these demands when investigating the effect of resources on well-being or other domains of stress outcomes.

In addition to environmental demands, environmental resources must also be considered. Following the definition of Hobfoll (2001, p. 339), resources are "objects, personal characteristics, conditions, or energies that are valued in their own right, or that are valued because they act as conduits to the achievement or protection of valued resources." Hobfoll (2001) grouped resources into several categories: objects

(e.g., a house), conditions (e.g., marriage), personal characteristics (e.g., social skillfulness), and energies (e.g., education). Significant evidence exists that demonstrates the importance of considering environmental resources in successful adaptation to adversity (Hobfoll, 1998). A more thorough overview of how self-efficacy may modify the effects of all these kinds of resource on different aspects of humans functioning is beyond the scope of this chapter; the reader is referred to Benight and Bandura (2004) for a deeper analysis. Here some empirical evidence is presented that supports the notion of self-efficacy as a relevant mediator between stress characteristics, resources, and different outcomes, beginning first with traumatic stress.

Self-efficacy and traumatic demands

Research on coping self-efficacy perceptions as a predictor of psychological distress following trauma has found these perceptions to be predictive of psychological adjustment within a variety of traumatic contexts such as natural disasters (e.g., hurricanes, fires, floods, and earthquakes; Benight *et al.*, 1997, 1999a, 1999b; Cheever & Hardin, 1999; Benight & Harper 2002; Sumer *et al.*, 2005), motor vehicle trauma (Benight *et al.*, 2008), domestic violence (Benight *et al.*, 2004), death of a spouse (Lindstrom, l997; Benight *et al.*, 2001), terrorist attacks (Benight *et al.*, 2000), and military combat (Solomon *et al.*, 1988, 1991). Coping self-efficacy also predicted positive outcomes (e.g., post-traumatic growth) following Hurricane Katrina in a sample of HIV-positive survivors with significant post-traumatic stress symptoms (Cieslak *et al.*, 2009).

Data also support the role of coping self-efficacy as a mediator between negative post-trauma cognitions (such as negative beliefs about self and the world) and psychological distress among survivors of child sexual abuse and motor vehicle trauma (Cieslak *et al.*, 2008). A recent meta-analysis indicated that self-efficacy has medium to large effects on post-traumatic adaptation indices (Luszczynska *et al.*, 2009), a testament to the importance of this construct.

Collectively, these studies demonstrate that the level of self-perceptions of coping capability following a trauma is important to consider. Positive coping self-efficacy (confidence) to manage stress adaptation demands provides an internal sense of control that promotes positive cognitions about the self, increases motivation to respond to ongoing demands, assists in self-management of emotions, and promotes effective decision making, in other words "resilience" (Bandura, 1997; Carver, 1998). Alternatively, lower levels of coping self-efficacy beliefs (i.e., confidence) lead survivors of trauma into a sense of increasing despair as recovery demands accumulate, leading to flooding of uncontrolled emotions, significant negative self-scrutiny, avoidance, and eventual capitulation (Carver, 1998). Turning attention now to general stress adaptation rather than traumatic stress, the results continue to be consistent.

Self-efficacy and other stressful demands

The above-mentioned studies provide evidence that high coping self-efficacy beliefs might reduce the deleterious effects of trauma-related demands on psychological distress. Outside the realm of trauma, a similar effect might be observed when other types of stressor are concerned (e.g., demands at work). Indeed, recent results provide evidence for the crucial role of self-efficacy when added to well-known models of work stress and burnout.

The job demands–control model is probably one of the most frequently tested models in occupational health psychology. In this model, work strain (i.e., work stress) is a result of working in the conditions where job demands are high and the latitude of control over the job is low (Karasek, 1979). In more recent developments of this model (i.e., in the demands–control–support model), social support (i.e., social resource) has moderated the interaction of high demands and low control on job strain (Johnson & Hall, 1988; Karasek & Theorell, 1990). Importantly,

self-efficacy perceptions may also be important in this context. Research indicates that the same moderating effect could be ascribed to self-efficacy. Results have shown that self-efficacy perceptions appear to buffer the effects of high job demands and low levels of control on important occupational outcomes such as physiological reactivity (Schaubroeck & Merritt, 1997) and job burnout (Salanova *et al.*, 2002). In addition, the match between level of self-efficacy and environmental control may also be important to consider. Among workers who report high self-efficacy, for example, low levels of control (under highly demanding conditions) have also increased blood pressure (Schaubroeck & Merritt, 1997) and increased symptoms of burnout (Salanova *et al.*, 2002).

Although these studies tested the moderating effects of self-efficacy, it may be that self-efficacy perceptions serve as a mediating mechanism rather than as a moderator (i.e., the cognitive mechanism through which these other variables influence important outcomes). Several workplace stress studies testing the mediating role of self-efficacy perceptions have been supportive. Brouwers and Tomic (2000) tested longitudinal relationships between teachers' burnout and work-related self-efficacy and found that perceived self-efficacy mediated the effects of emotional exhaustion on personal accomplishment and depersonalization (important occupational outcomes). Further, among teachers working in stressful conditions caused by recent organizational changes, self-efficacy in dealing with organizational changes was found to predict burnout symptoms, even after controlling for demographic variables (Evers *et al.*, 2002). Self-efficacy also mediated the effects of work stressors on job dissatisfaction and turnover intention (Jex & Gudanowski, 1992). Finally, in probably the most extensive study to date testing self-efficacy as a prime work stress mediator, Perrewé *et al.* (2002) conducted a study in nine countries and found that work role stress (i.e., role conflict and role ambiguity) was indirectly related to burnout through self-efficacy perceptions. Although these studies speak to the challenges of occupational stress, the focus has been on negative outcomes such as burnout or physiological stress markers. Future research is necessary to identify positive outcomes relating to resilience or thriving in these contexts.

The reviewed evidence on level of self-efficacy perceptions is supportive of the importance of these beliefs in managing environmental demands and effectively utilizing critical adaptational resources (Figure 3.3).

Yet this view fails to take into account the dynamic nature of human resilience. Also in Figure 3.3, one can see that changes in critical factors across time are vital to consider. Attention is now given to evidence testing the value of changes in self-efficacy perceptions across time in understanding resilience.

Changes in self-efficacy beliefs and psychological outcomes

Whereas the literature described above supports the role of levels of coping self-efficacy, there is also some evidence that the dynamic changes in self-perceptions are also important to consider in psychological adaptation. Indeed, if self-efficacy increases through positive management of resources in response to critical demands, it would suggest an *increasing* sense of mastery over the adaptation process. A decrease in self-efficacy beliefs would suggest an increasing sense of defeat and self-doubt.

In a study examining recovery after motor vehicle accident trauma (Benight *et al.*, 2008), early changes in coping self-efficacy perceptions (within the first month following an accident) were predictive of lower post-traumatic distress three months later, even after controlling for the other predictors of distress (such as responsibility for accident, involvement in litigation, peritraumatic dissociation, seven-day post-traumatic distress, and coping self-efficacy level). Based on these results, future investigations should consider changes in self-efficacy perceptions over time when attempting to model the resilience process following trauma. The model depicted in Figure 3.3 shows that both levels of and changes in self-efficacy may predict resilient functioning after a traumatic event.

Evidence for the importance of changes in self-efficacy outside the trauma realm also exists. For example, one study experimentally manipulated self-efficacy perceptions related to managing a phobic threat and found that change in coping self-efficacy perceptions (resulting from this manipulation) was a significant predictor of immunological functioning (Wiedenfeld *et al.*, 1990). In another study, the effectiveness of a group intervention for coping with HIV depended on changes in self-efficacy, namely changes in coping self-efficacy following a 10-week intervention mediated the effects of the intervention on stress and burnout (Chesney *et al.*, 2003). Among patients with another chronic illness (multiple sclerosis), both changes in efficacy perceptions and baseline levels of efficacy were

predictive of physical and psychological improvements (Riazi *et al.*, 2004).

In conclusion, research has supported the assumption that mastery experiences in high-anxiety environments translate into an increase of coping self-efficacy perceptions across time, which, in turn, results in important positive biopsychosocial implications. However, self-efficacy beliefs do not exist suspended in a shell of a human being void of characteristic traits. Personality interacts with self-regulatory processing during times of adversity.

Personality factors, self-efficacy, and resilience

Personality traits (e.g., hardiness, internal locus of control, etc.) are often regarded as an important resource in determining coping responses to adversity. There is a link between personality traits and self-efficacy. A meta-analysis that tested the relationship between the "big five" traits (extraversion, neuroticism, agreeableness, conscientiousness, and openness) and self-efficacy demonstrated that these personality traits may explain up to 49% of self-efficacy variance (Judge & Ilies, 2002). Another meta-analysis showed that general self-efficacy (a more trait-like construct) is related to job performance and job satisfaction (average corrected correlations were 0.23 and 0.45, respectively). These results suggest that people with more resilient personalities may appraise adverse events as less stressful and may have stronger beliefs about their capabilities to cope with these events, which, in turn, affects their behaviors and well-being (i.e., a mediating model).

This mediating effect of self-efficacy related to personality, stress, and its health outcomes can be supported. For example, the effect of personality factors (self-esteem, optimism, and control) on adjustment after abortion (i.e., distress, well-being, and decision satisfaction) was mediated by pre-abortion stress appraisals and self-efficacy (Major *et al.*, 1998). Similarly, Chen *et al.* (2000) found the effect of state-like factors, such as general self-efficacy and cognitive ability, on learning performance was mediated by specific self-efficacy beliefs. Benight *et al.* (1999b) found that coping self-efficacy perceptions mediated between optimism and psychological adjustment following Hurricane Opal.

Within the workplace environment, self-efficacy (together with optimism and self-esteem) mediated the effects of job resources (e.g., autonomy and social support) on work engagement, a positive dimension of work-related well-being (Xanthopoulou *et al.*, 2007). Job-related self-efficacy fully mediated the relationship between support from the organization and work–home conflict (Erdwins *et al.*, 2001). Self-efficacy also significantly predicted psychological detachment (a positive outcome) from work during off-work hours (Sonnentag & Kruel, 2006).

These studies suggest that a multifactorial model is necessary that includes trait factors and the mechanisms that translate these characteristics into effective adaptation (i.e., effective utilization of resources in managing stressful environmental demands). Although the presented empirical evidence for a model of this type is compelling, significant challenges lie ahead for advancing our understanding of the mechanisms involved in promoting resilience.

Challenges for cognitive approaches to investigating resilience

This chapter has emphasized the role of self-efficacy cognitions in coping with adversities, a concept derived from SCT and its recent developments. A theoretical framework for future research has also been proposed (Figures 3.2 and 3.3), emphasizing the mediating role of domain-specific self-efficacy and the need for a multifactorial model. It has been argued that both demands and resources should be considered when testing the mediating effect of self-efficacy. Further, a variety of aspects of human functioning should be considered among the outcomes variables. To understand the role of cognitive resilience factors in more detail, longitudinal and experimental studies testing aspects of this dynamic model of adaptation are necessary. Only these designs will allow for testing how changes in, and levels of, critical catalyst variables promote optimal adaptation in the fact of adversities in different domains of functioning.

Although this chapter targeted the role of self-regulation cognition in understanding resilience, we acknowledge that studying other motivational processes may lead to a more comprehensive picture of factors contributing to human resilience. The influential work leading to the learned helplessness theory (Seligman, 1975), the attribution theory (Weiner, 1974), the modified attribution theory (Abramson *et al.*, 1978), and the self-determination theory (Deci & Ryan, 1985) may elucidate our understanding of

the human process of perseverance or its counterpart "giving up." More recently, Ford and Smith (2007) outlined the benefit of utilizing an integrated or unified approach to understanding optimal human functioning by including key components of motivation: goals, self-efficacy, emotions, and environmental context. However, resilience cannot be separated from self-regulatory mechanisms. It is our suggestion that resilience research would greatly benefit from multiple theoretical approaches that elucidate how critical cognitive self-regulatory processes such as self-efficacy serve as catalysts for successful managing of environmental demands and available resources.

References

Abramson, L. Y., Seligman, M. E. P., & Teasdale, J. D. (1978). Learned helplessness in humans: Critique and reformulation. *Journal of Abnormal Psychology*, **87**, 49–74.

Antonovsky, A. (1987). *Unravelling the mystery of health: How people manage stress and stay well*. San Francisco, CA: Jossey-Bass.

Bandura, A. (1997). *Self-efficacy. The exercise of control*. New York: Freeman.

Benight, C. C. & Bandura, A. (2004). Social cognitive theory of posttraumatic recovery: The role of perceived self-efficacy. *Behaviour Research and Therapy*, **42**, 1129–1148.

Benight, C. C. & Harper, M. L. (2002). Coping self-efficacy perceptions as a mediator between acute stress response and long-term distress following natural disasters. *Journal of Traumatic Stress*, **15**, 177–186.

Benight, C. C., Antoni, M. H., Kilbourn, K., & Ironson, G. (1997). Coping self-efficacy buffers psychological and physiological disturbances in HIV-infected men following a natural disaster. *Health Psychology*, **16**, 248–255.

Benight, C. C., Ironson, G., Klebe, K., *et al.* (1999a). Conservation of resources and coping self-efficacy predicting distress following a natural disaster: A causal model analysis where the environment meets the mind. *Anxiety, Stress, and Coping*, **12**, 107–126.

Benight, C. C., Swift, E., Sanger, J., Smith, A., & Zeppelin, D. (1999b). Coping self-efficacy as a prime mediator of distress following a natural disaster. *Journal of Applied Social Psychology*, **29**, 2443–2464.

Benight, C. C., Freyaldenhoven, R. W., Hughes, J., *et al.* (2000). Coping self-efficacy and psychological distress following the Oklahoma City bombing. *Journal of Applied Social Psychology*, **30**, 1331–1344.

Benight, C. C., Flores, J., & Tashiro, T. (2001). Bereavement coping self-efficacy in cancer widows. *Death Studies*, **25**, 97–125.

Benight, C. C., Harding-Taylor, A., Midboe, A. M., & Durham, R. (2004). Development and psychometric validation of a Domestic Violence Coping Self-Efficacy Measure (DV-CSE). *Journal of Traumatic Stress*, **17**, 505–508.

Benight, C. C., Cieslak, R., Molton, I. R., & Johnson, L. E. (2008). Self-evaluative appraisals of coping capability and posttraumatic distress following motor vehicle accidents. *Journal of Consulting and Clinical Psychology*, **76**, 677–685.

Bonanno, G. A. (2004). Loss, trauma, and human resilience: Have we underestimated the human capacity to thrive after extremely aversive events? *American Psychologist*, **59**, 20–28.

Brouwers, A. & Tomic, W. (2000). A longitudinal study of teacher burnout and perceived self-efficacy in classroom management. *Teaching and Teacher Education*, **16**, 239–253.

Carver, C. S. (1998). Resilience and thriving. Issues, models, and linkages. *Journal of Social Issues*, **54**, 245–266.

Carver, C. S. & Scheier, M. F. (1981). *Attention and self-regulation: A control-theory approach to human behavior*. New York: Springer.

Cervone, D. (1997). Social-cognitive mechanisms and personality coherence: Self-knowledge, situational beliefs and cross-situational coherence in perceived self-efficacy. *Psychological Science*, **8**, 43–50.

Cervone, D. (2000). Thinking about self-efficacy. *Behavior Modification*, **24**, 30–56.

Cheever, K. H. & Hardin, S. B. (1999). Effects of traumatic events, social support, and self-efficacy on adolescents' self-health assessments. *Western Journal of Nursing Research*, **21**, 673–684.

Chen, G., Gully, S. M., Whiteman, J. A., & Kilcullen, B. N. (2000). Examination of relationships among trait-like individual differences, state-like individual differences, and learning performance. *Journal of Applied Psychology*, **85**, 835–847.

Cheng, C. (2003). Cognitive and motivational processes underlying coping flexibility: A dual-process model. *Journal of Personality and Social Psychology*, **84**, 425–435.

Chesney, M. A., Chambers, D. B., Taylor, J. M., Johnson, L. M., & Folkman, S. (2003). Coping effectiveness training for men living with HIV: Results from a randomized clinical trial testing a group-based intervention. *Psychosomatic Medicine*, **65**, 1038–1046.

Cieslak, R., Benight, C. C., & Lehman, V. C. (2008). Coping self-efficacy mediates the effects of negative cognitions on traumatic distress. *Behaviour Research and Therapy*, **46**, 788–798.

Cieslak, R., Benight, C. C., Schmidt, N., *et al.* (2009). Predicting posttraumatic growth among Hurricane Katrina survivors living with HIV: the role of self-efficacy, social support, and PTSD symptoms. *Anxiety, Stress, and Coping*, **22**, 449–462.

Compeau, D. R. & Higgins, C. (1995). Computer self-efficacy: Development of a measure and initial test. *MIS Quarterly*, **19**, 189–211.

Davidson, L. M., Baum, A., & Collins, D. L. (1982). Stress and control-related problems at Three Mile Island. *Journal of Applied Social Psychology*, **12**, 349–359.

Deci, E. L. & Ryan, R. M. (1985). *Intrinsic motivation and selfdetermination in human behavior*. New York: Plenum Press.

Demerouti, E., Bakker, A. B., Nachreiner, F., & Schaufeli, W. B. (2001). The Job Demands–Resources Model of burnout. *Journal of Applied Psychology*, **86**, 499–512.

Epel, E. S., McEwen, B. S., & Ickovics, J. R. (1998). Embodying psychological thriving: Physical thriving in response to stress. *Journal of Social Issues*, **54**, 301–322.

Erdwins, C. J., Buffardi, L. C., Casper, W. J., & O' Brien, A. S. (2001). The relationship of women's role strain to social support, role satisfaction, and self-efficacy. *Family Relations*, **50**, 230–238.

Evers, W. J. G., Brouwers, A., & Tomic, W. (2002). Burnout and self-efficacy: A study on teachers' beliefs when implementing an innovative educational system in the Netherlands. *British Journal of Educational Psychology*, **72**, 227–243.

Fiori, K. L., Antonucci, T. C., & Cortina, K. S. (2006). Social network typologies and mental health among older adults. *Journal of Gerontology: Psychological Sciences*, **61B**, 25–32.

Folkman, S. & Moskowitz, J. T. (2004). Coping: Pitfalls and promise. *Annual Review of Psychology*, **55**, 745–774.

Ford, M. E. & Smith, P. R. (2007). Thriving with social purpose: An integrative approach to the development of optimal human functioning. *Educational Psychologist*, **42**, 153–171.

Frankl, V. (1962). *Man's search for meaning: An introduction to logotherapy*. Boston, MA: Beacon Press.

Gaab, J., Rohleder, N., Nater, U. M., & Ehlert, U. (2005). Psychological determinants of the cortisol stress response: The role of anticipatory cognitive appraisals. *Psychoneuroendocrinology*, **30**, 599–610.

Hobfoll, S. (1998). *Stress, culture, and community: The psychology and philosophy of stress*. New York: Plenum Press.

Hobfoll, S. E. (1989). Conservation of resources: A new attempt at conceptualizing stress. *American Psychologist*, **44**, 513–524.

Hobfoll, S. E. (2001). The influence of culture, community, and the nested-self in the process: Advancing conservation of resources theory. *Applied Psychology: An International Review*, **50**, 337–421.

House, J. S. (1981). *Work stress and social support*. Reading, MA: Addison-Wesley.

Jex, S. M. & Gudanowski, D. M. (1992). Efficacy beliefs and work stress. An exploratory study. *Journal of Organizational Behavior*, **13**, 509–517.

Johnson, J. V. & Hall, E. M. (1988). Job strain, work place social support and cardiovascular disease: A cross-sectional study of a random sample of the Swedish working population. *American Journal of Public Health*, **78**, 1336–1342.

Judge, T. A. & Ilies, R. (2002). Relationship of personality to performance motivation: A meta-analytic review. *Journal of Applied Psychology*, **87**, 797–807.

Karasek, R. (1979). Job demands, job decision latitude, and mental strain: Implications for job redesign. *Administrative Science Quarterly*, **24**, 285–308.

Karasek, R. & Theorell, T. (1990). *Healthy work*. New York: Basic Books.

Kobasa, S. Q. (1979). Stressful life events, personality, and health: An inquiry into hardiness. *Journal of Personality and Social Psychology*, **37**, 1–11.

Lazarus, R. S. (1966). *Psychological stress and the coping process*. New York: McGraw-Hill.

Lazarus, R. S. & Folkman, S. (1984). *Stress, appraisal, and coping*. New York: Springer.

Lindstrom, T. C. (1997). Immunity and health after bereavement in relation to coping. *Scandinavian Journal of Psychology*, **38**, 253–259.

Lua, H. J. (2008). The mediating role of work stress and burnout management self-efficacy in the Job Demand-Resources model. Master's thesis, Warsaw School of Social Psychology, Warsaw.

Luszczynska, A. & Schwarzer, R. (2003). Planning and self-efficacy in the adoption and maintenance of breast self-examination: A longitudinal study on self-regulatory cognitions. *Psychology and Health*, **18**, 93–108.

Luszczynska, A., Benight, C. C., & Cieslak, R. (2009). Self-efficacy, psychological, and somatic health-related outcomes of collective trauma: A systematic review. *European Psychologist* **14**, 51–62.

Luthar, S. S. Cicchetti, D., & Becker, B. (2000). The construct of resilience: A critical evaluation and guidelines for future work. *Child Development*, **71**, 543–562.

Major, B., Richards, C., Cooper, M. L., Cozzarelli, C., & Zubek, J. (1998). Personal resilience, cognitive appraisals, and coping: An integrative model of adjustment to abortion. *Journal of Personality and Social Psychology*, **74**, 735–752.

Mischel, W. & Shoda, Y. (1995). A cognitive-affective system theory of personality: Reconceptualizing situations, dispositions, dynamics, and invariance in personality structure. *Psychological Review*, **102**, 246–268.

Perrewé, P. L., Hochwarter, W. A., Rossi, A. M., *et al.* (2002). Are work stress relationships universal? A nine-region examination of role stressors, general self-efficacy, and burnout. *Journal of International Management*, **8**, 163–187.

Riazi, A., Thompson, A. J., & Hobart, J. C. (2004). Self-efficacy predicts self-reported health status in multiple sclerosis. *Multiple Sclerosis*, **10**, 61–66.

Salanova, M., Peiró, J. M., & Schaufeli, W. B. (2002). Self-efficacy specificity and burnout among information technology workers. An extension of the job demand-control model. *European Journal of Work and Organizational Psychology*, **11**, 1–25.

Schaubroeck, J. & Merritt, D. E. (1997). Divergent effects of job control on coping with work stressors: The key role of self-efficacy. *Academy of Management Journal*, **40**, 738–754.

Scheier, M. F. & Carver, C. S. (1985). Optimism, coping, and health: Assessment and implications of generalized outcome expectancies. *Health Psychology*, **4**, 219–247.

Schyns, B. & von Collani, G. (2002). A new occupational self-efficacy scale and its relation to personality constructs and organizational variables. *European Journal of Work and Organizational Psychology*, **11**, 219–241.

Seligman, M. E. P. (1975). *Helplessness: On depression, development, and death*. San Francisco, CA: Freeman.

Selye, H. (1936). A syndrome produced by diverse nocuous agents. *Nature*, **138**, 32.

Siegrist, J., Starke, D., Chandola, T., *et al.* (2004). The measurement of effort–reward imbalance at work: European comparisons. *Social Science and Medicine*, **58**, 1483–1499.

Skaalvik, E. M. & Skaalvik, S. (2007). Dimensions of teacher self-efficacy and relations with strain factors, perceived collective teacher efficacy, and teacher burnout. *Journal of Educational Psychology*, **99**, 611–625.

Solomon, Z., Weisenberg, M., Schwarzwald, J., & Mikulincer, M. (1988). Combat stress reaction and posttraumatic stress disorder as determinants of perceived self-efficacy in battle. *Journal of Social and Clinical Psychology*, **6**, 356–370.

Solomon, Z., Benbenishty, R., & Mikulincer, M. (1991). The contribution of wartime, pre-war and post-war factors to self-efficacy: A longitudinal study of combat stress reaction. *Journal of Traumatic Stress*, **4**, 345–361.

Sonnentag, S. & Kruel, U. (2006). Psychological detachment from work during off-job time: The role of job stressors, job involvement, and recovery-related self-efficacy. *European Journal of Work and Organizational Psychology*, **15**, 197–205.

Strelau, J. (1998). *Temperament: A psychological perspective*. New York: Plenum Press.

Sumer, N., Karanci, A. N., Berument, S. K., & Gunes, H. (2005). Personal resources, coping self-efficacy, and quake exposure as predictors of psychological distress following the 1999 earthquake in Turkey. *Journal of Traumatic Stress*, **18**, 331–342.

Weiner, B. (1974). *Achievement motivation and attribution theory*. Morristown, NJ: General Learning Press.

Wiedenfeld, S. A., O'Leary, A., Bandura, A., *et al.* (1990). Impact of perceived self-efficacy in coping with stressors on components of the immune system. *Journal of Personality and Social Psychology*, **59**, 1082–1094.

Xanthopoulou, D., Bakker, A. B., Demerouti, E., & Schaufeli, W. (2007). The role of personal resources in the Job Demands–Resources model. *International Journal of Stress Management*, **14**, 121–141.

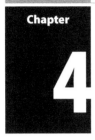

Personality factors in resilience to traumatic stress

Mark W. Miller and Kelly M. Harrington

Introduction

The study of individual differences in resilience to traumatic stress has received unprecedented attention in recent years from investigators in the field of post-traumatic stress disorder (PTSD) but there remains a lack of consensus regarding the definition, measurement, and conceptualization of the construct. Trait personality psychologists have grappled with similar issues since the seminal work of Jack Block (1961) on the construct of ego resilience over 50 years ago. In the process, they have developed comprehensive models of personality and psychometrically sophisticated tools for the measurement of its traits that can potentially inform and advance the study of resilience. The primary purpose of this chapter is to review the literature on personality factors involved in resilience to traumatic stress and to outline a model for conceptualizing this interface.

Contemporary models of personality aim to identify the structure and basis for behavioral traits – defined as individual differences in patterns of thoughts, feelings, and actions that are consistent across developmental periods and environmental contexts. Personality models differ considerably with regard to the factor structure, number, and definition of specific traits. Because of this, research on personality traits that confer risk or resilience to the development of post-traumatic psychopathology has yielded a complicated collection of studies examining disparate constructs and measures. To provide coherence and organization to this literature, this chapter will focus on three broadband personality dimensions described by Tellegen (1985, 2000) that are also represented with subtle definitional variations in most other contemporary trait models of personality. For this reason, they are known as the "big three" personality factors: positive emotionality/extraversion (PEM), negative emotionality/neuroticism (NEM), and constraint/impulsivity (CON).

Positive emotionality/extraversion refers to individual differences in the capacity to experience positive emotions and tendencies towards active involvement in the social and work environments and it is represented in other models as extraversion (Eysenck & Eysenck, 1975; Costa & McCrae, 1985). Occurrence of PEM has been linked conceptually to individual differences in sensitivity to signals of reward and to functioning of the neurobiological system underlying appetitive-approach behavior (i.e., the behavioral activation system) (Zuckerman, 1983; Gray, 1987; Panksepp, 1992), including the midbrain dopamine system (Berridge, 2003). Because of this, individuals high in PEM (extraverts) are more susceptible to the experience of positive affect than their low PEM counterparts (introverts). In line with this, trait measures of PEM/extraversion have been found to predict self-ratings of positive mood and the strength of responses to positive mood manipulations in the laboratory (Costa & McCrae, 1980; Larsen & Ketelaar, 1991; Gross & John, 1995). Low trait PEM has been shown to prospectively predict the development of major depression/dysthymia (e.g., Holohan & Moos, 1991; Verkerk et al., 2005) and is widely conceptualized as the personality vulnerability factor that distinguishes depression from anxiety (Watson et al., 1988a, 2005; Brown et al., 1998). High PEM, by comparison, is associated with higher levels of happiness and life satisfaction (Schimmack et al., 2004), greater achievement and leadership (Ross et al., 2003; Bono & Judge, 2004), and diminished risk for the development of social phobia and/or cluster C personality disorders (Jylhä et al., 2009).

Negative emotionality/neuroticism refers to dispositions toward negative mood and emotion and a tendency towards conflictual interactions with others. It is

Resilience and Mental Health: Challenges Across the Lifespan, ed. Steven M. Southwick, Brett T. Litz, Dennis Charney, and Matthew J. Friedman. Published by Cambridge University Press. © Cambridge University Press 2011.

statistically and conceptually orthogonal to PEM, synonymous with neuroticism (Eysenck & Eysenck, 1975; Costa & McCrae, 1985), and subsumes traits that relate to anxiety, alienation, and aggression. Occurrence of NEM is thought to be linked to sensitivity of the neurobiological system underlying defensive behavior (the behavioral inhibition system) (Zuckerman, 1983; Gray, 1987; Panksepp, 1992; Tellegen, 2000), including the central nucleus of the amygdala and bed nucleus of the stria terminalis (Davis & Lee, 1998; LeDoux, 2000). Theorists have reasoned that "because signals of punishment are the source of negative affect, and because neurotics are sensitive to signals of punishment, neurotics should therefore be more susceptible than stable or non-neurotic individuals to negative affect" (Larsen & Ketelaar, 1991, p. 134). Evidence for the validity of this proposition comes from multiple sources including studies showing that individuals with high NEM report more frequent and intense negative moods (e.g., Costa & McCrae, 1980) as well as heightened emotional reactivity to negative laboratory mood inductions (e.g., Larsen & Ketelaar, 1991). The trait NEM is ubiquitous in the field of personality assessment, has been represented in every major model of personality, and is conceptualized as the primary personality vulnerability for the development of a spectrum of problems variously referred to as the "internalizing" (Krueger, 1999), "distress" (Clark & Watson, 1991; Mineka et al., 1998), or "emotional" (Watson, 2005) disorders (i.e., the anxiety and depressive diagnoses in DSM-IV [American Psychiatric Association, 1994]).

Most models of personality also posit the existence of a separate disinhibition–constraint dimension – referred to here as CON – that involves tendencies anchored by planfulness versus spontaneity, restraint versus recklessness, and harm avoidance versus risk taking. The trait CON has been labeled by other theorists as psychoticism (Eysenck & Eysenck, 1975), novelty seeking (Cloninger, 1987), and impulsivity (Buss & Plomin, 1975), and it is thought to reflect individual differences in functioning of the brain regulatory system that governs behavioral restraint, including the prefrontal cortex and anterior cingulate cortex (Miller & Cohen, 2001). Numerous studies have implicated low CON as the primary personality risk factor for the development of "externalizing" or impulse control disorders, including substance-related problems, antisocial personality disorder, and attention-deficit hyperactivity disorder (Krueger, 1999; Krueger et al., 2001; Patrick & Bernat, 2006).

Additional support for the validity of these higher-order personality dimensions comes from evidence that they correspond closely to dimensions of temperament identified in studies on infancy and early childhood (Rothbart et al., 1994). Behavior genetics studies have shown them to have substantial heritabilities (e.g., heritability estimates in the 0.40–0.60 range [Tellegen et al., 1988; Robinson et al., 1992]) and scales measuring these constructs evidence long-term stability in adulthood (e.g., 6- to 12-year test–re-test reliability after age 30 on the order of 0.70–0.80 [Costa & McCrae, 1977, 1992; Watson & Walker, 1996]). Cross-cultural studies and research on the behavior of non-human primates also support the universality and evolutionary foundation of these traits (McCrae & Costa, 1997; Capitanio, 1999; Capitanio & Widaman, 2005).

Conceptual and methodological challenges

The existing body of research on personality factors involved in resilience to traumatic stress is limited by the fact that studies have focused primarily on PTSD and other measures of psychopathological adjustment as the outcome of interest, so relatively little is known about factors that may predict resilient or non-pathological outcomes. However, since the personality constructs of interest are conceptualized as bipolar dimensions, it is logical to view personality resilience factors as the polar opposites of established vulnerability factors. That is, if high NEM is identified as a PTSD vulnerability factor, then, by inference, low NEM can be conceptualized as a resilience factor. An important caveat to this assumption is that it is predicated on the notion that resilience is the absence of post-traumatic psychopathology; however, this basic definitional matter remains a source of controversy among resilience researchers (c.f. Bonanno, 2004; Agaibi & Wilson, 2005).

A number of methodological issues unique to the study of personality and resilience to traumatic stress present formidable obstacles to research in this area. Prospective longitudinal studies employing pre- and post-trauma assessments are the method of choice for studying personality and resilience because they permit examination of whether traits existed differentially between individuals with resilient versus non-resilient outcomes prior to trauma exposure. Unfortunately, obtaining an adequate sample of individuals who did not have PTSD at an initial assessment, but who developed the disorder by a second point in response to an interim event, necessitates a very large sample followed over an extended period of time, making this type of research expensive, time consuming, and rare. Because of this, some investigators have resorted to studying populations at high risk for trauma exposure (e.g., active duty military personnel [Bramsen *et al.*, 2000]), but this approach has its own limitations involving the external generalizability of study findings to other populations and the validity of baseline assessments obtained during stressful baseline (e.g., pre-deployment) intervals.

Post-trauma prospective designs in which trauma-exposed individuals are assessed shortly after trauma exposure and followed longitudinally to examine factors that affect the course of the post-traumatic adjustment (e.g., who recovers versus who develops a chronic condition) are becoming more common. Recent studies have followed trauma-exposed individuals over intervals ranging from months to years following motor vehicle accidents (e.g., Koren *et al.*, 1999; Bryant *et al.*, 2000), sexual assaults (e.g., Zoellner *et al.*, 1999), and combat (Wolfe *et al.*, 1999). The advantage of this approach is that it permits investigators to identify variables present immediately after trauma exposure that precede the onset of symptoms and/or that predict the course of the disorder. The drawback is that scores on personality measures administered post-trauma may be contaminated by transient correlates of the acute traumatic reaction and it may be impossible to differentiate phasic adjustment reactions from traits that existed prior to the trauma.

The latter issue is the primary problem with cross-sectional studies – by far the most common in the field. Personality traits measured post-trauma may reflect (1) enduring characteristics that were evident prior to the event, (2) correlates of transient stress-related symptomatology, (3) permanent alterations in personality that occur as a consequence of trauma exposure, or (4) any combination of these. Although there is substantial evidence for the longitudinal stability of personality (e.g., Costa & McCrae, 1977, 1992; Watson & Walker, 1996), trait scales are also known to be susceptible to contamination by mental health state at the time of measurement (Kerr *et al.*, 1970; Bianchi & Fergusson, 1977; Ingham *et al.*, 1986; Duncan-Jones *et al.*, 1990), and patients with anxiety and depressive disorders have been shown to respond differently to personality inventories during the experience of a disorder compared with after the remission of symptoms (Hirschfeld *et al.*, 1983; Reich *et al.*, 1986). As a result,

it is impossible to draw etiological inferences from cross-sectional studies of personality traits measured post-trauma. For this reason, the review that follows will focus primarily on studies that used pre- and post-trauma prospective designs.

Research on personality and resilience to trauma

Pre-trauma prospective studies

Table 4.1 lists prospective longitudinal studies that compared the pre-trauma personality traits of individuals who exhibited resilient versus psychopathological outcomes following exposure to a traumatic event. All of them found significant associations between characteristics linked to NEM measured prior to trauma exposure and the subsequent development of PTSD in samples ranging from combat veterans to civilians. O'Toole *et al.* (1998) examined the military records of 641 Vietnam veterans and found that those who developed combat-related PTSD scored significantly higher on a measure of neuroticism administered at the time of enlistment than those who never developed the disorder. Similarly, Bramsen *et al.* (2000) assessed 572 soldiers before and after deployment on a peacekeeping operation and found that a pre-deployment measure of NEM (i.e., negativism or "a negative, dissatisfied, and hostile attitude toward others and life in general" [Bramsen *et al.*, 2000, p. 1116]) predicted scores on a self-report measure of PTSD symptomatology post-deployment, even after statistically controlling for the severity of peacekeeping stressors, demographic variables, and other pre-morbid personality characteristics.

Studies with civilian samples have yielded similar findings. In the largest such study, 2085 participants in an Australian epidemiological survey were assessed before and after a disastrous bushfire (Parslow *et al.* 2006). Results showed that individuals who screened positive for PTSD after the fire had produced significantly higher scores on the Neuroticism Scale of the Eysenck Personality Questionnaire-Revised (Eysenck *et al.*, 1985) at the initial assessment several years before. Similarly, in a study of 81 university students exposed to a terrorist attack, Gil (2005) found that scores on the Harm Avoidance Scale (Cloninger, 1992) (which is highly [$r = 0.68$] correlated with NEM/neuroticism; e.g., Stewart *et al.*, 2005) measured two weeks before the trauma were positively associated with the presence of PTSD symptoms six months after the attack.

Table 4.1 Pre-trauma prospective studies of personality and post-traumatic adjustment.

Study	Sample	Personality assessment	PTSD assessment	Method	Findings
Bramsen et al., 2000	572 male military peacekeepers	Dutch version of the MMPI	Self-Rating Inventory for PTSD	Dutch MMPI administered prior to deployment on a peacekeeping mission; PTSD assessed less than 3 years later	Pre-deployment neuroticism and paranoia/psychotic ideation predicted post-deployment PTSD
Engelhard et al., 2003	118 women with recent pregnancy loss	Neuroticism Scale from EPQ	PSS-SR	Scale mailed within 12 weeks of pregnancy; PTSD assessed ~1 month after pregnancy loss	Pre-trauma neuroticism predicted PTSD symptoms, particularly arousal symptoms, after pregnancy loss; this relation between neuroticism and PTSD symptoms was no longer significant after controlling for pre-trauma arousal levels
Gil, 2005	81 male and female survivors of a terrorist explosion	TPQ	SCID	TPQ administered 2 weeks prior to and 1 month after a terrorist bus explosion; PTSD assessed 6 months after explosion	Pre-trauma harm avoidance (~high NEM) was positively associated with risk for PTSD; pre-trauma novelty seeking was negatively associated with risk for PTSD
Gil & Caspi, 2006	180 male and female survivors of a terrorist explosion	TPQ	SCID	TPQ administered 2 weeks prior to and 1 month after a terrorist bus explosion; PTSD assessed 6 months after explosion	Participants with PTSD scored higher on harm avoidance (~NEM) and lower on novelty seeking than participants without the disorder both before and after the terrorist attack
Lee et al., 1995	150 male veterans of World War II	Psychosomaticism Scale developed for this study	DSM-III-referenced rating and self-report measures developed for this study	Psychosomaticism assessed prior to military enlistment; PTSD assessed in 1946 and 1988	Pre-war psychosomaticism (NEM) predicted the development of PTSD in veterans exposed to low levels of combat intensity

Table 4.1 (*cont.*)

Study	Sample	Personality assessment	PTSD assessment	Method	Findings
O'Toole *et al.*, 1998	641 male Vietnam veterans	Self-description Inventory (highly correlated with Eysenck's neuroticism)	AUSCID-IV (interview derived from the SCID PTSD module)	Personality data drawn from enlistment records; PTSD assessed ~20 years after the war	Participants with combat-related PTSD scored higher than participants without the disorder on a measure of neuroticism administered at the time of entry into the service
Parslow *et al.*, 2006	2085 male and female Australian civilians	EPQ-R	TSQ	EPQ-R administered 3–4 years before the Canberra bushfires; PTSD assessed 12–82 weeks after the bushfires	Pre-trauma neuroticism predicted PTSD symptoms following the bushfires
Schnurr *et al.*, 1993	131 male Vietnam and Vietnam-era veterans	MMPI	MISS and SCID	MMPI administered prior to military enlistment; MISS and SCID collected ~20 years after the war	Pre-war scores on the MMPI Hypochondriasis, and Paranoia Scales (high NEM) as well as psychopathic deviate (low CON) predicted those who went on to develop PTSD symptoms

DSM-III, *Diagnostic and Statistical Manual of Mental Disorders*, 3rd edn (American Psychiatric Association, 1980); EPQ, Eysenck Personality Questionnaire (Eysenck & Eysenck, 1975); EPQ-R, Eysenck Personality Questionnaire-Revised (Eysenck *et al.*, 1985); MISS, Mississippi Scale for Combat-related PTSD (Keane *et al.*, 1988); MMPI, Minnesota Multiphasic Personality Inventory (Hathaway & McKinley, 1967); PSS-SR, Posttraumatic Symptom Scale self-report version (Foa *et al.*, 1993); SCID, Structured Clinical Interview for DSM (Spitzer *et al.*, 1987); TPQ, Tridimensional Personality Questionnaire (Cloninger, 1987); TSQ, Trauma Screening Questionnaire (Brewin *et al.*, 2002); CON, constraint/impulsivity; NEM, negative emotionality/neuroticism; PTSD, post-traumatic stress disorder.

Two significant limitations of these studies should be noted. First, most of them only measured a single dimension of personality so little is known about the possible direct or interactive effects of other dimensions. Second, it is plausible that the presence of pre-trauma anxiety or mood disorders at the first assessment may have contributed to the observed associations between measures of NEM and the subsequent development of PTSD.

Post-trauma prospective studies

As summarized in Table 4.2, post-trauma prospective studies suggest a possible role for not only NEM but also PEM in resilience to traumatic stress. Fauerbach *et al.* (2000) found that burn survivors characterized by elevated neuroticism and introversion at the time of hospital discharge were more likely to be diagnosed with PTSD at 4 and 12 months post-discharge. Similarly, Carlier *et al.* (1997) assessed the personality characteristics of police officers two weeks after traumatic exposure in the line of duty and found that introversion, but in this case not neuroticism, predicted the presence of PTSD symptoms three months later, even after controlling for trauma severity, emotional exhaustion during the trauma, social support, and emotional expressivity. Holeva and Tarrier (2001) reported that neuroticism scores on the Eysenck Personality Questionnaire obtained within one month of a traumatic motor vehicle accident predicted PTSD definition four to six months later, even

Table 4.2 Post-trauma prospective studies of personality and post-traumatic stress disorder.

Study	Sample	Personality assessment	PTSD assessment	Method	Personality-PTSD findings
Bennett *et al.*, 2002	89 male and female patients with recent myocardial infarction	PANAS-NA (trait)	PDS	Negative effect measured in hospital; PDS completed 3 months later	Negative effect trait at time 1 predicted PTSD symptom severity at time 2
Carlier *et al.*, 1997	262 male and female police officers	Sensation-seeking, neuroticism and, extraversion	SI-PTSD	Participants assessed 2 weeks, 3 months, and 12 months following traumatic events experienced on the job	Introversion measured 2 weeks post-trauma was a significant predictor of the presence of PTSD symptom severity at 3 months
Fauerbach *et al.*, 2000	70 male and female burn survivors	NEO-FFI	SCID	Participants completed the NEO at hospital discharge; PTSD assessed at discharge, and 4 and 12 months later	Neuroticism and introversion at time 1 predicted subsequent PTSD diagnosis
Holeva & Tarrier, 2001	265 male and female survivors of a motor vehicle accident	EPQ	Penn Inventory	EPQ was administered 2–4 weeks after the accident and PTSD was assessed 4–6 months after	Neuroticism and psychoticism at time 1 predicted PTSD symptom severity at time 2
Lawrence & Fauerbach, 2003	158 male and female burn survivors	NEO-FFI	DTS	NEO was administered during hospitalization; DTS administered at 1 and 6 months after discharge	Higher neuroticism scores at time 1 predicted PTSD diagnosis at time 2 (statistical trend); extraversion, openness, agreeableness, and conscientiousness at time 1 were not significant predictors of PTSD at time 2
McFarlane, 1992	290 male firefighters	EPQ	DIS	EPQ was completed 29 months after the fire and the DIS was administered 13 months later	Neuroticism at time 1 predicted PTSD diagnosis at time 2

Table 4.2 (cont.)

Study	Sample	Personality assessment	PTSD assessment	Method	Personality-PTSD findings
Nightingale & Williams, 2000	39 male and female survivors of a motor vehicle accident	NEO-FFI	Self-report inventory	Participants were assessed 1 and 6 weeks after the accident	Although analyses did not directly address the relationship between the NEO and PTSD, openness, extraversion, and agreeableness were shown to be associated with attitudes towards emotional expression, which, in turn, predicted PTSD symptom severity at time 2
Punamaki *et al.*, 2001	86 male and female Palestinian children exposed to political violence	Arabic translation of EPQ (Neuroticism Scale) (El Khalek, 1978)	CPTSD-RI	EPQ administered during the Intifada in 1993 (time 1) and at 3-year follow-up (time 2); CPTSD-RI administered at time 2	Higher neuroticism symptoms at time 1 predicted PTSD at 3-year follow-up; neuroticism symptoms decreased significantly from time 1 to time 2
Qouta *et al.*, 2007	65 male and female Palestinian adolescents exposed to military violence	Arabic translation of EPQ (Neuroticism Scale) (El Khalek, 1978)	CPTSD-RI	EPQ administered during the Intifada in 1993 (time 1); CPTSD-RI administered at 7-year follow-up (time 3)	Higher neuroticism at time 1 (middle childhood) predicted PTSD severity at time 3 (adolescence)
Roca *et al.*, 1992	29 male and female burn survivors	NEO-FFI	SCID	NEO was administered near the time of hospital discharge; SCID administered 4 months later	Individuals who endorsed re-experiencing symptoms at follow-up had lower openness scores at discharge

CPTSD-RI, Children's Post-traumatic Stress Disorder Reaction Index (Frederick *et al.*, 1992); DIS, DSM-III-R Diagnostic Interview Schedule (Robins *et al.*, 1989); DTS, Davidson Trauma Scale (Fontana & Rosenheck, 1994); EPQ, Eysenck Personality Questionnaire (Eysenck & Eysenck, 1975); NEO-FFI, NEO Five Factor Inventory (Costa & McCrae, 1992); PANAS-NA, Positive and Negative Affect Schedule, negative affect (Watson *et al.*, 1988b); PDS, Post-traumatic Diagnostic Scale (Foa *et al.*, 1997); SCID, Structured Clinical Interview for DSM (Spitzer *et al.*, 1987); SI-PTSD, Structured Interview for PTSD (Davidson *et al.*, 1989); PTSD, post-traumatic stress disorder.

after controlling for the influence of variables such as previous accident history, accident severity, the presence of acute stress disorder, and peritraumatic dissociation.

In one of the more sophisticated studies of this type, Lawrence and Fauerbach (2003) used structural equation modeling to examine the relationship between several predictor variables (i.e., personality measured with the NEO Five Factor Inventory [NEO-FFI; Costa & McCrae, 1992], coping strategies, social support, and chronic stress) and PTSD symptoms in a sample of male and female burn survivors. Results showed that higher neuroticism scores during hospitalization predicted greater PTSD symptoms at one month post-discharge, and avoidant coping was found to mediate roughly half of the variance of this association. Also of note, extraversion (PEM) was found to influence PTSD symptoms through indirect effects mediated by active coping and social support. Finally, in two related studies (Punamaki *et al.*, 2001; Qouta *et al.*, 2007), Palestinian children were followed prospectively after exposure to military violence. The Arabic translation of the Junior Eysenck Personality Questionnaire Neuroticism Scale (El Khalek, 1978) was administered to a group of Palestinian children during the height of the Intifada violence and PTSD symptoms were assessed at follow-up visits after three and seven years during more peaceful conditions. Results showed that higher neuroticism symptoms at baseline predicted the development of PTSD at the three-year follow-up (Punamaki *et al.*, 2001) and at the seven-year follow-up (Qouta *et al.*, 2007).

Hardiness

Although not derived from the tradition of trait personality research, an important subset of resilience studies has focused on a related construct termed *hardiness*, developed originally by Kobasa (1979). Hardiness is conceptualized as a constellation of personality characteristics that function as a resilience resource during encounters with stressful life events and it relates to how individuals perceive and cope with such events. Although it has not generally been conceptualized as a temperament-based dimension of behavior, there is a theoretical and empirical basis for relating it to PEM and NEM.

Hardiness is thought to reflect a combination of adaptive personality characteristics complemented by an early learning history characterized by rich, rewarding, and varied experiences and includes three facets: *commitment*, the sense of meaning, purpose, and perseverance attributed to one's existence; *control*, one's sense of autonomy and perceived ability to influence one's destiny and manage experiences; and *challenge,* one's tendency to perceive change as an exciting opportunity for growth. Hardy individuals tend to view potentially stressful situations as meaningful and

interesting (commitment, as opposed to alienation), appraise stressors as changeable (control, as opposed to powerlessness), and see change as a normal aspect of life and an opportunity for growth (challenge, as opposed to threat). Hardiness is thought to moderate the impact of stress on physical health, mental health, and other indices of stress adaptation and has been shown to predict (1) the physical health of men (Kobasa *et al.*, 1981) and women (Lawler & Schmied, 1992) over a five year period of time, (2) the mental health, performance, and probability of graduating from stressful military training programs (Westman, 1990; Florian *et al.*, 1995), and (3) the mental health of disaster assistance workers (Bartone *et al.*, 1989).

Many cross-sectional studies of trauma-exposed individuals have reported significant associations between hardiness and PTSD symptoms. For example, King and colleagues used structural equation modeling to analyze data from 1632 veterans collected for the National Vietnam Veterans Readjustment Study (Kulka *et al.*, 1990) in a pair of studies that examined the relative impact on the development of PTSD of hardiness, pre-war risk factors, war-zone stressors, post-war life stressors, and other post-war recovery and resilience factors. In both studies, hardiness was indexed by an 11-item scale constructed from the Readjustment Study's interview items. The structural equation model in the first study (King *et al.*, 1998) revealed evidence of a direct negative association between hardiness and PTSD symptom severity as well as an indirect effect of hardiness on PTSD mediated by social support. In other words, hardy individuals showed less-severe PTSD and were more likely to effectively utilize support from others, which, in itself, was associated with lower PTSD severity. Similar results were observed in a second study using a different combination of predictor variables (King *et al.*, 1999). Other work suggests that the influence of hardiness may be conditional on the severity of trauma exposure. For example, Bartone (1999) assessed hardiness, combat exposure, and PTSD symptoms in Gulf War veterans shortly after the war. Multiple regression analyses were used to predict PTSD severity, revealing a main effect of hardiness and a significant interaction between hardiness and combat exposure. These results indicated that highly hardy veterans were less symptomatic than those with low hardiness overall, and this difference was more pronounced for individuals reporting the highest levels of combat exposure.

Several recent studies have employed more informative longitudinal designs to study the influence of hardiness on the adaptation to stress. For example, Adler and Dolan (2006) assessed deployment stressors, hardiness, and depression in a large sample of military peacekeepers during and after deployment to a crisis in Kosovo. As in Bartone's (1999) study, analyses showed that hardiness moderated the influence of deployment-related stress on depression symptoms, with these effects evident only for soldiers exposed to high levels of deployment stress. Only one published study has measured hardiness at more than one time point, which is useful because it permits examination of the stability of the construct. Vogt *et al.* (2008) assessed US marine recruits at the beginning and end of basic training and found that men who were hardier at time 1 reported lower stress reactions at time 2, while men who reported more stress reactions at time 1 were less hardy at time 2, which points to the malleability of the construct.

Relating hardiness to the big three personality dimensions

Investigators who have examined the relationship between hardiness and trait measures of omnibus personality inventories have suggested that hardiness represents the inverse of NEM (Funk & Houston, 1987; Rhodewalt & Zone, 1989; Funk, 1992), or a combination of low NEM and high PEM (Parkes & Rendall, 1988). Evidence for the latter comes from several sources. For example, Maddi and colleagues (2002) investigated the construct validity of the Hardiness Scale by examining its relationship to the Minnesota Multiphasic Personality Inventory-2 (MMPI-2) and the NEO-FFI and found negative correlations greater than 0.6 between hardiness and several MMPI-2 scales including the Infrequency (F), Social Introversion (Si), Posttraumatic Stress (PK), Low Self-esteem (LSE), and Welsh Anxiety Scales (A; Maddi *et al.*, 2002). This study also found that the NEO Neuroticism and Extraversion Scales were correlated with total hardiness at levels of −0.46 and +0.47, respectively, and similar results have been reported by other investigators (Parkes & Rendall, 1988; Ramanaiah *et al.*, 1999). Other work has shown that the relationship between hardiness and health outcomes disappears when measures of NEM are removed (Funk & Houston, 1987; Rhodewalt & Zone, 1989). These findings suggest collectively that individuals who obtain low scores on hardiness tend to feel alienated from themselves and others, powerless, and in need of security – characteristics that are strongly associated with NEM and general measures of maladjustment. Further research is needed to specifically address the extent to which measures of hardiness provide incremental validity beyond personality traits (or vise versa) in predicting post-traumatic adjustment.

A conceptual model for the interface between personality and post-traumatic adjustment

This chapter has examined the literature on personality factors involved in resilience to traumatic stress. Studies have been discussed in relation to the "big three" dimensions of personality – PEM, NEM, and CON – that are represented in most contemporary trait models of personality. Numerous studies support the conclusion that NEM/neuroticism is the primary personality risk/resilience factor influencing post-traumatic adjustment. Individuals high in NEM describe themselves as nervous, tense, and easily upset. They are prone to worry, report feeling vulnerable and sensitive, and experience negative emotional states such as anger, distress, and guilt at a high frequency and intensity even under everyday life conditions. On the other end of the spectrum, individuals low in NEM describe themselves as emotionally stable, rarely nervous or anxious, and with the capacity to remain calm in stressful situations and to recover quickly from negative experiences. When these characteristics are combined with a disposition to be cheerful and enthusiastic, take pleasure in and value close interpersonal ties, and to be assertive, hardworking, and influential (i.e., high PEM), the profile that emerges is that of an individual who is highly resilient to stress, loss, adversity, trauma, and the development of post-traumatic psychopathology.

Figure 4.1 illustrates the big three dimensions of personality and their hypothesized relations with resilience versus vulnerability to the development of post-traumatic psychopathology. All three form the foundation of the model. The median of each dimension is located in the center of the figure; high and low extremes on each dimension are toward the periphery of the figure. Characteristics associated with vulnerability to the development of psychopathology are located in the upper (i.e., high NEM) part of the figure, while factors associated with resilience are in the lower

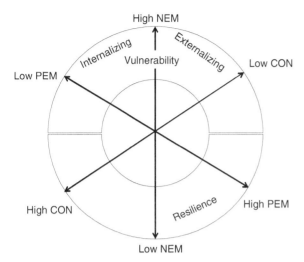

Figure 4.1 The hypothesized interactive model of relationships between the "big three" dimensions of personality and resilience versus vulnerability to the development of post-traumatic psychopathology. NEM, negative emotionality; PEM, positive emotionality; CON, constraint/impulsivity.

part. While NEM is viewed as the primary personality risk/resilience factor for post-traumatic psychopathology, low PEM and low CON are conceptualized as *moderating* factors that influence the form and expression of the post-traumatic adaptation (c.f. Miller, 2003, 2004). Individuals characterized prior to trauma by high NEM combined with low PEM are thought to be predisposed towards an *internalizing* form of post-traumatic response, characterized by marked anhedonia, depression, and social withdrawal. In contrast, pre-morbid high NEM combined with low CON is expected to predict an *externalizing* form of post-traumatic response, characterized by tendencies towards impulsivity, aggression, antisociality, substance-related disorders, and higher rates of the "dramatic–emotional" Cluster B personality disorders.

Results from a recent series of cluster-analytic studies of personality profiles of combat veterans and sexual assault survivors provide preliminary support for these propositions (Miller *et al.*, 2003, 2004; Miller & Resick, 2007). In each of these studies, cluster analyses of personality profiles of individuals with PTSD yielded evidence for a three-group typology. The first subgroup was a lower pathology or "simple PTSD" cluster comprising individuals with less-severe PTSD symptoms, low levels of co-morbidity, and normal-range personality profiles compared with individuals in the other two clusters. The other two more pathological or "complex PTSD" clusters differed on variables related to externalizing

versus internalizing co-morbidity (c.f. Krueger *et al.*, 1998). Across these studies, externalizers produced personality profiles defined by low CON coupled with high NEM. Individuals in this subgroup were characterized by the tendency to express post-traumatic distress outwardly through antagonistic interactions with others and behavior that conflicts with societal norms and values. They endorsed elevated levels of anger and aggression, substance-related disorders, and DSM-IV Cluster B personality disorder features. In contrast, internalizers were characterized by personality profiles defined by high NEM combined with low PEM and tendencies to direct their post-traumatic distress inwardly through shame, self-defeating/deprecating and anxious processes, avoidance, depression, and withdrawal. Individuals of this type were characterized by high rates of co-morbid major depression and panic disorder, and schizoid and avoidant personality disorder features. Although etiological inferences about the extent to which these subtypes reflect the influence of pre-morbid personality were limited by the cross-sectional methods employed in these studies, evidence for the longitudinal stability of personality traits in other research (e.g., Costa & McCrae, 1977, 1992; Watson & Walker, 1996) and indications of greater pre-military delinquency in the externalizing group in two of the studies (Miller *et al.*, 2003, 2004) are consistent with the notion that these subtypes reflect the influence of pre-morbid traits on the expression of post-traumatic symptomatology.

It is also possible, however, that these subtypes represent the manifestation of personality traits that were altered as a consequence of the development of PTSD. Successful personality development requires learning to inhibit pathological dispositional tendencies, including dispositions towards the internalization versus externalization of distress. For the individual with elevated trait NEM, this necessitates developing the capacity to regulate and inhibit the expression of intense negative affectivity. We hypothesize that under periods of intense stress, and during the experience of PTSD, these normal self-regulatory processes are compromised. This results in an unrestrained system driven by basic dispositional tendencies and impaired in the ability to adjust effectively to ongoing social and environmental demands. Individuals with a disposition towards internalization (i.e., low PEM combined with high NEM) resort to withdrawing from the world through social avoidance and passivity, and their post-traumatic adjustment is characterized by negative self-referential or ruminative thoughts, guilt, anxiety, and depression. In contrast, individuals with a propensity towards externalizing behaviors (i.e., low CON combined with high NEM) move against the world becoming at odds with others through antisocial behavior, antagonism, hostility, and aggression.

Consistent with this alternative hypothesis, prior theorists have conjectured that personality traits are most influential and evident in circumstances involving stress and significant life re-adjustment (Caspi & Bem, 1990). Prior studies have shown that the negative traits of irritable and explosive men were intensified during the severe economic stress of the Great Depression (Elder & Caspi, 1988), and the coping styles of entrepreneurs whose businesses were destroyed by natural disaster were accentuated during the aftermath (Anderson, 1977). Similarly, Allport *et al.* (1941), who studied the experiences of individuals during the Nazi revolution, concluded (pp. 7–8) that "very rarely does catastrophic… change produce catastrophic alterations in personality… Where change does take place it seems invariably to accentuate trends clearly present in the pre-[trauma] personality."

High positive emotionality/extraversion and resilience

The orientation of Figure 4.1 emphasizes low NEM as the primary personality resilience factor, but what role might high PEM play in also conferring resilience to traumatic stress? In the model proposed by Tellegen (1985, 2000), PEM is composed of four traits. The first two are associated with communal positive emotionality: *well-being*, the tendency to be optimistic, hopeful, cheerful, and interested and engaged in one's activities; and *social closeness*, the disposition toward social communion and interpersonal connectedness. Individuals with high levels of these traits attract and maintain close relationships with family, friends, and coworkers, and they experience greater perceived social support. This, in turn, has been shown repeatedly to be one of the most robust psychosocial moderators of post-traumatic adjustment (Connell & D'Augelli, 1990; King *et al.*, 1998; Lawrence & Fauerbach, 2003).

Tellegen's two other PEM traits involve tendencies towards agency and efficacy in the social and work domains (i.e., agentic positive emotionality): *social potency* is the tendency towards being persuasive, influential, enjoying social visibility, and being in charge; *achievement* relates to being ambitious, persistent, enjoying challenging tasks, and working

hard. When these traits co-occur with low NEM the result is a combination of characteristics that resemble both hardiness and a related construct termed *mental toughness* (Clough *et al.*, 2002). Clough and colleagues (sports psychologists) developed the construct of mental toughness to capture the personality attributes of elite athletes, who tend to be social and outgoing, calm and relaxed, with low anxiety and "an unshakeable faith that they control their own destiny" (Clough *et al.*, 2002, p. 38). Mental toughness has been shown to predict physical endurance (Crust & Clough, 2005) and achievement in professional sports (Golby & Sheard, 2004). Like hardiness, mental toughness is highly correlated with neuroticism and extraversion ($r = -0.64$, 0.45, respectively [Horsburgh *et al.*, 2009]). Not surprisingly, these traits are also the personality characteristics selected for in elite military units (e.g., US Navy SEALS [Braun *et al.*, 1994]) and have been found to predict leadership across a wide range of military and other professional settings (for a comprehensive review, see Judge *et al.* [2002]). Finally, analyses in the study of Horsburgh *et al.* (2009), which compared the similarity of mono- and dizygotic twins on a measure of mental toughness, showed that 52% of variability in this trait could be attributed to genetic effects, underscoring the role of temperament and constitutional factors in the etiology of resilience-related traits. These findings also beg the question, what are the mechanisms by which these genetic effects confer risk/resilience to the development of post-traumatic psychopathology? Findings from three extant areas of research – conditionability, coping style, and social support – provide possible answers to this question and are reviewed below.

Mediators of the link between personality and resilience

Conditionability

Low NEM has been conceptualized as a relative insensitivity of the neurobiological system underlying defensive behavior (the behavioral inhibition system [Gray, 1987], see also Zuckerman, 1983; Panksepp, 1992; Tellegen, 2000) and evidence points to the central nucleus of the amygdala and bed nucleus of the stria terminalis as integral components of this system (Davis & Lee, 1998; LeDoux, 2000). One manifestation of variation in functioning of this system is individual differences in *conditionability* – individuals who are most susceptible to aversive conditioning may be predisposed to acquire the intense and persistent conditioned emotional responses that are central to the psychopathology of PTSD (Keane *et al.*, 1985; Foa *et al.*, 1989). Evidence in support of this hypothesis comes from many sources. First, aversive conditioning and the acquisition of punishment expectancies has been shown to be enhanced in individuals high in trait anxiety (i.e., NEM) (Spence & Taylor, 1951; Spence & Farber, 1953; Spence & Beecroft, 1954; Spence *et al.*, 1954; Zinbarg & Mohlman, 1998) and introversion (i.e., low PEM) (Franks, 1957; Shagass & Kerenyi, 1958; Costello, 1967; Mangan, 1967; Kantorowitz, 1978; Paisey & Mangan, 1988; Gupta & Shukla, 1989; Weyer, 1989). Second, by definition, high NEM is associated with enhanced reactions to negative affect-evoking situations, which, in turn, facilitates conditioning. For example, high NEM has been shown to be associated with greater nervousness/negative affectivity during stressful laboratory procedures (e.g., Carver & White, 1994; Miller & Patrick, 2000) and enhanced acoustic startle reflex potentiation (an index of defensive emotional responding) during processing of threatening stimuli when compared with subjects with low NEM (Wilson *et al.*, 2000; Craske *et al.*, 2009). Finally, to the extent that individual differences in conditionability reflect an enduring characteristic, evidence that patients with PTSD are more conditionable than trauma-exposed individuals without the disorder (Orr *et al.*, 2000) would also support this hypothesis.

Coping style

Another mechanism by which personality can translate into resilience to traumatic stress is via coping style. Coping has been defined as the cognitions and behaviors that a person uses to reduce stress (Billings *et al.*, 1983; Folkman, 1984) and habitual coping strategies are believed to moderate the impact of stressful life events on functioning (Pearlin & Schooler, 1978; Billings & Moos, 1981). Although coping is conceptualized as a process that varies as a function of contextual demands, there is also evidence that coping styles tend to be consistent over time and predicted by personality traits (McCrae & Costa, 1986; Volrath *et al.*, 1995).

Many investigators have distinguished between *problem-focused* or *approach coping* (the channeling of resources to solving the stress creating problem), *emotion-focused coping* (the easing of tension though denial or changing one's attitude towards it), and

avoidance coping (behaviors or emotions that avoid or ignore the source of the stress) (Folkman & Lazarus, 1980; Folkman, 1984; Herman-Stahl *et al.*, 1995). Individuals high in NEM (or with the high NEM/low PEM combination) have been found to be more likely to utilize the latter two, less adaptive, forms of coping and are less likely to employ problem-focused/approach coping strategies (e.g., McCrae & Costa, 1986; Parkes, 1986; Bolger, 1990; Endler & Parker, 1990; Gomez *et al.*, 1999; Volrath & Torgersen, 2000).

Investigators have also identified a link between dysfunctional coping and the development and/or maintenance of PTSD. For example, in one longitudinal study of combat-exposed Israeli soldiers, Solomon *et al.* (1988) showed that PTSD symptomatology was predicted by the over-utilization of emotion-focused coping and underutilization of problem-focused coping strategies. Along the same lines, Morgan *et al.* (1995) found that neuroticism (NEM) was positively associated with use of emotion-focused coping strategies and that both predicted PTSD severity in a sample of civilian flood survivors. Similar findings have been observed in other samples of civilians (Amir *et al.*, 1997) and combat veterans (Nezu & Carnevale, 1987; Blake *et al.*, 1992) with PTSD. The implication of these findings is that individuals with high NEM who experience a traumatic event may have a stronger disposition towards avoidance of trauma-related stimuli than others. As a result, they would be expected to have fewer opportunities to experience the benefits of exposure to corrective information (Foa & Kozak, 1986) and other cognitive–affective processing of the traumatic experience that is believed to be essential for positive post-traumatic adjustment.

Social support

Other research suggests that social support plays a key role in mitigating the negative effects of stress on mental health (e.g., Cohen & Wills, 1985). Low PEM and high NEM have both been associated with low scores on measures of social support (e.g., Bolger & Eckenrode, 1991; Morgan *et al.*, 1995; Lara *et al.*, 1997; Caspi, 2000) and evidence suggests that each characteristic may be associated with a unique form of social impairment. Specifically, investigators have suggested that PEM, but not NEM, is associated with measures of actual number of social contacts (Bolger & Eckenrode, 1991), whereas high NEM relates to a tendency to underestimate the amount of social support that is available (Stokes & McKirnan, 1989) and is associated with a propensity to experience conflict with members of the social network (Caspi, 2000).

Research on psychosocial factors that contribute to the development of PTSD has shown that social support buffers the adverse psychological effects of stressful life events in combat veterans (Stretch, 1985, 1986) and sexual assault survivors (e.g., Ruch & Leon, 1983; Popiel & Susskind, 1985; Golding *et al.*, 1989). Conversely, inadequate social support has been implicated in the etiology of delayed-onset PTSD (Buckley *et al.*, 1996). Impaired social support is known to co-occur with PTSD (Kulka *et al.*, 1990; Boscarino, 1995; King *et al.*, 1998) and a meta-analysis of 14 separate risk factors for PTSD showed that lack of social support was second only to trauma severity in the proportion of variance accounted for in predicting concurrent PTSD symptomatology (Brewin *et al.*, 2000). Consequently, social support may represent a third mechanism by which these personality characteristics translate into risk versus resilience to the development of PTSD following trauma exposure.

Conclusions and future directions

Although this chapter has focused primarily on the influence of personality factors it is important to recognize that post-traumatic adaptations reflect the confluence of an array of environmental and individual difference factors and that personality traits account for only a portion of the variance in any outcome. One crucial etiological factor is the nature and severity of the trauma exposure, and in future work it will be important to develop models that better account for the interaction between personality and trauma intensity. In such work, it may be useful to draw from the models of diathesis–stress influences in depression outlined by Monroe and Simons (1991) and to examine whether the personality–trauma interaction is best represented by an additive or interactive model. In an additive model, trauma severity and the loading of the personality trait (i.e., the diathesis) summate to determine the probability of developing PTSD. Two independent effects are postulated: (1) the likelihood of PTSD increases with the severity of the trauma, and (2) the probability of developing the disorder increases as a function of the vulnerability. In this model individuals with a low diathetic loading (e.g., low NEM) would require more extreme levels of stress to achieve the same likelihood of developing the disorder as someone with higher levels of the diathesis, and vice versa.

Alternatively, in an interactive model, personality traits would interact with the stressor to determine the probability of developing PTSD such that at certain levels of trauma intensity vulnerable individuals would be at disproportionately high risk for the disorder. Figure 4.2 depicts such a model. At low levels of NEM, PTSD is unlikely to occur in response to even high levels of trauma severity. However, with high NEM, individuals are at high risk for the development of the disorder across levels of trauma intensity. The slopes of

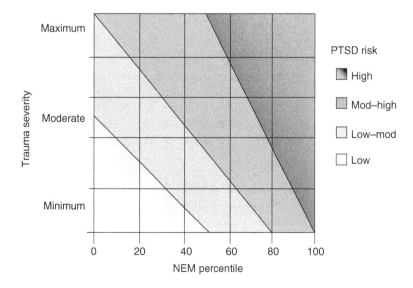

Figure 4.2 An interactive model of the relationship between negative emotionality (NEM) and the intensity of a traumatic stressor. PTSD, post-traumatic stress disorder; Mod, moderate.

the demarcation lines diverge across increasing levels of the *x*-axis indicating a synergistic, as opposed to additive, relationship between the variables. Individual differences in the response to trauma are most apparent at low levels of stress. Extreme levels of stress place virtually anyone at a moderate-high or high risk for PTSD, regardless of what temperamental resources exist. At the lowest levels of traumatic stress, however, there is a much wider range in the probability of developing PTSD.

At this early stage in the development of research in this area, it is unclear whether personality trait differences in resilience are more likely to be observed in response to low or high levels of stress. Some investigators have suggested that individual characteristics can be expected to play a greater role in influencing the nature and severity of stress reaction under conditions of lower stress intensity (e.g., Rabkin & Struening, 1976; Foy *et al.*, 1987; McCranie *et al.*, 1992; Lee *et al.*, 1995) and that extreme degrees of stress should produce symptoms of psychiatric disability in virtually all who are exposed to them (Hocking, 1970). Others have suggested that the influence of individual differences on the development of PTSD may be more pronounced at high levels of stress exposure (e.g., Bartone, 1999; Casella & Motta, 1990). Clearly more work is needed in this area to test these alternative hypotheses.

Evidence that certain combinations of personality traits (i.e., high PEM with low NEM) may be most reliably linked to resilience underscores the importance of moving beyond single-scale assessments of individual traits towards more comprehensive multidimensional assessments of personality. It would also be beneficial for investigators interested in constructs such as conditionability, coping, and social support to examine the extent to which these behaviors reflect the influence of higher-order personality traits and to attempt to relate these more specific constructs to a broader understanding of individuals' personality functioning across social, cognitive, affective, and biological levels of analysis.

Acknowledgement

This work was supported in part by a VA Merit Review Award to Dr. Miller.

References

Adler, A. B. & Dolan, C. A. (2006). Military hardiness as a buffer of psychological health on return from deployment. *Military Medicine*, **171**, 93–98.

Agaibi, C. E. & Wilson, J. P. (2005). Trauma, PTSD, and resilience. *Trauma, Violence, and Abuse*, **6**, 195–216.

Allport, G. W., Bruner, J. S., & Jandorf, E. M. (1941). Personality under social catastrophe: Ninety life-histories of the Nazi revolution. *Character and Personality: A Quarterly for Psychodiagnostic and Allied Studies*, **10**, 1–22.

American Psychiatric Association (1980). *Diagnostic and statistical manual of mental disorders,* 3rd edn. Washington, DC: American Psychiatric Press.

American Psychiatric Association (1994). *Diagnostic and statistical manual of mental disorders,* 4th edn. Washington, DC: American Psychiatric Press.

Amir, M., Kaplan, Z., Efroni, R., *et al.* (1997). Coping styles in post-traumatic stress disorder (PTSD) patients. *Personality and Individual Differences*, **23**, 399–405.

Anderson, C. R. (1977). Locus of control, coping behaviors, and performance in a stress setting: A longitudinal study. *Journal of Applied Psychology*, **62**, 446–451.

Bartone, P. T. (1999). Hardiness protects against war-related stress in army reserve forces. *Consulting Psychology Journal: Practice and Research*, **51**, 72–82.

Bartone, P. T., Ursano, R. J., Wright, K. M., & Ingraham, L. H. (1989). The impact of a military air disaster on the health of assistance workers: A prospective study. *Journal of Nervous and Mental Disease*, **177**, 317–328.

Bennett, P., Owen, R. L., Koutsakis, S., & Bisson, J. (2002). Personality, social context and cognitive predictors of post-traumatic stress disorder in myocardial infarction patients. *Psychology and Health*, **17**, 489–500.

Berridge, K. C. (2003). Pleasures of the brain. *Brain and Cognition*, **52**, 106–128.

Bianchi, G. N. & Fergusson, D. M. (1977). Short term mental state and scores on the Eysenck Personality Inventory. *British Journal of Psychiatry*, **131**, 306–309.

Billings, A. G. & Moos, R. H. (1981). The role of coping responses and social resources in attenuating the stress of life events. *Journal of Behavioral Medicine*, **4**, 139–157.

Billings, A. G., Cronkite, R. C., & Moos, R. H. (1983). Social-environmental factors in unipolar depression: Comparisons of depressed patients and nondepressed controls. *Journal of Abnormal Psychology*, **92**, 119–133.

Blake, D. D., Cook, J. D., & Keane, T. M. (1992). Post-traumatic stress disorder and coping in veterans who are seeking medical treatment. *Journal of Clinical Psychology*, **48**, 695–704.

Block, J. (1961). Ego identity, role variability, and adjustment. *Journal of Consulting Psychology*, **25**, 392–397.

Bolger, N. (1990). Coping as a personality process: A prospective study. *Journal of Personality and Social Psychology*, **59**, 525–537.

Bolger, N. & Eckenrode, J. (1991). Social relationships, personality, and anxiety during a major stressful event. *Journal of Personality and Social Psychology*, **61**, 440–449.

Bonanno, G. A. (2004). Loss, trauma, and human resilience: Have we underestimated the human capacity to thrive after extremely aversive events?. *American Psychologist*, **59**, 20–28.

Bono, J. E. & Judge, T. A. (2004). Personality and transformational and transactional leadership: A meta-analysis. *Journal of Applied Psychology*, **89**, 901–910.

Boscarino, J. A. (1995). Post-traumatic stress and associated disorders among Vietnam veterans: The significance of combat exposure and social support. *Journal of Traumatic Stress*, **8**, 317–336.

Bramsen, I., Dirkzwager, A. J. E., & van der Ploeg, H. M. (2000). Predeployment personality traits and exposure to trauma as predictors of posttraumatic stress symptoms: A prospective study of former peacekeepers. *American Journal of Psychiatry*, **157**, 1115–1119.

Braun, D. E., Prusaczyk, W. K., Goforth, H. W., & Pratt, N. C. (1994). *Personality profiles of US Navy sea–air–land (SEAL) personnel.* [US Naval Health Research Center Technical Report NHRC 94-8.] San Diego, CA: US Naval Health Research Center.

Brewin, C. R., Andrews, B., & Valentine, J. D. (2000). Meta-analysis of risk factors for posttraumatic stress disorder in trauma-exposed individuals. *Journal of Consulting and Clinical Psychology*, **68**, 748–766.

Brewin, C. R., Rose, S., Andrews, B., *et al.* (2002). Brief screening instrument for post-traumatic stress disorder. *British Journal of Psychiatry*, **181**, 158–162.

Brown, T. A., Chorpita, B. F., & Barlow, D. H. (1998). Structural relationships among dimensions of the DSM-IV anxiety and mood disorders and dimensions of negative affect, positive affect, and autonomic arousal. *Journal of Abnormal Psychology*, **107**, 179–192.

Bryant, R. A., Harvey, A. G., Guthrie, R. M., & Moulds, M. L. (2000). A prospective study of psychophysiological arousal, acute stress disorder, and posttraumatic stress disorder. *Journal of Abnormal Psychology*, **109**, 341–344.

Buckley, T. C., Blanchard, E. B., & Hickling, E. J. (1996). A prospective examination of delayed onset PTSD secondary to motor vehicle accidents. *Journal of Abnormal Psychology*, **105**, 617–625.

Buss, A. H. & Plomin, R. (1975). *A temperament theory of personality development.* New York: Wiley.

Capitanio, J. P. (1999). Personality dimensions in adult male rhesus macaques: Prediction of behaviors across time and situation. *American Journal of Primatology*, **47**, 299–320.

Capitanio, J. P. & Widaman, K. F. (2005). Confirmatory factor analysis of personality structure in adult male rhesus monkeys (*Macaca mulatta*). *American Journal of Primatology*, **65**, 289–294.

Carlier, I. V. E., Lamberts, R. D., & Gersons, B. P. R. (1997). Risk factors for posttraumatic stress symptomatology in police officers: A prospective analysis. *Journal of Nervous and Mental Disease*, **185**, 498–506.

Carver, C. S. & White, T. L. (1994). Behavioral inhibition, behavioral activation, and affective responses to impending reward and punishment: The BIS/BAS scales. *Journal of Personality and Social Psychology*, **67**, 319–333.

Casella, L. & Motta, R. W. (1990). Comparison of characteristics of Vietnam veterans with and without posttraumatic stress disorder. *Psychological Reports*, **67**, 595–605.

Caspi, A. (2000). The child is father of the man: Personality continuities from childhood to adulthood. *Journal of Personality and Social Psychology*, **78**, 158–172.

Caspi, A. & Bem, D. J. (1990). Personality continuity and change across the life course. In L. A. Pervin (ed.), *Handbook of personality: Theory and research* (pp. 549–575). New York: Guilford Press.

Clark, L. A. & Watson, D. (1991). Tripartite model of anxiety and depression: Psychometric evidence and taxonomic implications. *Journal of Abnormal Psychology*, **100**, 316–336.

Cloninger, C. R. (1987). A systematic method for clinical description and classification of personality traits. *Archives of General Psychiatry*, **44**, 573–588.

Cloninger, C. R. (1992). *The Temperament and Character Inventory.* (Available from C. R. Cloninger, Washington University School of Medicine, Department of Psychiatry, PO Box 8134, St. Louis, MO, 63110, USA.)

Clough, P. J., Earle, K., & Sewell, D. (2002). Mental toughness: The concept and its measurement. In I. Cockerill (ed.), *Solutions in sport psychology* (pp. 32–45). London: Thomson.

Cohen, S. & Wills, T. A. (1985). Stress, social support, and the buffering hypothesis. *Psychological Bulletin*, **98**, 310–357.

Connell, C. M. & D'Augelli, A. R. (1990). The contribution of personality characteristics to the relationship between social support and perceived physical health. *Health Psychology*, **9**, 192–207.

Costa, P. T. & McCrae, R. R. (1977). Age differences in personality structure revisited: Studies in validity, stability, and change. *Aging and Human Development*, **8**, 261–275.

Costa, P. T. & McCrae, R. R. (1980). Influence of extraversion and neuroticism on subjective well-being: Happy and unhappy people. *Journal of Personality and Social Psychology*, **38**, 668–678.

Costa, P. T. & McCrae, R. R. (1985). *The NEO Personality Inventory Manual.* Odessa, Fl: Psychological Assessment Resources.

Costa, P. T. & McCrae, R. R. (1992). Trait psychology comes of age. In T. B. Sonderegger (ed.), *Nebraska symposium on motivation 1991: Psychology and aging. Current theory and research in motivation, 39* (pp. 169–204). Lincoln, NE: University of Nebraska Press.

Costello, C. G. (1967). Extraversion, neuroticism, and the classical conditioning of word meaning. *Psychonomic Science*, **8**, 307–308.

Craske, M. G., Waters, A. M., Nazarian, M., *et al.* (2009). Does neuroticism in adolescents moderate contextual and explicit threat cue modulation of the startle reflex? *Biological Psychiatry*, **65**, 220–226.

Crust, L. & Clough, P. J. (2005). Relationship between mental toughness and physical endurance. *Perceptual and Motor Skills*, **100**, 192–194.

Davidson, J. T. R., Smith, R., & Kudler, H. S. (1989). Validity and reliability of the DSM-III criteria for post-traumatic stress disorder: Experience with a structured interview. *Journal of Nervous and Mental Disease*, **177**, 336–341.

Davis, M. & Lee, Y. (1998). Fear and anxiety: Possible roles of the amygdala and bed nucleus of the stria terminalis. *Cognition and Emotion*, **12**, 277–305.

Duncan-Jones, P., Fergusson, D. M., Ormel, J., & Horwood, L. J. (1990). A model of stability and change in minor psychiatric symptoms: Results from three longitudinal studies. *Psychological Medicine, Monograph Supplement* **18**, iii–28.

Elder, G. H. & Caspi, A. (1988). Economic stress in lives: Developmental perspectives. *Journal of Social Issues*, **44**, 25–45.

El Khalek, A. S. B. G. (1978). *Eysenck personality inventories.* [In Arabic.] Alexandria: Dar El Maaref.

Endler, N. S. & Parker, J. D. A. (1990). Multidimensional assessment of coping: A critical evaluation. *Journal of Personality and Social Psychology*, **58**, 844–854.

Engelhard, I. M., van den Hout, M. A., & Kindt, M. (2003). The relationship between neuroticism, pre-traumatic stress, and post-traumatic stress: A prospective study. *Personality and Individual Differences*, **35**, 381–388.

Eysenck, H. J. & Eysenck, S. B. G. (1975). *Eysenck Personality Questionnaire manual.* San Diego, CA: Educational and Industrial Testing Service.

Eysenck, S. B. G., Eysenck, H. J., & Barratt, P. (1985). A revised version of the psychoticism scale. *Personality and Individual Differences*, **6**, 21–29.

Fauerbach, J. A., Lawrence, J. W., Schmidt, C. W., Munster, A. M., & Costa, P. T. (2000). Personality predictors of injury-related posttraumatic stress disorder. *Journal of Nervous and Mental Disease*, **188**, 510–517.

Florian, V., Mikulincer, M., & Taubman, O. (1995). Does hardiness contribute to mental health during a stressful real-life situation? The roles of appraisal and coping. *Journal of Personality and Social Psychology*, **68**, 687–695.

Foa, E. B. & Kozak, M. J. (1986). Emotional processing of fear: Exposure to corrective information. *Psychological Bulletin*, **99**, 20–35.

Foa, E. B., Steketee, G., & Rothbaum, B. O. (1989). Behavioral/cognitive conceptualizations of post-traumatic stress disorder. *Behavior Therapy*, **20**, 155–176.

Foa, E. B., Riggs, D. S., Dancu, C. V., & Rothbaum, B. O. (1993). Reliability and validity of a brief instrument for assessing post-traumatic stress disorder. *Journal of Traumatic Stress*, **6**, 459–473.

Foa, E., Cashman, L., Jaycox, L., & Perry, K. (1997). The validation of a self-report measure of post-traumatic stress disorder: The Posttraumatic Diagnostic Scale. *Psychological Assessment*, **9**, 445–451.

Folkman, S. (1984). Personal control and stress and coping processes: A theoretical analysis. *Journal of Personality and Social Psychology*, **46**, 839–852.

Folkman, S. & Lazarus, R. S. (1980). An analysis of coping in a middle-aged community sample. *Journal of Health and Social Behavior*, **21**, 219–239.

Fontana, A. & Rosenheck, R. (1994). Posttraumatic stress disorder among Vietnam theater veterans: A causal model of etiology in a community sample. *Journal of Nervous and Mental Disease*, **182**, 677–684.

Foy, D. W., Resnick, H. S., Sipprelle, R. C., & Carroll, E. M. (1987). Premilitary, military, and postmilitary factors in the development of combat-related posttraumatic stress disorder. *Behavior Therapist*, **10**, 3–9.

Franks, C. M. (1957). Personality factors and the rate of conditioning. *British Journal of Psychology*, **48**, 119–126.

Frederick, C., Pynoos, R. S., & Nader, K. (1992). *Child Post-Traumatic Stress Disorder Reaction Index (CPTSD-RI).* Los Angeles, CA: University of California at Los Angeles Department of Psychiatry.

Funk, S. C. (1992). Hardiness: A review of theory and research. *Health Psychology*, **11**, 335–345.

Funk, S. C. & Houston, B. K. (1987). A critical analysis of the Hardiness Scale's validity and utility. *Journal of Personality and Social Psychology*, **53**, 572–578.

Gil, S. (2005). Pre-traumatic personality as a predictor of post-traumatic stress disorder among undergraduate students exposed to a terrorist attack: A prospective study in Israel. *Personality and Individual Differences*, **39**, 819–827.

Gil, S. & Caspi, Y. (2006). Personality traits, coping style, and perceived threat as predictors of posttraumatic stress disorder after exposure to a terrorist attack: A prospective study. *Psychosomatic Medicine*, **68**, 904–909.

Golby, J. & Sheard, M. (2004). Mental toughness and hardiness at different levels of rugby league. *Personality and Individual Differences*, **37**, 933–942.

Golding, J. M., Siegel, J. M., Sorenson, S. B., Burnam, M. A., & Stein, J. A. (1989). Social support following sexual assault. *Journal of Community Psychology*, **17**, 92–107.

Gomez, R., Holmberg, K., Bounds, J., Fullarton, C., & Gomez, A. (1999). Neuroticism and extraversion as predictors of coping styles during early adolescence. *Personality and Individual Differences*, **27**, 3–17.

Gray, J. A. (1987). *The psychology of fear and stress,* 2nd edn. Cambridge, UK: Cambridge University Press.

Gross, J. J. & John, O. P. (1995). Facets of emotional expressivity: Three self-report factors and their correlates. *Personality and Individual Differences*, **19**, 555–568.

Gupta, S. & Shukla, A. P. (1989). Verbal operant conditioning as a function of extraversion and reinforcement. *British Journal of Psychology*, **80**, 39–44.

Hathaway, S. R. & McKinley, J. C. (1967). *MMPI manual,* revised edn. New York: Psychological Corporation.

Herman-Stahl, M. A., Stemmler, M., & Peterson, A. C. (1995). Approach and avoidance coping: Implications for adolescent mental health. *Journal of Youth and Adolescence*, **24**, 649–665.

Hirschfeld, R. M. A., Klerman, G. L., Clayton, P. J., *et al.* (1983). Assessing personality: Effects of the depressive state on trait measurement. *American Journal of Psychiatry*, **140**, 695–699.

Hocking, F. (1970). Extreme environmental stress and its significance for psychopathology. *American Journal of Psychotherapy*, **24**, 4–26.

Holeva, V. & Tarrier, N. (2001). Personality and peritraumatic dissociation in the prediction of PTSD in victims of road traffic accidents. *Journal of Psychosomatic Research*, **51**, 687–692.

Holohan, C. J. & Moos, R. H. (1991). Life stressors, personal and social resources, and depression: A 4-year structural model. *Journal of Abnormal Psychology*, **100**, 31–38.

Horsburgh, V. A., Schermer, J. A., Veselka, L., & Vernon, P. A. (2009). A behavioural genetic study of mental toughness and personality. *Personality and Individual Differences*, **46**, 100–105.

Ingham, J. G., Kreitman, N. B., McMiller, P., Sashidharan, S. P., & Surtrees, P. G. (1986). Self-esteem, vulnerability, and psychiatric disorder in the community. *British Journal of Psychiatry*, **148**, 175–185.

Judge, T. A., Bono, J. E., Ilies, R., & Gerhardt, M. W. (2002). Personality and leadership: A qualitative and quantitative review. *Journal of Applied Psychology*, **87**, 765–780.

Jylhä, P., Melartin, T., & Isometsä, E. (2009). Relationships of neuroticism and extraversion with axis I and II comorbidity among patients with DSM-IV major depressive disorder. *Journal of Affective Disorders* **114**, 110–121.

Kantorowitz, D. A. (1978). Personality and conditioning of tumescence and detumescence. *Behaviour Research and Therapy*, **16**, 117–123.

Keane, T. M., Zimering, R. T., & Caddell, J. M. (1985). A behavioral formulation of posttraumatic stress disorder in Vietnam veterans. *Behavior Therapist*, **8**, 9–12.

Keane, T. M., Caddell, J. M., & Taylor, K. L. (1988). The Mississippi Scale for combat-related posttraumatic stress disorder: Three studies in reliability and validity. *Journal of Consulting and Clinical Psychology*, **56**, 85–90.

Kerr, T. A., Schapira, K., Roth, M., & Garside, R. F. (1970). The relationship between the Maudsley Personality Inventory and the course of affective disorders. *British Journal of Psychiatry*, **116**, 11–19.

King, D. W., King, L. A., Foy, D. W., Keane, T. M., & Fairbank, J. A. (1999). Posttraumatic stress disorder in a national sample of female and male Vietnam veterans: Risk factors, war-zone stressors, and resilience-recovery variables. *Journal of Abnormal Psychology*, **108**, 164–170.

King, L. A., King, D. W., Fairbank, J. A., Keane, T. M., & Adams, G. A (1998). Resilience-recovery factors in post-traumatic stress disorder among female and male Vietnam veterans: Hardiness, postwar social support, and additional stressful life events. *Journal of Personality and Social Psychology*, **74**, 420–434.

Kobasa, S. C. (1979). Stressful life events, personality, and health: An inquiry into hardiness. *Journal of Personality and Social Psychology*, **37**, 1–11.

Kobasa, S. C., Maddi, S. R., & Courington, S. C. (1981). Personality and constitution as mediators in the stress–illness relationship. *Journal of Health and Social Behavior*, **22**, 368–378.

Koren, D., Arnon, I., & Klein, E. (1999). Acute stress response and posttraumatic stress disorder in traffic accident victims: A one-year prospective, follow-up study. *American Journal of Psychiatry*, **156**, 367–373.

Krueger, R. F. (1999). The structure of common mental disorders. *Archives of General Psychiatry*, **56**, 921–926.

Krueger, R. F., Caspi, A., Moffitt, T. E., & Silva, P. A. (1998). The structure and stability of common mental disorders (DSM-III-R): A longitudinal-epidemiological study. *Journal of Abnormal Psychology*, **107**, 216–227.

Krueger, R. F., McGue, M., & Iacono, W. G. (2001). The higher-order structure of common DSM mental disorders: Internalization, externalization, and their connections to personality. *Personality and Individual Differences*, **30**, 1245–1259.

Kulka, R. A., Schlenger, W. E., Fairbank, J. A., *et al.* (1990). *Trauma and the Vietnam War generation: Report on the findings from the National Vietnam Veterans Readjustment Study.* New York: Brunner/Mazel.

Lara, M. E., Leader, J., & Klein, D. N. (1997). The association between social support and course of depression: Is it confounded with personality? *Journal of Abnormal Psychology*, **106**, 478–482.

Larsen, R. J. & Ketelaar, T. (1991). Personality and susceptibility to positive and negative emotional states. *Journal of Personality and Social Psychology*, **61**, 132–140.

Lawler, K. A. & Schmied, L. A. (1992). A prospective study of women's health: The effects of stress, hardiness, locus of control, type A behavior, and physiological reactivity. *Women and Health*, **19**, 27–41.

Lawrence, J. W. & Fauerbach, J. A. (2003). Personality, coping, chronic stress, social support and PTSD symptoms among adult burn survivors: A path analysis. *Journal of Burn Care and Rehabilitation*, **24**, 63–72.

LeDoux, J. E. (2000). Emotion circuits in the brain. *Annual Review of Neuroscience*, **23**, 155–184.

Lee, K. A., Vaillant, G. E., Torrey, W. C., & Elder, G. H. (1995). A 50-year prospective study of the psychological sequelae of World War II combat. *American Journal of Psychiatry*, **152**, 516–522.

Maddi, S. R., Khoshaba, D. M., Persico, M., *et al.* (2002). The personality construct of hardiness II: Relationships with comprehensive tests of personality and psychopathology. *Journal of Research in Personality*, **36**, 72–85.

Mangan, G. L. (1967). Studies of the relationship between neo-pavlovian properties of higher nervous system activity and western personality dimensions: IV. A factor analytic study of extraversion and flexibility and the sensitivity and mobility of the nervous system. *Journal of Experimental Research in Personality*, **2**, 124–127.

McCrae, R. R. & Costa, P. T. (1986). Personality, coping and coping effectiveness in an adult sample. *Journal of Personality*, **54**, 385–405.

McCrae, R. R. & Costa, P. T. (1997). Personality trait structure as a human universal. *American Psychologist*, **52**, 509–516.

McCranie, E. W., Hyer, L. A., Boudewyns, P. A., & Woods, M. G. (1992). Negative parenting behavior, combat exposure, and PTSD symptom severity: Test of a person–event interaction model. *Journal of Nervous and Mental Disease*, **180**, 431–438.

McFarlane, A. C. (1992). Avoidance and intrusion in posttraumatic stress disorder. *Journal of Nervous and Mental Disease*, **180**, 439–445.

Miller, M. W. (2003). Personality and the etiology and expression of PTSD: a three-factor model perspective. *Clinical Psychology: Science and Practice*, **10**, 373–393.

Miller, M. W. (2004). Personality and the development and expression of PTSD. *PTSD Research Quarterly*, **15**, 1–7.

Miller, E. K. & Cohen, J. D. (2001). An integrative theory of prefrontal cortex function. *Annual Review of Neuroscience*, **24**, 167–202.

Miller, M. W. & Patrick, C. J. (2000). Trait differences in affective and attentional responding to threat revealed by emotional Stroop interference and startle reflex modulation. *Behavior Therapy*, **31**, 757–776.

Miller, M. W. & Resick, P. A. (2007). Internalizing and externalizing subtypes in female sexual assault survivors: Implications for the understanding of complex PTSD. *Behavior Therapy*, **38**, 58–71.

Miller, M. W., Greif, J. L., & Smith, A. A. (2003). Multidimensional Personality Questionnaire profiles of veterans with traumatic combat exposure: Internalizing and externalizing subtypes. *Psychological Assessment*, **15**, 205–215.

Miller, M. W., Kaloupek, D. G., Dillon, A. L., & Keane, T. M. (2004). Externalizing and internalizing subtypes of combat-related PTSD: A replication and extension using the PSY-5 scales. *Journal of Abnormal Psychology*, **113**, 636–645.

Mineka, S., Watson, D., & Clark, L. A. (1998). Comorbidity of anxiety and unipolar mood disorders. *Annual Review of Psychology*, **49**, 377–412.

Monroe, S. M. & Simons, A. D. (1991). Diathesis-stress theories in the context of life stress research: Implications for the depressive disorders. *Psychological Bulletin*, **110**, 406–425.

Morgan, I. A., Matthews, G., & Winton, M. (1995). Coping and personality as predictors of posttraumatic intrusions, numbing, avoidance and general distress: A study of victims of the Perth flood. *Behavioural and Cognitive Psychotherapy*, **23**, 251–264.

Nezu, A. M. & Carnevale, G. J. (1987). Interpersonal problem solving and coping reactions of Vietnam veterans with posttraumatic stress disorder. *Journal of Abnormal Psychology*, **96**, 155–157.

Nightingale, J. & Williams, R. M. (2000). Attitudes to emotional expression and personality in predicting post-traumatic stress disorder. *British Journal of Clinical Psychology*, **39**, 243–254.

Orr, S. P., Metzger, L. J., Lasko, N. B., *et al.* (2000). De novo conditioning in trauma-exposed individuals with and without posttraumatic stress disorder. *Journal of Abnormal Psychology*, **2**, 290–298.

O'Toole, B. I., Marshall, R. P., Schureck, R. J., & Dobson, M. (1998). Risk factors for posttraumatic stress disorder in Australian Vietnam veterans. *Australian and New Zealand Journal of Psychiatry*, **32**, 21–31.

Paisey, T. J. & Mangan, G. L. (1988). Personality and conditioning with appetitive and aversive stimuli. *Personality and Individual Differences*, **9**, 69–78.

Panksepp, J. (1992). A critical role for "affective neuroscience" in resolving what is basic about basic emotions. *Psychological Review*, **99**, 554–560.

Parkes, K. R. (1986). Coping in stressful episodes: The role of individual differences, environmental factors, and situational characteristics. *Journal of Personality and Social Psychology*, **51**, 1277–1292.

Parkes, K. R. & Rendall, D. (1988). The hardy personality and its relationship to extraversion and neuroticism. *Personality and Individual Differences*, **9**, 785–790.

Parslow, R. A., Jorm, A. F., & Christensen, H. (2006). Associations of pre-trauma attributes and trauma exposure with screening positive for PTSD: Analysis of a community-based study of 2085 young adults. *Psychological Medicine*, **36**, 387–395.

Patrick, C. J. & Bernat, E. M. (2006). The construct of emotion as a bridge between personality and psychopathology. In R. F. Krueger & J. L. Tackett (eds.), *Personality and psychopathology* (pp. 174–209). New York: Guilford Press.

Pearlin, L. I. & Schooler, C. (1978). The structure of coping. *Journal of Health and Social Behavior*, **19**, 2–21.

Popiel, D. A. & Susskind, E. C. (1985). The impact of rape: Social support as a moderator of stress. *American Journal of Community Psychiatry*, **13**, 645–676.

Punamaki, R., Qouta, S., & El- Sarraj, E. (2001). Resiliency factors predicting psychological adjustment after political violence among Palestinian children. *International Journal of Behavioral Development*, **25**, 256–267.

Qouta, S., Punamaki, R., Montgomery, E., & El Sarraj, E. (2007). Predictors of psychological distress and positive resources among Palestinian adolescents: Trauma, child, and mothering characteristics. *Child Abuse and Neglect*, **31**, 699–717.

Rabkin, J. G. & Struening, E. L. (1976). Life events, stress, and illness. *Science*, **194**, 1013–1020.

Ramanaiah, N. V., Sharpe, J. P., & Byravan, A. (1999). Hardiness and major personality factors. *Psychological Reports*, **84**, 497–500.

Reich, J., Noyes, R., Coryell, W., & O'Gorman, T. W. (1986). The effect of state anxiety on personality measurement. *American Journal of Psychiatry*, **143**, 760–763.

Rhodewalt, F. & Zone, J. B. (1989). Appraisal of life change, depression, and illness in hardy and nonhardy women. *Journal of Personality and Social Psychology*, **56**, 81–88.

Robins, L. N., Helzer, J. E., Cottler, L. B., & Goldring, E. (1989). *National Institute of Mental Health Diagnostic Interview Schedule*, version 3, revised. St. Louis, MO: Washington University Department of Psychiatry,

Robinson, J. L., Kagan, J., Reznick, J. S., & Corley, R. (1992). The heritability of inhibited and uninhibited behavior: A twin study. *Developmental Psychology*, **28**, 1030–1037.

Roca, R. P., Spence, R. J., & Munster, A. M. (1992). Posttraumatic adaptation and distress among adult burn survivors. *American Journal of Psychiatry*, **149**, 1234–1238.

Ross, S. R., Rausch, M. K., & Canada, K. E. (2003). Competition and cooperation in the five-factor model: individual differences in achievement orientation. *Journal of Psychology*, **137**, 323–337.

Rothbart, M. K., Derryberry, D., & Posner, M. I. (1994). A psychobiological approach to the development of temperament. In J. E. Bates & T. D. Wachs (eds.), *Temperament: Individual differences at the interface of biology and behavior* (pp. 83–117). Washington, DC: American Psychological Association.

Ruch, L. O. & Leon, J. J. (1983). Sexual assault trauma and trauma change. *Women and Health*, **8**, 5–21.

Schimmack, U., Oishi, S., Furr, R. M., & Funder, D. C. (2004). Personality and life satisfaction: A facet-level analysis. *Personality and Social Psychology Bulletin*, **30**, 1062–1075.

Schnurr, P. P., Friedman, M. J., & Rosenberg, S. D. (1993). Premilitary MMPI scores as predictors of combat-related PTSD symptoms. *American Journal of Psychiatry*, **150**, 479–483.

Shagass, C. & Kerenyi, A. B. (1958). Neurophysiologic studies of personality. *Journal of Nervous and Mental Disease*, **126**, 141–147.

Solomon, Z., Mikulincer, M., & Flum, H. (1988). Negative life events, coping responses, and combat-related psychopathology: A prospective study. *Journal of Abnormal Psychology*, **97**, 302–313.

Spence, K. W. & Beecroft, R. S. (1954). Differential conditioning and level of anxiety. *Journal of Experimental Psychology*, **48**, 399–403.

Spence, K. W. & Farber, I. E. (1953). Conditioning and extinction as a function of anxiety. *Journal of Experimental Psychology*, **45**, 116–119.

Spence, K. W. & Taylor, J. (1951). Anxiety and strength of the UCS as determiners of the amount of eyelid conditioning. *Journal of Experimental Psychology*, **42**, 183–188.

Spence, K. W., Farber, I. E., & Taylor, E. (1954). The relation of electric shock and anxiety to level of performance in eyelid conditioning. *Journal of Experimental Psychology*, **48**, 404–408.

Spitzer, R. L., Williams, J. B., & Gibbon, M. (1987). *Structured clinical interview for DSM-III-R*, version NP-V. New York: New York State Psychiatric Institute, Biometrics Research.

Stewart, M. E., Ebmeier, K. P., & Deary, I. J. (2005). Personality correlates of happiness and sadness: EPQ-R and TPQ compared. *Personality and Individual Differences*, **38**, 1085–1096.

Stokes, J. P. & McKirnan, D. J. (1989). Affect and the social environment: The role of social support in depression and anxiety. In P. C. Kendall & D. Watson (eds.), *Anxiety and depression: Distinctions and overlapping features* (pp. 253–284). New York: Academic Press.

Stretch, R. H. (1985). Posttraumatic stress disorder among US Army reserve Vietnam and Vietnam-era veterans. *Journal of Consulting and Clinical Psychology*, **53**, 935–936.

Stretch, R. H. (1986). Incidence and etiology of post-traumatic stress disorder among active duty personnel. *Journal of Applied Social Psychology*, **16**, 464–481.

Tellegen, A. (1985). Structures of mood and personality and their relevance to assessing anxiety with an emphasis on self-report. In A. H. Tuma & J. D. Maser (eds.), *Anxiety and the anxiety disorders* (pp. 681–706). Hillsdale, NJ: Erlbaum.

Tellegen, A. (2000). *Manual for the Multidimensional Personality Questionnaire*. Minneapolis, MN: University of Minnesota Press.

Tellegen, A., Lykken, D. T., Bouchard, T. J., *et al.* (1988). Personality similarity in twins reared apart and together. *Journal of Personality and Social Psychology*, **54**, 1031–1039.

Verkerk, G. J., Denollet, J., van Heck, G. L., van Son, M. J., & Pop, V. J. (2005). Personality factors as determinants of depression in postpartum women: A prospective 1-year follow-up study. *Psychosomatic Medicine*, **67**, 632–637.

Vogt, D. S., Rizvi, S. L., Shipherd, J. C., & Resick, P. A. (2008). Longitudinal investigation of reciprocal relationship between stress reactions and hardiness. *Personality and Social Psychology Bulletin*, **34**, 61–73.

Volrath, M. & Torgersen, S. (2000). Personality types and coping. *Personality and Individual Differences*, **29**, 367–378.

Volrath, M., Torgersen, S., & Alnaes, R. (1995). Personality as a long-term predictor of coping. *Personality and Individual Differences*, **18**, 117–125.

Watson, D. (2005). Rethinking the mood and anxiety disorders: A quantitative hierarchical model for DSM-V. *Journal of Abnormal Psychology*, **114**, 522–536.

Watson, D. & Walker, L. M. (1996). The long-term stability and predictive validity of trait measures of affect. *Journal of Personality and Social Psychology*, **70**, 567–577.

Watson, D., Clark, L. A., & Carey, G. (1988a). Positive and negative affect and their relation to anxiety and depressive disorders. *Journal of Abnormal Psychology*, **97**, 346–353.

Watson, D., Clark, L. A., & Tellegen, A. J. (1988b). Development and validation of brief measures of positive and negative affect: the PANAS scales. *Personality and Social Psychology*, **54**, 1063–1070.

Watson, D., Gamez, W., & Simms, L. J. (2005). Basic dimensions of temperament and their relation to anxiety and depression: A symptom-based perspective. *Journal of Research in Personality*, **39**, 46–66.

Westman, M. (1990). The relationship between stress and performance: The moderating effect of hardiness. *Human Performance*, **3**, 141–155.

Weyer, G. (1989). Conditioned and unconditioned cardiovascular reactivity: Predictability and stability over time. *Personality and Individual Differences*, **10**, 633–652.

Wilson, G. D., Kumari, V., Gray, J. A., & Corr, P. J. (2000). The role of neuroticism in startle reactions to fearful and disgusting stimuli. *Personality and Individual Differences*, **29**, 1077–1082.

Wolfe, J., Erickson, D. J., Sharkansky, E. J., King, D. W., & King, L. A. (1999). Course and predictors of posttraumatic stress disorder among Gulf War veterans: A prospective analysis. *Journal of Consulting and Clinical Psychology*, **67**, 520–528.

Zinbarg, R. E. & Mohlman, J. (1998). Individual differences in the acquisition of affectively valenced associations. *Journal of Personality and Social Psychology*, **74**, 1024–1040.

Zoellner, L. A., Foa, E. B., & Brigidi, B. D. (1999). Interpersonal friction and PTSD in female victims of sexual and nonsexual assault. *Journal of Traumatic Stress*, **12**, 689–700.

Zuckerman, M. (1983). *Biological bases of sensation seeking, impulsivity, and anxiety*. Hillsdale, NJ: Erlbaum.

Social ties and resilience in chronic disease

Denise Janicki-Deverts and Sheldon Cohen

Introduction

Social ties are thought to affect mental and physical health by influencing emotions, cognitions, and behavior (Cohen, 1988, 2004). In the case of mental health, the hypothesis is that aspects of social relationships regulate these three response systems by preventing the occurrence of the kinds of extreme response that are associated with dysfunction. This regulation occurs through communication of social expectations, of appropriate norms, of rewards and punishments, and through the provision of coping assistance (Caplan, 1974; Cassel, 1976; Thoits, 1986). In the case of physical health, the hypothesis is that social ties influence behaviors with implications for health such as diet, exercise, smoking, alcohol consumption, sleep, and adherence to medical regimens. Moreover, the failure to regulate emotional responses can trigger health-relevant changes in the responses of the neuroendocrine, immune, and cardiovascular systems (Cohen, 1988; Cohen et al., 1994; Uchino, 2006).

During times of stress, social ties can be thought to operate by these same mechanisms to promote resilience, or positive adaptation in the face of adversity (Cohen & Wills, 1985; Luthar, 2006). People undergoing the stress of being diagnosed with a serious chronic illness are vulnerable to both physical and psychological adversity. Patients with chronic disease must cope with the physical threats of worsening health, loss of physical function, and the potential of a reduced lifespan, as well as with psychological threats such as feelings of isolation, loss of self-esteem, and loss of social and occupational role function.

This chapter focuses on resilience as it pertains to psychological and physiological adjustment to chronic disease. *Psychological adjustment* is taken to mean "adaptation to disease without continued elevations of psychological distress (e.g., anxiety, depression) and loss of role function (i.e., social, sexual, vocational)" (Helgeson & Cohen, 1996, p. 136). *Physiological adjustment* is taken to mean slowed biological progression of disease, with progression being operationalized as the reappearance of manifest disease expression (e.g., cancer recurrence, second heart attack in those with heart disease) and disease-related mortality.

The chapter will begin by introducing two important components of social relationships – social support and social integration – describing approaches that have been taken for their measurement and discussing models that have been proposed to describe the manner by which these components of social relationships deliver their beneficial effects. The subsequent discussion will focus on potential psychological, behavioral, and physiological mechanisms by which social ties might be translated into better adjustment, using studies from chronic disease research as specific examples. Then, evidence will be presented suggesting that social ties promote individuals' physical and psychological adjustments to chronic disease. Finally, the chapter will end with a brief discussion of the literature on social relationship interventions designed to promote adjustment in persons with chronic disease, as well as possible future directions for social ties and resilience research.

Social support and social integration: definitions and measurement

Social support

Social support refers to a social network's provision of psychological and material resources *intended to benefit an individual's ability to cope with stress* (Cohen, 2004). Support is often differentiated in terms of three

Resilience and Mental Health: Challenges Across the Lifespan, ed. Steven M. Southwick, Brett T. Litz, Dennis Charney, and Matthew J. Friedman. Published by Cambridge University Press. © Cambridge University Press 2011.

types of resource: instrumental, informational, and emotional (e.g., House & Kahn, 1985). Instrumental support involves the provision of material aid, for example financial assistance or help with daily tasks. Informational support refers to the provision of relevant information intended to help the individual to cope with current difficulties and typically takes the form of advice or guidance in dealing with one's problems. Emotional support involves the expression of empathy, caring, reassurance, and trust and provides opportunities for emotional expression and venting. Such typologies of support provide a basis for determining whether the effectiveness of different kinds of support differs by the nature of stressful events or by the characteristics of persons suffering adversity.

In general, measures of social support focus either on individuals' *perceptions* of available support from members of their social networks or on individuals' accounts of support that was *actually* provided by/received from their network members. Interestingly, measures of received support tend to correlate poorly with perceived support measures. Moreover, perceived support has been associated with greater benefits than support that was actually received. Explanations for this phenomenon include the fact that support generally is sought during times of stress and that asking for or simply needing support may be detrimental to one's self-esteem (Cohen & Wills, 1985; Uchino, 2004). An additional explanation is that the support provided by one's network members may not meet the individual's specific needs. Hence the *matching hypothesis*, which proposes that support will be most effective if the support provided matches the needs of the recipient (Cohen & McKay, 1984; Cutrona & Russell, 1990). On the one hand, for example, an individual who recently experienced the death of a close other would benefit more from receiving emotional or belonging support than from receiving material assistance. On the other hand, although emotional support tends to be well received in most circumstances, for an individual who has just lost his or her job, instrumental support in the form of financial assistance may prove to be a more effective support provision.

Social integration

Social integration is a multidimensional construct thought to include a behavioral component – active engagement in a wide range of social activities or relationships – and a cognitive component – a sense of communality and identification with one's social roles (Brissette *et al.*, 2000). The concept of social integration is rooted in the seminal work of Durkheim (1951), originally published in 1897, on social conditions and suicide. Durkheim proposed that stable social structure and widely held norms are protective and serve to regulate behavior.

Measures of social integration can be categorized according to whether they are role based (focus on *number* of relationships), participation based (focus on *frequency* of interaction or engagement with social network members), or perception based (focus on extent to which individuals *perceive* that they are embedded in a stable social structure and *identify* with network members and social positions) (Brissette *et al.*, 2000). Some social integration measures (e.g., Berkman & Syme, 1979) are complex and include two or even all of the types of assessment described above.

Main effects and buffering effects

Two models have been proposed to describe how social ties confer benefits on mental and physical health outcomes: the *main effects model* and the *buffering model* (House, 1981; Cohen & Wills, 1985; Cohen, 1988). The main effects model purports that social ties have an overall positive effect on health regardless of the support recipient's current stress level. The buffering model suggests that social ties confer positive effects for health by protecting individuals from the potentially detrimental effects of stress during times of adversity (Cohen & Wills, 1985). Which model more accurately describes the association of social ties with health outcomes depends on the component of social relationships that is being measured. Reviews of the research on social ties and psychological distress among physically healthy individuals suggest that main effects emerge when social ties are being measured in terms of social integration and that buffering effects are observed when social ties are being measured in terms of perceived availability of social support (Cohen & Wills, 1985). However, whether it is appropriate to test for buffering effects when examining the potential benefits of social ties for persons with chronic disease may be subject to question, as all participants are experiencing high levels of stress related to their illness.

Summary

Two important features of social relationships – social support and social integration – factor importantly in individuals' abilities to cope with stressful situations. Social support can be distinguished according to whether the support provision is informational, instrumental, or emotional in nature. Social integration can be categorized in terms of the number of social relationships in which one is involved, the frequency by which one interacts, or the number of types of relationship in which one participates. Social support is thought to buffer individuals from the negative effects of stressor exposure, whereas social integration is thought to operate according to a main effects model wherein being more highly integrated results in better adjustment, regardless of one's current stress levels. In both cases, just the perception that one is supported and/or is embedded in a diverse social network may be sufficient for the positive effects of social ties to be observed.

Mechanisms by which social ties promote adjustment to stress

Psychological mechanisms

There are several theoretical perspectives suggesting that social integration increases feelings of self-esteem, of self-identity, and of control over one's environment. Social integration is presumed to provide a source of generalized positive affect, a sense of predictability and stability in one's life situation, and recognition of self-worth because of demonstrated ability to meet normative role expectations (e.g., Thoits, 1985; Cohen, 1988). These positive psychological states are presumed to be facilitative because they lessen psychological despair (e.g., Thoits, 1985), result in greater motivation to care for oneself (e.g., Cohen & Syme, 1985), or result in a benign neuroendocrine response (e.g., Uchino, 2006).

A related psychological model assumes that it is social isolation that causes disease, rather than social integration that enhances health (House *et al.*, 1988). This approach assumes that isolation increases negative affect and feelings of alienation, and decreases feelings of control. Alternatively, one can merely view social isolation as a stressor in and of itself.

In regard to social support, availability of aid or of tangible or economic resources from one's social network could reduce the probability of potentially stressful events being appraised as threatening or harmful and hence could reduce the behavioral and affective concomitants of a more negative appraisal.

Others' willingness to help and/or the enhanced ability to cope that results from receiving help increases feelings of personal control and self-esteem. As noted above, such feelings may influence health through increased motivation to perform health behaviors or through suppression of neuroendocrine responses and enhanced immune function. Even the mere perception that help is available may similarly trigger these processes. Findings from several studies of persons facing life-threatening diseases such as cancer have demonstrated a positive association between social relationships and psychological factors. For example, Crothers and colleagues (2005), in a sample of patients receiving treatment for various types of cancer, found that greater satisfaction with social support and greater perceived closeness with the primary support provider were associated with higher levels of positive relative to negative affect and higher levels of hope. Similarly, Schroevers and colleagues (2003), also in a sample of persons with various types of cancer, found that greater perceived emotional and informational support was positively related to higher self-esteem. In a sample of patients after surgery for gastrointestinal cancer, Schulz and Mohamed (2004) examined whether received support during the period surrounding tumor removal surgery would be associated with greater self-efficacy and greater cancer-related benefit finding. Having received higher relative to lower levels of support during the period surrounding the surgery was associated with greater benefit finding 11 months later. However, received support was only weakly and non-significantly correlated with concurrent self-efficacy (Schulz & Mohamed, 2004).

Though not as extensive as the research on social ties and psychological outcomes in cancer patients, research conducted in samples of persons with other serious diseases also has provided evidence for the psychological benefits of social relationships. For example, among recent heart transplant recipients, those who reported stronger attachments to their social network members within the first few days after surgery also reported lower levels of anger and depression, and higher levels of optimism and life satisfaction six months later (Bohachick *et al.*, 2002). Similarly, in a sample of older men with HIV, Chesney and colleagues (2003) found that higher levels of perceived social support, operationalized as a composite of emotional and tangible support, were associated cross-sectionally with less psychological distress, and greater positive affect.

Behavioral mechanisms

Several models have been proposed to describe how social relationships might influence individuals' stress-coping behaviors (Cohen *et al.*, 1994). These influence processes carry the potential to affect the behaviors of individuals with chronic disease in such a way as to promote both physiological and psychological adjustment.

In regard to social integration, one possibility is that having a wide range of network ties presumably provides multiple sources of information and hence an increased probability of having access to an appropriate information source. Information could influence health-relevant behaviors or help in avoiding stressful or high-risk situations. For example, network members could provide information regarding access to medical services or regarding the benefits of behaviors that positively influence health and well-being. Another possibility is that socially integrated persons are subject to social controls and peer pressures that promote health behaviors (e.g., exercise, better diet, not smoking, moderating alcohol intake). Being embedded in a social network also increases individuals' motivation to care for themselves.

Social controls and peer pressures also might constitute a pathway by which social support could influence individuals' coping behaviors. Such influence processes would promote health to the extent that normative coping behaviors are effective in reducing perceptions of stress, non-adjustive behavioral adaptations, and negative affective responses. Inappropriate norms, however, could lead to less-effective coping and hence greater risk of poor psychological and physical adjustment. In so far as social coping norms have been internalized, or that individuals expect others to encourage them to behave in a socially appropriate and healthful manner, the mere perception of such encouragement could influence coping behaviors in the same manner as actually receiving it.

In their review of psychosocial factors and health behaviors in cancer survivors, Park and Gaffey (2007) concluded that social relationships positively influence health behavior change following a diagnosis of cancer. However, findings are not consistent across categories of health behaviors. More precisely, higher levels of social support consistently predict increases in exercise among cancer survivors but show little association with dietary changes. The positive influence of support on exercise levels is important, as regular exercise in cancer survivors has been associated with greater levels of physical and psychological well-being (reviewed by Pinto & Trunzo, 2005). In regard to the lack of association with dietary changes, this finding among cancer patients contrasts with findings from studies conducted with other patient populations, such as people with diabetes (reviewed by Gallant, 2003) and people with heart failure (e.g., Sayers *et al.*, 2008), wherein presence of support has been found to correlate with maintaining a better diet. It is possible that the null effect of social support on dietary changes in cancer patients may reflect the nature of the disease and its treatment. Because of the nausea frequently experienced while undergoing chemotherapy, the goal of support providers may be to encourage the patient to eat anything at all, regardless of healthfulness.

In addition to social ties promoting healthful behaviors among persons with chronic disease, social ties have been shown to increase patients' adherence to medical regimens. DiMatteo (2004) conducted a meta-analysis of 122 correlational studies conducted between 1948 and 2001 that examined the association of social support and social integration with patient adherence to medical regimens. The results suggested that social ties were associated with better adherence. A comparison of effects for social support versus social integration indicated that support correlated better with adherence than did integration.

Physiological mechanisms

In addition to having an indirect effect on physiological resilience via behavioral mechanisms, it also is possible that social ties influence health outcomes directly via three major physiological pathways: cardiovascular, immune, and neuroendocrine (Uchino, 2006).

Cardiovascular system

The cardiovascular system responds to stress by increasing heart rate and blood pressure. Physiological evidence suggests that exaggerated cardiovascular responses to stress are associated with the development of hypertension and cardiovascular disease (Manuck, 1994). Moreover, among persons with coronary heart disease (CHD), heightened cardiovascular reactivity in response to acute stress has been associated with brief episodes of cardiac ischemia (i.e., reduced oxygen supply to the heart through constriction or blockage of coronary arteries [Rozanski *et al.*, 1988]). Therefore, one mechanism by which social ties may protect individuals from development or progression of cardiovascular disease is by dampening the cardiovascular stress response.

This proposal has been tested in the laboratory by assigning individuals to an experimental condition, wherein they complete a stressful task in the presence of a supportive friend or confederate, or to a control condition, wherein individuals complete the same task but in the absence of a supportive other. The expectation is that individuals in the support condition would show reduced cardiovascular reactivity (i.e., smaller increases in blood pressure and heart rate) relative to those in the control condition. Findings from this literature have been mixed, with some studies showing lower reactivity in the support condition (e.g., Kamarck et al., 1990), some showing higher reactivity (e.g., Allen et al., 1991), and some showing no difference between conditions (e.g., Anthony & O'Brien, 1999). Methodological differences are thought to explain much of the inconsistency between studies (Kamarck et al., 1998). For example, social support has a greater attenuating effect on reactivity when it is received from a friend rather than a stranger (Christenfeld et al., 1997) or from a woman rather than a man (Glynn et al., 1999). Moreover, social support appears to be most effective in dampening cardiovascular reactivity to acute stress when the stressor is associated with high social threat (Kamarck et al., 1995).

In addition to influencing cardiovascular *reactivity* to stress, social ties may affect the cardiovascular system's capacity to *recover* from stress. Comparatively little research has been done in the area of cardiovascular recovery, and even less on the influence of social ties on recovery. However, existing evidence provides some indication that higher levels of perceived social support from one's existing network may promote better recovery from acute laboratory stressors (e.g., Roy et al., 1998).

Immune system

The inability of the immune system to mount an appropriate response to infection or injury has been implicated in the pathophysiology of several chronic diseases including cardiovascular disease (Libby, 2002), type 1 diabetes mellitus (Knip & Siljander, 2008), and some types of cancer (Dunn et al., 2002). A growing body of research provides suggestive evidence of a link between greater social support and social integration and better immune function (reviewed by Uchino [2006] and Uchino et al. [1996]).

One frequently employed assessment of immune function involves measuring the amount of antibody an individual produces in response to being inoculated with an inactive virus (i.e., receiving a vaccination). Production of more antibodies to the inoculated virus strain signifies a better functioning of the immune system. Glaser and colleagues (1992) adopted this technique to examine whether social support was associated with immune function in second year medical students, a group generally found to report elevated levels of stress. Students who reported higher levels of perceived social support developed more specific antibody in response to a hepatitis B vaccination relative to those reporting less support (Glaser et al., 1992). Similarly, college freshmen who reported smaller social networks mounted lower antibody responses to a component of the influenza vaccine relative to freshman with larger social networks (Pressman et al., 2005).

Cohen and colleagues (1997) took a different approach to examining the association of social ties with immune function by exposing 276 healthy men and women to a common cold virus and then examining whether extent of social integration assessed at the beginning of the study predicted the likelihood of developing a clinical cold during the five days following virus exposure. The presence of a cold was determined by the amount of mucus production and the nasal mucociliary clearance time (i.e., the length of time necessary for the upper respiratory tract to clear itself of inhaled particles). Those individuals who reported having a more diverse social network (i.e., greater number of different *types* of relationship) were less likely to develop a cold relative to those who reported less diverse networks.

Neuroendocrine system

Neuroendocrine activity is estimated primarily by measuring end-products of the hypothalamic–pituitary–adrenal axis (HPA) and the sympathetic–adrenomedullary system. The products of these two neuroendocrine systems function as mediators of *allostasis*, the active process by which the body maintains a state of internal balance in response to a changing environment (McEwen & Stellar, 1993); that is, the two systems function to promote physiological resilience in the face of potentially adverse environmental stimuli. The "fight or flight" response, a constellation of behavioral and biological adaptations that are directed toward promotion of survival in the face of an acute aversive stimulus, is one example of a function that depends upon activation of these systems. In the short term, then, excitation of these systems clearly is adaptive. Over longer periods of time, however, prolonged or repeated activation of these two systems can lead to *allostatic load*, the wear and tear on the body and brain that results from dysregulation of allostatic mechanisms (McEwen, 2007). Allostatic load has been thought to contribute to the pathophysiology of many if not most chronic diseases, and it has been suggested to be a pathway through which psychosocial factors, including social support, might influence susceptibility to and exacerbation of disease (McEwen, 2007).

Despite the fact that cardiovascular and immune activities are thought to be regulated in part by neuroendocrine mediators, research on social ties and neuroendocrine activity is relatively limited in comparison with that on social ties and cardiovascular and immune functions (Uchino, 2006). Findings from the few existing studies in this area suggest that supportive social relationships may have a positive influence on neuroendocrine regulation, but these effects may be moderated by other factors, including gender (Seeman & McEwen, 1996; Uchino, 2006). For example, social support has been associated with lower levels of plasma and urinary epinephrine and norepinephrine, hormones that are secreted in response to activation of the sympathetic–adrenomedullary system. In a study of married and cohabiting couples, self-reported support from one's partner was associated with lower plasma norepinephrine in women but not men (Grewen *et al.*, 2005). In healthy older adults, both social support (emotional, instrumental) and social integration (number of social ties) were associated with lower levels of urinary epinephrine and norepinephrine among men but not women (Seeman *et al.*, 1994). Social support also has been associated with lower levels of cortisol, the primary effector of the hypothalamic–pituitary–adrenal axis. Among women with metastatic breast cancer, salivary cortisol concentrations were found to decrease with increasing perceived social support (Turner-Cobb *et al.*, 2000). Both Grewen *et al.* (2005) and Seeman *et al.* (1994) measured cortisol in addition to epinephrine and norepinephrine. Findings for cortisol mirrored those for epinephrine and norepinephrine: social support was associated with lower cortisol concentrations in married/cohabiting women but not men (Grewen *et al.*, 2005) and in healthy older men but not women (Seeman *et al.*, 1994).

Summary

Three mechanisms by which social ties have been proposed to influence adjustment to stress involve psychological, behavioral, and physiological factors, respectively. Psychological mechanisms include enhancement of self-esteem, self-identity, and control over one's environment, as well as reduction in the probability of appraising a stressful event as threatening or harmful. Behavioral mechanisms include encouragement to engage in health-promoting behaviors and discouragement from engaging in risky behaviors. Physiological mechanisms include decreased stress responsivity of the cardiovascular, immune, and neuroendocrine systems.

Social ties and resilience: the evidence

The role of social ties in the promotion of psychological and physiological adjustment to chronic disease has been examined extensively in individuals with CHD, those with cancer, and to a lesser extent, those infected with HIV. The following section provides a brief overview of the association of social ties, measured in multiple ways, to psychological and physiological adjustment to chronic disease.

Social support and psychological adjustment

Coronary heart disease

Across CHD studies, adjustment has been operationalized in terms of depression (e.g., Brummett *et al.*, 1998; Frasure-Smith *et al.*, 2000), quality of life (Bennett *et al.*, 2001), and anxiety (reviewed by Duits *et al.*, 1997). Significant interest has surrounded predictors of depression in patients with CHD because depression, which has a prevalence rate of approximately 19.8% in heart attack survivors (Thombs *et al.*, 2006), has been found to predict re-hospitalization (Levine *et al.*, 1996) and shorter survival times (Frasure-Smith *et al.*, 1993; Barth *et al.*, 2004). In a sample of patients with CHD who had been hospitalized for cardiac catheterization (a medical procedure used to diagnose and treat some heart conditions), Brummett and colleagues (1998) examined whether in-hospital measures of perceived social support predicted depression symptoms one month later. Using structural equation modeling, the authors detected a direct path between social support (a composite of instrumental, informational, and emotional support) and later depression symptoms, such that higher levels of support were associated with fewer symptoms. This association remained significant when in-hospital measures of depression were included in the model. Similarly, Frasure-Smith and colleagues (2000) found that among heart attack survivors at one year who were depressed at baseline (i.e., when in hospital), higher levels of perceived social support at baseline predicted greater declines in depression symptoms assessed one year later. Interestingly, when the authors included two measures of social integration (frequency of social interaction and living alone or not) into their regression model, all three social relationship measures emerged as independent predictors of changes in depression symptoms (Frasure-Smith *et al.*, 2000).

Cancer

Helgeson and Cohen (1996) reviewed the extant research examining the role of social relationships in the promotion of psychological adjustment among persons with cancer. From their review of existing correlational research, the authors concluded that emotional support is both the type of support that is most desired by cancer patients and the type that has the strongest associations with psychological adjustment. More recent research is consistent with these findings. For example, Helgeson *et al.* (2004) followed a sample of women with breast cancer from 4 to 55 months after diagnosis and examined whether the patients fell into distinct trajectories of social–psychological and physical adjustment, and whether social resources (among other variables) assessed at four months after diagnosis could distinguish between adjustment trajectories. Social resources in this study were operationalized as a composite of two measures: perceived availability of emotional, informational, and tangible support from friends, family, and partner; and frequency of negative interactions with friends, family, and partner (reverse-scored). Findings indicated that social resources differentiated between two trajectories. Women with higher levels of social support followed a trajectory characterized by high levels of psychological adjustment at four months that were maintained throughout the follow-up period; whereas women with lower levels of social support followed a trajectory characterized by lower levels of adjustment at four months and that continued to decline throughout the follow-up (Helgeson *et al.*, 2004).

Human immunodeficiency virus

A few studies that were conducted in the early 1990s examined the association between social ties and psychological adjustment among persons with HIV. Findings from these studies were generally supportive of the hypothesis that social ties promote psychological adjustment to the stress of living with HIV-positive status. For example, higher levels of perceived social support were found to be related cross-sectionally to lower levels of depression (Hays *et al.*, 1992) and psychological distress (Blaney *et al.*, 1991) and to higher levels of social adjustment (Pakenham *et al.*, 1994). Similar evidence was reported in a recent prospective study. Johnson and colleagues (2001) examined whether perceived social support could predict subsequent changes in psychological adjustment among HIV-positive men. Lower levels of perceived support at baseline were related to higher concurrent helplessness and symptoms of depression and to greater *increases* in hopelessness and depression six months later. Moreover, additional analyses indicated that the changes in hopelessness over time mediated the association between baseline social support and changes in depression symptoms (Johnson *et al.*, 2001).

Summary

Existing literature on social ties and psychological adjustment to CHD, cancer, and HIV strongly suggest that perceived social support promotes psychological resilience to chronic physical disease. That social ties should protect individuals with chronic disease from developing depression symptoms, specifically, may have important implications for physical as well as psychological well-being.

Social support and physiological adjustment

Coronary heart disease

Lett and colleagues (2005) reviewed the existing literature on social ties and disease progression in patients with CHD, and concluded that social ties exert a positive main effect on progression of CHD such that patients with deficient social relationships are two to four times more likely to experience a second heart attack or CHD-related death relative to persons with adequate social relationships. Findings were consistent across various indicators of perceived social support (i.e., emotional support, marital quality, instrumental support, general availability of needed support) and social integration (i.e., social network size, marital status, participation in clubs or social/recreational activities), with neither social relationship domain emerging as the more prognostic.

By comparison, tests of whether social support is beneficial to patients with CHD because it buffers the negative effects of CHD-related depression have provided mixed results. In a study of social support and mortality in patients with cardiac disease, Frasure-Smith and colleagues (2000) found an interaction between perceived social support and depression such that high levels of perceived support were protective against mortality only in those patients who also were depressed. Contrariwise, Lett and colleagues (2007) found that higher levels of perceived support predicted longer survival times among patients with CHD who had lower rather than higher levels of depression symptomatology, thus suggesting that the moderating effect of depression on the association of perceived support and CHD survival is complex and in need of further examination.

Cancer

Helgeson *et al.* (1998) reviewed studies examining the association of social ties with cancer survival and recurrence. The authors identified three types of social relationship measure that were examined in this literature: marital status, social integration, and emotional support. The marital status literature was inconsistent, with some studies reporting increased survival time among married persons, some reporting decreased survival time, and some reporting no effect of marital status. Studies that examined recurrence as the outcome were similarly inconsistent. Findings for studies that either focused on perceived emotional support or on characteristics of the social network were more encouraging, with various markers of social integration (e.g., frequency of engagement in activities involving social interaction) showing a positive association with recurrence and survival time.

A well-controlled prospective study by Kroenke and colleagues (2006) found a link between social integration and survival among women with breast cancer. Specifically, women with more social ties (i.e., close relatives, friends, or living children) exhibited increased survival relative to women with fewer ties. Interestingly, the authors found no association between their measure of socioemotional support (frequency of communication with a confidant) and survival. One

explanation for this unexpected finding may be that their emotional support measure might be interpreted as a measure of *received* rather than *perceived* support. For example, an individual may talk to her confidant (e.g., a sister who lives out of town) only a few times per year. However, if she feels that her sister is always available to provide her with a sense of caring or reassurance, her levels of perceived support may match or even exceed those of someone who interacts with her confidant more frequently.

Human immunodeficiency virus

Ironson and Hayward (2008) examined 11 prospective social relationship studies in their review of positive psychosocial factors and disease progression in persons infected with HIV. Disease progression was defined as development of AIDS, appearance of AIDS-related disease complications, or physiological evidence of worsening immune function (e.g., declines in CD4 T-cell numbers, immune cells that are affected by HIV). Of these studies, five found that having social ties was predictive of less-severe disease progression, whereas the remaining six found no significant effect of social ties. Of the positive studies, two reported buffering effects of social ties in that effects were observed only among those with more severe disease. In one case, having a larger social network was associated with increased survival among men who had progressed to AIDS, but not among other HIV-infected men (Patterson *et al.*, 1996). In the second case, perceived social support interacted with CD4 T-cell levels, such that higher levels of perceived support was associated with less disease progression one year later only among men who were the most immunocompromised at the beginning of the study (Solano *et al.*, 1993).

Summary

Findings across three different chronic diseases provide suggestive evidence of a role for social ties in promoting physiological resilience to disease progression. Moderating factors such as disease severity or depression may influence the effectiveness of social relationship factors on physiological outcomes.

Promoting resilience through social relationship interventions

Despite the suggestive evidence that social relationships may play an important role in promoting psychological and physiological resilience in the face of chronic disease, there are surprisingly few experimental studies testing the possibility that interventions aimed at improving social relationships, either by increasing the diversity of individuals' social networks or by increasing their levels of perceived functional support, would be beneficial to persons with chronic diseases. Moreover, the intervention studies that do exist seldom draw inspiration from the evidence reported in the correlational literature described in the preceding sections. Specifically, while the correlational studies have found that characteristics of *natural social networks* were protective, intervention studies have generally manipulated support by facilitating interactions with strangers (Helgeson & Cohen, 1996; Cohen & Janicki-Deverts, 2009).

Psychological adjustment

Most of the intervention studies aimed at improving psychological adjustment to chronic disease have been carried out with cancer patients, comparing participation in therapy groups together with other cancer patients to usual care. Because the therapy is conducted in groups, these studies are generally referred to as tests of the effectiveness of social support. Evidence to support the effectiveness of social support interventions on psychological adjustment to cancer has been inconsistent (Helgeson & Cohen, 1996; Ross *et al.*, 2002), with recommendations for their use largely being tentative (Newell *et al.*, 2002). In many cases, studies that have demonstrated positive effects of social support on psychological adjustment have done so only for certain subsets of the studied populations. For example, results from a supportive–expressive group intervention trial found that patients with breast cancer who had been randomized to the support condition showed lower levels of negative affect following the intervention than women randomized to the control condition (Goodwin *et al.*, 2001). However, this association was qualified by a significant group-by-distress interaction such that only women reporting the highest levels of distress at baseline benefited from the support intervention. Similar evidence for social support benefiting only certain individuals is provided by two studies conducted by Helgeson and colleagues (Helgeson *et al.*, 2000, 2006). In the first study, women with early-stage breast cancer received benefit from support groups designed to provide informational and emotional support only if they were lacking strong external support networks (Helgeson *et al.*, 2000). In the second study,

which was conducted with patients with prostate cancer, only those men with the lowest self-esteem, the lowest prostate-specific self-efficacy, and the highest depression symptoms at baseline showed improved psychological adjustment after participating in a psychoeducational support group intervention (Helgeson *et al.*, 2006).

Physiological adjustment

Coronary heart disease

The very few studies that have attempted to curb CHD progression (i.e., recurrent cardiac event or mortality) by improving patients' perceptions of social support have, for the most part, been unsuccessful. One multisite trial in which nurses regularly called and visited patients to provide social support actually found *negative* effects of the intervention on women and no benefit to men (Frasure-Smith *et al.*, 1997). Another trial conducted with heart attack survivors used cognitive-behavioral therapy in an attempt to increase patients' perceptions of social support from existing natural networks (Berkman *et al.*, 2003). Although patients in the intervention group reported greater support than those in the control group, there was no effect on subsequent heart attacks or mortality.

Cancer

In regard to disease progression, although two early studies did find beneficial effects of group psychotherapy on cancer survival (Spiegel *et al.*, 1989; Fawzy *et al.*, 1993), this work has been criticized in terms of design and data interpretation (Fox, 1998; Coyne *et al.*, 2007). Moreover, more recent work (Ilnyckyj *et al.*, 1994; Cunningham *et al.*, 1998) including studies conducted at multiple sites with larger samples (Goodwin *et al.*, 2001; Spiegel *et al.*, 2007), failed to replicate the early results. Goodwin and colleagues (2001), for example, examined whether supportive–emotional group therapy would improve survival among women with metastatic breast cancer. Although the intervention improved mood among the women who were the most distressed at the beginning of the study, the intervention had no effect on length of survival (Goodwin *et al.*, 2001).

Human immunodeficiency virus

To date, only one published study has examined whether a social support intervention can influence disease progression among persons with HIV. Simoni and colleagues (2007) examined whether participation in a peer-support intervention would be associated with less-severe declines in immune function among HIV-positive patients who were receiving highly active antiretroviral therapy. The intervention influenced neither immune function nor the secondary outcomes of adherence to the therapy regimen and satisfaction with received social support. The null findings of this study are difficult to interpret. In the broadest sense, one might argue that, based on the findings of this study, social support interventions are not effective in attenuating HIV progression. However, because the intervention was not successful at improving patients' satisfaction with their social support, it cannot be known whether a more effective support intervention might have had a greater impact on HIV progression.

Summary

At present, evidence for social support interventions providing psychological and physiological benefits to persons with chronic disease is less than convincing. However, there are relatively few studies, and many of these may have employed inadequate interventions or failed to account for confounding influences. Given that voluntary social ties have been related more consistently to better psychological well-being than have obligatory ties (Helgeson & Cohen, 1996; Uchino, 2004), the contrived nature of social support manipulations may be the fundamental reason for their apparent lack of effectiveness. Consequently, developing and testing interventions designed to improve patients' existing social networks and perceptions of available support from existing networks seems the next logical step. However, with the exception of the study of Berkman *et al.* (2003), the effectiveness of interventions of this sort on improving psychological and physical outcomes among persons with chronic disease remains relatively unexplored.

Conclusions and future directions

Whether measured in terms of the size and diversity of one's social network or in terms of the specific resources provided by one's social network members, social relationships are associated with the promotion of resilience in persons with chronic diseases, as indicated by the beneficial effects of social ties on psychological and physiological adjustment. In contrast to the literature on social support and psychological distress among physically healthy persons, the association of social integration with main effects and social support with buffering effects appears not to be as reliable among persons with chronic disease. However, it is likely that tests for buffering effects may not be appropriate when examining the effects of social ties among persons with chronic disease, as all participants are experiencing high levels of stress associated with their illness.

Potential mechanisms through which social ties might influence adjustment include promotion of positive psychological states, encouragement of healthy behaviors and adherence to medical regimens, and attenuation of excessive physiological responses to stress. Though discussed separately, psychological, behavioral, and physiological pathways are far from mutually exclusive. One could envision a situation wherein the boost to self-esteem received from a supportive social network could motivate a cancer patient to engage in more health-promoting behaviors. Having a companion available to exercise with might encourage better adherence to an exercise regimen in a person with CHD. Appraisal support or even the perception that social support of any kind is available can act to reduce the perceived stressfulness associated with disease-related adversity, and this, in turn, could result in a dampening of physiological reactivity that otherwise might contribute to further progression of disease processes.

Although the association between social support and better adjustment is readily observed when support is naturally occurring, attempts at producing similar beneficial effects through social support interventions have largely been unsuccessful, particularly when physiological adjustment is the outcome of interest. Perhaps the key to improving the effects of support interventions is for future research to enhance the existing natural support resources of patients with chronic disease rather than to introduce new sources of support that may not be easily assimilated into these individuals' lives. Emphasis might be placed, for example, on encouraging chronically ill persons to recognize the breadth and diversity of their existing networks and the extent to which they feel they have been supported by network members *before* they became ill. Creating an association between social support resources and a time when ill persons were healthier may reduce potential losses in self-esteem often associated with receiving help, increase feelings of self-worth and self-efficacy, and ultimately promote resilience.

References

Allen, K. M., Blascovich, J., Tomaka, J., & Kelsey, M. (1991). Presence of human friends and pet dogs as moderators of autonomic responses to stress in women. *Journal of Personality and Social Psychology*, **61**, 582–589.

Anthony, J. L. & O' Brien, W. H. (1999). An evaluation of the impact of social support manipulations on cardiovascular reactivity to laboratory stressors. *Behavioral Medicine*, **25**, 78–87.

Barth, J., Schumacher, M., & Herrmann-Lingen, C. (2004). Depression as a risk factor for mortality in patients with coronary heart disease: A meta-analysis. *Psychosomatic Medicine*, **66**, 802–813.

Bennett, S. J., Perkins, K. A., Lane, K. A., *et al.* (2001). Social support and health-related quality of life in chronic heart failure patients. *Quality of Life Research*, **10**, 671–682.

Berkman, L. F. & Syme, L. S. (1979). Social networks, host resistance, and mortality: A nine-year follow-up study of Alameda County residents. *American Journal of Epidemiology*, **109**, 186–204.

Berkman, L. F., Blumenthal, J., Burg, M., *et al.* (2003). Effects of treating depression and low perceived social support on clinical events after myocardial infarction: The Enhancing Recovery in Coronary Heart Disease Patients (ENRICHD) randomized trial. *Journal of the American Medical Association*, **289**, 3106–3116.

Blaney, N. T., Goodkin, K., Morgan, R. O., *et al.* (1991). A stress-moderator model of distress in early HIV-1 infection: Concurrent analysis of life events, hardiness and social support. *Journal of Psychosomatic Research*, **35**, 297–305.

Bohachick, P., Taylor, M. V., Sereika, S., Reed, S., & Anton, B. B. (2002). Social support, personal control, and psychosocial recovery following heart transplantation. *Clinical Nursing Research*, **11**, 34–51.

Brissette, I., Cohen, S., & Seeman, T. E. (2000). Measuring social integration and social networks. In S. Cohen, L. Underwood, & B. Gottlieb (eds.), *Measuring and intervening in social support: A guide for social and health scientists* (pp. 53–85). New York: Oxford University Press.

Brummett, B. H., Babyak, M. A., Barefoot, J. C., *et al.* (1998). Social support and hostility as predictors of depressive symptoms in cardiac patients one month following hospitalization: A prospective study. *Psychosomatic Medicine*, **60**, 707–713.

Caplan, G. (1974). *Support systems and community mental health*. New York: Behavioral Publications.

Cassel, J. (1976). The contribution of the social environment to host resistance. *American Journal of Epidemiology*, **104**, 107–123.

Chesney, M. A., Chambers, D. B., Taylor, J. M., & Johnson, L. M. (2003). Social support, distress, and well-being in older men living with HIV infection. *Journal of Acquired Immunodeficiency Syndromes*, **33**(Suppl. 2), s185–s193.

Christenfeld, N., Gerin, W., Linden, W., & Pickering, T. G. (1997). Social support effects on cardiovascular reactivity: Is a stranger as effective as a friend? *Psychosomatic Medicine*, **59**, 388–398.

Cohen, S. (1988). Psychosocial models of social support in the etiology of physical disease. *Health Psychology*, 7, 269–297.

Cohen, S. (2004). Social relationships and health. *American Psychologist*, **59**, 676–684.

Cohen, S. & Janicki-Deverts, D. (2009). Can we improve our physical health by altering our social networks? *Perspectives in Psychological Science*, **4**, 375–378.

Cohen, S. & McKay, G. (1984). Social support, stress, and the buffering hypothesis: A theoretical analysis. In A. Baum, J. E. Singer, & S. E. Taylor (eds.), *Handbook of psychology and health*, Vol. IV (pp. 253–267). Hillsdale, NJ: Erlbaum.

Cohen, S. & Syme, S. L. (1985). Issues in the study and application of social support. In S. Cohen & S. L. Syme (eds.), *Social support and health* (pp. 3–22). San Diego, CA: Academic Press.

Cohen, S. & Wills, T. A. (1985). Stress, social support, and the buffering hypothesis. *Psychological Bulletin*, **98**, 310–357.

Cohen, S., Kaplan, J. R., & Manuck, S. B. (1994). Social support and coronary heart disease: Underlying psychologic and biologic mechanisms. In S. A. Shumaker & S. M. Czajkowski (eds.), *Social support and cardiovascular disease* (pp. 195–221). New York: Plenum Press.

Cohen, S., Doyle, W. J., Skoner, D. P., Rabin, B. S., & Gwaltney, J. M. Jr. (1997). Social ties and susceptibility to the common cold. *Journal of the American Medical Association*, **277**, 1940–1944.

Coyne, J. C., Stefanek, M., & Palmer, S. C. (2007). Psychotherapy and survival in cancer: The conflict between hope and evidence. *Psychological Bulletin*, **133**, 367–394.

Crothers, M. K., Tomter, H. D., & Garske, J. P. (2005). The relationships between satisfaction with social support, affect balance, and hope in cancer patients. *Journal of Psychosocial Oncology*, **23**, 103–118.

Cunningham, A. J., Edmonds, C. V., Jenkins, G. P., *et al.* (1998). A randomized controlled trial of the effects of group psychological therapy on survival in women with metastatic breast cancer. *Psycho-Oncology*, 7, 508–517.

Cutrona, C. E. & Russell, D. W. (1990). Type of social support and specific stress: Toward a theory of optimal matching. In I. G. Sarason, B. R. Sarason, & G. R. Pierce (eds.), *Social support: An interactional view* (pp. 319–366). New York: Wiley.

DiMatteo, M. R. (2004). Social support and patient adherence to medical treatment: A meta-analysis. *Health Psychology*, **23**, 207–218.

Duits, A. A., Boeke, S., Taams, M. A., Passchier, J., & Erdman, R. A. (1997). Prediction of quality of life after coronary artery bypass graft surgery: A review and evaluation of multiple, recent studies. *Psychosomatic Medicine*, **59**, 257–268.

Dunn, G. P., Bruce, A. T., Ikeda, H., Old, L. J., & Schreiber, R. D. (2002). Cancer immunoediting: From immunosurveillance to tumor escape. *Nature Immunology*, **3**, 991–998.

Durkheim, E. (1951). *Suicide*. New York: Free Press (originally published in 1897).

Fawzy, F. I., Fawzy, N. W., Hyun, C. S., *et al.* (1993). Malignant melanoma: Effects of an early structured psychiatric intervention, coping, and affective state on recurrence and survival 6 years later. *Archives of General Psychiatry*, **50**, 681–689.

Fox, B. H. (1998). A hypothesis about Spiegel *et al.*'s 1989 paper on psychosocial intervention and breast cancer survival. *Psycho-Oncology*, **7**, 361–370.

Frasure-Smith, N., Lesperance, F., & Talajic, M. (1993). Depression following myocardial infarction. *Journal of the American Medical Association*, **270**, 1819–1825.

Frasure-Smith, N., Lesperance, F., Prince, R. H., *et al.* (1997). Randomised trial of home-based psychosocial nursing intervention for patients recovering from myocardial infarction. *Lancet*, **350**, 473–479.

Frasure-Smith, N., Lesperance, F., Gravel, G., *et al.* (2000). Social support, depression, and mortality during the first year after myocardial infarction. *Circulation*, **101**, 1919–1924.

Gallant, M. P. (2003). The influence of social support on chronic illness self-management: A review and directions for research. *Health Education and Behavior*, **30**, 170–195.

Glaser, R., Kiecolt-Glaser, J. K., Bonneau, R., Malarkey, W., & Hughes, J. (1992). Stress-induced modulation of the immune response to recombinant hepatitis B vaccine. *Psychosomatic Medicine*, **54**, 22–29.

Glynn, L. M., Christenfeld, N., & Gerin, W. (1999). Gender, social support, and cardiovascular responses to stress. *Psychosomatic Medicine*, **61**, 234–242.

Goodwin, P. J., Leszcz, M., Ennis, M., *et al.* (2001). The effect of group psychosocial support on survival in metastatic breast cancer. *New England Journal of Medicine*, **345**, 1719–1726.

Grewen, K. M., Girdler, S. S., Amico, J., & Light, K. C. (2005). Effects of partner support on resting oxytocin, cortisol, norepinephrine, and blood pressure before and after warm partner contact. *Psychosomatic Medicine*, **67**, 531–538.

Hays, R. B., Turner, H., & Coates, T. J. (1992). Social support, AIDS-related symptoms, and depression among gay men. *Journal of Consulting and Clinical Psychology*, **60**, 463–469.

Helgeson, V. S. & Cohen, S. (1996). Social support and adjustment to cancer: Reconciling descriptive, correlational, and intervention research, *Health Psychology*, **15**, 135–148.

Helgeson, V. S., Cohen, S., & Fritz, H. L. (1998). Social ties and cancer. In J. C. Holland & W. Breitbart (eds.), *Psycho-Oncology* (pp. 99–109). New York: Oxford University Press.

Helgeson, V. S., Cohen, S., Schulz, R., & Yasko, J. (2000). Group support interventions for women with breast cancer: Who benefits from what? *Health Psychology*, **19**, 107–114.

Helgeson, V. S., Snyder, P., & Seltman, H. (2004). Psychological and physical adjustment to breast cancer over 4 years: Identifying distinct trajectories of change. *Health Psychology*, **23**, 3–15.

Helgeson, V. S., Lepore, S. J., & Eton, D. T. (2006). Moderators of the benefits of psychoeducational interventions for men with prostate cancer. *Health Psychology*, **25**, 348–354.

House, J. S. (1981). *Work stress and social support*. Reading, MA: Addison-Wesley.

House, J. S. & Kahn, R. L. (1985). Measures and concepts of social support. In S. Cohen & S. L. Syme (eds.), *Social support and health* (pp. 83–108). New York: Academic Press.

House, J. S., Landis, K. R., & Umberson, D. (1988). Social relationships and health. *Science*, **241**, 540–545.

Ilnyckyj, A., Farber, J., Cheang, M., & Weinerman, B. (1994). A randomized controlled trial of psychotherapeutic intervention in cancer patients. *Annals of the Royal College of Physicians and Surgeons of Canada*, **272**, 93–96.

Ironson, G. & Hayward, H. (2008). Do positive psychosocial factors predict disease progression in HIV-1? *Psychosomatic Medicine*, **70**, 546–554.

Johnson, J. G., Alloy, L. B., Panzarella, C., *et al.* (2001). Hopelessness as a mediator of the association between social support and depressive symptoms: Findings of a study of men with HIV. *Journal of Consulting and Clinical Psychology*, **69**, 1056–1060.

Kamarck, T. W., Manuck, S. B., & Jennings, J. R. (1990). Social support reduces cardiovascular reactivity to psychological challenge: A laboratory model. *Psychosomatic Medicine*, **52**, 42–58.

Kamarck, T. W., Annunziato, B., & Amateau, L. M. (1995). Affiliation moderates the effects of social threat on stress-related cardiovascular responses: Boundary conditions for a laboratory model of social support. *Psychosomatic Medicine*, **57**, 183–194.

Kamarck, T. W., Peterman, A. H., & Raynor, D. A. (1998). The effects of the social environment on stress-related cardiovascular activation: Current findings, prospects, and implications. *Annals of Behavioral Medicine*, **20**, 247–256.

Knip, M. & Siljander, H. (2008). Autoimmune mechanisms in type 1 diabetes. *Autoimmunity Reviews*, 7, 550–557.

Kroenke, C. H., Kubzansky, L. D., Schernhammer, M. D., Holmes, M. D., & Kawachi, I. (2006). Social networks, social support, and survival after breast cancer diagnosis. *Journal of Clinical Oncology*, **24**, 1105–1111.

Lett, H. S., Blumenthal, J. A., Babyak, M. A., *et al.* (2005). Social support and coronary heart disease: Epidemiologic evidence and implications for treatment. *Psychosomatic Medicine*, **67**, 869–878.

Lett, H. S., Blumenthal, J. A., Babyak, M. A., *et al.* (2007). Social support and prognosis in patients at increased psychosocial risk recovering from myocardial infarction. *Health Psychology*, **26**, 418–427.

Levine, J. B., Covino, N. A., Slack, W. V., *et al.* (1996). Psychological predictors of subsequent medical care among patients hospitalized with cardiac disease. *Journal of Cardiopulmonary Rehabilitation*, **16**, 109–116.

Libby, P. (2002). Atherosclerosis: The new view. *Scientific American*, **286**, 47–55.

Luthar, S. S. (2006). Resilience in development: A synthesis of research across five decades. In D. Cicchetti & D. J. Cohen (eds.), *Developmental psychopathology, Vol. 3: Risk, disorder, and adaptation*, 2nd edn (pp. 740–795). New York: Wiley.

Manuck, S. B. (1994). Cardiovascular reactivity in cardiovascular disease: "Once more unto the breach." *International Journal of Behavioral Medicine*, **1**, 4–31.

McEwen, B. S. (2007). Physiology and neurobiology of stress and adaptation: Central role of the brain. *Physiological Reviews*, **87**, 873–904.

McEwen, B. S. & Stellar, E. (1993). Stress and the individual. Mechanisms leading to disease. *Archives of Internal Medicine*, **153**, 2093–2101.

Newell, S. A., Sanson-Fisher, R. W., & Savolainen, N. J. (2002). Systematic review of psychological therapies for cancer patients: Overview and recommendations for future research. *Journal of the National Cancer Institute*, **94**, 558–584.

Pakenham, K. I., Dadds, M. R., & Terry, D. J. (1994). Relationships between adjustment to HIV and both social support and coping. *Journal of Consulting and Clinical Psychology*, **62**, 1194–1203.

Park, C. L. & Gaffey, A. E. (2007). Relationships between psychosocial factors and health behavior change in cancer survivors: An integrative review. *Annals of Behavioral Medicine*, **34**, 115–134.

Patterson, T. L., Shaw, W. S., Semple, S. J., *et al.* (1996). Relationship of psychosocial factors to HIV disease progression. *Annals of Behavioral Medicine*, **18**, 30–39.

Pinto, B. M. & Trunzo, J. J. (2005). Health behaviors during and after a cancer diagnosis. *Cancer*, **104**(Suppl. 11), 2614–2623.

Pressman, S. D., Cohen, S., Miller, G. E., *et al.* (2005). Loneliness, social network size, and immune response to influenza vaccination in college freshmen. *Health Psychology*, **24**, 297–306.

Ross, L., Boesen, E., Dalton, S., & Johansen, C. (2002). Mind and cancer. Does psychosocial intervention improve survival and psychological well-being? *European Journal of Cancer*, **38**, 1447–1457.

Roy, M. P., Steptoe, A., & Kirschbaum, C. (1998). Life events and social support as moderators of individual differences in cardiovascular and cortisol reactivity. *Journal of Personality and Social Psychology*, **75**, 1273–1281.

Rozanski, A., Bairey, N., Krantz, D. S., *et al.* (1988). Mental stress and the induction of silent myocardial ischemia in patients with coronary artery disease. *New England Journal of Medicine*, **318**, 1005–1012.

Sayers, S. L., Riegel, B., Pawlowski, S., Coyne, J. C., & Samaha, F. F. (2008). Social support and self-care of patients with heart failure. *Annals of Behavioral Medicine*, **35**, 70–79.

Schroevers, M. J., Ranchor, A. V., & Sanderman, R. (2003). The role of social support and self-esteem in the presence and course of depressive symptoms: A comparison of cancer patients and individuals from the general population. *Social Science and Medicine*, **57**, 375–385.

Schulz, U. & Mohamed, N. E. (2004). Turning the tide: Benefit finding after cancer surgery. *Social Science and Medicine*, **59**, 653–662.

Seeman, T. E. & McEwen, B. S. (1996). Impact of social environment characteristics on neuroendocrine regulation. *Psychosomatic Medicine*, **58**, 459–471.

Seeman, T. E., Berkman, L. F., Blazer, D., *et al.* (1994). Social ties and support and neuroendocrine function, MacArthur Studies of Successful Aging. *Annals of Behavioral Medicine*, **16**, 95–106.

Simoni, J. M., Pantalone, D. W., Plummer, M. D., & Huang, B. (2007). A randomized controlled trial of a peer support intervention targeting antiretroviral medication adherence and depressive symptomatology in HIV-positive men and women. *Health Psychology*, **26**, 488–495.

Solano, L., Costa, M., Salvati, S., *et al.* (1993). Psychosocial factors and clinical evolution in HIV-infection: A longitudinal study. *Journal of Psychosomatic Research*, **37**, 39–51.

Spiegel, D., Bloom, J., Kraemer, H., & Gottheil, E. (1989). Effect of psychosocial treatment on survival of patients with metastatic breast cancer. *Lancet*, **ii**, 888–891.

Spiegel, D., Butler, L. D., Giese-Davis, J., *et al.* (2007). Effects of supportive-expressive group therapy on survival of patients with metastatic breast cancer: A randomized prospective trial. *Cancer*, **110**, 1130–1138.

Thoits, P. A. (1985). Social support processes and psychological well-being: Theoretical possibilities. In I. G. Sarason & B. Sarason (eds.), *Social support: Theory, research, and applications* (pp. 51–72). The Hague: Martinus Nijhoff.

Thoits, P. A. (1986). Social support as coping assistance. *Journal of Consulting and Clinical Psychology*, **54**, 416–423.

Thombs, B. D., Bass, E. B., Ford, D. E., *et al.* (2006). Prevalence of depression in survivors of acute myocardial infarction. *Journal of General Internal Medicine*, **21**, 30–38.

Turner-Cobb, J. M., Sephton, S. E., Koopman, C., Blake-Mortimer, J., & Spiegel D. (2000). Social support and salivary cortisol in women with metastatic breast cancer. *Psychosomatic Medicine*, **62**, 337–345.

Uchino, B. N. (2004). *Social support and physical health: Understanding the health consequences of relationships* (pp. 9–32). New Haven, CT: Yale University Press.

Uchino, B. N. (2006). Social support and health: A review of physiological processes potentially underlying links to disease outcomes. *Journal of Behavioral Medicine*, **29**, 377–387.

Uchino, B. N., Cacioppo, J. T., & Kiecolt-Glaser, J. K. (1996). The relationship between social support and physiological processes: A review with emphasis on underlying mechanisms and implications for health. *Psychological Bulletin*, **119**, 488–531.

Chapter

6

Religious and spiritual factors in resilience

David W. Foy, Kent D. Drescher, and Patricia J. Watson

Introduction

This chapter will examine how religion/spirituality plays an important role as a resource used by most people in coping with the immediate, as well as longer-term, consequences of highly stressful or traumatic experiences. First, working definitions of the key concepts of resilience and religion/spirituality will be given. Distinctions are made between definitions for general communications and operational definitions suitable for clinical and research purposes. Spirituality is conceptualized as a dynamic process that is an integral and inseparable part of humanity. A current conceptual model of spirituality as being multidimensional in nature is presented, and core dimensions are described. Findings from a selective review of current studies on religion and/or spirituality and resilience are presented. Four key obstacles, or "spiritual red flags," are identified, and a group therapy module for addressing them is presented. Finally, conclusions about our current knowledge, as well as recommendations for future clinical and research applications are made.

Spirituality is acknowledged as an important part of life by most individuals. Annual Gallup polls consistently show that more than 90% of the US population report a "belief in God," and approximately 70% report affiliation with a faith community and attending religious services. In addition, religion or spirituality has been consistently linked to positive mental (Nooney & Woodrum, 2002) and physical (Powell *et al.*, 2003) health functioning, as well as increased longevity (Oxman *et al.*, 1995). When mental health services are sought, clergy are most frequently the first point of contact, with more than 40% seeking counseling from them rather than mental health providers (Weaver *et al.*, 1997). In the immediate aftermath of the terrorist

attacks of September 11 2001, more than 90% of those surveyed reported that they coped by "turning to religion," second only to "talking with others," which was endorsed by 98% (Schuster *et al.*, 2001). However, despite the widely recognized positive aspects of religion or spirituality, there are large gaps in our scientific knowledge of the dynamic processes of spirituality that could explain these relationships.

As a starting point, promising areas for empirical inquiry have been identified. It has been suggested that spirituality offers a positive meaning-making framework for coping (Park, 2005). In addition, enhanced social support and effective cognitive processing of stressful events have also been proposed as mechanisms by which one's spirituality might be involved (McIntosh *et al.*, 1993).

General definitions of religion/spirituality and resilience

Religion has long been a topic of discussion and research within the field of psychology, dating back to William James' writings in the twentieth century (James, 1997). Pargament, a prominent researcher in the field, has put forth a brief and powerful definition of religion as, "a search for significance in ways related to the sacred" (Pargament, 1997). Relatedly, Larson and colleagues (1997), defined spirituality as the "multidimensional space in which everyone can be located." A core element of transcendence is found in these definitions for both religion and spirituality. A definition of spirituality that we have found useful in clinical work is that of Drescher and colleagues (2004): "an individual's understanding of, experience with, and connection to that which transcends the self." In popular usage, distinctions are often made such that many people may profess to be "spiritual, but not religious." An individual's

---

spirituality may be realized in a religious context or it may be highly personalized and entirely distinct from religion of any sort. Of the two, spirituality is broader and more individual, while religion contains within it the element of a shared understanding within a group/community context.

One way of seeing religion might be as a corporate/community expression of individual spiritual experience. Our preferred definition of religion is "a system of beliefs, values, rituals, and practices shared in common by a social community as a means of experiencing and connecting with the sacred or divine" (Drescher *et al.*, 2004). While there are meaningful distinctions between religion and spirituality, and while they are not synonymous, there is also much overlap. Accordingly, for purposes of this chapter, religion and spirituality will be considered as a single construct, religion/spirituality (RS).

Resilience generally refers to the human ability to withstand stressful challenges and retain or regain normal functioning. Consequently, individuals display resilience when they manifest positive adaptation under extenuating circumstances. The American Psychological Association Task Force on Promoting Resilience in Response to Terrorism defines it as "the process of adapting well in the face of adversity, trauma, tragedy, threats, or even significant sources of stress." It is generally accepted that resilience is common and derives from the basic human ability to adapt to new situations (Masten, 2001).

Spirituality and resilience as dynamic processes

Individuals' experiences of RS are often described as part of a "spiritual journey" that involves a lifelong quest for meaning and direction. A physical journey is dynamic because it occurs across both space and time. Similarly, a spiritual journey occurs throughout the course of a person's life, across whatever stages of physical or emotional development that occur, and it may involve multiple and changing dimensions of spiritual experience. From a research perspective, this means a unidimensional measurement of spirituality captured during a cross-sectional (i.e., single time point) period of data collection may miss an enormous wealth of information about the interaction of individual life history and spirituality, some of which may be predictive of important outcomes in the physical, emotional, or psychological arenas. Recently, a

six-stage model of spiritual development has been described (Hagberg & Guelich, 2005) that identifies the following key stages:

Stage 1: The recognition of the divine or transcendence
Stage 2: Joining the religious or spiritual community
Stage 3: Leading the community
Stage 4: Inward journey, re-evaluation of personal spirituality
Stage 5: Journey outward, reclaim service based on internal connection
Stage 6: Life of connection to divine.

In using this model, it should not be assumed that stages are attained in a straightforward, linear fashion. Rather, the starting point, movement in a forward or backward direction, and the ultimate end point, may vary from person to person depending on biological limiting factors, familial and relational history, life experiences, and, probably, other factors.

During the first stage, there is the initial connection with God or the divine, where the sense of awe and divine sovereignty is experienced. Learning the language, beliefs, and traditions of a faith community compose key elements of the second stage. The third stage involves personal productivity within the faith community, often including teaching and other service roles. Re-examining personal beliefs and connection with the divine characterize the "inward journey," or fourth stage. Maturing in spiritual development marks the final two stages, during which individuals may reassess and internalize their connections to the divine. In these later stages, relationships with religious communities may be re-evaluated and redefined in ways that reflect and promote more mature spirituality, reaching beyond narrow constraints dictated by a faith community. Along the course of individuals' spiritual journeys, life experiences represent opportunities for challenge and doubt, as well as meaning and support, and these experiences are well documented across both Western and Eastern traditions (Eriksson, 2008).

The varying facets of trauma exposure include (1) the nature and intensity of the trauma (i.e., natural versus human caused, intentional versus accidental), (2) the personal risk and resilience characteristics of the victim, (3) the emotional and instrumental support context before, during, and after the event, and (4) the level of predictability and controllability perceived by the victim. These facets may all interact differently with the victim's spirituality depending on the stage of spiritual development and on the available spiritual support and familiar spiritual coping behaviors utilized. This interaction will then produce unique appraisals about the trauma itself and the individual's degree of self-efficacy in managing its effects, and it may result in varying levels of need to reconstruct core beliefs, values, meanings, and assumptions about the world and the individual's place in it. The ultimate impact of the trauma may lead to either maturation or disintegration of the person's spiritual development, which may, in turn, result in either resilient personal growth or development of physical or psychological difficulties.

Resilience is also currently conceptualized in a more dynamic perspective (e.g., Richardson, 2002). The study of resilience has evolved through three phases of inquiry, starting with a basic search for resilient qualities: that is those traits, assets, and protective factors associated with positive outcomes. A second phase introduced a dynamic view that featured resilience as both a disruptive and a re-integrative process that involves using resilient qualities. The third phase (current) defines resilience as "the force that drives a person to grow through adversity and disruptions" (Richardson, 2002).

Many empirical studies of resilience exemplify the first phase in attempting to identify qualities that distinguish resilient from non-resilient individuals in the wake of a destabilizing experience. Well-designed longitudinal studies of high-risk children in diverse geographic locations have been very influential in identifying characteristics of resilient individuals (Werner, 1982; Rutter, 1985; Garmezy, 1991). More recently, studies in the field of positive psychology have identified several RS-related factors associated with resilience, including morality and self-control (Baumeister & Exline, 2000), forgiveness (McCullough, 2000), and hope (Snyder, 2000).

Developmentally, resilience is not fixed in time and is not exhibited in the same way at different developmental stages. For example, resilient toddlers would show behaviors that reflect mastery of that psychosocial stage of development, such as a strong autonomy as well as secure attachment to their mothers, whereas resilient school-age children would show a capacity to master educational skills and interact well with their peers and adults in the school setting. Furthermore, resilient adolescents would show facility with multiple roles and activities and a strong self-image in the face of peer pressure. Children might excel at a given point in time, but with trauma, continuing adversities, or without adequate supports to deal with such occurrences, they can show developmental deterioration or gaps in key resilient capacities that continue throughout life (Rutter, 1998).

While developmental approaches view current adaptive capacities as a function of an individual's history of successful adaptations to stressful conditions (i.e., successful coping with earlier mild stressors can serve to inoculate children against the effects of later major stressors), contextual factors play an equally large role in producing positive outcomes. For example, high-competence children raised in high-risk environments do worse than low-competence children raised in low-risk environments (Sameroff et al., 1998). Therefore, resilience is also a function of the family's ability, and other aspects of the social environment's ability, to buffer the effects of high-risk, adverse circumstances. For example, a core theme in resilient children under diverse risk conditions is the presence of a strong, supportive relationship with at least one adult that shows a sustained degree of continuity and consistency (Werner, 2000). While resilience is not "fixed" forever, in order to achieve and sustain resilient adaptation, children must receive support from adults in their environments.

Not surprisingly, this finding is reflected as well in the literature on spiritual development, with a number of studies showing a relationship between early attachment to primary caregivers and later quality of relationship with God. Whereas secure attachments tend to lead to stronger, more positive internalized images of God, insecure attachments in childhood lead to either an insecure attachment to God or a need to depend on God strongly under adverse situations (Hall, 2007). Garbarino and Bedard (1996, p. 467) additionally described that "the experience of childhood traumatization functions as a kind of 'reverse religious experience', a process combining overwhelming arousal and overwhelming cognitions that threatens core 'meaningfulness' for the child" and can create spiritual crisis. This trauma can conceivably impact the child's resilience primarily in the mastery of tasks at their particular developmental stage. For example, trauma literature emphasizes that very early childhood trauma has the most profound effects on trust. However, the type and extent of the trauma, if severe enough, can also overwhelm and deteriorate previously mastered stages (Perry & Pollard, 1998; Anda et al., 2006). The recent convergence in developmental research on competence, resilience, trauma, behavioral and emotional problems, brain development, and prevention science underscores the importance for building resilience into human development in multiple stages, levels, and contexts: within the child, the family, the community, and their interactions. Young children who have attachment bonds with competent and loving caregivers, the stimulation and nutrition required for healthy brain development, opportunities to learn and experience the pleasure of mastering new skills, and the limit setting or structure needed to develop self-control typically manifest resilience in the face of adversity, as long as their fundamental protective skills and relationships continue to operate and develop (Luthar, 2005).

Certain types of trauma, as well as unique aspects of the traumatic experience, may create developmental barriers to resilience. Early childhood abuse, for example, particularly when perpetrated within the family, can dramatically change a child's ability to engage in future loving and trusting relationships, and thus diminish the possibility of the social support needed for resilient responding. Such trauma can also damage the child's view of him/herself as a worthwhile and competent person and thus impair the ability to experience self-confidence and ultimately resilience. Traumas that involve personal violation such as rape and battering can also damage self-esteem and self-efficacy. Combat is unique as a traumatic experience in that it involves not only direct experience of trauma and witnessing but also calls for inflicting trauma upon an enemy. These combat-specific factors can introduce strong elements of guilt and shame, which may warp an individual's self-esteem and cause them to withdraw from social relationships.

The process by which resilience is achieved has been the focus of many studies, from which five key factors have been identified. The findings of these studies show that primary factors in resilience are (1) caring relationships within and outside the family that create love and trust, provide role models, and encourage and reassure; (2) the capacity to make realistic plans and implement them; (3) self-confidence; (4) communication and problem-solving skills; and (5) the capacity to manage emotions (Masten, 2001).

It is notable that RS presents aspects that are easily found in each of the five resilience factors. For example, scientists have recently begun to map the brain regions related to both well-being and positive emotions such as empathy. They have found that individuals evidencing tonic left frontal activation are more apt than individuals showing tonic right frontal activation to "organize limited resources in support of goal-approaching behaviors" (Sutton & Davidson, 1997). They also suggest that taking an active role in life and appropriately engaging sources of motivation, behaviors that are characteristic of those involved in active religious and spiritual programs, may contribute to higher levels of well-being, sense of meaning, and self-confidence (Urry et al., 2004). Moreover, they have found that seasoned Buddhist monks who are meditating on compassion while hooked up to electroencephalography sensors show a striking increase in gamma waves in the left prefrontal cortex, an area correlated with reported feelings of well-being (Lutz et al., 2004). When applying these findings to a training program, they found that workers in a high-technology company who took a two-month training program in meditation showed significant changes in brain activity, declines in anxiety, beneficial changes in immune function, as well as positive impact on emotional regulation (Davidson et al., 2003). Along another line, research has shown that caring relationships, such as those found among members of faith communities, can provide essential social support in recovery from life crises (Charuvastra & Cloitre, 2008).

Multidimensional representation of religion/spirituality

Major obstacles in the advancement of the scientific study of RS have included lack of interest in RS as a primary study variable by researchers, and, in the relatively few studies that did include it as a variable, the use of non-standard, single-item measures of RS. Reviews of studies published during the 1980s and 1990s found that only 1–3% of scholarly journal articles in psychology, psychiatry, and medicine included spiritual variables (Larson et al., 1986; Weaver et al., 1997). Additionally, within this small body of literature, the majority of studies utilized ad hoc, non-standard RS measures, or used a single item as the measure of religious or spiritual experience. These limitations constrict scientific study of RS by impeding replication of findings across studies through problems with basic measurement.

To address these measurement limitations, a national work group was formed, with its members selected because of their expertise and prominence in measurement of religious or spiritual constructs. The group was supported by the Fetzer Institute in collaboration with the National Institute of Aging, part of the US National Institutes of Health. Based on the consensus that RS was best represented as a multidimensional construct, the group developed a measure, the Brief Multidimensional Measure of Religion/Spirituality (BMMRS), which taps into 12 domains of religion and spirituality that have been empirically linked to mental and physical health. These domains include daily spiritual experience, meaning, values, beliefs, forgiveness, private religious practices, RS coping, religious support, RS history, commitment, organizational religiousness, and religious preference. During the creation of the measure, care was taken in conceptualization and wording to maximize its potential use with a wide variety of religious groups. Whenever possible, use of the specific term God was avoided. When it was unavoidable, the instructions direct individuals uncomfortable with the term God to replace it with their own transcendent or higher power. Preliminary studies support the theoretical basis for the BMMRS and indicate acceptable findings for its measures of reliability and validity. What remains is for future studies to use it to improve understanding of the complex relationship between religion, spirituality, and adjustment or health (Idler *et al.*, 2003).

Selective review of studies on religion/spirituality and resilience

While the study of RS and resilience is still in an early phase of development, there have been a growing number of studies represented in the literature since the late 1990s. Here we will focus initially on findings from a meta-analytic study (Ano & Vasconcelles, 2005) that incorporated results from 49 studies meeting inclusion criteria from the 109 studies initially identified. In this study, Pargament's (1997) model of religious coping was used to distinguish between positive and negative uses of RS to deal with life crises. Ten positive strategies were identified, ranging from forgiveness and seeking spiritual direction, to finding spiritual connection and benevolent religious reappraisal. Examples of negative strategies included spiritual discontent, demonic reappraisal, passive deferral, interpersonal religious discontent, and reappraisal of God's powers. Psychological adjustment was also dichotomized into positive and negative categories. Examples of positive indicators included acceptance, emotional

well-being, hope, happiness, self-esteem and quality of life. Measures for negative adjustment ranged from anxiety, depression, and symptoms of post-traumatic stress disorder (PTSD) to social dysfunction, suicidality, and trait anger.

Bivariate correlations between religious coping (positive and negative) measures and psychological adjustment (positive and negative) were averaged to obtain effect size estimates for findings for the four key relationships: positive religious coping and positive adjustment; positive coping and negative adjustment; negative coping and positive adjustment; and negative coping and negative adjustment. The strongest average effect size estimate (0.33) was obtained for the 29 studies examining the relationship between positive coping and positive adjustment. From 38 studies examining correlations between positive coping and negative adjustment, a small, yet significant, effect size estimate of −0.12 was obtained. For the 16 studies of negative coping and positive adjustment, a non-significant effect size estimate (0.02) was found. Finally, the 22 studies of negative coping and negative adjustment produced a significant moderate effect size estimate of 0.22. Taken together, findings from this meta-analysis (Ano & Vasconcelles, 2005) showed that both forms of religious coping are related to psychological adjustment to stress. Positive religious coping is related to both positive and negative forms of adjustment in the directions expected, whereas negative coping is only significantly related to negative adjustment.

Findings from more recent studies were consistent with those of Ano and Vasconcelles (2005). For example, a study of help-seeking military veterans found significant associations between lack of forgiveness (along with negative religious coping) and worse mental health outcomes (PTSD and depression) (Witvliet *et al.*, 2004). Similarly, loss of faith was found to be associated with worse mental health outcomes (i.e., greater utilization of mental health services) among military veterans in treatment for PTSD (Fontana & Rosenheck, 2004). Most recently still, in a study of religiously active trauma survivors, positive relationships were found between a measure of positive religious coping, seeking spiritual support, and post-traumatic growth. In the same study, a negative religious coping indicator, religious strain, was significantly related to post-traumatic symptoms (Harris *et al.*, 2008). Therefore, there is consistency of findings of a complex relationship between religious coping and psychological adjustment following stress, such that positive religious coping is related to both positive adjustment and lower levels of negative adjustment, while negative religious coping is related to negative adjustment.

Spiritual "red flags"

Under ideal circumstances, one's spiritual beliefs and practices would be ready resources in coping with life crises. They would help to buffer the immediate effects of severely stressful experiences, promote cognitive processing of their meaning, and facilitate finding their appropriate place in one's life narrative. Unfortunately, surviving trauma often results in shattering of adaptive illusions and sustaining beliefs, along with intense emotions and arousal, and an endangered sense of agency and control. Survivors may feel like strangers to themselves and the world around them. The very core or sustaining elements of the self may have been severely threatened. Consequently, key aspects of survivors' spirituality may become casualties of the traumatic experience, rendering them unavailable for use as coping resources.

Given the findings regarding negative religious coping and negative psychological adjustment, what elements of spirituality may be responsible for this relationship? The use of the term spiritual "red flags" dates back to a seminal study by Pargament and colleagues (1998). In their original study, three problematic domains or "red flags" were identified in the context of religious coping with life crises: choosing inappropriate goals or ends, using inappropriate means, and conflict with one's spiritual beliefs and values. In their original terminology, "wrong direction," "wrong road," and "against the wind" were used to describe the "red flags" (Pargament *et al.*, 1998). Here we have extended the use of the term to refer to four specific RS-related obstacles or difficulties frequently encountered by trauma survivors during their recovery (Drescher & Foy, 2008). These obstacles may be problematic as RS issues per se, and/or they may impede progress toward more general psychological trauma processing and recovery. The "red flags" we have identified are loss of faith, negative religious coping, guilt, and lack of forgiveness. These indices of spiritual struggling or "stuck points" are empirically based, having been identified by studies of trauma survivors, many of which were cited in the previous section of this chapter.

Loss of faith refers to a crisis-related reaction that initially involves confusion or disillusionment about one's spiritual beliefs in light of the significant life crisis just encountered. When the experience cannot be readily assimilated by the individual's existing cognitive interpretive framework or schema, then accommodation, or change in the schema, is required. Frequently, individuals resolve such a spiritual struggle by over-accommodation, a process of discarding or setting aside their previously held spiritual beliefs. In the short term, the cognitive conflict is resolved; however, a longer-term consequence is the loss of the positive coping potential found in spiritual beliefs and faith practices. Among combat veterans in treatment for PTSD, "difficulty reconciling my faith with combat experiences" was endorsed by more than 75% of respondents (Drescher & Foy, 1995).

Negative religious coping, as we have used the term, is characterized by questions or tensions about God's presence, power, and character; strong anger at God; discontent with one's faith community and its clergy; and punitive appraisals of negative experiences (e.g., God is punishing me for my sins) (Drescher & Foy, 2008).

Guilt is represented in three forms: acts of commission, acts of omission, and survivor guilt experienced when others are killed and the survivor is spared. Survivor guilt often involves unresolved issues of perceived randomness and fairness, as well as the persistent belief that others who died were more deserving of life or had more to live for. In addition, cognitive distortions about the degree of personal culpability for tragic outcomes are often critical elements that may serve to exacerbate and perpetuate this particular spiritual "red flag."

Lack of forgiveness represents the inability to positively resolve perceptions of having forgiven others, feeling forgiven by God, and having forgiven oneself for acts of omission or commission related to life experiences with tragic outcomes. As noted above, lack of forgiveness has been found to be associated with more severe PTSD and depression among combat veterans in treatment for PTSD (Witvliet *et al.*, 2004). The four "red flags" often co-occur and so they are more frequently found in combination than in isolation (Drescher & Foy, 2008). In a sense, trauma survivors who exhibit spiritual "red flags" may appear to be "stuck" or "derailed" in their journey of trauma processing and recovery.

Spirituality group therapy module

What systematic efforts have been made to address the spiritual "red flags" found so frequently among trauma survivors receiving mental health services? A concerted effort has been made to develop a standardized group therapy or modular approach to incorporate RS issues into combat PTSD treatment (Drescher *et al.*, 2004). The Trauma and Spirituality group at the Menlo Park treatment program, under the auspices of the US Department of Veterans Affairs (VA), has its roots in the rich clinical expertise of highly experienced psychotherapists in that program working with combat veterans with PTSD. The Menlo Park program features a group therapy approach, employing a variety of therapy groups aimed at the specific treatment and rehabilitation issues presented by many veterans with chronic PTSD. Earlier experiences in other treatment groups had shown that many veterans expressed a great deal of rage when religious or spiritual topics were mentioned. Some veterans reported feeling that military chaplains had deceived or let them down during their war zone service, and consequently, they had been reticent to seek counsel from VA chaplains or other clergy since then. Data collected in the PTSD residential program indicated that 74% of residents reported having difficulty reconciling their religious beliefs with the traumatic events they saw and experienced in the war zone and 51% reported that they abandoned their religious faith in the war zone (Drescher & Foy, 1995). Consequently, several spirituality-related issues relevant to treatment had been identified that were not being addressed by other treatment groups.

Pilot work on the Trauma and Spirituality Group Module began in 2000. The format was designed to balance educational presentation of content with group discussion and interactive small-group opportunities to enhance interpersonal sharing among the members. A guiding principle in designing the group experience was that it would be a forum for the safe discussion and interpersonal processing of difficult and emotionally laden issues related to spirituality, broadly defined. In that respect, it was to be different from other groups in the program that relied upon a psychoeducational format (i.e., teaching "correct" ways to view relevant issues). In order to standardize group procedures, the plan was to develop a manual set (module) consisting of a facilitator's guide, a member's workbook, and an evaluation packet.

Throughout the pilot testing process, several main themes emerged, from which the current eight sessions in the module were drawn.

- What is spirituality? How can I find connection within and beyond myself?
- Theodicy: how does one think about God and the world around after trauma?
- Forgiveness: of self and others; feeling forgiven by God.
- Pursuit of what matters. Where do I find my values?
- How can I find meaning as a trauma survivor?

Feedback received over time from group members and staff suggested that these themes were important and were not being addressed in other groups within the program at that time. Therefore, the clinical aims of the intervention were to help veterans to understand better how their spirituality was affected by their traumatic life experiences, and to promote awareness of their spirituality as a potential healing resource.

From a research and dissemination perspective, it was important to standardize the group intervention and evaluate its effectiveness. Accordingly, three primary components of a manual set were planned, including a facilitator's manual, a participant's workbook, and an assessment packet to evaluate the module. The primary purpose of creating the manual set was to provide a systematic approach to incorporating spirituality into trauma treatment, while allowing for the empirical investigation of this group treatment. This also provides a guideline for other treatment programs or individual clinicians to incorporate spirituality into their interventions with trauma survivors. The purpose of the facilitator's manual is to provide group leaders with clinical strategies and guidelines for implementing the group treatment. The facilitator's manual details the eight-session group intervention using a predominantly present-centered approach. The eight session themes are:

1. What is spirituality?
2. Building connections (including spiritual practices)
3. Spiritual practices
4. Theodicy (the "problem of evil")
5. Hostility and forgiveness
6. Forgiveness of self
7. Values
8. Making meaning.

The participant's workbook is a session-by-session guide designed to accompany the facilitator's manual. The organization of the workbook follows the facilitator's manual outline. It is a practically oriented volume that serves several purposes. First, it provides systematic and consistent implementation. Second, it establishes a framework of practical applications for group participation and support, guiding group members through their treatment process. Third, the workbook provides members with practical information about the use of spirituality as a healing resource. Finally, the materials presented can be used as a reference that includes spiritual readings, healing stories, relevant definitions and a journal for their own spiritual experiences.

The assessment packet includes measures for three components. The first component evaluates each member's knowledge gain for the material presented in each session. A second component assesses the facilitator's adherence to the session guidelines in the facilitator's manual. The third component measures members' changes in religiosity and spirituality, and it is administered before the first group session and after the final session. More detailed descriptions of the Trauma and Spirituality Group Module development have been provided by Drescher *et al.* (2004). The facilitator's manual, participant's workbook, and assessment packet are available in electronic form and may be requested from the authors.

Why might a group approach to address trauma and spirituality be especially appropriate? Along with its core symptoms, chronic PTSD frequently involves social disconnection and isolation. Using a group format provides positive social supports for its members while stimulating the use and further development of their interpersonal connections and skills. Members are accountable to their peers, the other group members, for providing a therapeutically safe and respectful group environment where diversity in religious backgrounds and spiritual beliefs and practices is encouraged. Using a group format is also consistent with current concepts about how spirituality might promote trauma recovery.

For example, McIntosh *et al.* (1993) suggested three potential healing pathways through which spirituality could ameliorate some of the impact of a traumatic event. These pathways were enhanced social support, changed cognitive processing of the event, and enhanced sense of meaning attached to the traumatic event. Therapeutically safe groups can provide opportunities for members to receive support and encouragement while they take on the challenges of trauma processing work.

Other notable religion/spirituality interventions

A review and meta-analysis of 14 forgiveness intervention studies found that those receiving a process-based form of intervention showed significant improvements by forgiving more, increasing their positive affect and self-esteem, and reducing their negative affect (Lundahl *et al.*, 2008). The review suggested that results were better for individually administered interventions than for a group format. Additionally, multiple sessions, administered over a sustained period of time, were associated with better outcomes. Most of the studies in the review were conducted with individuals reporting interpersonal betrayal. The applicability of these interventions for more severe trauma survivors has not been established, nor has the specific issue of self-forgiveness been addressed (Lundahl *et al.*, 2008).

Another example of a mental health treatment based upon principles of Eastern spirituality is the work being done utilizing the construct of mindfulness. Kabat-Zinn (1990) introduced a commonly used definition of mindfulness as "intentional, nonjudgmental awareness." The mindfulness construct has been incorporated into several behavioral treatments for both PTSD and depression, including acceptance and commitment therapy and dialectical behavior therapy. Acceptance and commitment therapy has been identified as an empirically supported treatment for depression, and evaluation of its efficacy for PTSD is ongoing. Dialectical behavior therapy was originally created as a treatment for borderline personality disorder and has been utilized with several other disorders. There is empirical support for its use in combination with exposure treatment in effectively addressing issues related to PTSD (Cahill *et al.*, 2009). Two additional approaches using mindfulness have recently been reviewed. One is mindfulness-based cognitive therapy (Coelho *et al.*, 2007), which is a group treatment incorporating mindfulness meditation with elements of cognitive therapy for depression. After examining four relevant studies, including two randomized clinical trials and one non-randomized trial, the authors concluded that there is sufficient initial evidence to support the use of this therapeutic approach for individuals suffering recurrent bouts (more than three) of severe depression. Another approach is called mindfulness-based stress reduction, which is a group program running over 8–10 weeks and utilizing mindfulness meditation to alleviate suffering associated with a variety of physical effects associated with mental health problems. A recent meta-analysis of studies using mindfulness-based stress reduction (Grossman *et al.*, 2004) found a medium sized positive effect for mental health outcomes, including depression and anxiety.

Conclusions

It is encouraging that progress is being made with respect to identifying key RS elements associated with resilience. Recent studies have shown that positive religious coping consistently shows a strong relationship to positive adjustment after crises. Progress has also been made in operationally defining positive religious coping. Examples of positive religious coping activities significantly linked to positive psychological adjustment in the Western traditions include religious purification, forgiveness, seeking support from clergy and/or faith community members, collaborative religious coping, religious surrender, and benevolent religious reappraisal (Ano & Vasconcelles, 2005). Universal compassion, self-reflection, mindfulness, and detachment from desire and negative emotion have been linked to well-being in Eastern traditions (Davidson *et al.*, 2003). Equally important is the empirical identification of spiritual obstacles or "red flags" – loss of faith, guilt, and lack of forgiveness – that are correlated with negative psychological adjustment. Although the importance of RS as a resource in coping with life crises is widely acknowledged, the dynamic processes by which the coping is accomplished remain to be identified and understood.

With the exception of studies of forgiveness and mindfulness/compassion interventions, the empirical validation of RS-specific interventions to promote trauma recovery or resilience is in its infancy. To date, there are no published controlled trials. Considerable progress has been made, however, on the development of a testable intervention, a Trauma and Spirituality Group Module. Standardized elements for the module are available, including a facilitator's manual, a participant's workbook, and an assessment packet for evaluating each session and the overall module.

Implications for future clinical and research applications

There is a very clear clinical implication that can be drawn from the current scientific knowledge about RS and resilience: clinicians need to promote the use of positive religious coping methods by those clients whose religious backgrounds and practices are consistent with them. A first step for trauma clinicians is learning what the positive religious coping methods actually are. Much of the empirical work on identifying these practices has been accomplished by Pargament and his colleagues (1998), where a full explanation of each positive practice is given. Examples of these practices include *benevolent reappraisal*, or seeking a lesson from God in the event; *seeking spiritual support*, or searching for comfort in God's care; *active religious surrender*, or coping as one can and then leaving the outcome with God; and *seeking spiritual connection*, or recognizing that one is part of a larger spiritual force (Peres *et al.*, 2007). Description of Eastern practices related to well-being, such as compassion, mindfulness, and challenging one's source of identity, can also be found (Ricard, 2007).

A second clinical implication is also clear: clinicians need to be aware of spiritual "red flags" that may be part of the problem their clients are experiencing in their recovery attempts. Loss of faith and cognitive distortions about lack of forgiveness and guilt per se may present formidable obstacles in the path to trauma recovery, and they may disallow the use of positive religious and other coping practices that might otherwise promote recovery. For clients mired in these "red flags," clinicians might consider referral to a member of the clergy for help in their resolution.

More generally, trauma clinicians need to inquire about their clients' religious backgrounds and spiritual beliefs and practices as part of their intake assessment. Clients' RS strengths and resources can be identified, as well as possible spiritual "red flags." Clinicians need not share their clients' religious backgrounds, practices, and beliefs, but they do need to be aware of them, show respect for them, and encourage the use of positive coping practices associated with them.

Several pressing research implications are also apparent. Perhaps the most important research issue for future studies concerns measurement of RS. There needs to be consistency across studies employing operational measures of RS. In this area as well, Pargament and his colleagues (2000) have made a major contribution by developing a standardized measure of positive and negative religious coping (RCOPE) that can be adjusted for various needs. The BMMRS (Idler *et al.*, 2003) is another well-designed and standardized instrument that taps 12 RS dimensions, including short versions of Pargament's positive and negative religious coping questionnaire. Beyond the use of standardized instruments that provide consistent operational definitions for RS, future studies also need to assess both positive and negative aspects of religious coping, as well as other dimensions of RS. Designing studies to include multiple dimensions of RS will allow relationships between RS dimensions to be empirically examined directly.

Regarding the experimental designs of future studies, there needs to be an emphasis on using longitudinal designs that allow temporal and causal relationships between study variables to be addressed. Most currently published studies are cross-sectional in design and can provide no information about temporality and causality in the relationships found between variables of interest. However, the consistent findings across these preliminary studies can inform the hypotheses to be tested in more rigorously designed future studies.

A final research implication regards the need for studies to evaluate the efficacy of RS interventions for trauma survivors. Ultimately, randomized controlled trials, comparing different forms of intervention (or wait-list controls), are needed. In the interim, manualized interventions can be developed and pilot tested. As a start, pre-treatment and post-treatment measures can be administered to treatment groups as they are conducted. When possible, untreated similar groups could receive the same assessments to provide scores to compare with those in the treatment group.

References

Anda, R. F., Felitti, V. J., Bremner, J. D., *et al.* (2006). The enduring effects of abuse and related adverse experiences in childhood: A convergence of evidence from neurobiology and epidemiology. *European Archives of Psychiatry and Clinical Neuroscience*, **256**, 174–186.

Ano, G. G. & Vasconcelles, E. B. (2005). Religious coping and psychological adjustment distress: A meta-analysis. *Journal of Clinical Psychology*, **61**, 461–480.

Baumeister, R. F. & Exline, J. J. (2000). Self-control, morality, and human strength. *Journal of Social and Clinical Psychology*, **19**, 29–42.

Cahill, S. P., Rothbaum, B. O., Resick, P. A., & Follette, V. M. (2009). Cognitive behavioral therapy for adults. In E. B.

Foa, T. M. Keane, M. J. Friedman, & J. A. Cohen (eds.), *Effective treatments for PTSD: Practice guidelines from the International Society for Traumatic Stress Studies,* 2nd edn. New York: Guilford Press.

Charuvastra, A. & Cloitre, M. (2008). Social bonds and posttraumatic stress disorder. *Annual Review of Psychology*, **59**, 301–328.

Coelho, H. F., Canter, P. H., & Ernst, E. (2007). Mindfulness-based cognitive therapy: Evaluating current evidence and informing future research. *Journal of Consulting and Clinical Psychology*, **75**, 1003–1005.

Davidson, R. J., Kabat-Zinn, J., Schumacher, J., *et al.* (2003). Alterations in brain and immune function produced by mindfulness meditation. *Psychosomatic Medicine*, **65**, 564–570.

Drescher, K. D. & Foy, D. W. (1995). Spirituality and trauma treatment: Suggestions for including spirituality as a coping resource. *National Center for PTSD Clinical Quarterly*, **5**, 4–5.

Drescher, K. D. & Foy, D. W. (2008). When they come home: Posttraumatic stress, moral injury, and spiritual consequences for veterans. *Reflective Practice: Formation and Supervision in Ministry*, **28**, 85–102.

Drescher, K. D., Ramirez, G., Leoni, J. J., *et al.* (2004). Spirituality and trauma: Development of a group therapy module. *Group Journal*, **28**, 71–87.

Eriksson, C. B. (2008). Religion as a risk and resilience factor. In *Proceedings of the Annual Conference of the International Society for Traumatic Stress,* Chicago, November, 2008.

Fontana, A. & Rosenheck, R. (2004). Trauma, change in strength of religious faith, and mental health service use among veterans treated for PTSD. *Journal of Nervous and Mental Disease*, **192**, 579–584.

Garbarino, J. & Bedard, C. (1996). Spiritual challenges to children facing violent trauma. *Childhood: A Global Journal of Child Research*, **3**, 467–478.

Garmezy, N. (1991). Resiliency and vulnerability to adverse developmental outcomes associated with poverty. *American Behavioral Scientist*, **34**, 416–430.

Grossman, P., Niemann, L., Schmidt, S., & Walach, H. (2004). Mindfulness-based stress reduction and health benefits: A meta-analysis. *Journal of Psychosomatic Research*, **57**, 35–43.

Hagberg, J. O. & Guelich, R. A. (2005). *The critical journey: Stages in the life of faith,* 2nd edn. Salem, WI: Sheffield Publishing.

Hall, T. (2007). Psychoanalysis, attachment, and spirituality. Part I: The emergence of two relational traditions. *Journal of Psychology and Theology*, **3**, 14–28.

Harris, J. I., Erbes, C. R., Engdahl, B. E., *et al.* (2008). Christian religious functioning and trauma outcomes. *Journal of Clinical Psychology*, **64**, 17–29.

Idler, E. L., Musick, M. A., Ellison, C. G., *et al.* (2003). Measuring multiple dimensions of religion and spirituality for health research: Conceptual background and findings from the 1998 General Social Survey. *Research on Aging*, **25**, 327–365.

James, W. (1997). *The varieties of religious experience.* New York: Touchstone.

Kabat-Zinn, J. (1990). *Full catastrophe living: Using the wisdom of your body and mind to face stress, pain, and illness.* New York: Delacorte.

Larson, D. B., Pattison, E. M., Blazer, D. G., Omran, A. R., & Kaplan, B. H. (1986). Systematic analysis of research on religious variables in four major psychiatric journals, 1978–1982. *American Journal of Psychiatry*, **143**, 329–334.

Larson, D. B., Swyers, J. P., & McCullough, M. E. (1997). *Scientific research on spirituality and health: A consensus report.* Rockville, MD: National Institute for Healthcare Research.

Lundahl, B. W., Taylor, M. J., Stevenson, R., & Roberts, K. D. (2008). Process-based forgiveness interventions: A meta-analytic review. *Research on Social Work Practice*, **18**, 465–478.

Luthar, S. S. (2005). Resilience at an early age and its impact on child psychosocial development. In R. E. Tremblay, R. G. Barr, & R. De V. Peters (eds.), *Encyclopedia on early childhood development* (pp. 1–6). Montreal: Centre of Excellence for Early Childhood Development, http://www.child-encyclopedia.com/documents/LutharANGxp.pdf (accessed February 26, 2011).

Lutz, A., Greischar, L. L., Rawlings, N. B., Ricard, M., & Davidson, R. J. (2004). Long-term meditators self-induce high-amplitude gamma synchrony during mental practice. *Proceedings of the National Academy of Sciences of the USA*, **101**, 16369–16373.

Masten, A. S. (2001). Ordinary magic: Resilience processes in development. *American Psychologist*, **56**, 227–238.

McCullough, M. E. (2000). Forgiveness as a human strength: Theory, measurement, and links to well-being. *Journal of Social and Clinical Psychology*, **19**, 43–55.

McIntosh, D. N., Silver, R. C., & Wortman, C. B. (1993). Religion's role in adjustment to a negative life event: coping with the loss of a child. *Journal of Personality and Social Psychology*, **65**, 812–821.

Nooney, J. & Woodrum, E. (2002). Religious coping and church-based social support as predictors of mental health outcomes: Testing a conceptual model. *Journal for the Scientific Study of Religion*, **41**, 359–368.

Oxman, T. E., Freeman, D. H., & Manheimer, E. D. (1995). Lack of social participation or religious strength and comfort as risk factors for death after cardiac surgery in the elderly. *Psychosomatic Medicine*, **57**, 5–15.

Pargament, K. I. (1997). *The psychology of religion and coping: Theory, research, practice.* New York: Guilford Press.

Pargament, K. I., Zinnbauer, B. J., Scott, A. B., *et al.* (1998). Red flags and religious coping: Identifying some religious warning signs among people in crisis. *Journal of Clinical Psychology*, **54**, 77–89.

Pargament, K. I., Koenig, H. G., & Peres, L. M. (2000). The many methods of religious coping: Development and initial validation of the RCOPE. *Journal of Clinical Psychology*, **56**, 519–543.

Park, C. L. (2005). Religion as a meaning-making framework in coping with life stress. *Journal of Social Issues*, **61**, 707–730.

Peres, J. F. P., Moreira-Almeida, A., Nasello, A. G., & Koenig, H. G. (2007). Spirituality and resilience in trauma victims. *Journal of Religion and Health*, **46**, 343–350.

Perry, B. D. & Pollard, R. (1998). Homeostasis, stress, trauma, and adaptation: A neurodevelopmental view of childhood trauma. *Child and Adolescent Psychiatric Clinics of North America*, 7, 33–51.

Powell, L. H., Shajhabi, L., & Thoresen, C. E. (2003). Religion and spirituality: Linkages to physical health. *American Psychologist*, **58**, 36–52.

Ricard, M. (2007). *Happiness: A guide to developing life's most important skill.* New York: Little Brown.

Richardson, G. E. (2002). The metatheory of resilience and resiliency. *Journal of Clinical Psychology*, **58**, 307–321.

Rutter, M. (1985). Resilience in the face of adversity: Protective factors and resistance to psychiatric disorder. *British Journal of Psychiatry*, **147**, 598–611.

Rutter, M. (1998). Developmental catch-up, and deficit, following adoption after severe global early privation. *Journal of Child Psychology and Psychiatry and Allied Disciplines*, **39**, 465–476.

Sameroff, A. J., Bartko, W. T., Baldwin, A., Baldwin, C., & Seifer, R. (1998). Family and social influences on the development of child competence. In M. Lewis & C. Feiring (eds.), *Families, risk, and competence* (pp. 161–185). Mahwah, NJ: Erlbaum.

Schuster, M. A., Stein, B. D., Jaycox, L. H., *et al.* (2001). A national survey of stress reactions after the September 11, 2001, terrorist attacks. *New England Journal of Medicine*, **345**, 1507–1512.

Snyder, C. R. (2000). The past and possible futures of hope. *Journal of Social and Clinical Psychology*, **19**, 11–28.

Sutton, S. K. & Davidson, R. J. (1997). Prefrontal brain asymmetry: A biological substrate of the behavioral approach and inhibition systems. *Psychological Science*, **8**, 204–210.

Urry, H. L., Nitschke, J. B., Dolski, I., *et al.* (2004). Making a life worth living: neural correlates of well-being. *Psychological Science*, **15**, 367–372.

Weaver, A. J., Samford, J., Kline, A. E., *et al.* (1997). What do psychologists know about working with the clergy? An analysis of eight APA journals: 1991–1994. *Professional Psychology: Research & Practice*, **28**, 471–474.

Werner, E. E. (1982). *Vulnerable but invincible: A longitudinal study of resilient children and youth.* New York: McGraw-Hill.

Werner, E. E. (2000). Protective factors and individual resilience. In J. P. Shonkoff & S. J. Meisels (eds.), *Handbook of early childhood intervention.* 2nd edn, (pp. 115–132). New York: Cambridge University Press.

Witvliet, C. V. O., Phillips, K. A., Feldman, M. E., & Beckham, J. C. (2004). Posttraumatic mental and physical health correlates of forgiveness and religious coping in military veterans. *Journal of Traumatic Stress*, **17**, 269–273.

Chapter

7

Resilience in children and adolescents

Ann S. Masten, Amy R. Monn, and Laura M. Supkoff

Introduction

In the sciences concerned with human development, resilience can be defined as the capacity of a dynamic, living system to endure or recover from a major disturbance and continue to develop in healthy ways. Resilience is a broad systems concept that generally refers to the capacity of any dynamic system to adapt or recover from a significant threat to its function or viability. It can be applied to an individual, a family, an organization, or an ecosystem. Interest in resilience emerged independently in the ecological and social sciences around the same time (late 1960s and early 1970s), probably as a result of common roots in general systems theory (Masten & Obradović, 2008).

Judging from ancient tales of young heroes and heroines, people have been intrigued with the idea of overcoming adversity for millennia. The science of resilience in children, however, emerged in the 1960s as investigators, searching for the causes of mental illnesses such as schizophrenia and behavioral problems such as delinquency, began to study children at risk for psychopathology (Luthar, 2006; Masten, 2007, 2011). The rationale behind this approach was to begin research before disorders were evident in order to study their causes and course of development (Garmezy & Streitman, 1974; Watt et al., 1984; Obradović et al., 2011). When investigators began to study groups of children believed to be at risk, the striking variability in the life course among the individual children became apparent. The diversity in outcomes of children who shared risk factors was impressive, particularly when followed forward in time. Investigators were confronted with the puzzle of numerous young people in "high-risk" groups who were showing positive mental health and development.

A small but highly influential group of scientists in child development, clinical psychology, and psychiatry recognized the potential importance of understanding such resilience in high-risk children, both for theory and practice. These pioneers, including Norman Garmezy, Lois Murphy, Michael Rutter, and Emmy Werner, inspired the descriptive first wave of resilience research, which focused on defining and measuring resilience to identify the most promising factors associated with the phenomena that fell under this rather large conceptual umbrella (Masten & Wright, 2009). Subsequent waves of research have focused on explanatory processes, with the goals of understanding the processes by which resilience occurs (wave two), whether it can be promoted through intervention (wave three), and how it works across levels of human function (wave four), from the molecular level of cells to the macro level of societies (Masten, 2007; Masten & Wright, 2009).

The early work on resilience in children and youth was part of a broader movement that has revolutionized theory and practice in mental health, contributing to the emergence of the integrative perspective of developmental psychopathology in the 1970s (Cicchetti, 1984, 2006; Masten, 2006a). The developmental psychopathology framework represented a synthesis of two great traditions in science, one focused on problems and mental illness and the other focused on normal development (Masten, 2006a). Longitudinal studies of children at risk required ideas, methods, and investigators from both traditions. Soon a synergistic merger was underway, with the promise of bridging developmental and clinical perspectives to improve the understanding of pathways toward and away from psychopathology over the life course. New textbooks and journals followed, with a focus on delineating the new conceptual approach of developmental psychopathology.

Resilience and Mental Health: Challenges Across the Lifespan, ed. Steven M. Southwick, Brett T. Litz, Dennis Charney, and Matthew J. Friedman. Published by Cambridge University Press. © Cambridge University Press 2011.

A central tenet of the new framework was the idea that contrasting variations in adaptation – successful and unsuccessful, normal and deviant, resilient and maladaptive – are mutually informative for understanding the course of human development in its varying forms, pathological and healthy (Sroufe *et al.*, 2005; Cicchetti, 2006; Masten, 2006a). In developmental psychopathology, it was just as important to understand pathways to competence and positive mental health as it was to understand the pathways to problems and disorders. Proponents of this approach argued that the study of competence and positive development, particularly among those at risk for psychopathology, was informative for understanding, preventing, and treating symptoms and disorders. They also argued that a developmental perspective was essential for understanding adaptation and behavior in a developing organism. Thus, the developmental psychopathology movement strongly supported research on positive aspects of development, including resilience.

This chapter highlights the concepts and findings from the developmental research on resilience in young people, spanning childhood to adulthood. The first section describes how resilience has been defined in developmental research, including discussion of salient controversies and issues in defining resilience for research. The second section highlights core models and approaches that guided the developmental research on resilience. The third section highlights findings from the broad literature on resilience in children and youth, discussing the "short list" of widely reported protective factors for resilience and what this list may signify about the core adaptive systems for resilience in human development. The fourth section presents a resilience framework for intervention based on the main evidence, with general guidelines for applying current evidence to help young people who are suffering now and cannot wait for scientists to learn all the answers. The resilience framework includes the five "Ms" of mission, models, measures, methods, and multiple levels. Concluding comments highlight new horizons of research on resilience in the early decades of life.

Defining resilience from a developmental perspective

Resilience broadly refers to good adaptation in the context of significant threats to the development or viability of a dynamic system. It is an inferential concept because the definition is conditional with respect to two major stipulations: there must be "good adaptation" by some definition and there must have been exposure to "serious risk" of some kind. Judging or assessing good adaptation is typically based on expectations for developmental level. Expectations for infant and adult behavior clearly differ. However, the threat side of the equation also has a developmental context because the nature of threat exposure and the perception of threat also vary with developmental level. Infants and adolescents experience different kinds of adversity and experience the same objective threat in different ways.

Resilience also is a dynamic concept, which means that it refers to how well a system is (or has been) actively adapting or developing in relation to a significant challenge. Definitions variously refer to the capacity for, outcomes of, or processes involved in the dynamics of resilience. Generally, resilience must be manifested (i.e., there is an observable track record of doing alright during or after adversity), although presumably it is possible to predict resilience based on evidence from other people. In other words, investigators typically are reluctant to identify people as "resilient" who have never been exposed to serious adversity, although they might be willing to predict better odds for resilience based on similarities to other people who have manifested resilience.

The overarching goal of research on resilience in children has been to understand how resilience happens, with an eye toward promoting and protecting positive adaptation in development. Identifying resilience is a key first step, but it is also important to work out what makes a difference for better adaptation and how. Consequently, it is also important to attend to the predictors of resilience among those exposed to hazards: the promotive and protective factors associated with good adaptation during or following serious threats. The predictors of resilience also would be expected to change with development, as resources and adaptive systems develop, mature, and decline.

This section of the chapter discusses developmental approaches to the definition of resilience, including the two core components of *adaptation* and *threat* that are required to identify resilience, as well as the meaning of *promotive* and *protective* influences that are invoked to explain how resilience comes about. Key definitional issues and controversies are also discussed.

Defining good adaptation in developmental resilience research

In research on human development, good adaptation is often defined from a normative perspective, with respect to typical development and expected achievements across the lifespan for people of a given age, gender, culture, and period in history (Masten & Coatsworth, 1998). These expectations for competence based on normative development have been termed *developmental tasks* (Havighurst, 1972; Masten *et al.*, 2006a). For a school-age child, these expectations might include obedience to parents, following community norms for public conduct, going to school and behaving appropriately in the classroom, learning what is being taught in school, and getting along with other people, including peers and teachers. As children mature, developmental tasks also change. School work is more challenging and children are expected to follow societal rules without constant supervision. In adolescence and early adulthood, there are new domains of developmental tasks, including expectations for work, romantic relationships, parenting, and civic engagement.

In psychiatry, good adaptation might be judged in reference to normal mental health or the absence of mental health disorders or impairment. In this case too, judgments about adaptive function take developmental expectations into account, often in the form of diagnostic criteria that consider impairment in life tasks (e.g., going to school or learning to read) and developmental level (see Masten *et al.*, 2006a). In the diagnostic criteria for attention-deficit hyperactivity disorder, for example, an individual must show symptoms of inattention or hyperactivity–impulsivity "to a degree that is maladaptive and inconsistent with developmental level" (American Psychiatric Association, 2000, p. 92).

Good adaptation or healthy function is not enough to define resilience, however. There also must be some kind of challenge to the organism with the potential to disrupt or destroy normative function or development.

Defining threats in developmental resilience research

Many kinds of potential threat to the lives of children and youth have been studied under the rubric of resilience, including well-established risk factors for normal development (such as low birth weight or neglect), individual traumatic experiences (such as abuse), and mass disasters (such as hurricanes or war). What all of these various risk factors have in common is their established potential to disrupt or harm normal function or development.

It was quickly apparent to the researchers examining early risk that risk factors or negative life experiences often pile up in the lives of children and youth (Obradović *et al.*, 2011). Divorce, for example, was not a simple event but a complex sequence of experiences often accompanied by chronic family conflict, economic hardship, moving, and loss. Children with one major risk factor, such as an abusive parent, often faced other risks too. As a result, attention shifted away from the study of isolated risk factors to concentrate on *cumulative risk*. Methods of tallying or combining risk factors were developed, ranging from simple counts of negative life events to complex ratings of adversity based on clinical interviews (e.g., Obradović *et al.*, 2011).

Risk gradients were created by plotting adaptive function (positive or negative) as a function of risk level. As risk level rises, the average level of positive adaptive behavior declines and problems rise (depending on what is being plotted). Consequently, studies of stressful life events and disaster often find a *dose gradient* where the children who were more highly exposed (more adversity) show more problems (Pine *et al.*, 2005; Masten & Osofsky, 2010; Obradović *et al.*, 2011). Risk gradients have been illustrated for many health and behavior outcomes plotted as a function of various indicators of cumulative risk (Obradović *et al.*, 2011).

Resilience theorists have pointed out that it is often arbitrary to designate these gradients as "risk gradients" because, in many cases, high risk also indicates low assets or resources (Masten A.S. *et al.*, 2009a). A high-risk score, for example, might be based on the following risk factors: single-parent household, a parent who is poorly educated, low birth weight, poor parenting skills, low income, and a disadvantaged neighborhood with high unemployment. A low-risk score, in this case, is likely to indicate that a child has more resources in the form of two better educated parents, more family income, and a neighborhood with more social capital, better schools, and greater safety.

Also of greatest interest to resilience investigators was the striking variability in adaptive function *within levels of risk*. They observed individuals exposed to high levels of risk or adversity who showed good adaptive behavior, thus appearing to be "off gradient" cases in terms of prediction. These resilient individuals were doing better than expected based on their level of risk, or "beating the odds." Similarly, there were individuals who were doing worse than expected at low levels of risk, although these "vulnerable" individuals (poor adaptation in the context of low risk) appear to be less common than the resilient individuals (see Masten *et al.*, 1999).

The risk side of the resilience equation also must be considered from a developmental perspective because the nature of exposure and the repercussions of the threat are influenced by the development of the individual. For example, younger children are less likely to be kidnapped and forced to be a child soldier and less likely to understand the full import of war (Masten & Osofsky, 2010). The loss of parents in a war zone, however, may have much greater significance for a young child who is unable to survive without the care of others than it may have for an older youth. Responses to threat also are influenced by development because the capacities of individuals for adaptation also change with development.

Promotive and protective factors in developmental resilience research

From the outset, resilience investigators were looking for factors that might counteract, buffer, or ameliorate the effects of adversity and other kinds of threat – whatever made it possible for some young people to overcome adversity when others did not. Promotive factors or influences encompass those assets, resources, relationships, or strengths that appear to contribute in positive ways to good adaptation and development, regardless of risk level. Protective factors, by comparison, show a special effect in the context of high threat, moderating the consequences of threat for adaptation or development. Sometimes it is difficult to tell the difference between these two types of effect, either because the low-risk groups are missing (only high-risk groups are studied) or because the same factor (e.g., an effective parent) seems to have both types of effect. The difference between promotive and protective functions is most striking for the protective factors that *only are functional when risk is high*. Airbags in automobiles and antibodies to infectious agents that form with vaccination are classic examples of protective effects that work only in specific high-risk conditions. Crisis nursery services are designed to operate in a similar way,

protecting children when risk is high for child maltreatment or neglect. In contrast, good parents may take all kinds of routine action to raise healthy children under normal conditions, but also spring into emergency action when a child's life is threatened. Parents are a multipurpose adaptive system for child rearing, with many promotive and protective roles.

Under circumstances of threat, individual people may call on or attract help and resources from self, other people, community organizations, and the environment. These resources and access to them all change as a function of development and as contexts change across the life course. For example, the individual problem-solving capabilities of children improve as the brain matures and they learn more cognitive skills (i.e., *human capital* develops). Older children and youth also develop connections and friendships in the community that extend the resources they have to call upon in times of threat (*social capital* develops). At the same time, older children and youth have greater mobility and access to more extensive networks of information. All of these changes have the potential to alter the resources and tools available for adaptation in the face of threat. However, it is important to remember that sometimes development brings greater vulnerability to threat as well as greater exposure to adversity. Development can be a two-edged sword when it comes to adaptive behavior. In adolescence, greater awareness of threats and greater exposure to adversity may accompany developmentally based improvements in thinking abilities, knowledge, physical skills, and mobility.

Definitional issues and controversies

There have been a number of issues and controversies about the meaning of resilience in research on human development. Consideration of these issues generally has had a positive effect on the quality of the science, often clarifying confusing variations in terminology from meaningful differences in substance. Several key examples are highlighted here.

Who decides on the criteria for resilience?

To study resilience, it was necessary to define and measure both "good adaptation" and "threat," as noted above. Resilience research has been criticized for inconsistencies across studies of these criteria and measures, which does make it difficult to aggregate findings. These definitions by different investigators, both conceptual and operational, involved many decisions and, in the end, judgment calls about the best criteria and measures for the purpose at hand. Many issues are embedded in these decisions. Should resilience be defined in terms of developmental task achievement or subjective well-being, or both? If a person does not have a diagnosable mental illness, does this mean they are doing well? When young people live in bicultural contexts (e.g., immigrant youth), should bicultural criteria be applied in defining resilience? Should the criteria for resilience vary as a function of the severity of adversity exposure? What does resilience mean in a child soldier? What are the best ways to composite risk factors and stressful life experiences? Is subjective stress appraisal more important than objective exposure?

These are just a small sample of questions that convey some of the issues involved in defining and measuring the adaptive behavior and risk components of resilience. Given the potential for confusion, the conclusions in this literature have shown remarkable consistency, as discussed in a subsequent section.

Specificity issues: narrow versus broad definitions?

A related set of issues were focused on whether to define resilience in narrow or broad ways, in one domain or in multiple domains simultaneously. Variable-focused approaches (discussed below) tended to focus on one particular outcome domain and its predictors (e.g., school achievement and the predictors of "academic resilience"), whereas person-focused approaches (also discussed below), such as case studies and the identification of resilient subgroups of children in high-risk samples, tended to consider multiple domains of function in identifying resilient people. Variable-focused studies highlighted the fact that doing well can be domain specific and that a given protective factor may be more important in one domain than another. The specificity of this approach can be illuminating for closing in on clues to the processes involved in specific aspects of adaptation. In person-focused studies, resilience was akin to a diagnosis of doing well in spite of risk or adversity. As in other kinds of diagnosis, multiple criteria made sense. A child who excelled in one domain (e.g., having friends) but failed miserably in other domains (e.g., school achievement) was not usually identified as resilient. Resilience in person-focused work typically meant that the person was doing adequately well across all the domains that matter to stakeholders such as parents or society. Not surprisingly, these broad approaches to the definitions of resilience, focused on multiple criteria, tend to identify the protective factors with the broadest effects, such as parenting or general intellectual skills.

Time issues: resilience versus recovery and resistance

The time frame for defining resilience also has generated some debate. Some would argue that when recovery from a traumatic disturbance takes a long time, it should be called recovery and not resilience (e.g., Bonanno, 2004), while others encompass a wide range of resistance and recovery patterns under the conceptual umbrella of resilience (e.g., Masten, 2001, 2011). Still others differentiate resistance (maintaining good function despite trauma exposure) from resilience (disturbance in function followed by rapid recovery) from recovery (when the return to good function takes longer). Norris *et al.* (2008) have provided an overview of such differences. The important point is probably to note that defining resilience requires a time perspective. The nature of the risk or adversity also may be important, since some adversities have acute onset and short duration while others are chronic and extended over time. Many investigators note that the same person may appear to be maladaptive at one point in life and doing well at a different point. Consequently, it could depend on when the assessment of adaptive function is done as to whether a person is viewed as resilient or maladaptive. In any event, there is considerable interest in the possibilities of "late emerging resilience" or "late bloomers" in developmental resilience research, reflecting dramatic turnarounds in the life course. Clearly, there are individual cases of young people whose lives were going in a bad direction in adolescence who become successful young adults (Werner & Smith, 1992; Masten *et al.*, 1999, 2006b). It also is clear that there are dramatic declines in some areas of bad behavior during the transition from adolescence to adulthood after a sharp increase in the same behaviors during the adolescent years; such behaviors include antisocial behavior, alcohol use and dependence, or risk-taking behavior (Miller *et al.*, 1998; Masten *et al.*, 2008; Steinberg, 2008).

System issues: capacity, process, or outcome; internal or external adaptation; resiliency or resilience?

Other definitional issues in resilience science probably have their origins in the challenges of defining properties of dynamic systems. Definitions of resilience vary, for example in referring to resilience in terms of capacity, process, or outcome, or all three aspects. In ecology theory, where resilience is strongly embedded in systems theory, resilience nearly always refers to the capacity of a system for change and resuming development after a disturbance. Definitions of resilience in the social sciences also vary in their focus on internal versus external adaptation or both, a variation that likely reflects another systems issue. Living systems have a dual nature with respect to adaptation, in that they must maintain internal coherence or equilibrium while growing and developing and they must also adapt to the environments in which they live, which are also continually changing (Masten *et al.*, 2006a). Some investigations have defined resilience strictly in terms of external adaptation (e.g., how well a child is functioning in the family, school, and with peers) while others focus only on internal well-being (e.g., how well the child is feeling and thinking) and still others on both aspects of adaptation. Some investigators define resilience in terms of internal and external symptoms rather than competence (e.g., the absence of internalizing and externalizing disorders or clinical levels of these symptom dimensions). Finally, there has been considerable controversy about the use of the term "resiliency" and whether resilience can be considered a trait of the individual. We would concur with those who object to this term, and argue that resilience usually involves drawing on resources or systems that extend well beyond the individual, embedded in attachment relationships, family systems, and emergency response systems in the community. The capacity for resilience in human function, as in other dynamic living systems, is far more complex than the property of a material (e.g., a rubber band or steel) to withstand stress and recover its form without breaking.

Models and methods in developmental research on resilience

The goals of resilience research called for new models, measures, and methods because positive aspects of adaptation and assessment had been relatively neglected in the early research on psychopathology and risk, while normative studies of child development had largely ignored individual differences. Among the important contributions of resilience research was a renewed interest in the concepts and tools for assessing competence, environmental assets, and adaptive systems, as well as promotive and protective effects (Masten & Obradović, 2006).

Person-focused and variable-focused models of resilience

Resilience investigators often combined person-focused with variable-focused approaches in their studies. Person-focused approaches initially included case examples of individuals judged to be resilient and also studies that compared resilient subgroups of high-risk children with their less adaptive peers with similar risk level. Such people inspired the pioneers to study resilience. Person-focused approaches also included analyses of individual pathways over time and studies of groups of children with life patterns or trajectories that illustrated good function during or following adversity exposure. Recent advances in multivariate statistics and growth models have made it possible to identify such patterns in longitudinal data. Figure 7.1 illustrates a variety of resilience pathways, representing various pathways in the course of adaptive behavior over time before, during, and after a significant threat to development, both for an acute disturbance (a traumatic experience or disaster) and for an extended, chronic period of adversity.

Variable-focused approaches concentrated on the relation among measured variables in the lives of individuals, often linking adaptive outcome measures to risk or adversity measures, with analyses centered on identifying other variables that helped to predict better outcomes in relation to risk posed by the measured adversities. Analytically, these approaches often relied on multivariate statistics, such as regression analysis or structural equation modeling, that attempted to test hypotheses about potential contributors to resilience and their role.

Figure 7.2 illustrates some of the major effects tested in studies of resilience, including intervention effects. Risk factors are defined as direct, negative predictors of adaptive behavior. In Figure 7.2, several risk effects are illustrated. Risk 0, which normally has a negative effect on adaptive behavior, is totally prevented by some intervention (e.g., premature birth is prevented by good prenatal care). Risk 1 has a direct, negative effect on adaptive behavior (e.g., child abuse predicts worse mental health and school function). The effect of risk 2 is moderated (reduced) by a naturally occurring protective factor while the effect of risk 3 is attenuated or eliminated by an intervention that also functions as a moderator of risk. Risk 4 has an indirect effect on adaptive behavior by undermining an important asset (asset 2) for adaptive behavior (e.g., economic hardship or divorce undermines

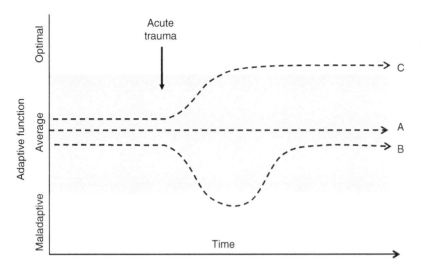

Figure 7.1 Examples of resilience pathways in the context of acute trauma or chronic adversity. In acute trauma (top), pathway A shows resistance, B shows breakdown and recovery, and C shows post-traumatic growth. In chronic adversity (bottom), pathway A shows resistance, B shows breakdown and rapid recovery, and C shows breakdown with later recovery.

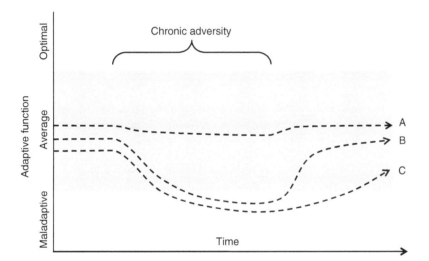

good parenting, which, in turn, affects adaptive behavior). In this case, asset 2 is said to function as a *mediator* of risk 4 effects on adaptive behavior. Interventions can be designed to protect asset 2 (e.g., providing support for parents under economic stress or in the course of divorce). Interventions also can be designed to increase the assets available; asset 3 (e.g., a tutor) has been added through intervention in Figure 7.2.

Often, what is called a risk factor or a promotive factor (asset) is arbitrary, because the actual variable that is measured is a continuously distributed bipolar indicator of variation, with a negative and positive pole. Intelligence quotient (IQ) test scores provide a classic example, in that high IQ can be viewed as a promotive factor for learning in school while low IQ can be viewed

as a risk factor for school achievement. A child's IQ is a good predictor of school achievement, probably along a continuum that extends from low to high scores.

In contrast, there are some experiences and resources that appear to function only in one way. Negative life experiences such as injury in a car accident are generally viewed only as a risk factor. Genetic anomalies that alter development only in negative ways also could be viewed as pure risk factors. Infections similarly are viewed as risk factors for health. Positive examples of pure assets or promotive factors – those when present seem to confer advantages in life but when lacking are not necessarily harmful – might include non-essential talents (e.g., musical or athletic talent), a good sense of humor, a helpful neighbor, or a nearby library.

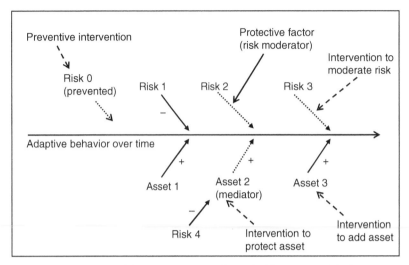

Figure 7.2 Resilience models showing potential effects of risk factors, assets (also known as promotive factors), protective factors (moderating risk effects), and interventions strategies that target risks or assets. Risk 0 is prevented by intervention. Risk 1 has a direct negative effect on adaptive behavior while asset 1 has a direct positive effect. The risk 2 effect is reduced or eliminated by a naturally occurring protective factor that functions as a moderator of risk for the adaptive behavior under study. Risk 3 is moderated by an intervention designed to reduce the effects of risk 3. Risk 4 has a negative effect on adaptive behavior through its effects on asset 2 (which is a mediator of risk 4 effects on adaptive behavior). Intervention can be directed at protecting asset 2 in the context of risk 4. Asset 3 is added through intervention and has a positive effect on adaptive behavior.

Variables that appear to moderate risk also frequently work both ways and so could be viewed as vulnerability or protective factors in the context of an interaction model, depending on the emphasis or perspective. Intellectual skills and parenting quality, both widely implicated as key moderators of risk in the lives of children, probably work both ways, conferring greater vulnerability when they are low or poor and greater protection when they are high (Masten, 2001, 2011; Luthar, 2006).

Other multivariate models focus attention on *mediating effects*, where risk factors damage children through their effects on key promotive or protective factors. For example, if a life event such as a car accident or assault causes brain damage in a child (lowering IQ) or in a parent (lowering the quality of parenting available), the developmental outcomes that depend on good IQ or good parenting may be harmed as well.

Intervention models are also built around these basic models of resilience, as noted in Figure 7.2. Intervention effects can be aimed to build up assets or resources in an attempt to counterbalance risks; they can target risk factors by preventing them from happening or they can target key promotive or protective factors (such as parenting) in an effort to protect these key advantages for development (see Masten & Shaffer

[2006] for a more extended discussion of these models with respect to parenting). Some of the most effective intervention programs to promote achievement and prevent antisocial behavior in child development have focused on parent education or training (Patterson *et al.*, 2004). Recent efforts to apply this approach to disaster planning have argued for targeting parents and teachers as "first responders" who could learn to mitigate the consequences of disasters on children through advance training (Pine *et al.*, 2005; Masten & Obradović, 2008).

Resilience models have had a transformative effect on intervention, by underscoring the significance of positive influences on adaptive behavior and development. Positive models have great appeal to stakeholders, which may explain why these positive models are taking hold in school counseling (Galassi & Akos, 2007), prevention science (Miller *et al.*, 1998), social welfare (Flynn *et al.*, 2006), and other areas of intervention and policy (Luthar & Cicchetti, 2001).

Research on competence and cascades

Another key contribution of the resilience researchers was the attention they brought to theory and assessment of individual differences in positive adaptation and development (Masten & Obradović, 2006). Such

Table 7.1 Examples of widely reported resilience factors for children and implicated adaptive systems.

Promotive/protective factors	Implicated adaptive systems
Good caregiving	Attachment, family
Close relationships with other competent and prosocial people	Attachment
Intelligence and problem-solving skills	Learning and cognition systems of the brain
Self-regulation skills	Regulatory systems for self-control, executive functions of the brain
Self-efficacy and positive self-perceptions	Mastery motivation
Hope, faith, and religious affiliations	Meaning-making systems of belief, religion
Effective schools	Community education system

variations in positive function had been neglected in favor of methods to study either typical (normative or average) development or problems and symptoms. Methods for assessing and tracking competence in age-salient developmental tasks were developed and greater attention was given to the variability in the normal range for social competence, work or romantic competence, civic engagement, and other domains of competence across the lifespan. Renewed attention was given to theories about adaptation, developmental tasks, and competence, which had roots deep in the history of science (Masten *et al.*, 2006a).

The complex conceptual and empirical connections between competence and psychopathology in development was re-examined (Masten *et al.*, 2006a). With powerful new statistical tools and longitudinal data on positive development as well as symptoms, it was possible to test ideas about *developmental cascades*, or the spreading effects of good and poor adaptation from one domain to another over time (Masten *et al.*, 2005; Masten & Cicchetti, 2010). Longitudinal data clearly indicated the high return on investment in programs in early childhood that promoted competence as these programs prevented problems developing (Heckman, 2006).

Highlights of the research findings on resilience in children and youth

In light of the extraordinary range in resilience research with respect to the populations and adversities studied, as well as conceptual and methodological variations, the findings have been remarkably consistent (Garmezy, 1985; Luthar, 2006; Masten, 2001, 2011). Many studies converge on a "short list" of factors with strong ties to resilience in children and youth, affording

important clues to the adaptive tools and systems for resilience (Masten, 2001). Table 7.1 provides examples of the factors often found in resilience studies and also the adaptive systems that may explain the power of these factors to facilitate adaptive behavior or recovery in the context of challenge.

Masten (2001) concluded that, in most situations, resilience depends on the operation of fundamental adaptive systems that are the legacy of biological and cultural evolution, rather than rare or extraordinary talents, resources, or efforts. Masten hypothesized that the capacity for resilience is generated by the "ordinary magic" of these systems when they are operating normally and, therefore, that the greatest lasting threats to children occur when the capacity of these protective systems is damaged, impaired, or destroyed. Catastrophic adversity can overwhelm all human adaptive capacity, even on a regional scale, as happens in major disasters. As the threat subsides and adaptive capacity is restored, adaptive processes begin to support recovery.

The basic adaptive systems that support individual resilience extend well beyond the individual. All living systems are interdependent with respect to the functioning of the systems in their environments. Moreover, humans are highly social, with lives embedded in many levels of social and cultural organization to enhance adaptability and the quality of life.

Each of these adaptive systems implicated for human development and resilience has a long history of research, in some cases across disciplines and levels of analysis, although there is less study of exactly how they work in the context of varying threats. Only a few of the adaptive systems are described here, with a focus on those that are being targeted in interventions to promote resilience.

Attachment relationships in resilience

From the earliest days of resilience science, investigators noted the essential role of close relationships for resilience, including the attachments among family members, romantic partners, friends, and also spiritual relationships. Every review of the evidence since then has corroborated the central importance of relationships for resilience. The role of these relationships appears to be multifaceted, providing emotional security, arousal regulation, practical help, physical defense, and access to resources through additional relationships (social capital). A powerful biological system is implicated by the data on relationships, initially delineated by John Bowlby (1969) in his attachment theory on the bonds that form between a caregiving parent figure and a child during infancy. This system has effects on behavior of both the caregiver and the child. Once an attachment bond has formed, for example, the child and the parent will both respond to perceived danger by seeking proximity and experience anxiety or panic if contact is blocked. An attachment figure can provide comfort to a frightened child and also serves as a secure emotional base for venturing out in the world when there is no danger. If a toddler ventures too far or becomes frightened for some reason, the child will rush back to the secure base for comfort. Children typically form attachment bonds with other family members and caregivers, pets, or snuggly objects; when they grow older, people form strong attachment relationships with friends, romantic partners, and spiritual figures. Loss of attachment figures can induce profound grief, but also can leave a young child unprotected from threats. When the primary caregiver of a child is lost or injured, it is crucial that someone else takes on the protective roles of the primary attachment figure. As people mature, they form attachment bonds with friends and partners that are more symmetrically balanced with respect to mutual comforting and care than the relationships of a parent with a child. Much of the research on the role of close relationships for adults in resilience has focused on the role of "social support," but the fundamental nature of the adaptive system underlying the protective effects of relationships is likely to be a mature form of attachment.

Intelligence and problem-solving systems of the human central nervous system

Another widely implicated system (or set of systems) for human adaptation is the central nervous system and its thinking capabilities for solving problems. Historically, intelligence has been described as the mental or cognitive activity associated with effective adaptation (Masten *et al.*, 2006a). It is not surprising from this perspective to observe that good cognitive skills have been implicated in many resilience studies of both children and adults (Masten, 2001; Luthar, 2006). The capabilities of the human brain to learn, think, and come up with solutions to problems about what is going on and what to do clearly improve with brain development, education, and experience. Until this adaptive tool is fully grown and operational, attachment relationships with adults and social organizations function to extend the cognitive capacities for resilience of an individual. Books, computers, and information processing on the Internet also have expanded human capacity for problem solving and finding adaptive solutions to specific threats.

Motivation to adapt: agency, self-efficacy, and the mastery motivation system

In 1959, Robert White published a now classic paper on competence, positing a motivation system that rewards and reinforces adaptive behavior leading to competence, thus yielding pleasure for perceived success in efforts to adapt. Pleasure in mastery, he argued, can be observed in humans and other similar species as they explore the world and try to solve problems or make things happen. White posited that humans are motivated to adapt to the environment and experience pleasure when they succeed. Later scholars elaborated on reward systems for adaptive behavior in theories about self-efficacy (Bandura, 1997) and intrinsic motivation (Ryan & Deci, 2000). People enjoy learning to walk, to throw a ball, to solve riddles, and to get jokes. Very powerful reward systems motivate and reinforce efforts to adapt and people who believe they will be successful can anticipate these rewards and also tend to persist in the face of failure. Parents and teachers are well aware of mastery motivation for learning and performance, and they often seek to provide small experiences of success to enhance the motivation for effort and achievement. Studies in resilience research of late bloomers, individuals who turn their lives in better directions in late adolescence or early adulthood, suggest that the motivation to change plays a key initiating role in change (Masten *et al.*, 2006b). This system may be shut down by neglect or adversity, particularly experiences that remove any sense of control over the environment and opportunities to experience agency in the world. The apathy observed among infants with neglect in orphanages or among animals in early learned helplessness experiments may be related to the extinction of this motivational system (Seligman & Beagley, 1975; Zeanah *et al.*, 2006). Interventions that provide opportunities for children and youth to experience success, or to help or lead others in recovery efforts after disaster, may have positive effects on the mastery motivation system.

Self-regulation systems

Effective responses to challenges often require the capacity to regulate and coordinate one's own behavior in the interest of adaptive goals, including the regulation of attention, arousal, emotions, and impulses. Self-regulation skills have been widely implicated in resilience studies. In the early history of psychology, the capacity to regulate oneself in the interest of adaptive behavior was described as a major function of the "ego" in psychoanalytic theory (Masten *et al.*, 2006a). More recently, self-regulation has been examined in theories about *executive function* and the underlying neural systems associated with the capacity and skills to control and coordinate one's own attention, thinking, planning, and actions (Rothbart *et al.*, 2007). Self-regulation systems develop over time with brain maturation (particularly as the prefrontal cortex develops), socialization, and experience. Self-regulatory skills are widely viewed as important tools for successful school entry in young children (Blair, 2002), and interventions to improve these skills with high-risk children show very promising effects (Diamond *et al.*, 2007). Evidence supports the developmental hypothesis that parents play an important role in the development of self-regulation, including their functioning as co-regulators of infant and child behavior until children develop the capabilities for self-regulation (Ainsworth *et al.*, 1978; Brody *et al.*, 2002; Eisenberg *et al.*, 2005). As noted above, attachment relationships, and particularly parent–child bonds in childhood, serve many regulatory functions in child development, helping children to learn impulse control and modulate their emotions. Later, peers influence self-regulation as they support or discourage risk-taking behaviors, thrill seeking, or self-control (Steinberg, 2008). There appears to be integral connections between self-regulation and social regulation over the life course. Similarly, institutions, religions, and other cultural practices also influence the development, reinforcement, and support of self-regulation in adaptive behavior.

Cultural systems in resilience

The rituals, routines, values, and practices of religions and other cultural systems that have evolved around the world appear to play many roles in potential support of resilience. The great religions of the world, through their values, rituals, and practices, appear to engage and nurture many of the fundamental protective systems for individual resilience. These include attachment relationships (both human and spiritual), emotion or arousal regulation (e.g., through rules for living, prayer, or meditation practices, and rituals for major life passages), and they also imbue life with meaning and value (Crawford *et al.*, 2006). Cultural groups based on ethnicity or nationality also have developed values, advice, wisdom, rituals, and practices to support adaptive responses to adversity, although culturally based protective systems have been relatively neglected in the research on individual resilience (Luthar, 2006; Masten & Wright, 2009). There is growing interest in adaptive systems embedded in cultural practices that serve to support the development of resilience capacity in communities, families, and individuals.

Other adaptive systems

Many other adaptive systems have evolved in human life, ranging from schools to emergency services, and it is not feasible to consider all the possibilities here. Effective schools and good teachers have been widely implicated as protective for high-risk children. Schools provide an important context for promoting the capacity for resilience in children because schools are charged with educational goals that enhance the development of fundamental protective systems such as problem solving and self-regulation systems (Masten *et al.*, 2008; Masten & Motti-Stefanidi, 2009). Schools also afford many opportunities for the development of protective relationships and mastery motivation. The Strength-Based School Counseling movement (Galassi & Akos, 2007) has the goal of enhancing the role of schools in building resilience capacity. Additionally, because children spend so much time in school, members of staff must be viewed as first responders in disaster planning. Social welfare systems also play a large role in the lives of some children, and some of these systems now actively have the goal of promoting resilience in human development (see Flynn *et al.*, 2006). There also is growing discussion of building resilient communities (Norris *et al.*, 2008), along with increasing interest in a more integrated approach to resilience that brings together knowledge from biological, social, communication, organizational, and large-scale ecosystem sciences to address problems that cut across traditional disciplinary boundaries, such as preparing for large-scale natural or human-generated disasters (Masten & Obradović, 2008; Longstaff, 2009).

A resilience framework for practice and policy

The study of resilience always had the ultimate goal of helping people faced with adversities and challenges that had the potential to undermine healthy function and development. As knowledge about resilience expanded, the complexity and enormity of the scientific quest became more apparent. Clearly, there remains much research ahead to understand the processes that result in resilience. Yet there are children and adults who are suffering now in the wake of disasters and other kinds of adversity. They cannot wait for a more complete explication of resilience. Therefore, it is reasonable to consider an evidence-informed, resilience-guided framework for practice and policy, while acknowledging that further research will undoubtedly improve the knowledge base about how resilience works and how to effectively promote resilience.

The ideas, results, and perspectives from research on resilience in children has had a transformative influence on theories and practices for intervention, shifting the paradigm for intervention away from deficit-focused models to more positive and strength-focused approaches (Cicchetti *et al.*, 2000; Luthar & Cicchetti, 2001; Nation *et al.*, 2003; Akos & Galassi, 2008; Masten & Wright, 2009).

Components of a resilience framework: the five Ms

The core features of a resilience-oriented approach to intervention can be described in terms of five "Ms"

mission: frame positive goals

models: include strengths, promotive and protective processes in models of change

measures: include assessments of positive predictors, outcomes, and change

methods: consider strategies that reduce risk, boost resources, mobilize/protect fundamental adaptive systems, and generate positive cascades

multilevel approaches: consider multiple systems that may influence human resilience.

These features reflect lessons gleaned from the study of resilience that can be applied to practice or programs aimed at promoting competence, preventing psychopathology, or planning for disaster response (Masten & Powell, 2003; Masten, 2006b; Masten & Wright, 2009). Each of these features also is enhanced by an understanding of development.

Mission

At the heart of a resilience-oriented approach is the concept of promoting positive outcomes. Positive goals and achievements are not only appealing to stakeholders and congruent with reward systems (e.g., mastery motivation) but also marking progress on such goals may improve morale, build self-efficacy of the young people and those implementing the program, and document progress that might be missed with a singular focus on symptoms or problems. Problems and suffering are not ignored, but the goals are defined in positive terms of promoting or supporting health, competence, achievements, or other positive objectives. Ideally, these goals are guided by a solid understanding of developmental pathways, tasks, and progressions related to the desired outcomes.

Models

Resilience research has generated new models of behavior and change that place greater emphasis on positive components and processes that had been overlooked in earlier models of intervention focusing exclusively on risks, vulnerabilities, symptoms, and disorders. More inclusive models can generate more complete measurement strategies and lead to new theories and strategies for change that can be tested in intervention experiments. Prevention science and programs aimed at positive youth development among high-risk youth have adopted these broader models in experimental designs that serve to test resilience theory about protective or promotive effects (e.g., Beardsley *et al.*, 1997; Forgatch & DeGarmo, 1999; Cicchetti *et al.*, 2000; Wolchik *et al.*, 2002; Greenberg, 2006; Masten A.S. *et al.*, 2006a, 2009a). Prevention and intervention strategies based on developmentally informed resilience-oriented models have proven to be effective not only for promoting competence and resilience but also for preventing and treating problems. Measures and methods of intervention often parallel models of change and, therefore, the new look of these models resulted in different strategies of intervention and assessment.

Measures

When the pioneers began their studies of resilience, they faced the challenge of inadequate measures, because the emphasis had been on assessing the problem side of behavior. Resilience research focused greater attention on reliable, valid, and developmentally attuned assessment of positive behavior and outcomes (Masten & Obradović, 2006). As a result, new and improved methods for assessing competence and positive aspects of development were developed. Nonetheless, there continues to be insufficient attention to culturally suitable measures of competence over the life course for assessing achievements and progress in development.

Methods

Resilience models and findings suggested several basic strategies for resilience promotion and also underscored the important of developmental perspectives on change. *Preventing risk factors* from occurring or lowering cumulative risk exposure was a basic strategy, and the stunning success of efforts to prevent premature birth and low birth weight in the twentieth century showed what risk-focused efforts could achieve. This strategy also reflects the recognition of "safety first" priorities; it does not make sense to build a new school if there are still landmines in the ground from war. Targeting risk exposure can take many forms, ranging from treating depression in new mothers to averting multiple foster home placements. The second basic resilience-oriented strategy of *boosting resources* or access to resources also takes many forms, from the provision of food and tutors to the building of schools and libraries or adding a case manager. The third strategy is focused on *mobilizing or improving fundamental adaptive systems*, in an effort to restore or boost the most powerful and universal protective systems for positive development and recovery. Again, this approach may take many forms, from adding parents or mentors to a child's life, providing opportunities to succeed or develop talent, to supporting cultural traditions that provide children with adaptive tools and opportunities for relationships with prosocial adults.

There is increasing interest in the possibility of "reprogramming" cognitive systems to improve executive function skills, discussed in the concluding section of this chapter. Finally, there is growing attention to strategic timing of interventions to increase the return on investment and the spread of positive effects, building on knowledge of development and the potential of cascading consequences of well-timed improvements in adaptive behavior. Developmental research shows that competence begets competence; this finding explain why early intervention focused on developmental task achievement has such lasting and cost-effective consequences (Heckman, 2006).

Multilevel approaches

The nature of dynamic, developing systems and the evidence on resilience converge on the conclusion that resilience can be studied and promoted across many levels of analysis and also that a multidisciplinary and multiple-level perspective may be necessary to harness the full potential for change in human development (Masten, 2007). Theoretically, effective changes at one level or location in interdependent systems will reverberate through interactions to influence other levels and other systems. The leverage for change may be greater at one level or location than another, as well as at one time in development or history than another. The chapters of this volume attest to the multiple levels and disciplines of resilience science. Those developing policies and practices to promote resilience in young people at risk are beginning to consider the potential of multiple-level approaches, whether one is reforming the child welfare systems (e.g., Flynn *et al.*, 2006) or preparing for disaster (e.g., Masten & Obradović, 2008).

Conclusions and future directions

As the second decade of the century begins, the fourth wave of resilience science is swelling on the horizon and overtaking earlier waves of research (Masten, 2007). The new wave is characterized by integrative goals and methodological advances that are opening new opportunities for studying the processes of resilience across an unprecedented range of levels, from the molecular to the global. In studies of resilience in human development, there is keen interest in neural plasticity and the possibility of interventions to alter how the brain develops and functions in processing information and responding to stress (Curtis & Cicchetti, 2003; Cicchetti & Curtis, 2006; Gunnar *et al.*, 2006; Lester *et al.*, 2006;

Belsky & Pluess, 2009). The idea that "plasticity" or "sensitivity to context" develops and changes, and may be shaped by nurture and reshaped by intervention, is opening new avenues of theory and empirical investigation with profound implications for interventions to promote resilience (Boyce & Ellis, 2005; Belsky & Pluess, 2009; Obradović & Boyce, 2009). With new tools to measure genes and their status ("on" or "off"), investigators are searching for genetic moderators of risk with protective effects, with an eye to future interventions that may facilitate resilience through preventing or promoting gene expression (Kim-Cohen & Gold, 2009).

At the level of social interaction, new methodologies are also making it possible to study social experience at the level of neural function (e.g., social neuroscience studies of peer rejection with brain imaging technology [Masten & Eisenberger, 2009; Masten C.L. *et al.*, 2009b]). In addition, the dynamics of dyadic interaction (among peers or parent–child) can be studied through "state-space grids" that depict the reciprocal interaction in relationships based on observational coding (Dishion & Piehler, 2007; Lewis, 2000). Through the use of this and other new tools that allow for observation and analysis at the micro-social level, it is becoming possible to examine in detail how parents may scaffold the development of self-regulation through the co-regulation they provide. It is also possible to study how prosocial peers may shape their mutual social competence by the positive modeling and reinforcement they provide each other. These methodological advances that capture social dynamics are producing new insights into the ways that relationships influence the development of competence and resilience.

Developmental scientists also are beginning to connect with investigators who study the behavior of much larger systems, such as communities and ecosystems, to tackle common conceptual and methodological issues and also to address problems like disaster or pandemics where many systems are involved in the effects or resilience in individuals, families, and communities (Masten & Obradović, 2008). Integrating resilience science across scale and disciplines is just at early stages. Disciplinary "cross-talk" has the potential to bring innovative ideas and methods across fields to accelerate progress. The first international conference on resilience science with a broad, integrative agenda across disciplines and scale was held in 2008 in Stockholm (known as "Resilience2008")

and a second is planned for 2011. Ecology and social sciences share a focus on resilience in developing, living systems.

In short, there remains much to do. Nonetheless, the compelling regularities in the findings on resilience in human development to date are encouraging in two ways. First, the findings offer a strong set of clues about "hot spots" for integration and further study of processes in the fourth wave of research (Masten, 2007). Second, the findings provide guidance for policy makers and those charged with helping young people in the near future, while further evidence on resilience accrues. Children and youth cannot wait for all the data. It is encouraging to know that there are robust findings in the initial waves of data collection that point to reasonable strategies for action in promoting resilience. It is also reassuring that resilience does not seem to require rare and extraordinary capabilities, but instead depends on common and ordinary human adaptive systems that develop and change, and can be nurtured, protected, and restored, with impressive power for recovery and resilience.

Acknowledgements

Preparation of this chapter was supported in part by the National Science Foundation with a grant to Ann Masten (No. 0745643) and Graduate Fellowships to Amy Monn and Laura Supkoff. Any opinions, conclusions, or recommendations expressed in this chapter are those of the authors and do not necessarily reflect the views of the National Science Foundation.

References

Ainsworth, M. D. S., Blehar, M., Waters, E., & Wall, S. (1978). *Patterns of attachment*. Hillsdale, NJ: Erlbaum.

Akos, P. & Galassi, J. P. (2008). Strengths-based school counseling. *Professional School Counseling*, Special issue **12**.

American Psychiatric Association (2000). *Diagnostic and statistical manual of mental disorders,* 4th edn, text revision. Washington, DC: American Psychiatric Press.

Bandura, A. (1997). *Self-efficacy: The exercise of control*. New York: Freeman.

Beardsley, W. R., Salt, P., Versage, E. M., *et al.* (1997). Sustained change in parents receiving preventive interventions for families with depression. *American Journal of Psychiatry*, **154**, 510–515.

Belsky, J. & Pluess (2009). The nature (and nurture?) of plasticity in early human development. *Perspectives on Psychological Science*, **4**, 345–351.

Blair, C. (2002). School readiness: Integrating cognition and emotion in a neurobiological conceptualization of child functioning at school entry. *American Psychologist*, **57**, 111–127.

Bonanno, G. A. (2004). Loss, trauma, and human resilience: Have we under-estimated the human capacity to thrive after extremely aversive events? *American Psychologist*, **59**, 20–28.

Bowlby, J. (1969). *Attachment and loss*. New York: Basic Books.

Boyce, W. T. & Ellis, B. J. (2005). Biological sensitivity to context: I. An evolutionary-developmental theory of the origins and functions of stress reactivity. *Development and Psychopathology*, **17**, 271–301.

Brody, G. H., Murry, V. M., Kim, S., & Brown, A. C. (2002). Longitudinal pathways to competence and psychological adjustment among African-American children living in rural single-parent households. *Child Development*, **73**, 1505–1516.

Cicchetti, D. (1984). The emergence of developmental psychopathology. *Child Development*, **55**, 1–7.

Cicchetti, D. (2006). Development and psychopathology. In D. Cicchetti & D. Cohen (eds.), *Developmental psychopathology*, Vol. 1: *Theory and method,* 2nd edn (pp. 1–23). Hoboken, NJ: Wiley.

Cicchetti, D. & Curtis, W. J. (2006). The developing brain ad neural plasticity: Implications for normality, psychopathology, and resilience. In D. Cicchetti & D. Cohen (eds.), *Developmental psychopathology,* Vol. 2: *Developmental neuroscience,* 2nd edn (pp. 1–64). Hoboken, NJ: Wiley.

Cicchetti, D., Rappaport, J., Sandler, I., & Weissberg, R. P. (eds.) (2000). *The promotion of wellness in children and adolescents*. Washington, DC: CWLA Press.

Crawford, E., Wright, M. O. D., & Masten, A. S. (2006). Resilience and spirituality in youth. In P. L. Benson, E. C. Roehlkepartain, P. E. King & L. Wagener (eds.), *The handbook of spiritual development in childhood and adolescence* (pp. 355–370). Newbury Park, CA: Sage.

Curtis, J. & Cicchetti, D. (2003). Moving resilience on resilience into the 21st century: Theoretical and methodological considerations in examining the biological contributors to resilience. *Development and Psychopathology*, **15**, 773–810.

Diamond, A., Barnett, W. S., Thomas, J. & Munro, S. (2007). Preschool program improves cognitive control. *Science*, **318**, 1387–1388.

Dishion, T. J. & Piehler, T. F. (2007). Peer dynamics in the development and change of child and adolescent problem behavior. In A. S. Masten (ed.), *Multilevel dynamics in developmental psychopathology: Pathways to the future* (pp. 151–180). Mahwah, NJ: Erlbaum.

Eisenberg, N., Zhou, Q., Spinrad, T. L., *et al.* (2005). Relations among positive parenting, children's effortful

control, and externalizing problems: A three-wave longitudinal study. *Child Development*, **76**, 1055–1071.

Flynn, R. J., Dudding, P. M., & Barber, J. G. (eds.) (2006). *Promoting resilience in development: A general framework for systems of care*. Ottawa: University of Ottawa Press.

Forgatch, M. S. & DeGarmo, D. S. (1999). Parenting through change: An effective prevention program for single mothers. *Journal of Consulting and Clinical Psychology*, **67**, 711–724.

Galassi, J. P. & Akos, P. (2007). *Strength-based school counseling: Promoting student development and achievement*. Mahway, NJ: Earlbaum.

Garmezy, N. (1985). Stress-resistant children: The search for protective factors. In J. E. Stevenson (ed.), *Recent research in developmental psychopathology* (pp. 213–233). [*Journal of Child Psychology and Psychiatry* Book Supplement 4.] Oxford: Pergamon Press.

Garmezy, N. & Streitman, S. (1974). Children at risk: the search for the antecedents to schizophrenia: Part 1. Conceptual models and research methods. *Schizophrenia Bulletin*, **8**, 14–90.

Greenberg, M. T. (2006). Promoting resilience in children and youth: Preventive interventions and their interface with neuroscience. *Annals of the New York Academy of Sciences*, **1094**, 139–150.

Gunnar, M. R. & Fisher, P. A. for the The Early Experience, Stress, and Prevention Network (2006). Bringing basic research on early experience and stress neurobiology to bear on preventive interventions for neglected and maltreated children. *Development and Psychopathology*, **18**, 651–677.

Havighurst, R. J. (1972). *Developmental tasks and education*, 3rd edn. New York: McKay.

Heckman, J. J. (2006). Skill formation and the economics of investing in disadvantaged children. *Science*, **312**, 1900–1902.

Kim-Cohen, J. & Gold, A. L. (2009). Measured gene–environment interactions and mechanisms promoting resilient development. *Current Directions in Psychological Science*, **18**, 138–142.

Lester, B. M., Masten, A., & McEwen, B. (eds.) (2006). Resilience in children. *Annals of the New York Academy of Sciences*, **1094**, 139–150.

Lewis, M. D. (2000). The promise of dynamic systems approaches for an integrated account of human development. *Child Development*, **71**, 36–43.

Longstaff, P. H. 2009. Managing surprises in complex systems: Multidisciplinary perspectives on resilience. *Ecology and Society*, **14**, 49, http://www.ecologyandsociety.org/vol14/iss1/art49/ (accessed February 24, 2011).

Luthar, S. S. (2006). Resilience in development: A synthesis of research across five decades. In D. Cicchetti &

D. J. Cohen (eds.), *Developmental psychopathology,* Vol. 3: *Risk, disorder, and adaptation,* 2nd edn (pp. 739–795). New York: Wiley.

Luthar, S. S. & Cicchetti, D. (2001). The construct of resilience: Implications for interventions and social policies. *Development and Psychopathology,* **12**, 857–885.

Masten, A. S. (2001). Ordinary magic: Resilience processes in development. *American Psychologist,* **56**, 227–238.

Masten, A. S. (2006a). Developmental psychopathology: Pathways to the future. *International Journal of Behavioral Development,* **31**, 47–54.

Masten, A. S. (2006b). Promoting resilience in development: A general framework for systems of care. In R. J. Flynn, P. Dudding, & J. G. Barber (eds.), *Promoting resilience in child welfare* (pp. 3–17). Ottawa: University of Ottawa Press.

Masten, A. S. (2007). Resilience in developing systems: Progress and promise as the fourth wave rises. *Development and Psychopathology,* **19**, 921–930.

Masten, A. S. (2011). Risk and resilience in development. In P. D. Zelazo (ed.), *Oxford handbook of developmental psychology.* New York: Oxford University Press, in press.

Masten, A. S. & Cicchetti, D. (2010). Editorial: Developmental cascades. *Development and Psychopathology,* **22**, 491–495.

Masten, A. S. & Coatsworth, J. D. (1998). The development of competence in favorable and unfavorable environments: Lessons from successful children. *American Psychologist,* **53**, 205–220.

Masten, A. S. & Motti-Stefanidi, F. (2009). Understanding and promoting resilience in children: Promotive and protective processes in schools. In T. B. Gutkin & C. R. Reynolds (eds.), *The handbook of school psychology,* 4th edn (pp. 721–738). New York: Wiley.

Masten, A. S. & Obradović, J. (2006). Competence and resilience in development. *Annals of the New York Academy of Sciences,* **1094**, 13–27.

Masten, A. S. & Obradović, J. (2008). Disaster preparation and recovery: Lessons from research on resilience in human development. *Ecology and Society,* **13**, 9, http://www.ecologyandsociety.org/vol13/iss1/art9/ (accessed February 26, 2011).

Masten, A. S. & Osofsky, J. (2010). Disasters and the impact on child development: Introduction to the special section. *Child Development,* **81**, 1029–1039.

Masten, A. S. & Powell, J. L. (2003). A resilience framework for research, policy, and practice. In S. S. Luthar (ed.), *Resilience and vulnerabilities: Adaptation in the context of childhood adversities* (pp. 1–25). New York: Cambridge University Press.

Masten, A. S. & Shaffer, A. (2006). How families matter in child development: Reflections from research on risk and resilience. In A. Clarke-Stewart & J. Dunn (eds.), *Families count: Effects on child and adolescent development* (pp. 5–25). New York: Cambridge University Press.

Masten, A. S. & Wright, M. O'D. (2009). Resilience over the lifespan: Developmental perspectives on resistance, recovery, and transformation. In J. W. Reich, A. J. Zautra, & J. S. Hall (eds.), *Handbook of adult resilience* (pp. 213–237). New York: Guilford Press.

Masten, A. S., Hubbard, J. J., Gest, S. D., *et al.* (1999). Competence in the context of adversity: Pathways to resilience and maladaptation from childhood to late adolescence. *Development and Psychopathology,* **11**, 143–169.

Masten, A. S., Roisman, G. I., Long, J. D., *et al.* (2005). Developmental cascades: Linking academic achievement, externalizing and internalizing symptoms over 20 years. *Developmental Psychology,* **41**, 733–746.

Masten, A. S., Burt, K. B., & Coatsworth, J. D. (2006a). Competence and psychopathology in development. In D. Ciccheti & D. J. Cohen (eds.), *Developmental psychopathology,* Vol. 3: *Risk, disorder and adaptation,* 2nd edn (pp. 696–738). New York: Wiley.

Masten, A. S., Obradović, J., & Burt, K. (2006b). Resilience in emerging adulthood: Developmental perspectives on continuity and transformation. In J. J. Arnett & J. L. Tanner (eds.), *Emerging adults in America: Coming of age in the 21st century* (pp. 173–190). Washington, DC: American Psychological Association Press.

Masten, A. S., Herbers, J. E., Cutuli, J. J., & Lafavor, T. L. (2008). Promoting competence and resilience in the school context. *Professional School Counseling,* **12**, 76–84.

Masten, A. S., Cutuli, J. J., Herbers, J. E., & Gabrielle-Reed, M. J. (2009a). Resilience in development. In C. R. Snyder, & S. J. Lopez (eds.), *The handbook of positive psychology,* 2nd edn (pp. 117–131). New York: Oxford University Press.

Masten, C. L. & Eisenberger, N. I. (2009). Exploring the pain of social rejection in adults and adolescents: A social cognitive neuroscience perspective. In M. Harris (ed.), *Bullying, rejection, and peer victimization: A social cognitive neuroscience perspective* (pp. 53–78). New York: Springer.

Masten, C. L., Eisenberger, N. I., Borofsky, L. A., *et al.* (2009b). Neural correlates of social exclusion during adolescence: Understanding the distress of peer rejection. *Social Cognitive and Affective Neuroscience,* **4**, 143–157.

Miller, G. E., Brehm, K., & Whitehouse, S. (1998). Reconceptualizing school-based prevention for antisocial behavior within a resiliency framework. *School Psychology Review,* **27**, 364–379.

Nation, M., Crusto, C., Wandersman, A., *et al.* (2003). What works in prevention: Principles of effective prevention programs. *American Psychologist*, **58**, 449–456.

Norris, F. H., Stevens, S. P., Pfefferbaum, B., Wyche, K. F., & Pfefferbaum, R. L. (2008). Community resilience as a metaphor, theory, set of capacities and strategy for disaster readiness. *American Journal of Community Psychology*, **41**, 127–150.

Obradović, J. & Boyce, W. T. (2009). Individual differences in behavioral, physiological, and genetic sensitivities to contexts: Implications for development and adaptation. *Developmental Neuroscience*, **31**, 300–308.

Obradović, J., Shaffer, A., & Masten, A. S. (2011). Risk in developmental psychopathology: Progress and future directions. In L. C. Mayes & M. Lewis (eds.), *The environment of human development: A handbook of theory and measurement*. New York: Cambridge University Press, in press.

Patterson, G. R., DeGarmo, D. S., & Forgatch, M. S. (2004). Systematic changes in families following prevention trials. *Journal of Abnormal Child Psychology*, **32**, 621–633.

Pine, D. S., Costello, J., & Masten, A. S. (2005). Trauma, proximity, and developmental psychopathology: The effects of war and terrorism on children. *Neuropsychopharmacology*, **30**, 1781–1792.

Rothbart, M. K., Sheese, B. E., & Posner, M. I. (2007). Executive attention and effortful control: Linking temperament, brain networks, and genes. *Child Development Perspectives*, **1**, 2–7.

Ryan, R. M. & Deci, E. L. (2000). Self-determination theory and the facilitation of intrinsic motivation, social development, and well-being. *American Psychologist*, **55**, 68–78.

Seligman, M. E. P. & Beagley, G. (1975). Learned helplessness in the rat. *Journal of Comparative and Physiological Psychology*, **88**, 534–541.

Sroufe, L. A., Egeland, B., Carlson, E. A., & Collins, W. A. (2005). *The development of the person: The Minnesota Study of Risk and Adaptation from birth to adulthood*. New York: Guilford Press.

Steinberg, L. (2008). A social neuroscience perspective on adolescent risk-taking. *Developmental Review*, **28**, 78–106.

Watt, N. F., Anthony, E. J., Wynne, L. C., & Rolf, J. E. (eds.) (1984). *Children at risk for schizophrenia: A longitudinal perspective*. Cambridge, UK: Cambridge University Press.

Werner, E. E. & Smith, R. S. (1992). *Overcoming the odds: High risk children from birth to adulthood*. Ithaca, NY: Cornell University Press.

White, R. W. (1959). Motivation reconsidered: The concept of competence. *Psychological Review*, **66**, 297–333.

Wolchik, S. A., Sandler, I. N., Millsap, R. E., *et al.* (2002). Six-year follow-up of preventive interventions for children of divorce: A randomized controlled trial. *Journal of the American Medical Association*, **288**, 1874–1881.

Zeanah, C. H., Smyke, A. T., & Settles, L. D. (2006). Orphanages as a developmental context for early childhood. In K. McCartney & D. Phillips (eds.), *Blackwell handbook of early childhood development* (pp. 424–454). Malden, MA: Blackwell.

Toward a lifespan approach to resilience and potential trauma

George A. Bonanno and Anthony D. Mancini

Introduction

As much as we might wish it otherwise, bad things happen: war, natural disaster, the death of close friends and relatives, serious accidents, senseless abuse or violence at the hand of others, and so on. Any of these things can and all too often do happen, and at every stage of life. Epidemiological data indicate that most adults experience at least one and usually several potentially traumatic events (PTE) during the course of their lives (Norris, 1992; Kessler *et al.*, 1995; Breslau *et al.*, 2000), and that most children are also exposed to such experiences (Copeland *et al.*, 2007). It is important to note, however, that life event research typically relies on retrospective accounts, which more than likely *underestimate* the frequency of PTEs. Indeed, a recent study that measured life events among college students over a four-year period using a weekly internet survey reported an average of six PTEs per student (Lalande & Bonanno, 2011).

Perhaps because acutely aversive events are so dreaded, both clinicians and the lay public tend to assume that they will almost always result in lasting emotional damage. The available evidence, however, suggests a more complex and far more encouraging picture. To emphasize the pronounced individual differences in the way people react to adversity, we emphasize that such events are only "potentially traumatic" (Norris, 1992; Bonanno, 2004), for the simple reason that not everyone experiences them as traumatic. Most people in fact cope with PTEs remarkably well (Bonanno, 2004, 2005; Bonanno & Mancini, 2008). Although some do, in fact, endure lasting emotional difficulties, the vast majority of people exposed to extreme adversity recover a semblance of their normal level of functioning within several months to several years after the event, and many if not most show

little evidence of more than transient disruptions in functioning.

This chapter briefly traces the history of the construct of psychological trauma and then describes recent empirical research on individual variation. The most common or prototypical outcome trajectories that have been elucidated in recent longitudinal research on PTEs are considered and the growing evidence for the human capacity to thrive even after the most difficult of experiences is addressed. The chapter then moves on to enumerate both individual differences and contextual factors that have been associated with a resilient outcome among children and adults. This capacity is examined from a lifespan perspective, situating resilience in the context of developmental factors. Finally, the implications of resilience across the lifespan are consider for therapeutic intervention .

Historical conceptions of psychological trauma

Practically since the beginnings of psychology and psychiatry as formal disciplines, researchers, theorists, and practitioners have looked to violent or life-threatening events as antecedents to psychological and physiological dysfunction (Ellenberger, 1970; Lamprecht & Sack, 2002). However, the primary source of dysfunction, even in the case of extreme stressor events, was generally situated within the individual, as for example in Kardiner's (1941) concept of *traumatic neuroses*. The great wars of the twentieth century, and in particular the global conflicts surrounding World War II, brought increasing awareness of the caustic impact of extreme stress on human functioning (Keegan, 1976). Nevertheless, it was not until late in the twentieth century that consensus began to emerge that extremely aversive events by themselves could be

Resilience and Mental Health: Challenges Across the Lifespan, ed. Steven M. Southwick, Brett T. Litz, Dennis Charney, and Matthew J. Friedman. Published by Cambridge University Press. © Cambridge University Press 2011.

the primary source of trauma-related dysfunction. In 1980, the American Psychiatric Association (1980) first formalized post-traumatic stress disorder (PTSD) as a legitimate diagnostic category, filling an enormous gap in public health knowledge about the impact of trauma. At the same time, the PTSD category also helped to consolidate and promote a surge of new research on traumatic stress (McNally, 2003). As a result, our understanding of the neurobiology, etiology, and treatment of PTSD has advanced considerably (Foa & Rothbaum, 1998; Ozer *et al.*, 2003; Dalgleish, 2004).

The advances generated by the nearly exclusive emphasis on PTSD have, however, come at a cost. When viewed from the perspective of the lay and professional literatures, this emphasis has tended to obscure the diversity in people's responses to PTEs. Indeed, the impact of PTEs is still commonly seen in relatively simplistic terms as a binary distinction between pathology versus the absence of pathology. This simplified view has resonated, with lingering controversies about the sometimes elusive distinction between genuine psychological trauma and malingering, an issue with particular relevance to war-related PTSD. Throughout the twentieth century, warfare had been plagued by an enduring tension about the proper time and place for diagnosis or treatment (Shepard, 2001; Lamprecht & Sack, 2002). During the most recent Iraq war, these issues once again flared into the open. For example, one recent study of returning US Army and Marine Corps soldiers involved in combat operations in Iraq and Afghanistan reported that many soldiers wanted but did not seek treatment out of fear of the stigma still associated with treatment for psychological difficulties in the armed forces (Hoge *et al.*, 2004).

This same type of oversimplification has plagued our understanding of bereavement, where there has long been confusion over distinctions between grief, healthy functioning, and denial. As was the case for psychological trauma more broadly, bereavement researchers and theorists have tended to view acute and chronic grief reactions as normative while offering little insight about possible resilience to loss. This emphasis on dysfunction has perhaps grown out of wider cultural assumptions about the appropriate way to grieve (Archer, 2001; Bonanno *et al.*, 2005a). For example, a report summarizing the views of bereavement experts in the 1980s stated that it was commonly assumed, particularly by clinicians, "that the absence of grieving phenomena following bereavement represents some form of personality pathology"(Osterweis

et al., 1984, p. 18). In similar fashion, Bowlby (1980, p. 138) considered the "prolonged absence of conscious grieving" as a type of disordered mourning, while, according to Rando (1993, p. 158), bereaved individuals who do not experience intense distress following a loss are in a state of denial and have "a powerful ability to block out reality." Indeed, the failure to grieve in response to bereavement was thought to reflect underlying psychopathology, because it suggested that the person is inhibiting or dissociating from negative feelings (Middleton *et al.*, 1993) or lacked sufficient attachment to the deceased (Fraley & Shaver, 1999). Bereaved people who failed to display overt grief or distress were presumed to be avoiding the "tasks" of grieving (Worden, 1991; Rando, 1993) and were commonly expected to have more severe difficulties or otherwise delayed reactions.

Trajectories of individual differences following potentially traumatic events

The discrepancy between clinical/cultural expectations and the empirical reality of how people behave in the aftermath of acute adversity can be attributed at least in part to misunderstandings about the nature of the underlying variability in change across time. Most traditional approaches to trauma, including the binary distinction between pathology versus the absence of pathology, are couched in the broader assumption that aversive life events produce a single *homogeneous* distribution of change over time (Muthén, 2004; Duncan *et al.*, 2006). Indeed, even non-categorical approaches to trauma, such as those that assess variability in the average level of functioning over time, have continued to embody the assumption that the underlying distribution is homogeneous.

In stark contrast to this approach, recent conceptual (Bonanno, 2004; Mancini *et al.*, 2011a) and statistical (Curran & Hussong, 2003; Muthén, 2004; Jung & Wickrama, 2008) advances have dramatically underscored the natural *heterogeneity* of human stress response. Empirical studies using this approach indicate that most of the variability in response to PTEs can be captured by four prototypical trajectories of adjustment across time: chronic dysfunction, gradual recovery, delayed reactions, and a relatively stable trajectory of healthy functioning or resilience (Bonanno, 2004). These trajectories are illustrated in Figure 8.1 and elaborated below.

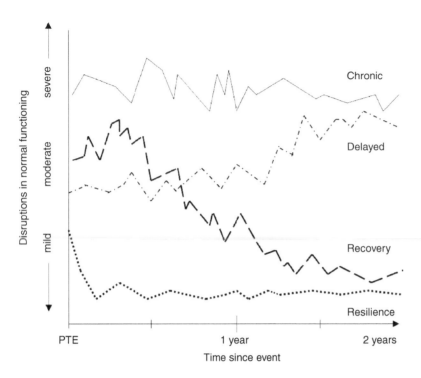

Figure 8.1 Prototypical patterns of disruption in normal functioning across time following potentially traumatic events (PTE). (Adapted with permission from Bonanno, 2004.).

The initial research in this area used relatively basic mathematical algorithms based on means and standard variation to assess individual differences in the trajectory of adjustment across time. Despite the simplicity of this approach, the same basic longitudinal and prospective trajectories have been identified across studies in response to bereavement (Bonanno *et al.*, 2002a, 2005b), disaster (Bonanno *et al.*, 2005c), and radiation treatment for breast cancer (Deshields *et al.*, 2006). More recent studies have benefited from advances in latent growth mixture modeling (LGMM; Muthén, 2004), a sophisticated statistical approach that is uniquely suited to identifying multiple unobserved trajectories in the data. The LGMM approach has been applied to a wide variety of longitudinal phenomena, including drinking among college students (Greenbaum *et al.*, 2005), childhood aggression (Schaeffer *et al.*, 2003, 2006), acclimation to retirement in late life (Pinquart & Schindler, 2007), and developmental learning trajectories (Boscardin *et al.*, 2008). The LGMM has also now been applied to the study of variability following PTEs, and has identified the same basic longitudinal trajectories in the aftermath of disease epidemic (Bonanno *et al.*, 2008), bereavement (Mancini *et al.*, 2011a), and traumatic injury (DeRoon-Cassini *et al.*, 2010).

Chronic dysfunction

It is well established that only a relatively small subset of those exposed to PTEs will eventually develop chronic pathological reactions. Post-traumatic stress disorder (American Psychiatric Association, 2000) is typically observed, for example, in only 5–10% of exposed individuals (Kessler *et al.*, 1995). The proportion of any sample will vary, of course, depending on the type and degree of exposure to PTEs. In exposure to exceptionally acute or corrosive events, the proportion of full-blown PTSD reactions may reach higher levels, sometimes as high as one third of the sample. For example, a survey of a population obtained by random-digit dialing one month after the September 11 2001 (9/11) terrorist attack in New York City estimated that 7.5% of Manhattan residents met criteria for PTSD and another 17.4% subsyndromal PTSD (Galea *et al.*, 2002). However, among those physically injured in the attack, PTSD prevalence rose to 26% (Bonanno *et al.*, 2006). In another study reanalyzing a representative sample of 1200 Vietnam veterans, chronic PTSD was estimated at 9% overall but among veterans with the highest levels of combat exposure the prevalence estimate rose to 28% (Dohrenwend *et al.*, 2006).

In studies of bereavement, the proportion of the individuals displaying more severe and chronic grief, or complicated grief, exhibits a similar bandwidth. Generally around 10% to 15% of those in bereaved samples will evidence complicated grief reactions (Bonanno & Kaltman, 2001). As was the case for PTEs in general, however, complicated grief tends to be more prevalent following more extreme losses, such as when the loss was from a violent cause (Zisook et al., 1998; Kaltman & Bonanno, 2003) or when the lost loved one was a child (Bonanno et al., 2005a).

There are relatively fewer data available on trauma and grief reactions among children. However, the data that are available suggest similar levels of complicated grief in children (Christ, 2000) but somewhat less PTSD in children than in adults (Copeland et al., 2007). As will be discussed in greater detail below, it is important to keep in mind that the question of adjustment is in many ways more complex among children. For example, children exposed to aversive events may fail to evidence PTSD or complicated grief but may manifest decrements in other areas, such as increased behavioral problems, substance use, academic problems, or peer conflict.

Delayed reactions

As mentioned above, one of the axiomatic assumptions in the bereavement literature has been that the absence of overt signs of grieving will eventually manifest as delayed grief reactions (Deutsch, 1937; Bowlby, 1980; Parkes & Weiss, 1980; Osterweis et al., 1984; Rando, 1993; Sanders, 1993). Despite the prevalence of this belief, solid empirical evidence for delayed grief has yet to be produced (Wortman & Silver, 1989; Bonanno & Kaltman, 1999), even in longitudinal studies explicitly designed to capture the phenomenon (Middleton et al., 1996; Bonanno & Field, 2001). By contrast, delayed PTSD reactions following PTEs have been detected, usually at low frequencies (e.g., Buckley et al., 1996; Bonanno et al., 2005c). The way delayed PTSD manifests, however, does not necessarily conform to the traditional idea of denied symptoms turning into full-blown pathology. Rather, delayed PTSD reactions are more accurately characterized as subthreshold PTSD that tends to worsen over time (Buckley et al., 1996; Brewin et al., 2008).

Resilience and recovery

Until recently, it was widely assumed that the enduring absence of trauma symptoms following exposure to a PTE was rare and would occur only in people with exceptional emotional strength (Casella & Motta, 1990; McFarlance & Yehuda 1996; Tucker et al., 2002). And as noted above, bereavement theorists have persistently regarded the relative absence of grief as a form of denial or hidden psychopathology (Middleton et al., 1993). There is now compelling evidence, however, that a genuine and enduring resilience is not rare but common and neither a sign of exceptional strength nor of psychopathology, but rather a fundamental feature of normal coping skills evident in both children and adults (Masten, 2001; Bonanno, 2004). Moreover, although resilience and recovery are sometimes conflated, the available longitudinal evidence, such as the LGMM analyses mentioned above, clearly demonstrate that resilience and recovery can be mapped as discrete and empirically separable outcome trajectories. Distinctions between resilience and recovery have been identified, for example, following loss (Bonanno et al., 2002a), treatment for neoplastic disease (Deshields et al., 2006), disease epidemic (Bonanno et al., 2008), terrorist attack (Bonanno et al., 2005c), and traumatic injury (DeRoon-Cassini et al., 2010).

Development of the construct of psychological resilience

Much of the original theorizing on resilience can be traced to developmental psychologists and psychiatrists during the 1970s. These pioneering researchers documented the large number of children who despite growing up in caustic socioeconomic circumstances (e.g., poverty, chronic abuse) nonetheless tended to reach normal healthy developmental milestones (Murphy & Moriarty, 1976; Rutter, 1979; Garmezy, 1991; Werner, 1995). A surprising feature of this work was that it showed resilience in children at risk to be common (Masten, 2001). Whereas traditional deficit-focused models of development had assumed that only children with remarkable coping ability could thrive in such adverse contexts, a growing body of evidence began to suggest that resilience is a result of normal human adaptational mechanisms (Masten, 2001). As noted above, however, most of this research focused on enduring aversive contexts, rather than isolated PTEs.

Although at the time of these studies the construct of resilience had not yet "trickled up" to the adult literature, the adult literature had periodically included reports of widespread resilience in the aftermath of isolated PTEs (e.g., Janis, 1951; Rachman, 1978). More recently, however, as the resilience construct has gained currency among trauma researchers, the differences between resilient outcomes in adults and children have begun to become apparent (Bonanno, 2004, 2005; Bonanno & Mancini, 2008). Some of the key differences seem to hinge on the temporal and sociocontextual characteristics of stress and adaptation at different points in the lifespan. For developing children, the definition of healthy adaptation is a complex issue (Luthar et al., 2000; Masten, 2001). For example, children at risk may evidence competence in one domain but fail to meet long-term developmental challenges in other domains (Luthar et al.,1993). By contrast, for adults exposed to a PTE this situation is arguably more straightforward (Bonanno, 2004, 2005).

Most but certainly not all of the PTEs adults might be confronted with can be classified as isolated stressor events (e.g., an automobile accident) that occur in a broader context of otherwise normative (i.e., low stress) circumstances. There may be concomitant stressors accompanying or extending the PTE (e.g., enduring health problems or change in financial situation), but this level of variability can typically be measured with a reasonable degree of reliability (e.g., Bonanno et al., 2005b, 2007). Finally, because developmental considerations are less pronounced in adults, responses to PTEs can usually be assessed in terms of deviation from or return to normative (baseline) functioning (Carver, 1998) rather than in terms of more abstract developmental milestones.

Based on these considerations, Bonanno (2004, pp. 20–21) defined *resilience* in adults as the ability of individuals "in otherwise normal circumstances who are exposed to an isolated and potentially highly disruptive event such as the death of a close relation or a violent or life-threatening situation to maintain relatively stable, healthy levels of psychological and physical functioning … as well as the capacity for generative experiences and positive emotions." By contrast, the more traditional *recovery* pathway is characterized by readily observable elevations in psychological symptoms that endure for at least several months before gradually returning to baseline, pre-trauma levels.

A key point is that even resilient individuals may experience at least some form of transient stress reaction. However, these reactions are usually mild to moderate in degree, relatively short term, and do not significantly interfere with their ability to continue functioning (Bonanno et al., 2002a, 2005b; Bisconti et al., 2006; Ong et al., 2006). For example, resilient individuals may have difficulty sleeping, or experience intrusive thoughts or memories of the event for several days or even weeks, but most can still manage to adequately perform the tasks of their daily life or career, or care for others. This is not to say, of course, that people showing resilient outcomes were not upset, disturbed, or unhappy about the occurrence of the event. Our point is merely that, as undesirable as PTEs might be, many people cope with such events extremely well and are able to continue meeting the normal daily demands of their lives.

Resilience across the lifespan

Despite the conceptual differences and similarities in the concept of resilience across the lifespan, there are surprisingly few comparative data on trauma and grief reactions among children and adults. Nonetheless, although there is variability across studies, the available data on the whole suggest that children cope as well if not better than adults. A study of children in the aftermath of Hurricane Andrew, a category 4 storm, observed elevated PTSD but at rates not dramatically dissimilar to those observed in adults: 39% of the children met PTSD criteria one month after the storm. Chronic PTSD measured 10 months after the storm was observed in 18% of the children (La Greca et al., 1996). Although this study did not report data on resilience, it can be surmised that approximately 44% of the children from the same sample evidenced minimal or a complete absence of PTSD symptoms at three months, suggesting that a substantial proportion most likely showed resilience. Consistent with the adult literature, the most robust predictor of PTSD scores at three months was an exposure variable, accounting for 15% of the variance. These findings would seem to suggest that children, when compared with adults, are equally and perhaps more vulnerable to PTSD. However, this study used a self-report measure that does not map directly onto a PTSD diagnosis. The researchers also employed a convenience sample.

By contrast, studies using representative samples and diagnostic interviews have suggested PTSD prevalence rates for children that are equal to if not substantially lower than adults. For example, another investigation of Hurricane Andrew found that among children aged 12 to 17 years, only 2.9% of males and 9.0% of females met criteria for a PTSD diagnosis (Garrison et al., 1995). Interestingly, increased age was associated with higher rates of PTSD, underlining the role of developmental factors. A similar prevalence of PTSD was observed (4.5%) in a study of child and adolescent survivors of the 1999 earthquake in Ano Liosia, Greece (Roussos et al., 2005). More recently, an epidemiological investigation of PTSD among children and young adults aged 9 to 16 years found even lower prevalence rates using a diagnostic interview measure and a representative probability sample (Copeland et al., 2007). In a longitudinal design spanning eight years and encompassing exposure to a variety of potentially extreme stressors (violence, interpersonal loss, sexual trauma), remarkably, less than 0.5% of children in the sample met full criteria for the PTSD diagnosis.

When considered together, these findings suggest, albeit preliminarily, that children cope extremely well with isolated PTEs. It remains to be determined, however, whether the phenomenology of PTSD in children is different from that in adults (Perrin et al., 2000). In addition, as noted above, the question of adjustment in children is in many ways more complex than among adults owing to the developmental issues involved. These conclusions, therefore, should be tempered with caution.

However, from the other end of the developmental continuum, older adulthood, we also find evidence of enhanced resilience. Again, while there is some variability across studies, the available evidence generally suggests that age buffers against harmful reactions to potential trauma. Phifer (1990) reported, for example, that after high exposure to a severe flood older adults were less vulnerable to psychological distress than were middle-aged adults with similar levels of exposure. Other studies have also suggested that older adults experience fewer symptoms than younger adults in response to various natural disasters, including a tornado (Bell, 1978) and the Buffalo Creek dam collapse (Green et al., 1990). In their meta-analysis of PTSD risk factors, Brewin and colleagues (2000) reported that older age is modestly associated with reduced PTSD. It is important to stress, however, that this effect showed heterogeneity across samples. As a counterexample, a comparison of the reactions of younger and older adults to the 1988 earthquake in Armenia failed to reveal differences in overall PTSD symptoms (Goenjian et al., 1994).

Few studies have explicitly examined resilience across adult and older adult groups. The available data, however, are partially consistent with the idea that age serves a buffering effect. Epidemiological data on reactions among New Yorkers to the 9/11 attacks indicated a nearly linear increase in resilience from younger to older adults (Bonanno et al., 2007). Moreover, in a full regression model that controlled for demographic and other predictor variables, adults 65 years of age or older were over three times as likely as young adults to be resilient after the 9/11 attacks. By contrast, a study of long-term adjustment of Hong Kong residents who had been hospitalized for severe acute respiratory syndrome (SARS) failed to find a link between resilience and age. It is not clear, however, whether the null effects of age reflected the nature of the stressor, or possible cultural variation.

One type of stressor that has consistently shown an age-related coping advantage is bereavement. Research on grief reactions in older adults indicate that they are generally less intense than those of younger adults (Sherbourne et al., 1992; Sanders, 1993; Nolen-Hoeksema & Ahrens, 2002); one obvious reason is that the loss may be viewed by older adults as a more normative, and hence less disturbing, consequence of the later stages of life (Neugarten, 1979). Indeed, other common late-life stressors, such as disability, appear to have more long-lasting and deleterious effects than bereavement (Reich et al., 1989).

An additional factor is that older bereaved persons are more likely to have provided high levels of care to a disabled spouse, resulting in increased caregiver strain but perhaps the opportunity for relief during bereavement (Bonanno et al., 2002a). Research by Schulz et al. (2001) has shown, in fact, that elderly bereaved people who experienced stressful caregiving reported *declines* in psychological distress after the spouse had died. However, spousal illness by itself, even in the absence of caregiver strain, may be enough to produce this pattern. In the Bonanno et al. (2002a) prospective study of conjugally bereaved older adults, mentioned above, 10% of the sample evidenced a similar trajectory of elevated depression prior to bereavement followed by improvement following the spouse's death loss. Although individuals showing the improved pattern did not report greater caregiving strain relative to other bereaved individuals, their spouses were nonetheless markedly more likely to have been ill in the years prior to their death. The depression–improvement pattern was also observed in a recent study of bereavement among HIV-positive gay men who had been caring for a partner who died of AIDS (Bonanno et al., 2005b). Again, the improvement pattern was associated spousal illness but not caregiver burden per se.

A more general mechanism that may inform resilience to PTEs among older adults is their increased ability to regulate emotion. The ratio of positive to negative affect, for example, has been shown to increase linearly with age (Mroczek & Kolarz, 1998; Charles *et al.*, 2001). In addition, older adults also generally show a superior capacity to regulate their own emotional experience (Lawton *et al.*, 1992) and report more complex or mixed emotional states (Labouvie-Vief *et al.*, 1989). These abilities, in turn, suggest that older adults may be particularly competent managers of their emotional states and may be better able to manage the distress related to loss or other PTEs.

A heterogeneous array of resilience-promoting factors

Research on the factors that promote resilient outcomes following PTEs is still in an embryonic stage. Yet, an emergent conclusion even at this early juncture is that resilience is multiply determined. In other words, there are not one or two dominant factors that might make a person resilient – nor does resilience appear to be an exclusive property of the individual. Rather, multiple, independent factors, some personal and some situational and contextual, contribute jointly to the development of resilient outcomes.

That a multiplicity of factors might promote resilience is not a new idea. This same conclusion was already evident decades earlier following the initial pioneering research into the nature of resilience in children. Among the factors implicated in that research were person-centered variables (e.g., temperament of the child) and sociocontextual factors (e.g., supportive relations, community resources) (Cowen, 1991; Werner, 1995; Rutter, 1999). Research on resilience in adults following PTEs has suggested a similar conclusion (Hobfoll, 2002; Bonanno, 2005; Bonanno & Mancini, 2008). Multivariate modeling of resilient outcomes has, for example, revealed upwards of 13 unique and independent predictive factors (e.g., Bonanno *et al.*, 2007).

Demographic and contextual factors

A prosaic group of predictors can be found in simple demographic variation. Resilience to trauma has been associated with male gender, older age, and greater education (Bonanno *et al.*, 2007). Racial/ethnic minority status is often considered as a risk factor for PTSD.

However, these effects usually disappear when socioeconomic status is statistically controlled. A recent exception, however, was a finding that among New Yorkers exposed to the 9/11 attacks, ethnic Chinese were considerably more likely to be resilient (Bonanno *et al.*, 2007).

Numerous theorists have delineated a crucial role for social and personal resources in the ways adults cope with stress (Murrell & Norris, 1983; Holahan & Moos, 1991; Hobfoll, 2002) There is also considerable research linking resources or change in resources with adjustment following PTEs (Freedy *et al.*, 1992; Kaniasty & Norris, 1993; Norris & Kaniasty, 1996; Ironson *et al.*, 1997). Recent research on resilience to trauma has further highlighted the particular importance of maintaining full-time employment and of a range of social resources (e.g., social support, social network size) (Bonanno *et al.*, 2007, 2008).

There is also strong evidence linking PTSD with increased life stress prior to and following the marker traumatic event (Brewin *et al.*, 2000; Kubiak, 2005). Recent evidence suggests an even stronger relationship between the relative absence of current and prior life stress and resilience to trauma (Bonanno *et al.*, 2007).

Personality: flexible and pragmatic coping

Perhaps the most imperative, but poorly understood conclusion from this emergent research is the idea that resilience does *not* depend solely on trait-like characteristics of the person. In part, the confusion arises from the fact that there are several unique person-centered factors that can be reliably associated with resilience. In attempting to place these findings in their proper perspective, however, we recall Mischel's (1969) famous if not timeless observation that personality rarely explains more than 10% of the actual variance in people's behavior across situations. And so is the case with the research on personality and resilience. What has yet to be done, and should be imperative for future research endeavors, is to examine the predictive role of personality in the context of broader, multivariate models that could help to ascertain the relative contribution of these measures.

In an attempt to move toward this type of integrative understanding, we have elsewhere parsed personality factors into two broad categories, which we have labeled *flexible adaptation* and *pragmatic coping* (Bonanno, 2005; Mancini & Bonanno, 2006; Bonanno & Mancini, 2008). The construct of pragmatic coping stems from the fact that highly stressful life events often pose very specific coping demands. Successfully meeting these demands may require a highly *pragmatic* or "whatever it takes" approach that is single minded and goal directed. Although pragmatic coping can arise in response to the situational demands, it has also been observed as a consequence of relatively rigid personality characteristics, such as repressive coping (Weinberger *et al.*, 1979) and the habitual use of self-enhancing attributions and biases, otherwise known as trait self-enhancement (Paulhus, 1998). A compelling finding with these pragmatic styles is that although they have been associated with some genuine costs (e.g., narcissism) they consistently predict superior adjustment in the face of loss or other PTEs (Bonanno *et al.*, 1995, 2002b, 2005c; Coifman *et al.*, 2007).

It should be stressed, however, that the majority of people who exhibit resilient outcomes are genuinely healthy people who appear to possess a capacity for behavioral elasticity or *flexible adaptation* to impinging challenges. A core aspect of this kind of flexibility is the capacity to shape and modify one's behavior to meet the demands of a given stressor event. This capacity can be observed early in development, yet can change over time as a result of the dynamic interplay of personality and social interactions with key attachment figures (Block & Block, 2006). Practically speaking, then, flexibility is a personality resource that helps to bolster resilience to aversive events, such as childhood maltreatment (Flores *et al.*, 2005), but it may also be enhanced or reduced by developmental experiences (Shonk & Cicchetti, 2001). Preliminary research on flexibility in adults suggests that the construct does eventually become stable and predicts resilience to PTEs (Fredrickson *et al.*, 2003; Bonanno *et al.*, 2004; Westphal *et al.*, 2010).

Worldviews (a-priori beliefs)

A broad-based predictor of resilient outcomes has to do with a-priori beliefs or worldviews. In the most general terms, worldviews form our most abstract and generalized conceptions of the extent that life is fair, benevolent, and predictable (Rubin & Peplau, 1975; Janoff-Bulman, 1992; Park & Folkman, 1997). Because worldviews are widely thought to be influenced by extremely stressful events (Schwartzberg & Janoff-Bulman, 1991; Janoff-Bulman, 1992), it has historically been difficult to untangle their direct effects on coping. The only feasible methodological solution to

this confound requires a design in which worldviews are assessed a priori, that is before the PTE occurs. For obvious reasons, this type of prospective design poses practical and methodological difficulties. Indeed, to our knowledge, only a few studies have as yet managed to meet such a condition. In the prospective study of spousal loss discussed above, Bonanno *et al.* (2002a) identified pre-loss predictors of a resilient outcome; among these were stronger a-priori beliefs in the world's justice and more accepting attitudes toward death. We recently provided additional confirmation for the role of a-priori beliefs by showing that favorable worldviews were related to adjustment over time only among bereaved persons and not among non-bereaved controls (Mancini *et al.*, 2011b). In one of the few investigations of PTSD to use pre-event data, Bryant and Guthrie (2007) assessed firefighters during their training and then collected a second wave of data four years later. Similar to the findings on bereavement, more negative pre-event beliefs, and in particular beliefs about the self, were associated with elevated PTSD symptoms four years later, accounting for 20% of the variance in those symptoms.

Positive emotions

One of the most robustly studied resilience factors in recent years has been positive emotion. It is widely acknowledged that positive emotions provide an array of adaptive benefits, both for everyday life and in response to stressful events (Lazarus *et al.*, 1980; Keltner & Bonanno, 1997; Tugade & Fredrickson, 2004; Fredrickson & Losada, 2005; but see also Bonanno *et al.*, 2007). However, the link between positive emotion and adjustment is particularly prominent in aversive contexts. In a recent experimental study (Papa & Bonanno, 2008), for example, the expression of positive emotion following exposure to a sad film predicted better psychological adjustment two years later. By contrast, positive emotional expressions following an amusing film were unrelated to long-term adjustment. Not surprisingly, then, the expression of positive emotions have consistently been shown to be a critical pathway toward healthy adaptation (Bonanno, 2004). For example, bereaved individuals who exhibited genuine laughs and smiles when describing a recent loss were found to be better adjusted over the first several years of bereavement (Bonanno & Keltner, 1997), and also evoked more favorable responses in observers (Keltner & Bonanno, 1997). Moreover, resilient bereaved people also reported the fewest regrets about their behavior with the spouse, or about things they may have done or failed to do when he or she was still alive. Finally, resilient individuals were less likely to search to make sense of or find meaning in the spouse's death, suggesting that they are less likely to engage in rumination, which has negative consequences for adjustment to loss (Nolen-Hoeksema *et al.*, 1997).

Positive emotions also serve a critical function in adapting to more extreme and acute events. In a prospective study on reactions to the 9/11 terrorist attacks among college students, Fredrickson *et al.* (2003) found that positive emotions, such as love, interest, and gratitude, fully mediated the relation between pre-event ego resilience, a trait-like personality characteristic, and post-event depression and growth experiences. In the study of Bonanno *et al.* (2005c) of high-exposure survivors of the 9/11 attacks, the trait self-enhancers who had coped so effectively in that study were also more likely to have experienced positive affect when talking about the event.

An ongoing and particularly compelling issue in this research pertains to the question of *how* positive emotions facilitate coping. The available empirical and theoretical literature suggests two independent but equally viable mechanisms may be at work. One is that positive emotions quiet or "undo" negative emotions, which, in turn, helps to reduce levels of distress following PTEs (Keltner & Bonanno, 1997; Fredrickson, 1998, 2001). A second mechanism is that positive emotions seem to facilitate coping by contagious influence on others and, more indirectly, by increasing the availability of social resources (Malatesta, 1990; Keltner & Bonanno, 1997; Fredrickson, 2001). There is consistent empirical support for the role of both of these mechanisms. However, what has not yet been clear is the extent to which each may be involved in coping with PTEs. Recently, Papa and Bonanno (2008) sought to clarify the issue using an unusual approach of embedding an experimental methodology within a broader, long-term field study of real-world adjustment among college students following the 9/11 terrorist attack. Their results showed clearly that *both* the undoing and social facilitation components of positive emotion each independently promoted adjustment over a two-year period following the attack (Papa & Bonanno, 2008).

Resilience factors specific to childhood

Given the paucity of research on trauma among children, relatively little progress has been made in identifying factors that might inform childhood resilience to isolated PTEs. In many cases, it may be possible to identify resilience factors as the inverse of identified risk factors (Bonanno, 2004). Indeed, as Masten (2001) has pointed out, risk and resilience factors often index a bipolar characteristic that can be either positive or negative, such as parenting (good or poor) or emotional stability (high or low). Although research on resilience in adults does not always conform to this simple bipolar scheme (e.g., Bonanno *et al.*, 2007), such a scheme may be more plausible in predicting childhood outcomes because of the longer-term developmental considerations. Proceeding in this way, some characteristics of children that are associated with better outcomes can be identified, although again we hasten to point out the paucity of prospective research in this area.

One study that met this criterion came from the programmatic investigation of children's responses to Hurricane Andrew carried out by La Greca and colleague (1998). These researchers had obtained data 15 months in advance of the hurricane and then at three and seven months after the hurricane. Among the predictors of positive post-hurricane outcome were low pre-hurricane anxiety and better pre-hurricane school performance, suggesting that emotional stability and academic achievement function as resilience factors.

Implications for intervention across the lifespan

The evolving literature on resilience in the face of PTEs holds important implications for possible intervention across the lifespan. Most prominent is the general rebuttal to the nearly axiomatic assumption that psychotherapeutic intervention for PTEs is invariably beneficial. The study of resilience advances the counterargument that such an assumption is misguided and that sweeping interventions can potentially even lead to harm (McNally *et al.*, 2003; Bonanno, 2004). For most people, intrinsic recovery processes will restore equilibrium relatively soon after exposure. Early interventions, such as critical incident stress debriefing, targeted indiscriminately at persons immediately after exposure to a PTE are not of questionable efficacy but have been shown in several studies to exacerbate trauma reactions, possibly by interfering with natural recovery processes (Mayou *et al.*, 2000; Litz *et al.*, 2002; McNally *et al.*, 2003). Although research on early interventions has up to now been confined to adults, we see no reason to think that children are more likely to benefit from such early interventions or that children would necessarily be inure to the potential iatrogenic effects of such interventions. Indeed, because children are more suggestible, it would appear likely that the processes that give rise to deterioration effects from early interventions may indeed be more and not less salient for children.

With regard to grief counseling, although opinion is somewhat mixed (Larson & Hoyt, 2007), we would maintain that the balance of evidence has not been favorable to traditional models of grief counseling (Bonanno, 2004; Bonanno & Lilienfeld, 2008). Meta-analyses of the effectiveness of grief counseling have consistently indicated small and often non-significant effects, which are substantially less than typically observed for other forms of psychotherapeutic intervention (Allumbaugh & Hoty, 1999; Kato & Mann, 1999; Currier *et al.*, 2008). Moreover, some studies have found no long-term benefits for grief counseling. Previously we have argued that, given the increasing awareness that resilience is the modal response to loss, grief-related interventions should only be targeted toward those who evidence obvious signs of enduring dysfunction and express a clear desire for help (Bonanno & Mancini, 2006; Mancini & Bonanno, 2006; Bonanno & Lilienfeld, 2008). Indeed, recent studies of grief interventions that adopted just such a targeted approach (e.g., Shear *et al.*, 2005; Boelen *et al.*, 2007) have shown markedly more promising results than were previously observed. We would suggest that similar guidelines should obtain when considering treatment for bereaved children. Indeed, a recent meta-analytic examination of grief counseling with children showed essentially the same pattern of overall poor effect sizes as observed with adults (Currier *et al.*, 2008). Consequently, rather than assuming that all children will benefit, it would seem to be the wiser course to reserve treatment for those children experiencing genuine and persistent difficulties and not just an expectable reaction to loss.

Although the story is somewhat more complicated for adults and children who have experienced other types of acutely aversive experience, the study of resilience makes it clear that PTSD afflicts only a small minority of those exposed. This appears to be the case in childhood, adulthood, and old age. For this reason, we would again argue that only those persons *at any age* who might evidence genuine dysfunction in the face of PTEs, as defined by recurring symptoms and interference with social roles and obligations, should

be candidates for treatment. It is inarguable that there are effective treatments for PTSD, particularly with respect to exposure treatment (Institute of Medicine, 2007). However, this fact does not preclude the possibility of iatrogenic effects, as witnessed in blanket early interventions following PTE.

Conclusions

It is our hope that continued research on resilience will foster an increased understanding of the normal human adaptability that characterizes all age groups, and focus on the factors that might both promote or prevent resilience at each stage of life. How resilience changes and how the factors that promote it might continue, disappear, or evolve across the lifespan are topics for future research. The study of resilience in the face of PTEs is nascent. Its promise, however, is enormous.

References

Allumbaugh, D. L. & Hoty, W. T. (1999). Effectiveness of grief therapy: A meta-analysis. *Journal of Counseling Psychology*, **46**, 370–380.

American Psychiatric Association (1980). *Diagnostic and statistical manual of mental disorders,* 3rd edn. Washington, DC: American Psychiatric Association.

American Psychiatric Association (2000). *Diagnostic and statistical manual*, 4th edn revised (DSM-IV-TR). Washington, DC: American Psychiatric Press.

Archer, J. (2001). Broad and narrow perspectives on grief: A commentary on Bonanno and Kaltman (1999). *Psychological Bulletin*, **127**, 554–560.

Bell, B. D. (1978). Disaster impact and response: Overcoming the thousand natural shocks. *Gerontologist*, **18**, 531–540.

Bisconti, T. L., Bergeman, C. S., & Boker, S. M. (2006). Social support as a predictor of variability: An examination of the adjustment trajectories of recent widows. *Psychology and Aging*, **21**, 590–599.

Block, J. & Block, J. H. (2006). Venturing a 30-year longitudinal study. *American Psychologist*, **61**, 315–327.

Boelen, P. A., de Keijser, J., van den Hout, M. A., & van den Bout, J. (2007). Treatment of complicated grief: A comparison between cognitive-behavioral therapy and supportive counseling. *Journal of Consulting and Clinical Psychology*, **75**, 277–284.

Bonanno, G. A. (2004). Loss, trauma, and human resilience: Have we underestimated the human capacity to thrive after extremely aversive events? *American Psychologist*, **59**, 20–28.

Bonanno, G. A. (2005). Resilience in the face of loss and potential trauma. *Current Directions in Psychological Science*, **14**, 135–138.

Bonanno, G. A. & Field, N. P. (2001). Examining the delayed grief hypothesis across 5 years of bereavement. *American Behavioral Scientist*, **44**, 798–816.

Bonanno, G. A. & Kaltman, S. (1999). Toward an integrative perspective on bereavement. *Psychological Bulletin*, **125**, 760–776.

Bonanno, G. A. & Kaltman, S. (2001). The varieties of grief experience. *Clinical Psychology Review*, **21**, 705–734.

Bonanno, G. A. & Keltner, D. (1997). Facial expressions of emotion and the course of conjugal bereavement. *Journal of Abnormal Psychology*, **106**, 126–137.

Bonanno, G. A. & Lilienfeld, S. O. (2008). Let's be realistic: When grief counseling is effective and when it's not. *Professional Psychology: Research and Practice*, **39**, 377–378.

Bonanno, G. A. & Mancini, A. D. (2006). Bereavement-related depression and PTSD: Evaluating interventions. In L. Barbanel & R. Sternberg (eds.), *Psychological interventions in times of crisis* (pp. 37–55). New York: Springer.

Bonanno, G. A. & Mancini, A. D. (2008). The human capacity to thrive in the face of potential trauma. *Pediatrics*, **121**, 369–375.

Bonanno, G. A., Keltner, D., Holen, A., & Horowitz, M. J. (1995). When avoiding unpleasant emotions might not be such a bad thing: Verbal–autonomic response dissociation and midlife conjugal bereavement. *Journal of Personality and Social Psychology*, **69**, 975–989.

Bonanno, G. A., Wortman, C. B., Lehman, D. R., *et al.* (2002a). Resilience to loss and chronic grief: A prospective study from preloss to 18-months postloss. *Journal of Personality and Social Psychology*, **83**, 1150–1164.

Bonanno, G. A., Field, N. P., Kovacevic, A., & Kaltman, S. (2002b). Self-enhancement as a buffer against extreme adversity: Civil war in Bosnia and traumatic loss in the United States. *Personality and Social Psychology Bulletin*, **28**, 184–196.

Bonanno, G. A., Papa, A., Lalande, K., Westphal, M., & Coifman, K. (2004). The importance of being flexible: The ability to both enhance and suppress emotional expression predicts long-term adjustment. *Psychological Science*, **15**, 482–487.

Bonanno, G. A., Papa, A., Lalande, K., Zhang, N., & Noll, J. G. (2005a). Grief processing and deliberate grief avoidance: A prospective comparison of bereaved spouses and parents in the United States and the People's Republic of China. *Journal of Consulting and Clinical Psychology*, **73**, 86–98.

Bonanno, G. A., Moskowitz, J. T., Papa, A., & Folkman, S. (2005b). Resilience to loss in bereaved spouses, bereaved parents, and bereaved gay men. *Journal of Personality and Social Psychology*, **88**, 827–843.

Bonanno, G. A., Rennicke, C., & Dekel, S. (2005c). Self-enhancement among high-exposure survivors of the September 11th terrorist attack: Resilience or social maladjustment? *Journal of Personality and Social Psychology*, **88**, 984–998.

Bonanno, G. A., Galea, S., Bucciarelli, A., & Vlahov, D. (2006). Psychological resilience after disaster: New York City in the aftermath of the September 11th terrorist attack. *Psychological Science*, **17**, 181–186.

Bonanno, G. A., Galea, S., Bucciarelli, A., & Vlahov, D. (2007). What predicts psychological resilience after disaster? The role of demographics, resources, and life stress. *Journal of Consulting and Clinical Psychology*, **75**, 671–682.

Bonanno, G. A., Ho, S. M. Y., Chan, J., *et al.* (2008). Psychological resilience and dysfunction among hospitalized survivors of the SARS epidemic in Hong Kong: A latent class approach. *Health Psychology*, **27**, 659–667.

Boscardin, C. K., Muthén, B., Francis, D. J., & Baker, E. L. (2008). Early identification of reading difficulties using heterogeneous developmental trajectories. *Journal of Educational Psychology*, **100**, 192–208.

Bowlby, J. (1980). *Attachment and loss,* Vol 3: *Loss: Sadness and depression*. New York: Basic Books.

Breslau, N., Davis, G. C., Peterson, E. L., & Schultz, L. R. (2000). A second look at comorbidity in victims of trauma: A posttraumatic stress disorder-major depression connection. *Biological Psychiatry*, **48**, 902–909.

Brewin, C. R., Andrews, B., & Valentine, J. D. (2000). Meta-analysis of risk factors for posttraumatic stress disorder in trauma-exposed adults. *Journal of Consulting and Clinical Psychology*, **68**, 748–766.

Brewin, C. R., Scragg, P., Robertson, M., *et al.* (2008). Promoting mental health following the London bombings: a screen and treat approach. *Journal of Traumatic Stress*, **21**, 3–8.

Bryant, R. A. & Guthrie, R. M. (2007). Maladaptive self-appraisals before trauma exposure predict posttraumatic stress disorder. *Journal of Consulting and Clinical Psychology*, **75**, 812–815.

Buckley, T. C., Blanchard, E. B., & Hickling, E. J. (1996). A prospective examination of delayed onset PTSD secondary to motor vehicle accidents. *Journal of Abnormal Psychology*, **105**, 617–625.

Carver, C. S. (1998). Resilience and thriving: Issues, models, and linkages. *Journal of Social Issues*, **54**, 245–266.

Casella, L. & Motta, R. W. (1990). Comparison of characteristics of Vietnam veterans with and without posttraumatic stress disorder. *Psychological Reports*, **67**, 595–605.

Charles, S. T., Reynolds, C. A., & Gatz, M. (2001). Age-related differences and change in positive and negative affect over 23 years. *Journal of Personality and Social Psychology*, **80**, 136–151.

Christ, G. H. (2000). *Healing children's grief: Surviving a parent's death from cancer*. New York: Oxford University Press.

Coifman, K. G., Bonanno, G. A., Ray, R. D., & Gross, J. J. (2007). Does repressive coping promote resilience? Affective–autonomic response discrepancy during bereavement. *Journal of Personality and Social Psychology*, **92**, 745–758.

Copeland, W. E., Keeler, G., Angold, A., & Costello, E. J. (2007). Traumatic events and posttraumatic stress in childhood. *Archives of General Psychiatry*, **64**, 577–584.

Cowen, E. L. (1991). In pursuit of wellness. *American Psychologist*, **46**, 404–408.

Curran, P. J. & Hussong, A. M. (2003). The use of latent trajectory models in psychopathology research. *Journal of Abnormal Psychology*, **112**, 526–544.

Currier, J. M., Neimeyer, R. A., & Berman, J. S. (2008). The effectiveness of psychotherapeutic interventions for bereaved persons: A comprehensive quantitative review. *Psychological Bulletin*, **134**, 648–661.

Dalgleish, T. (2004). Cognitive approaches to posttraumatic stress disorder: The evolution of multirepresentational theorizing. *Psychological Bulletin*, **130**, 228–260.

DeRoon-Cassini, T. A., Mancini, A. D., Rusch, M. D., & Bonanno, G. A. (2010). Psychopathology and resilience following traumatic injury: A latent growth mixture model analysis. *Rehabilitation Psychology*, **55**, 1–11.

Deshields, T., Tibbs, T., Fan, M. Y., & Taylor, M. (2006). Differences in patterns of depression after treatment for breast cancer. *Psycho-Oncology*, **15**, 398–406.

Deutsch, H. (1937). Absence of grief. *Psychoanalytic Quarterly*, **6**, 12–22.

Dohrenwend, B. P., Turner, J. B., Turse, N. A., *et al.* (2006). The psychological risks of Vietnam for US veterans: A revisit with new data and methods. *Science*, **313**, 979–982.

Duncan, T. E., Duncan, S. C., & Strycker, L. A. (2006). *An introduction to latent variable growth curve modeling: concepts, issues, and applications*, 2nd edn. Mahwah, NJ: Erlbaum.

Ellenberger, H. F. (1970). *The discovery of the unconscious: History and evolution of dynamic psychiatry*. New York: Basic Books.

Flores, E., Cicchetti, D., & Rogosch, F. A. (2005). Predictors of resilience in maltreated and nonmaltreated Latino children. *Developmental Psychology*, **41**, 338–351.

Foa, E. B. & Rothbaum, B. O. (1998). *Treating the trauma of rape: Cognitive behavioral therapy for PTSD*. New York: Guilford Press.

Fraley, R. C. & Shaver, P. R. (1999). Loss and bereavement: Attachment theory and recent controversies concerning "grief work" and the nature of detachment. In J. Cassidy & P. R. Shaver (eds.), *Handbook of attachment: Theory, research, and clinical applications* (pp. 735–759). New York: Guilford Press.

Fredrickson, B. L. (1998). What good are positive emotions? *Review of General Psychology*, **2**, 300–319.

Fredrickson, B. L. (2001). The role of positive emotions in positive psychology: The broaden-and-build theory of positive emotions. *American Psychologist*, **56**, 218–226.

Fredrickson, B. L. & Losada, M. F. (2005). Positive affect and the complex dynamics of human flourishing. *American Psychologist*, **60**, 678–686.

Fredrickson, B. L., Tugade, M. M., Waugh, C. E., & Larkin, G. R. (2003). What good are positive emotions in crisis? A prospective study of resilience and emotions following the terrorist attacks on the United States on September 11th, 2001. *Journal of Personality and Social Psychology*, **84**, 365–376.

Freedy, J. R., Shaw, D. L., Jarrell, M. P., & Masters, C. R. (1992). Towards an understanding of the psychological impact of natural disasters: An application of the conservation resources stress model. *Journal of Traumatic Stress*, **5**, 441–454.

Galea, S., Ahern, J., Resnick, H., *et al.* (2002). Psychologial sequelae of the September 11 terrorist attacks in New York City. *New England Journal of Medicine*, **346**, 982–987.

Garmezy, N. (1991). Resilience and vulnerability to adverse developmental outcomes associated with poverty. *American Behavioral Scientist*, **34**, 416–430.

Garrison, C. Z., Bryant, E. S., Addy, C. L., *et al.* (1995). Posttraumatic stress disorder in adolescents after Hurricane Andrew. *Journal of the American Academy of Child and Adolescent Psychiatry*, **34**, 1193–1201.

Goenjian, A. K., Najarian, L. M., Pynoos, R. S., *et al.* (1994). Posttraumatic stress disorder in elderly and younger adults after the 1988 earthquake in Armenia. *American Journal of Psychiatry*, **151**, 895–901.

Green, B. L., Lindy, J. D., Grace, M. C., *et al.* (1990). Buffalo Creek survivors in the second decade: Stability of stress symptoms. *American Journal of Orthopsychiatry*, **60**, 43–54.

Greenbaum, P. E., Del Boca, F. K., Darkes, J., Wang, C.-P., & Goldman, M. S. (2005). Variation in the drinking trajectories of freshmen college students. *Journal of Consulting and Clinical Psychology*, **73**, 229–238.

Hobfoll, S. E. (2002). Social and psychological resources and adaptation. *Review of General Psychology*, **6**, 307–324.

Hoge, C. W., Castro, C. A., Messer, S. C., *et al.* (2004). Combat duty in Iraq and Afghanistan, mental health problems, and barriers to care. *New England Journal of Medicine*, **351**, 13–22.

Holahan, C. J. & Moos, R. H. (1991). Life stressors, personal and social resources, and depression: A 4-year structural model. *Journal of Abnormal Psychology*, **100**, 31–38.

Institute of Medicine (2007). *Treatment of posttraumatic stress disorder: An assessment of the evidence*. Washington, DC: National Academies Press.

Ironson, G., Wynings, C., Schneiderman, N., *et al.* (1997). Posttraumatic stress symptoms, intrusive thoughts, loss, and immune function after Hurricane Andrew. *Psychosomatic Medicine*, **59**, 128–141.

Janis, I. L. (1951). *Air war and emotional stress*. New York: McGraw Hill.

Janoff-Bulman, R. (1992). *Shattered assumptions: towards a new psychology of trauma*. New York: Free Press.

Jung, T. & Wickrama, K. A. (2008). An introduction to latent class growth analysis and growth mixture modeling. *Social and Personality Psychology Compass*, **2**, 302–317.

Kaltman, S. & Bonanno, G. A. (2003). Trauma and bereavement: Examining the impact of sudden and violent deaths. *Journal of Anxiety Disorders*, **17**, 131–147.

Kaniasty, K. & Norris, F. H. (1993). A test of the social support deterioration model in the context of natural disaster. *Journal of Personality and Social Psychology*, **64**, 395–408.

Kardiner, A. (1941). *The traumatic neuroses of war*. New York: Paul B. Hoeber.

Kato, P. M. & Mann, T. (1999). A synthesis of psychological interventions for the bereaved. *Clinical Psychology Review*, **19**, 275–296.

Keegan, J. (1976). *The face of battle*. Harmondsworth, UK: Chaucer Press.

Keltner, D. & Bonanno, G. A. (1997). A study of laughter and dissociation: Distinct correlates of laughter and smiling during bereavement. *Journal of Personality and Social Psychology*, **73**, 687–702.

Kessler, R. C., Sonnega, A., Bromet, E., Hughes, M., & Nelson, C. B. (1995). Posttraumatic stress disorder in the National Comorbidity Survey. *Archives of General Psychiatry*, **52**, 1048–1060.

Kubiak, S. P. (2005). Trauma and cumulative adversity in women of a disadvantaged social location. *American Journal of Orthopsychiatry*, **75**, 451–465.

La Greca, A. M., Silverman, W. K., Vernberg, E. M., & Prinstein, M. J. (1996). Symptoms of posttraumatic stress in children after Hurricane Andrew: A prospective study. *Journal of Consulting and Clinical Psychology*, **64**, 712–723.

La Greca, A. M., Silverman, W. K., & Wasserstein, S. B. (1998). Children's predisaster functioning as a predictor of posttraumatic stress following Hurricane Andrew. *Journal of Consulting and Clinical Psychology*, **66**, 883–892.

Labouvie-Vief, G., DeVoe, M., & Bulka, D. (1989). Speaking about feelings: Conceptions of emotion across the life span. *Psychology and Aging*, **4**, 425–437.

LaLande, K. M. & Bonanno, G. A. (2011). Retrospective memory bias for the frequency of potentially traumatic events. *Psychological Trauma*, in press.

Lamprecht, F., & Sack, M. (2002). Posttraumatic stress disorder revisited. *Psychosomatic Medicine*, **64**, 222–237.

Larson, D. G. & Hoyt, W. T. (2007). What has become of grief counseling? An evaluation of the empirical foundations of the new pessimism. *Professional Psychology: Research and Practice*, **38**, 347–355.

Lawton, M., Kleban, M. H., Rajagopal, D., & Dean, J. (1992). Dimensions of affective experience in three age groups. *Psychology and Aging*, **7**, 171–184.

Lazarus, R. S., Kanner, A. D., & Folkman, S. (1980). Emotions: A cognitive–phenomenological analysis. In R. Plutchik & H. Kellerman (eds.), *Theories of emotion. Emotions: theory, research, and experience*, Vol. 1 (pp. 189–217). New York: Academic Press.

Litz, B. T., Gray, M. J., Bryant, R. A., & Adler, A. B. (2002). Early intervention for trauma: Current status and future directions. *Clinical Psychology: Science and Practice*, **9**, 112–134.

Luthar, S. S., Doernberger, C. H., & Zigler, E. (1993). Resilience is not a unidimensional construct: Insights from a prospective study of inner-city adolescents. *Development and Psychopathology*, **5**, 703–717.

Luthar, S. S., Cicchetti, D., & Becker, B. (2000). The construct of resilience: A critical evaluation and guidelines for future work. *Child Development*, **71**, 543–562.

Malatesta, C. Z. (1990). The role of emotions in the development and organization of personality. In R. A. Thompson (ed.), *Nebraska symposium on motivation*, Vol. 36 (pp. 1–56). Lincoln, NB: University of Nebraska Press.

Mancini, A. D. & Bonanno, G. A. (2006). Resilience in the face of potential trauma: Clinical practices and illustrations. *Journal of Clinical Psychology*, **62**, 971–985.

Mancini, A. D., Bonanno, G. A., & Clark, A. E. (2011a). Stepping off the hedonic treadmill: Individual differences in response to major life events. *Journal of Individual Differences*, in press.

Mancini, A. D., Prati, G., & Bonanno, G. A. (2011b). Do shattered worldviews lead to complicated grief? Prospective and longitudinal analyses. *Journal of Social and Clinical Psychology*, 30, 184–215.

Masten, A. S. (2001). Ordinary magic: Resilience processes in development. *American Psychologist*, **56**, 227–238.

Mayou, R. A., Ehlers, A., & Hobbs, M. (2000). Psychological debriefing for road traffic accident victims. *British Journal of Psychiatry*, **176**, 589–593.

McFarlane, A. C. & Yehuda, R. (1996). Resilience, vulnerability, and the course of posttraumatic reactions. In A. C. M. B. A. van der Kolk, & L. Weisaeth (eds.), *Traumatic stress* (pp. 155–181). New York: Guilford Press.

McNally, R. J. (2003). Progress and controversy in the study of posttraumatic stress disorder. *Annual Review of Psychology*, **54**, 229–252.

McNally, R. J., Bryant, R. A., & Elhers, A. (2003). Does early psychological intervention promote recovery from posttraumatic stress? *Psychological Science in the Public Interest*, **4**, 45–79.

Middleton, W., Moylan, A., Raphael, B., Burnett, P., & Martinek, N. (1993). An international perspective on bereavement related concepts. *Australian and New Zealand Journal of Psychiatry*, **27**, 457–463.

Middleton, W., Burnett, P., Raphael, B., & Martinek, N. (1996). The bereavement response: A cluster analysis. *British Journal of Psychiatry*, **169**, 167–171.

Mischel, W. (1969). Continuity and change in personality. *American Psychologist*, **24**, 1012–1018.

Mroczek, D. K. & Kolarz, C. M. (1998). The effect of age on positive and negative affect: A developmental perspective on happiness. *Journal of Personality and Social Psychology*, **75**, 1333–1349.

Murphy, L. B. & Moriarty, A. E. (1976). *Vulnerability, coping, and growth*. New Haven, CT: Yale University Press.

Murrell, S. A. & Norris, F. H. (1983). Resources, life events, and changes in psychological states: A prospective framework. *American Journal of Community Psychology*, **11**, 473–491.

Muthén, B. (2004). Latent variable analysis: Growth mixture modeling and related techniques for longitudinal data. In D. Kaplan (ed.), *Handbook of quantitative methodology for the social sciences* (pp. 345–368). Newbury Park, CA: Sage.

Neugarten, B. L. (1979). Time, age, and the life cycle. *American Journal of Psychiatry*, **136**, 887–894.

Nolen-Hoeksema, S. & Ahrens, C. (2002). Age differences and similarities in the correlates of depressive symptoms. *Psychology and Aging*, **17**, 116–124.

Nolen-Hoeksema, S., McBride, A., & Larson, J. (1997). Rumination and psychological distress among bereaved partners. *Journal of Personality and Social Psychology*, **72**, 855–862.

Norris, F. H. (1992). Epidemiology of trauma: Frequency and impact of different potentially traumatic events on different demographic groups. *Journal of Consulting and Clinical Psychology*, **60**, 409–418.

Norris, F. H. & Kaniasty, K. (1996). Received and perceived social support in times of stress: A test of the social support deterioration deterrence model. *Journal of Personality and Social Psychology*, **71**, 498–511.

Ong, A. D., Bergeman, C. S., Bisconti, T. L., & Wallace, K. A. (2006). Psychological resilience, positive emotions, and successful adaptation to stress in later life. *Journal of Personality and Social Psychology*, **91**, 730–749.

Osterweis, M., Solomon, F., & Green, F. (1984). *Bereavement: Reactions, consequences, and care*. Washington, DC: National Academies Press.

Ozer, E. J., Best, S. R., Lipsey, T. L., & Weiss, D. S. (2003). Predictors of posttraumatic stress disorder and symptoms in adults: A meta-analysis. *Psychological Bulletin*, **129**, 52–73.

Papa, A. & Bonanno, G. A. (2008). Smiling in the face of adversity: Interpersonal and intrapersonal functions of smiling. *Emotion*, **8**, 1–12.

Park, C. L. & Folkman, S. (1997). Meaning in the context of stress and coping. *Review of General Psychology*, **1**, 115–144.

Parkes, C. M. & Weiss, R. S. (1980). *Recovery from bereavement*. New York: Basic Books.

Paulhus, D. L. (1998). Interpersonal and intrapsychic adaptiveness of trait self-enhancement: A mixed blessing? *Journal of Personality and Social Psychology*, **74**, 1197–1208.

Perrin, S., Smith, P., & Yule, W. (2000). Assessment and treatment of PTSD in children and adolescents. *Journal of Child Psychiatry and Psychology*, **41**, 277–289.

Phifer, J. F. (1990). Psychological distress and somatic symptoms after natural disaster: Differential vulnerability among older adults. *Psychology and Aging*, **5**, 412–420.

Pinquart, M. & Schindler, I. (2007). Changes of life satisfaction in the transition to retirement: a latent-class approach. *Psychology and Aging*, **22**, 442–455.

Rachman, S. J. (1978). *Fear and courage*. New York: Freeman.

Rando, T. A. (1993). *Treatment of complicated mourning*. Champaign, IL: Research Press.

Reich, J. W., Zautra, A. J., & Guarnaccia, C. A. (1989). Effects of disability and bereavement on the mental health and recovery of older adults. *Psychology and Aging*, **4**, 57–65.

Roussos, A., Goenjian, A. K., Steinberg, A. M., *et al.* (2005). Posttraumatic stress and depressive reactions among children and adolescents after the 1999 earthquake in Ano Liosia, Greece. *American Journal of Psychiatry*, **162**, 530–537.

Rubin, Z. & Peplau, L. A. (1975). Who believes in a just world? *Journal of Social Issues*, **31**, 65–89.

Rutter, M. (1979). Protective factors in children's responses to stress and disadvantage. In M. W. Kent & J. E. Rolf (eds.), *Primary prevention of psychopathology: Social competence in children*, Vol. 3 (pp. 49–74). Lebanon, NH: University Press of New England.

Rutter, M. (1999). Resilience concepts and findings: Implications for family therapy. *Journal of Family Therapy*, **21**, 119–144.

Sanders, C. M. (1993). Risk factors in bereavement outcome. In M. S. Stroebe, W. Stroebe, & R. O. Hansson (eds.), *Handbook of bereavement: Theory, research, and intervention* (pp. 255–267). Cambridge, UK: Cambridge University Press.

Schaeffer, C. M., Petras, H., Ialongo, N., Poduska, J., & Kellam, S. (2003). Modeling growth in boys' aggressive behavior across elementary school: Links to later criminal involvement, conduct disorder, and antisocial personality disorder. *Developmental Psychology*, **39**, 1020–1035.

Schaeffer, C. M., Petras, H., Ialongo, N., *et al.* (2006). A comparison of girls' and boys' aggressive–disruptive behavior trajectories across elementary school: prediction to young adult antisocial outcomes. *Journal of Consulting and Clinical Psychology*, **74**, 500–510.

Schulz, R., Beach, S. R., Lind, B., *et al.* (2001). Involvement in caregiving and adjustment to death of a spouse: Findings from the caregiver health effects study. *Journal of the American Medical Association*, **285**, 3123–3129.

Schwartzberg, S. S. & Janoff-Bulman, R. (1991). Grief and the search for meaning: Exploring the assumptive worlds of bereaved college students. *Journal of Social and Clinical Psychology*, **10**, 270–288.

Shear, K., Frank, E., Houck, P. R., & Reynolds, C. F. (2005). Treatment of complicated grief: a randomized controlled trial. *Journal of the American Medical Association*, **293**, 2601–2608.

Shepard, B. (2001). *A war of nerves: Soldiers and psychiatrists in the twentieth century*. Cambridge, MA: Harvard University Press.

Sherbourne, C., Meredith, L., Rogers, W., & Ware, J. (1992). Social support and stressful life events: Age differences in their effects on health-related quality of life among the chronically ill. *Quality of Life Research*, **1**, 235–246.

Shonk, S. M. & Cicchetti, D. (2001). Maltreatment, competency deficits, and risk for academic and behavioral maladjustment. *Developmental Psychology*, **37**, 3–17.

Tucker, P., Pfefferbaum, B., Doughty, D. E., *et al.* (2002). Body handlers after terrorism in Oklahoma City: Predictors of posttraumatic stress and other symptoms. *American Journal of Orthopsychiatry*, **72**, 469–475.

Tugade, M. M. & Fredrickson, B. L. (2004). Resilient individuals use positive emotions to bounce back from negative emotional experiences. *Journal of Personality and Social Psychology*, **86**, 320–333.

Weinberger, D. A., Schwartz, G. E., & Davidson, R. J. (1979). Low-anxious, high-anxious, and repressive coping styles: Psychometric patterns and behavioral and physiological responses to stress. *Journal of Abnormal Psychology*, **88**, 369–380.

Werner, E. E. (1995). Resilience in development. *Current Directions in Psychological Science*, **4**, 81–85.

Westphal, M., Seivert, N., & Bonanno, G. A. (2010). Expressive flexibility. *Emotion*, **10**, 92–100.

Worden, J. W. (1991). *Grief counseling and grief therapy: A handbook for the mental health practitioner*, 2nd edn. New York: Springer.

Wortman, C. B. & Silver, R. C. (1989). The myths of coping with loss. *Journal of Consulting and Clinical Psychology*, **57**, 349–357.

Zisook, S., Chentsova-Dutton, Y., & Shuchter, S. R. (1998). PTSD following bereavement. *Annals of Clinical Psychiatry*, **10**, 157–163.

Resilience in older adults

Diane L. Elmore, Lisa M. Brown, and Joan M. Cook

Introduction

Older adulthood is a developmental stage at the end of the lifespan when an individual experiences a number of significant changes in life circumstances. These age-associated events include changes in physical appearance and body composition, which can result in increased vulnerability to both acute and chronic physical illness as well as functional limitations such as decreased mobility and diminished sensory capacities. In addition, older people generally experience numerous losses and stressors, such as moving to a fixed income, increasing expenses, and loss of retirement investments; death of family members, friends and loss of social network; alterations in social position; changes in housing and work; and spousal caregiving and widowhood. The ability to adapt positively to these types of stressful life event and to other adversities is likely an important factor in "successful" aging.

Currently, older adults are among the fastest growing subgroups of the population in the USA as in many other countries. Recent estimates suggest that there are approximately 37 million people aged 65 years and over in the USA, accounting for over 12% of the total population (US Federal Interagency Forum on Aging-Related Statistics, 2008). By the year 2030, the number of individuals age 65 years and over is expected to nearly double to 71.5 million, accounting for approximately 20% of the US population (US Federal Interagency Forum on Aging-Related Statistics, 2008).

In addition to the increase in size of the older adult population, the aging community is also becoming increasingly racially and ethnically diverse and is enjoying greater educational attainment than previous generations of older people (US Federal Interagency Forum on Aging-Related Statistics, 2008). Both the increase in number and the growing diversity of older adults makes this subgroup of the population exceedingly important to policy makers, service providers, clinicians, and researchers.

This chapter will focus on issues of resilience in older adults. First, definitions of resilience and historical perspectives on its investigation in older adults will be reviewed. Then, a brief general background regarding older adult mental health and aging will be presented. Next, an overview of the resilience of older adults in the face of stressful life events will be provided. Fourth, an overview of resilience and recovery from trauma in older adults will be discussed. Lastly, areas for continued scientific and clinical investigation related to resilience among older adults will be highlighted.

Definitions and historical perspectives

The impact of trauma on older adults appears to be a complicated relationship with a number of potentially exacerbating and buffering variables that can impact outcomes. While a great deal of work has been done to identify predictors of post-traumatic stress disorder (PTSD), few efforts have focused on predictors of resilience (Bonanno, 2004). A number of key variables have been discussed as potentially influencing the response to traumatic events, including gender; type of trauma; a history of prior trauma; personality traits; social support; interpersonal relationships; sense of purpose; humor; self-efficacy; and interactions of age with social, economic, cultural, and historical contexts (Breslau *et al.*, 1998; Norris *et al.*, 2002a; Boardman *et al.*, 2008). Bonanno (2004) suggested that more work was needed to assess whether the inversion of the predictors of PTSD may allow for the prediction of resilient functioning.

Resilience and Mental Health: Challenges Across the Lifespan, ed. Steven M. Southwick, Brett T. Litz, Dennis Charney, and Matthew J. Friedman. Published by Cambridge University Press. © Cambridge University Press 2011.

Since the late 1990s, the concept of resilience has received increasing attention, yet its exact definition is still being debated. Foster (1997) posited that one's ability to function in the face of stress and adversity is influenced by genetics, life experiences and learning, and individual differences in resources. Some of these genetic, environmental, and individual variables may be particularly important to older adults, including the trauma-specific variables (e.g., severity and duration), social support, and societal reaction to the particular trauma.

Hardy *et al.* (2004, p. 260) conceptualized resilience as a response to a stressful event, rather than a personality trait, and identified several possible resilient responses, including "a small initial decremental effect of the event, a rapid recovery, minimal negative long-term consequences, and positive long-term consequences of the event." Bonanno (2004, p. 20) theorized that resilience is the ability "to maintain relatively stable, healthy levels of psychological and physical functioning" in the face of loss and trauma. He described recovery as a distinct concept represented by a return to pre-event functioning following a period of clinical or subclinical psychopathology. He asserted that the distinctions between resilience and recovery are critical, as they can inform the appropriate need for and timing of clinical intervention (Bonanno, 2004).

Although the investigation of resilience and its potential correlates and predictors has received limited attention in older adults, the importance of related concepts in the early stages of the field of gerontology should be noted. These include successful aging, positive adjustment to aging, personality traits, and morale and life satisfaction. The relationship between these earlier age-related concepts and resilience will be discussed throughout this chapter.

Mental health and aging

In order to understand resilience in older adults, it is useful to be aware of some basic facts regarding aging and mental health. Community-based prevalence estimates suggest that approximately 5% of older adults meet criteria for either an anxiety or a depressive disorder (Gallo & Lebowitz, 1999). It is estimated that approximately 20% of those aged 55 years or older experience some type of mental disorder, and that 13% of those aged 65 years and over meet criteria for a mental disorder other than dementia (Robins & Regier, 1991; US Department of Health and Human

Services, 1999). Additionally, approximately 3% of older adults have PTSD, while the prevalence is 10% among middle-aged adults and 9% among younger adults (Norris, 1992).

While these data may imply that a majority of older adults enjoy good mental health, the existing literature suggests that the mental health problems of older adults are often underreported and, therefore, underdiagnosed (Brown *et al.*, 2007a). Further complicating detection is a subsyndromal presentation of symptoms in this population. Although the person's symptoms are not sufficient to warrant a formal psychiatric diagnosis, the presence of subthreshold symptoms can still adversely affect quality of life, morbidity, and mortality and may require clinical attention.

Resilience and recovery from trauma

Traumatic experiences can impact individuals across the lifespan. For some, such experiences are associated with negative psychological outcomes, such as PTSD (Norris, 1992; Norris *et al.*, 2002b, 2002c). While most attention in the loss and trauma literature has focused on the maladaptive outcomes associated with traumatic experiences, not all individuals experience significant negative psychosocial outcomes following trauma. In fact, a growing body of research suggests that most people are highly resilient and able to fully recover from serious adverse life events (US Department of Health and Human Services, 2001; Bonanno, 2004). A number of key variables have been discussed as potentially influencing the response to traumatic events, including age.

To date, relatively limited attention in the trauma literature has focused exclusively on older adults. What literature does exist identifies older adults as a group that is either primarily vulnerable or mainly resilient to the negative consequences of traumatic stressors (e.g. Kilijanek & Drabek, 1979). Further, most of the literature related to the impact of trauma on older adults focuses on psychopathology and the negative effects of such events; the small body of resilience research does present some possible explanations for resilient responses in the face of adversity.

Theories of resilience and aging

A number of theories have been developed to explain the response of older adults to traumatic events. Among the theories that may help in understanding resilience in older adults are those based on vulnerability, inoculation, burden, mortality effects, and maturation. A brief overview and critical summary of these theories in respect to their relevance to older adults are given below.

Vulnerability theory

Early research on trauma suggested that disasters had a disproportionate effect on older adults. It was hypothesized that this group experienced a greater sense of deprivation relative to their losses and, consequently, more psychological distress than younger adults (Kilijanek & Drabek, 1979). However, this was not borne out by other research (Fields, 1996). Some evidence finds support for the vulnerability hypothesis, in which older adult survivors of prolonged stress (e.g., Holocaust survivors, prisoners of war) are thought to be at greater risk because of their increasing age in conjunction with the accumulation of greater numbers of traumas resulting from their longer lives (Solomon & Prager, 1992; Danieli, 1997). Older adults have a varied and extensive accumulation of life experiences that affect short- and long-term vulnerability following exposure to traumas (Phifer & Norris, 1989; Brown *et al.*, 2007b).

Stress inoculation hypothesis

The stress inoculation hypothesis was posited by Eysenck (1983), who asserted that earlier trauma fosters resilience to subsequent traumas. Specifically, two paths were suggested: direct tolerance, in which prior exposure to a specific stressor may lessen the effect of that stressor in the future, and cross-tolerance, in which prior exposure to a particular stressor may lessen the effect of a different stressor in the future (Eysenck, 1983). According to Norris and Murrell (1988), the stress inoculation theory is particularly relevant to understanding the effects of trauma on older adults because of their rich history of experience. Evidence that supports the inoculation hypothesis suggests that older adults may respond better following traumatic events because of their experience with trauma earlier in life (Knight *et al.*, 2000). Despite a more severe or direct exposure to the event, poorer health status, and fewer social and economic resources, a lifetime of learning how to cope with taxing events as well as fewer currently unresolved stressful experiences are believed to promote adaptation to disasters in older adults (Phifer, 1990).

Several studies have found support for the inoculation hypothesis among aging survivors of trauma (Norris & Murrell, 1988; Knight *et al.*, 2000). In a study

of older adults following significant floods, Norris and Murrell (1988) examined the concepts of both direct tolerance and cross-tolerance in older adults. Their investigation suggested that prior experience with floods as well as prior exposure to other traumatic events moderated the impact of the event. Interestingly, stronger support was found for the relationship with direct tolerance than for cross-tolerance (Norris & Murrell, 1988). Similarly, in a study of adults aged 30 to 102 years following the 1994 Northridge earthquake, Knight *et al.* (2000) found that greater prior earthquake exposure was associated with lower post-earthquake depression scores. These findings are consistent with the inoculation hypothesis.

Norris and Murrell (1988) cautioned that, while the inoculation hypothesis may hold true for older adults who experience intermittent stressors, similar results may not be expected following prolonged or extended stress. In fact, other studies of aging survivors, which are discussed later in this chapter, have not found sufficient support for this hypothesis but instead have suggested that prior prolonged stressors may be associated with increased vulnerability to subsequent traumas (Bremner *et al.*, 1992; Solomon & Prager, 1992; Yehuda *et al.*, 1995; Breslau *et al.*, 1998; Green *et al.*, 2000; Nishith *et al.*, 2000).

Burden hypothesis

The burden perspective is another theory that may be relevant to understanding resilience among some older adults. This hypothesis posits that middle-aged individuals are the most affected by trauma because they experience the greatest disruptions and demands on their time as providers of care to both younger and older generations and as breadwinners. In a study of adults following Hurricane Hugo, Thompson *et al.* (1993) found a curvilinear interaction between post-disaster distress and age, with middle-aged adults experiencing the highest symptom levels. This study provides support for the burden hypothesis.

Maturation hypothesis

Another explanation for resilience among older adults is the maturation hypothesis, which suggests that older adults have more mature coping styles and this makes them less emotionally reactive to stressful events (Knight *et al.*, 2000). However, this theory was not supported by research that examined depressed mood prior to and after the 1994 Northridge earthquake. Age did not moderate the relationship between damage exposure and rumination. As noted above, the inoculation hypothesis was supported by the findings from this study.

The mortality effect

The mortality effect has also been posited as a possible explanation for the resilience that is observed among older adults who have experienced trauma. This effect refers to the fact that many of the less resilient survivors of trauma may have died before reaching older adulthood, thus leaving a healthier group of aging individuals behind (Creamer & Parslow, 2008).

Summary

While these hypotheses are important in understanding the possible relationships between age and trauma, overly simplistic explanations that characterize the entire population of older adults do not provide an accurate scientific or clinical picture. Recent reviews of the literature suggest that such differential classifications of older adults may be unhelpful and may have deleterious effects for older adults (Norris et al., 2002a; Cook & Elmore, 2009).

Bonanno (2004) suggested that individuals may be more resilient to extremely aversive events than commonly thought. He asserted that theorists in the loss and trauma fields may underestimate and misunderstand resilience, as most of the evidence in the field is derived from samples of individuals who have had negative outcomes following trauma. According to Bonanno (2004), most who experience a traumatic event will display healthy responses indicative of a resilience trajectory. Bonanno et al. (2005a) asserted that the resilient pathway is far more common than the recovery trajectory. Therefore, caution should be taken to ensure that clinical interventions do not interfere with or undermine the natural resilience of the majority of survivors (Bonanno, 2004).

Resilience in daily life and in the face of stressful events

In general, older adults experience stressful life events at a much greater frequency than younger adults (Hughes et al., 1988). Indeed, some events that were previously infrequent across the lifespan become increasingly normative. A review of the literature revealed that a growing number of researchers are examining the role of resilience and aging. Below is a brief synopsis of several studies that were published since the mid 1990s. In a sample of community-dwelling adults over 60 years of age, a self-rating of successful aging was significantly correlated with higher resilience, greater activity, and greater number of close friends – despite some having chronic physical illnesses and some type of disability (Montross et al., 2006).

In a sample of community-dwelling predominately Caucasian women over age 60 years, exploratory factor analysis using the Connor–Davidson Resilience Scale (Connor & Davidson, 2003) yielded four factors: (1) personal control and goal orientation, (2) adaptation and tolerance for negative affect, (3) leadership and trust in instincts, and (4) spiritual coping (Lamond et al., 2008). Consistent with the findings of Montross et al. (2006), self-rated successful aging was positively associated with resiliency. Other predictors of resiliency were higher emotional well-being, optimism, social engagement, and fewer cognitive complaints. These results are similar to those obtained in younger samples. However, the authors posited that the construct of resilience differs between younger and older adults (Lamond et al., 2008, p. 152): in younger adults resilience may be construed as "problem- or task-focused active coping" whereas in older adults it may be better characterized as "acceptance and toleration of negative affect."

In a sample of community-residing older adults, a wide range of reactions associated with resilience were displayed in response to a stressful event. Resilience was associated with a range of demographic, clinical, functional, and psychosocial factors (Hardy et al., 2004). In particular, high resilience was associated with male gender, living with others, high grip strength, independence in ability to perform instrumental activities of daily living, having few depressive symptoms, and having good to excellent self-rated health. The authors suggested that resilience is a key factor for older adults in maintaining their well-being as well as a potentially important predictor of recovery from future illness and disability (Hardy et al., 2004).

The relationship between resilience, sense of coherence, purpose in life, and self-transcendence to perceived physical and mental health was examined in individuals aged 85 years or older (Nygren et al., 2005). There was a high correlation between scores on several of the resilience-like scales suggesting some core dimension of inner strength.

In an examination of resilience in the face of daily stressors and recent widowhood, Ong and colleagues (2004, 2006) found that the occurrence of daily positive emotions moderated stress reactivity and mediated stress recovery. Just as the research conducted by Nygren *et al.* (2005) suggested that resilience was related to some aspect of inner strength, this study found that a stable facet of personality, sometimes referred to as stress tolerance or neuroticism, predicted a weaker association between negative and positive emotions during periods of heightened stress trait resilience. Their findings revealed that experiencing positive emotions over time helped high-resilient individuals to recover from daily stress.

Results from the population-based Heidelberg Centenarian Study challenged the concept that psychological resilience may end in very advanced age (Jopp & Rott, 2006). Indeed, centenarians reported high levels of happiness, a substantial proportion of which was accounted for by basic resources such as health and social network. Some resource effects were mediated through self-referent beliefs (e.g., self-efficacy) and attitudes toward life (e.g., optimistic outlook).

Qualitative research also yielded similar results to the quantitative studies described above. A series of interviews were conducted with women between the ages of 70 and 80 years to determine factors that contribute to resilience (Kinsel, 2005). Seven factors emerged as contributing to resilience, including social connectedness, facing challenges "head-on," spiritual grounding, curiosity, and helping others (Kinsel, 2005).

In addition to daily stressors, there are a number of specific stressors that are often increasingly encountered with age. These include caregiving and widowhood. Further, there are also traumatic stressors that are particularly salient for the current and emerging cohort of older adults, such as being a veteran of World War II, the Holocaust, and the Korean conflict. Consideration of such historical sociopolitical stressors may be helpful in identifying potential generational traumas. The following provides an overview of some key research findings associated with these events as they relate to resilience in older adults.

Caregiving and illness

Currently, approximately 80% of older adults live with at least one chronic health condition, which can often result in limitations in daily activities and health-related quality of life (Centers for Disease Control and Prevention & the Merck Company Foundation, 2007). The most likely caregiver of an impaired older adult

in the community is their aging spouse (American Psychological Association, 1997). While caregiving can be extremely stressful and result in negative outcomes for some, others appear to be quite resilient to the potential deleterious effects of caregiving (Schulz *et al.*, 1997; Beach *et al.*, 2000). The caregiving literature makes a unique contribution to our understanding of resilience. Several recent studies that examined resilience and caregiving are discussed.

In a longitudinal investigation of caregivers of someone with dementia, who were in various stages related to providing care (e.g., institutionalization, care-recipient death), high baseline resilience was associated with less-frequent institutionalization and loss to follow-up as well as more frequent care-recipient mortality (Gaugler *et al.*, 2007). High resilience at baseline was also associated with the following variables: female care recipients, providing care for a longer duration, spending more time providing care, and greater utilization of formal and informal resources (Gaugler *et al.*, 2007). Furthermore, contextual care-recipient status and resource indicators were also associated with stress resistance or resilience in caregivers for a person with dementia. In contrast, higher baseline resilience was associated with caregivers being white, having independent activities of daily living dependencies, living with care recipients, and having greater education and income; it was also associated with greater cognitive impairment in care recipients (Gaugler *et al.*, 2007).

Qualitative research has also examined aging, caregiving, and resilience. Three to five in-depth interviews were conducted over the course of several years with older African-Americans who had chronic illness (Becker & Newsom, 2005). Their experiences and perceptions of racism influenced how they viewed and coped with their illnesses. The cultural beliefs and mores held by the older women placed a high value on resilience, independence, and survival.

Interviews with women over the age of 85 years from various ethnic, racial, and socioeconomic backgrounds who were currently dealing with chronic illness revealed several factors that appeared to be related to the resilience (Felten, 2000). These included determination to overcome adversity and previous experience with hardship.

Widowhood

Not surprisingly, widowhood becomes increasingly prevalent as individuals age. For most older adults the death of a loved one is a significant loss and life stressor. Here three studies on widowhood are reviewed that examined resilience as it relates to bereavement. In a sample of middle-aged and older bereaved spouses, parents, and gay men who had lost a partner, the quality of their relationship with the deceased was not a factor that influenced resilience (Bonanno *et al.*, 2005b). Resilient people were rated as "well adjusted" prior to the person's death and as possessing positive traits.

In a prospective investigation of older adults who had experienced the death of a spouse, Bonanno *et al.* (2002) identified five unique trajectories of bereavement outcome, one of which was resilience. The resilient group showed remarkably healthy profiles in reacting to and processing the loss. In particular, resilient individuals showed differences in coping and meaning-making and showed little signs of struggling with or denying the loss.

In a sample of older bereaved spouses, five out of six people adjusted well over time, and one in three showed substantial resilience without negative consequences (Ott *et al.*, 2007). This resilient pattern was characterized by low levels of grief and depression and high quality of life.

Former combatants and prisoners of war

Recent estimates suggest that two of every three men aged 65 years and over in the USA and Puerto Rico are veterans (US Federal Interagency Forum on Aging-Related Statistics, 2008). Many of these men were likely exposed to stressors or traumas associated with war zone-related duty or other stressful aspects of their military service. Consequently, older veterans are a particularly valuable group from which to gather data on resilience.

In a large sample of aging veterans, 40% of whom had experienced combat, most identified more positive effects of their military service, including enhanced coping skills and self-esteem and increased independence and self-discipline, than undesirable effects (Aldwin *et al.*, 1994). In fact, in those who had experienced combat, perceiving positive benefits from this experience mitigated the deleterious effects. In essence, their positive perception buffered their experience of distress.

In a national sample of former American prisoners of war, Engdahl and colleagues (1993) examined psychosocial functioning as measured by positive and negative affect, somatic symptoms, captivity trauma, and resilience. Data were collected in 1967 and in 1985.

Affect and somatic symptoms were strongly associated with resilience.

Holocaust survivors

Much attention in the trauma literature has focused on the impact of the Holocaust on the health and well-being of the survivors, who would have had a wide range of ages at the time of the trauma. Today, the remaining survivors of the Holocaust are rapidly aging. Studies of Holocaust survivors provide unique insight into the effects of trauma on the normative aging process (Danieli, 1994). In a study of aging Israeli Holocaust survivors that was conducted during the Persian Gulf War, Solomon and Prager (1992) found that the study participants perceived higher levels of danger, reported more symptoms of acute distress, and displayed higher levels of both state and trait anxiety compared with non-survivors. This study did not support the inoculation hypothesis and instead suggested that these aging survivors may have been more vulnerable because of their prior trauma. Dougall *et al.* (2000) suggested that prior trauma history could sensitize the individual to new stressors, thus potentiating their effects. Exposure to prolonged, extreme stress at developmentally crucial points in time may result in permanent effects that increase vulnerability to future traumatic events throughout the lifespan.

Yehuda and colleagues (1995) investigated the impact of cumulative lifetime trauma and recent stress on current PTSD symptoms in Holocaust survivors. Greater cumulative trauma and recent stress was reported by survivors with PTSD than those without PTSD. In her work with Holocaust survivors and their families over several decades, Danieli (1994) found that adaptational styles and post-Holocaust adjustment differed substantially among survivor families. She identified four adaptational styles of survivor families: victim families, fighter families, numb families, and "those who made it." Families considered in the "those who made it" category appeared to display greater resilience than those in some of the other groups.

A recent study compared the responses of female survivors of the Holocaust with those of non-Holocaust survivor women following the September 11, 2001 (9/11) terrorist attacks (Lamet *et al.*, 2009). A non-linear relationship was found between stress and coping, with Holocaust survivors reporting both more symptoms of PTSD as well as higher levels of resilience compared with the non-Holocaust survivor group.

Other trauma groups

A phone survey conducted following the 9/11 attacks found that resilience was predicted by the age of the study participant (Bonanno *et al.*, 2007). Participants who were 65 years of age and older were three time more likely to be resilient than a younger cohort of participants (18–24 years), and less likely to have PTSD. Other factors associated with resilience included male gender, Asian race/ethnicity, and lack of major life stressors (i.e., that person had experienced no prior traumatic events or recent life stressors or additional traumas since 9/11). Higher levels of education were not predictive of resilience. Those who were less likely to be resilient included people who had experienced loss of income because of the terror attack, had a chronic disease, or reported lower levels of perceived social support. The authors noted that their findings were consistent with earlier work conducted by developmental theorists (Garmezy, 1991; Werner, 1995; Rutter, 1999) who posited that resilience results from a "cumulative mix of person-center variables (e.g., disposition, personality) and sociocontextual (e.g., family interaction, community support systems) risk and protective factors" (Bonanno *et al.*, 2007, p. 769).

In a qualitative investigation of coping strategies and mental health among low-income older African-Americans who experienced Hurricane Katrina, expressions of spirituality were found to buffer the aftermath and promote emotional resilience (Lawson & Thomas, 2007). Regular communication with a "Higher Power," daily reading of the Bible and various devotional materials, as well as helping others as a consequence of faith were spiritual coping strategies that promoted resilience.

Older adults and resilience

The empirical evidence specific to older adults and trauma reveals that most older adults, like their younger counterparts, will recover rapidly without intervention in the aftermath of trauma (Phifer & Norris, 1989; Norris, 1992; Norris *et al.*, 2002a; Shalev, 2002; Bonanno *et al.*, 2004; Boerner *et al.*, 2005). Unfortunately, because much of the research related to trauma and older adults has focused on clinical samples of individuals suffering from psychopathology or dysfunction, relatively little is known about the ways in which resilience is attained or fostered. The following section provides an overview of the current evidence related to resilience following trauma and describes how it may apply to the growing population of older adults.

Older adults who react to but quickly bounce back from traumatic stressors are sometimes considered to be responding in a maladaptive fashion. However, Boerner *et al.* (2005) contended that "doing well" following an event like the death of a loved one may be a normal response compared with the response that is a cause for concern and intervention. While it may be challenging for loss and trauma experts, as well as society as a whole, to fully understand rapid recoveries following tragic events, a growing body of research does support the occurrence of such outcomes.

Examples from the aging literature can also help us to understand resilience in older adults. In a study related to age and memory for positive, negative, and neutral images, Charles *et al.* (2003) found age-associated reductions in memory for negative images. The authors suggested that older adults put less effort into remembering negative information that was deemed less important to their everyday functioning, in order to reserve energy for other more central issues. Therefore, it is plausible that traumatized older adults may minimize the effects of the traumatic event and appear highly resilient when relaying their experience to others because they spent less time and effort encoding negative information. Further, social comparison theory suggests that older adults may compare themselves with age peers as a way to reinterpret their present situation in a more positive manner (Frieswijk *et al.*, 2004). In large-scale disasters, such as hurricanes and earthquakes, older adults may compare themselves with others and downplay the extent of trauma or disruption they are experiencing (Brown *et al.*, 2007b). Although this cognitive appraisal may be psychologically protective, minimizing or downplaying their losses and troubles may be problematic when needed services are not sought – or accepted when offered.

Additionally, the relationship between personality traits and resilience deserves attention in older adulthood. The "five factor model" is a personality inventory that is widely used by researchers to describe traits (John & Srivastava, 1999; Morey, 2007). The inventory encompasses five dimensional measures of personality traits: openness, conscientiousness, extraversion, agreeableness, and neuroticism (OCEAN). Neuroticism is closely associated with resilience across the lifespan (van Os *et al.*, 2001; Ong *et al.*, 2006). Neuroticism reflects a person's stress tolerance, stability of emotions, and ability to adapt in response to change and evolving environmental demands (Costa & McCrae, 1992). Not unexpectedly, current research indicates that people with poor stress tolerance are less resilient than those who are highly adaptive (van Os *et al.*, 2001; Ong & Bergeman, 2004; Ong *et al.*, 2006). McCrae and Costa (2003, pp. 218–219) noted that "Neuroticism is the aspect of personality most relevant to adjustment, and those high on this dimension are likely to show evidence of maladjustment at all ages… and more likely to use ineffective coping mechanisms such as hostile reactions, passivity, wishful thinking, and self-blame in dealing with stress."

A variety of pathways have been proposed that could result in resilience (Bonanno *et al.*, 2005a). Bonanno (2004) identified several distinct dimensions related to resilience: hardiness, self-enhancement, repressive coping, and positive emotions. He asserted that hardiness is characterized by three dimensions, including "being committed to finding meaningful purpose in life, the belief that one can influence one's surroundings and the outcome of events, and the belief that one can learn and grow from both positive and negative life experiences" (Bonanno, 2004, p. 25).

Self-enhancement was described as an overly positive and sometimes unrealistic self-perception (Bonanno, 2004). It has been suggested that self-bias may be helpful in promoting well-being following trauma, but that it is also associated with more negative qualities such as narcissism (Paulhus, 1998; Bonanno, 2004). As noted above, personality traits are relatively stable over the lifespan. Personality styles likely influence interactions with the social environment, coping, and adaptation. How one perceives or cognitively appraises a traumatic event can magnify or minimize the degree of stress and shape the meaning a person may attach to the event. It is a complex interaction among personal and environmental factors that evolve with life experience and aging.

Trauma-specific variables

There are a number of variables specific to the particular trauma that may lead to more or less favorable outcomes among older adults, including the timing and severity of the trauma. The type of trauma experienced may have an impact on the response of older adult survivors (e.g., elder abuse as opposed to vehicle accident). The severity of a trauma is thought to impact responses among survivors across the lifespan (Yehuda *et al.*, 1995). Some have suggested that emotional responses to single traumatic events (e.g., natural disaster) may differ from those experienced following more prolonged

trauma (e.g., incarceration in a concentration camp or prisoner of war camp) (Norris *et al.*, 2002b).

When seeking to understand the responses of older adults to traumatic events, it is also important to recognize that other stressful events may have occurred earlier in life and have adversely affected the person's developmental trajectory. Earlier traumatic events that can later increase vulnerability of older adults include those that occurred during childhood (e.g., child abuse), early in adulthood (e.g., military combat), or during older adulthood (e.g., elder abuse, traumatic loss). For the current cohort of older adults, the lack of knowledge regarding the potential psychological and developmental impact of traumatic events that occurred during their youth may have reduced the possibility of seeking and obtaining appropriate post-trauma attention and care. Older individuals may have been encouraged to minimize or keep their traumatic experiences private and may have been discouraged from positive opportunities to share, potentially recover, and to grow from their experiences.

If trauma was experienced during middle adulthood or older adulthood, the affected person may have encountered other benefits or challenges. For example, during middle adulthood, many people are at the height of their productivity as well as at their greatest burden threshold. Middle-aged adults are often working, caring for children, and sometimes assisting with the care needs of aging parents. A traumatic event during this time is often characterized by tremendous responsibility and demands that may lead to more negative responses. This experience is consistent with the burden hypothesis as described above.

Traumas during older adulthood bring yet another set of possible outcomes that may be influenced by the developmental characteristics of this time period. Consistent with hypotheses discussed above, individuals who experience trauma during older adulthood may respond resiliently or recover relatively rapidly as a result of their prior successful experience with such traumatic events. Others may be less likely to ward off the negative effects of trauma because of decreases in physical or cognitive functioning, which may be compounded by fewer social and economic resources.

Social support

A great deal of research has focused on the role of social support as an important factor related to an individual's ability to cope following stressful life events. The issue of social support may be particularly important when considering the impact of trauma on older adults, as much has been written about the effects of diminishing social networks as part of the aging process. Death, relocation (e.g., move to a nursing home or retirement community), and increased functional limitations (e.g., inability to drive or ambulate without assistance) may reduce contact with significant others and close friends.

Norris and Murrell (1990) found that social networks buffer the effects of bereavement in older adults. In a sample of community-residing older adults, formal volunteering was associated with more positive affect and moderated the negative effect of having role-identity absences in major life domains (e.g., partner, employment, and parental) on feelings of purpose in life (Greenfield & Marks, 2004). Therefore, appropriately seeking social support and formally volunteering may be ways to help older adults to feel engaged and connected and thus possibly more resilient.

Society's response to the trauma

The response of society to a particular traumatic event can significantly impact post-trauma outcomes. Although limited empirical research has focused on this particular topic, existing evidence suggests the potential importance of society's reaction in the aftermath of trauma (Danieli, 1994; Solomon, 1995). History attests to the fact that some survivors are revered and treated as heroes, while others receive societal disapproval or indifference. For example, World War II veterans were largely treated with admiration and respect by American society, even being referred to as "the greatest generation." In contrast, many of those who served in the Vietnam War returned to the USA to chanting protestors and an indifferent citizenry. Accounts from Holocaust survivors in both the USA and Israel indicate that they often encountered a disbelieving society and people who discouraged them from sharing the horrors of their experiences (Solomon, 1995).

Future research and clinical directions

A great deal of work remains to fully understand how resilience is manifested in older adults. Research needs to be conducted that investigates prevalence, phenomenology, and assessment and that determines the best methods for fostering resilience in an aging population.

Because it is likely that resilience is multifaceted and related to a number of variables, including genetic underpinnings, environmental context, personality, social support and relationships, and culture, a comprehensive biopsychosocial framework measured with multiple methods would likely yield the most fruitful information on resilience in older adults (Inui, 2003).

Understanding how to maintain and enhance resilience in the face of daily life hassles, stressful events, and major traumas is an important area to address in future investigations. Because recent research has suggested that some people may use maladaptive coping strategies to be resilient (Bonanno, 2004), it is important for clinical researchers to develop healthful interventions for use by at-risk populations. Lamond et al. (2008) suggested the need for investigations of psychosocial and behavioral interventions that may help to teach resilience in older adults. Specifically, they recommended that attention be paid to interventions aimed at enhancing problem-solving skills, such as problem-solving therapy.

Shortly after the 9/11 terror attacks, the American Psychological Association produced a fact sheet intended to assist psychologists who were seeking to foster resilience in older adults (Zeiss et al., 2003). Suggested tips for promoting resilience in critical times included maintaining a routine, taking good care of oneself, engaging in pleasurable activities, finding supportive people, setting a plan and following through, and finding meaning or purpose. Although it is important to teach older adults how to handle their reactions to a major catastrophic event, it is equally important to teach older adults how to be resilient when encountering everyday stressors.

Lastly, a concept that may be related to resilience is the notion of post-traumatic growth (Westphal & Bonanno, 2007). Unlike recovery, which is an eventual return to baseline functioning with or without intervention, or resilience, which is the capability to resist or remain undamaged by stressful or traumatic events, post-traumatic growth is defined by Tedeschi and Calhoun (2004) as a positive adaptation or development that results in event-related personal growth. They suggested that fewer changes in growth following trauma may be evident in older adults because they may be less open to change and may have already learned many life lessons. Additional research is needed to determine the conditions under which post-traumatic growth may occur in older adults.

Conclusions

During the course of a lifetime, most older adults will experience at least one stressful or traumatic event. At present, there is an emphasis on screening and treating those who have been exposed to a major stressor. However, recent research suggests that it may be beneficial to foster resilience in populations prior to a stressor (e.g., strengthening social support in preparing for the death of a loved one) and to create and support recovery environments after an event (e.g., assisting people with chronic health conditions who might be at greater risk for adverse outcomes). A hallmark of successful aging is the ability to adapt and recover from adverse life events. As the older adult population continues to grow and diversify, the need to enhance resilience in this subgroup of the population takes on new importance.

References

Aldwin, C. M., Levenson, M. R., & Spiro, A. (1994). Vulnerability and resilience to combat exposure: Can stress have lifelong effects? *Psychology and Aging*, **9**, 34–44.

American Psychological Association (1997). *What practitioners should know about working with older adults*. Washington, DC: American Psychological Association Press.

Beach, S. R., Schulz, R., Yee, J. L., & Jackson, S. (2000). Negative and positive health effects of caring for a disabled spouse: Longitudinal findings from the caregiver health effects study. *Psychology and Aging*, **15**, 259–271.

Becker, G. & Newsom, E. (2005). Resilience in the face of serious illness among chronically ill African Americans in later life. *Journals of Gerontology*, **60B**, S214–S223.

Boardman, J. D., Blalock, C. L., & Button, T. M. (2008). Sex differences in the heritability of resilience. *Twin Research and Human Genetics*, **11**, 12–27.

Boerner, K., Wortman, C. B., & Bonanno, G. A. (2005). Resilient or at risk? A 4-year study of older adults who initially showed high or low distress following conjugal loss. *Journals of Gerontology*, **60B**, 67–73.

Bonanno, G. A. (2004). Loss, trauma, and human resilience: Have we underestimated the human capacity to thrive after extremely aversive events? *American Psychologist*, **59**, 20–28.

Bonanno, G. A., Wortman, C. B., Lehman, D. R., *et al.* (2002). Resilience to loss and chronic grief: A prospective study from pre-loss to 18 months post-loss. *Journal of Personality and Social Psychology*, **83**, 1150–1164.

Bonanno, G. A., Wortman, C. B. & Nesse, R. M. (2004). Prospective patterns of resilience and maladjustment during widowhood. *Psychology and Aging*, **19**, 260–271.

Bonanno, G. A., Rennicke, C., & Dekel, S. (2005a). Self-enhancement among high-exposure survivors of the September 11th terrorist attack: Resilience or social maladjustment? *Journal of Personality and Social Psychology*, **88**, 984–998.

Bonanno, G. A., Moskowitz, J. T., Papa, A., & Folkman, S. (2005b). Resilience to loss in bereaved spouses, bereaved parents, and bereaved gay men. *Journal of Personality and Social Psychology*, **88**, 827–843.

Bonanno, G. A., Galea, S., Bucciarelli, A., & Vlahov, D. (2007). What predicts psychological resilience after disaster? The role of demographics, resources, and life stress. *Journal of Consulting and Clinical Psychology*, **75**, 671–682.

Bremner, J. D., Southwick, S., Brett, E., *et al.* (1992). Dissociation and posttraumatic stress disorder in Vietnam combat veterans. *American Journal of Psychiatry*, **149**, 328–332.

Breslau, N., Kessler, R. C., Chilcoat, H. D., *et al.* (1998). Trauma and posttraumatic stress disorder in the community: The 1996 Detroit area survey of trauma. *American Journal of Psychiatry*, **55**, 626–632.

Brown, L. M., Rothman, M., & Norris, F. (2007a). Issues in mental health care for older adults during disasters. *Generations*, **31**, 25–30.

Brown, L. M., Cohen, D., & Kohlmaier, J. (2007b). Older adults and terrorism. In B. Bongar, L. M. Brown., L. Beutler, P. Zimbardo, & J. Breckenridge (eds.), *Psychology of terrorism* (pp. 288–310). New York: Oxford University Press.

Centers for Disease Control and Prevention & the Merck Company Foundation (2007). Public health and aging: trends in aging: United States and worldwide. *Morbidity and Mortality Weekly Report*, **52**, 101–106.

Charles, S. T., Mather, M., & Carstensen, L. L. (2003). Aging and emotional memory: The forgettable nature of negative images for older adults. *Journal of Experimental Psychology*, **132**, 310–324.

Connor, K. M. & Davidson, J. R. T. (2003). Development of a new resilience scale: The Connor–Davidson Resilience Scale (CD-RISC). *Depression and Anxiety*, **18**, 76–82.

Cook, J. M. & Elmore, D. L. (2009). Disaster mental health in older adults: Symptoms, policy and planning. In Y. Neria, S. Galea, & F. Norris (eds.), *The mental health consequences of disasters* (pp. 233–263). New York: Cambridge University Press.

Costa, P. T. & McCrae, R. R. (1992). *Revised NEO Personality Inventory (NEO–PI–R) and NEO Five-Factor Inventory (NEO–FFI) professional manual*. Odessa, FL: Psychological Assessment Resources.

Creamer, M. & Parslow, R. (2008). Trauma exposure and posttraumatic stress disorder in the elderly: A community prevalence study. *American Journal of Geriatric Psychiatry*, **16**, 853–856.

Danieli, Y. (1994). As survivors age: Part 1. *National Center for PTSD Clinical Quarterly*, **4**, 1, 3–7.

Danieli, Y. (1997). As survivors age: An overview. *Journal of Geriatric Psychiatry*, **30**, 9–26.

Dougall, A. L., Herberman, H. B., Delahanty, D. L., Inslicht, S. S., & Baum, A. (2000). Similarity of prior trauma exposure as a determinant of chronic stress responding to an airline disaster. *Journal of Consulting and Clinical Psychology*, **68**, 290–295.

Engdahl, B. E., Harkness, A. R., Eberly, R. E., Page, W. F., & Bielinski, J. (1993). Structural models of captivity trauma, resilience, and trauma response among former prisoners of war 20 to 40 years after release. *Social Psychiatry and Psychiatric Epidemiology*, **28**, 109–115.

Eysenck, H. J. (1983). Stress, disease, and personality: The inoculation effect. In C. L. Cooper (ed.), *Stress research* (pp. 121–146). New York: Wiley.

Felten, B. S. (2000). Resilience in a multicultural sample of community-dwelling women older than age 85. *Clinical Nursing Research*, **9**, 102–123.

Fields, R. B. (1996). Severe stress in the elderly: Are older adults at increased risk for posttraumatic stress disorder? In P. E. Ruskin & J. A. Talbott (eds.), *Aging and posttraumatic stress disorder* (pp. 79–100). Washington, DC: American Psychiatric Press.

Foster, J. R. (1997). Successful coping, adaptation and resilience in the elderly: An interpretation of epidemiologic data. *Psychiatric Quarterly*, **68**, 189–219.

Frieswijk, N., Buunk, B. P., Steverink, N., & Slaets, J. P. J. (2004). the interpretation of social comparison and its relation to life satisfaction among elderly people: Does frailty make a difference? *Journal of Gerontology*, **59**, P250–P257.

Gallo, J. J. & Lebowitz, B. D. (1999). The epidemiology of common late-life mental disorders in the community: themes for the new century. *Psychiatric Services*, **50**, 1158–1168.

Gaugler, J. E., Kane, R. L., & Newcomer, R. (2007). Resilience and transitions from dementia caregiving. *Journals of Gerontology*, **62B**, P38–P44.

Garmezy, N. (1991). Resilience and vulnerability to adverse developmental outcomes associated with poverty. *American Behavioral Scientist*, **34**, 416–430.

Green, B. L., Goodman, L. A., Krupnick, J. L., *et al.* (2000). Outcomes of single versus multiple trauma exposure in a screening sample. *Journal of Traumatic Stress*, **13**, 271–286.

Greenfield, E. A. & Marks, N. F. (2004). Formal volunteering as a protective factor for older adults' psychological well-being. *Journals of Gerontology*, **59B**, S258–S264.

Hardy, S. E., Concato, J., & Gill, T. M. (2004). Resilience in community-dwelling older persons. *Journal of the American Geriatrics Society*, **52**, 257–262.

Hughes, D. C., Blazer, D. G., & George, L. K. (1988). Age differences in life events: A multivariate controlled analysis. *International Journal of Aging and Human Development*, **27**, 207–220.

Inui, T. S. (2003). The need for an integrated biopsychosocial approach to research on successful aging. *Annals of Internal Medicine*, **139**, 391–394.

John, O. P. & Srivastava, S. (1999). The big-five trait taxonomy: History, measurement, and theoretical perspectives. In L. A. Pervin & O. P. John (eds.), *Handbook of personality: Theory and research*, Vol. 2 (pp. 102–138). New York: Guilford Press.

Jopp, D. & Rott, C. (2006). Adaptation in very old age: Exploring the role of resources, beliefs, and attitudes for centenarians' happiness. *Psychology and Aging*, **21**, 266–280.

Kilijanek, T. S. & Drabek, T. E. (1979). Assessing long-term impacts of a natural disaster: A focus on the elderly. *Gerontologist*, **19**, 555–566.

Kinsel, B. (2005). Resilience as adaptation in older women. *Journal of Women and Aging*, **17**, 23–39.

Knight, B. G., Gatz, M., Heller, K., & Bengtson, V. L. (2000). Age and emotional response to the Northridge earthquake: A longitudinal study. *Psychology and Aging*, **15**, 627–634.

Lamet, A., Szuchman, L., Perkel, L., & Walsh, S. (2009). Risk factors, resilience, and psychological distress among holocaust and nonholocaust survivors in the post-9/11 environment. *Educational Gerontology*, **35**, 32–46.

Lamond, A. J., Depp, C. A., Allison, M., *et al.* (2008). Measurement and predictors of resilience among community-dwelling older women. *Journal of Psychiatric Research*, **43**, 148–154.

Lawson, E. J. & Thomas, C. (2007). Wading in the waters: Spirituality and older Black Katrina survivors. *Journal of Health Care for the Poor and Underserved*, **18**, 341–354.

McCrae, R. R. & Costa, P. T. (2003). *Personality in adulthood: A five-factor theory perspective.* New York: Guilford Press.

Montross, L. P., Depp, C., Daly, J., *et al.* (2006). Correlates of self-rated successful aging among community-dwelling older adults. *American Journal of Geriatric Psychiatry*, **14**, 43–51.

Morey, L. C. (2007). *Personality Assessment Inventory, professional manual.* Odessa, FL: Psychological Assessment Resources.

Nishith, P., Mechanic, M. B., &. Resnick, P. A. (2000). Prior interpersonal trauma: The contribution to current PTSD symptoms in female rape victims. *Journal of Abnormal Psychology*, **109**, 20–25.

Norris, F. H. (1992). Epidemiology of trauma: Frequency and impact of different potentially traumatic events on different demographic groups. *Journal of Consulting and Clinical Psychology*, **60**, 409–418.

Norris, F. H. & Murrell, S. A. (1988). Prior experience as a moderator of disaster impact on anxiety symptoms in older adults. *American Journal of Community Psychology*, **16**, 665–683.

Norris, F. H. & Murrell, S. A. (1990). Social support, life events, and stress as modifiers of adjustment to bereavement by older adults. *Psychology and Aging*, **5**, 429–436.

Norris, F. H., Kaniasty, K. Z., Conrad, M. L., Inman, G. L., & Murphy, A. D. (2002a). Placing age differences in cultural context: A comparison of the effects of age on PTSD after disasters in the United States, Mexico, and Poland. *Journal of Clinical Geropsychology*, **8**, 153–173.

Norris, F. H., Friedman, M. J., & Watson, P. J. (2002b). 60 000 disaster victims speak: Part II. Summary and implications of the disaster mental health research. *Psychiatry*, **65**, 240–260.

Norris, F. H., Friedman, M. J., Watson, P. J., *et al.* (2002c). 60 000 disaster victims speak: Part I. An empirical review of the empirical literature, 1981–2001. *Psychiatry*, **65**, 207–239.

Nygren, B., Alex, L., Jonsen, E., *et al.* (2005). Resilience, sense of coherence, purpose in life and self-transcendence in relation to perceived physical and mental health among the oldest old. *Aging and Mental Health*, **9**, 354–362.

Ong, A. D. & Bergeman, C. S. (2004). The complexity of emotions in later life. *Journals of Gerontology*, **59B**, P117–P122.

Ong, A. D., Bergeman, C. S., & Bisconti, T. L. (2004). The role of daily positive emotions during conjugal bereavement. *Journals of Gerontology*, **59B**, P168–P176.

Ong, A. D., Bergeman, C. S., Wallace, K. A., & Bisconti, T. L. (2006). Psychological resilience, positive emotions, and successful adaptation to the stress in later life. *Journal of Personality and Social Psychology*, **91**, 730–749.

Ott, C. H., Lueger, R. J., Kelber, S. T., & Prigerson, H. G. (2007). Spousal bereavement in older adults: Common, resilient, and chronic grief with defining characteristics. *Journal of Nervous and Mental Disease*, **195**, 332–341.

Paulhus, D. L. (1998). Interpersonal and intrapsychic adaptiveness of trait self-enhancement: A mixed blessing? *Journal of Personality and Social Psychology*, **74**, 1197–1208.

Phifer, J. F. (1990). Psychological distress and somatic symptoms after natural disaster: Differential vulnerability among older adults. *Psychology and Aging*, **5**, 412–420.

Phifer, J. F. & Norris, F. H. (1989). Psychological symptoms in older adults following natural disaster: Nature, timing, duration, and course. *Journals of Gerontology*, **44**, S207–S217.

Robins, L. N. & Regier, D. A. (1991). *Psychiatric disorders in America: The Epidemiologic Catchment Area Study*. New York: Free Press.

Rutter, M. (1999). Resilience concepts and findings: Implications for family therapy. *Journal of Family Therapy*, **21**, 119–144.

Schulz, R., Mittelmark, M., Burton, L., Hirsch, C., & Jackson, S. (1997). Health effects of caregiving: The caregiver health effects study: An ancillary study of the cardiovascular health study. *Annals of Behavioral Medicine*, **19**, 110–116.

Shalev, A. Y. (2002). Acute stress reactions in adults. *Biological Psychiatry*, **51**, 532–543.

Solomon, Z. (1995). From denial to recognition: Attitudes toward Holocaust survivors form World War II to the present. *Journal of Traumatic Stress*, **8**, 215–228.

Solomon, Z. & Prager, E. (1992). Elderly Israeli Holocaust survivors during the Persian Gulf War: A study of psychological distress. *American Journal of Psychiatry*, **149**, 1707–1710.

Tedeschi, R. G. & Calhoun, L. G. (2004). Posttraumatic growth: Conceptual foundations and empirical evidence. *Psychological Inquiry*, **15**, 1–18.

Thompson, M. P., Norris, F. H., & Hanacek, B. (1993). Age differences in the psychological consequences of Hurricane Hugo. *Psychology and Aging*, **8**, 606–616.

US Department of Health and Human Services (1999). *Mental Health: A report of the Surgeon General*. Rockville, MD: US Department of Health and Human Services.

US Department of Health and Human Services (2001). *Older adults and mental health: Issues and opportunities*. Washington, DC: US Department of Health and Human Services, Administration on Aging.

US Federal Interagency Forum on Aging-Related Statistics (2008). *Older Americans 2008: Key indicators of well-being*. Washington, DC: Government Printing Office.

van Os, J., Park, S. B. G., & Jones, P. B. (2001). Neuroticism, life events and mental health: Evidence for person–environment correlation. *British Journal of Psychiatry*, **178**, s72–s77.

Werner, E. E. (1995). Resilience in development. *Current Directions in Psychological Science*, **4**, 81–85.

Westphal, M. & Bonanno, G. A. (2007). Posttraumatic growth and resilience to trauma: Different sides of the same coin or different coins? *Applied Psychology: An International Review*, **56**, 416–426.

Yehuda, R., Kahana, B., Schmeidler, J., *et al.* (1995). Impact of cumulative lifetime trauma and recent stress on current posttraumatic stress disorder symptoms in Holocaust survivors. *American Journal of Psychiatry*, **152**, 1815–1818.

Zeiss, A. M., Cook, J. M., & Cantor, D. W. (2003). *Fostering resilience in response to terrorism: For psychologists working with older adults.* [Report to American Psychological Association Task Force on Resilience in Response to Terrorism.] Washington, DC: American Psychological Association Press, http://www.apa.org/pi/aging/older-adults.pdf (accessed March 12, 2011).

Family resilience: a collaborative approach in response to stressful life challenges

Froma Walsh

Introduction

Family resilience can be defined as the ability of families to withstand and rebound from disruptive life challenges, strengthened and more resourceful (Walsh, 2003, 2006). Building on studies of family stress, coping, and adaptation, and research on well-functioning family systems, family resilience is seen to involve dynamic processes that foster positive adaptation of the family unit and its members in the context of significant adversity (Walsh, 1996; Luthar *et al.*, 2000).

This chapter presents core principles of resilience derived from a family systems orientation, highlighting sociocultural and developmental perspectives. The assessment of family resilience is described, identifying key processes that can be targeted to strengthen family resilience in intervention and prevention efforts. Program applications in training and services are described briefly to illustrate the broad utility of this systemic approach for intervention and prevention efforts.

Individual resilience: a systemic perspective

Most resilience theory, research, and intervention approaches since the early 1980s have been individually focused, reflecting the dominant medical and mental health paradigm and the cultural ethos of the "rugged individual" (Walsh, 1996). Early studies of resilience sought to identify innate or acquired personal traits that made some children less vulnerable to the impact of extreme conditions or the damage of parental pathology.

An interactive view of resilience emerged as research was extended to a wide range of adverse conditions – such as growing up in impoverished circumstances, dealing with chronic illness, or recovering from catastrophic life events, trauma, and loss. Resilience came to be seen in terms of an interplay of multiple risk and protective processes over time, involving individual, family, and larger sociocultural influences (Rutter, 1987). Individual vulnerability or the impact of stressful conditions could be outweighed by mediating influences.

The crucial influence of significant relationships stood out across studies. Reports of children who thrived despite a parent's mental illness or maltreatment noted that their resilience was often nurtured in strong bonds with mentors, such as coaches and teachers, who had invested in the child. Yet, the narrow focus on parental deficits led many to dismiss the family as dysfunctional and to only consider outside resources. In mental health and child development literature, families were thought to contribute to risk, but not to resilience.

Family systems theory, research, and practice have broadened our recognition of the potential family resources for individual resilience in the network of relationships, from couple and sibling bonds to relationships with extended family members. Family assessment and intervention with troubled and at-risk youth aim to identify and involve family members who are invested in them and can support their best efforts, believe in their potential, and encourage them to make the most of their lives (Ungar, 2004). Even in multistressed families, strengths and potential can be found alongside vulnerabilities and limitations (Walsh, 2003, 2006).

The concept of family resilience

The concept of family resilience expands focus beyond a dyadic view – seeing a family member as a resource

---

Resilience and Mental Health: Challenges Across the Lifespan, ed. Steven M. Southwick, Brett T. Litz, Dennis Charney, and Matthew J. Friedman. Published by Cambridge University Press. © Cambridge University Press 2011.

for individual resilience – to a systemic perspective on risk and resilience in the family as a functional unit (Walsh, 1996). A basic premise is that stressful life challenges have an impact on the whole family and, in turn, key family processes mediate the recovery – or maladaptation – of all members *and* the family unit. The family response to adversity is crucial. Major stressors can derail the functioning of a family system, with ripple effects for all members and their relationships. Key processes and extrafamilial resources enable the family system to rally in times of crisis, to buffer stress, to reduce the risk of dysfunction, and to support optimal adaptation.

The concept of family resilience extends theory and research on family stress, coping, and adaptation (McCubbin & Patterson, 1983; Boss, 2001; Patterson, 2002). It entails more than managing stressful conditions, shouldering a burden, or surviving an ordeal. It involves the potential for personal and relational transformation and growth that can be forged out of adversity. Tapping into key processes for resilience, families that have been struggling can emerge stronger and more resourceful in meeting future challenges. Members may develop new insights and abilities. A crisis can be a wake-up call, heightening their attention to core values and important matters. It often becomes an opportunity for families to reappraise life priorities and stimulates greater investment in meaningful relationships. In studies of strong families (Stinnett & DeFrain, 1985), many report that through weathering a crisis together their relationships were enriched and became more loving than they might otherwise have been.

Sociocultural and developmental contexts of family resilience

A family resilience framework is grounded in family systems theory, combining ecological and developmental perspectives to view family functioning in relation to its broader sociocultural context and multigenerational family life cycle passage.

Risk and resilience are viewed in light of multiple, recursive influences involving individuals, families, and larger social systems. These can be seen from biological, psychological, social, or spiritual system orientation. Symptoms of distress may be primarily biologically based, as in serious illness or neurological vulnerabilities, but are also influenced by sociocultural variables, such as barriers of poverty and discrimination that

render some families or communities more at risk. Symptoms of family members may be generated by a crisis event, such as a sexual assault or a tragic loss, or by the wider impact of a large-scale disaster. Family distress is exacerbated by unsuccessful attempts to cope with an overwhelming situation, whatever its source. The family, peer group, community resources, school, work setting, and other social systems are seen as nested contexts for nurturing and sustaining resilience. A multidimensional, holistic approach addresses the varied contexts, identifies common elements in a crisis situation, and also takes into account each family's unique perspectives, resources, and challenges.

Family transformations in changing societies

The concept of family resilience is particularly timely as our world grows increasingly unpredictable and families face unprecedented challenges. With profound social, economic, and political upheavals over recent decades, families have been undergoing rapid transformation (Walsh, 2012a, 2012b). To understand family challenges and resources, it is important to consider the implications of the following trends: varied family structures and changing gender roles, increasing cultural diversity and economic disparity, and varying expanded family life course. Efforts to strengthen family resilience must be relevant to this growing diversity and complexity.

Varied family structures and gender roles

Over the past century, multigenerational kinship networks living in close proximity in traditional rural societies have fragmented with industrialization, urbanization, and modernization. Amidst economic and social changes of recent decades, the intact nuclear family with traditional gender roles, idealized in mid-twentieth century modern society, currently accounts for only a small band on the spectrum of contemporary families. Increasingly, individuals and couples construct a wide variety of household and kinship arrangements and eschew traditional patriarchal gender patterns in favor of a more egalitarian partnership in marriage, family life, and childrearing. Increasing rates of cohabitation, divorce, single-parent households, stepfamilies, and gay/lesbian-headed families has led to concerns about their pathogenic influence for children. However, since the late 1990s, research has clearly shown that families can function well and children can thrive in a variety of family structures that are stable, nurturing, and financially secure (Lansford *et al.*, 2001; Oswald, 2002; Johnson-Garner & Meyers, 2003; Green, 2004; Greene *et al.*, 2012). What matters most are effective family processes.

Cultural diversity and economic disparity

Cultural norms and values shape family belief systems, organization, and communication. McCubbin *et al.* (1998) have studied varied pathways in resilience in ethnic minority, native, and immigrant families. As societies become more culturally diverse, families are becoming increasingly multiethnic, multiracial, and multifaith, requiring mutual understanding and acceptance of differences (Walsh, 2009a). Socioeconomic conditions strongly impact family risk and resilience. A wide disparity between the rich and the poor have severe consequences for the welfare of growing numbers of families worldwide. Declining economic conditions, job dislocation, and persistent unemployment have a devastating impact on family functioning and stability, fueling conflict, violence, divorce, and homelessness. Conditions of discrimination, neighborhood decay, poor schools, crime, violence, and inadequate healthcare worsen life chances for parents and their children.

Varying, expanded life course

Medical advances and the aging of societies have increased the number of four- and five-generation families, with concomitant challenges of chronic illness and caregiving (Walsh, 2011). Two or more committed couple relationships are increasingly common over time, with periods of cohabitation and single living. Children and their parents are likely to transition in and out of several household and kinship arrangements over their life course. For resilience, families need to buffer transitions and learn how to live successfully in complex arrangements.

Stressful events in the broader social context: family impact and resilience

In the early study of family stress, the family impact of combat-related trauma in returning military veterans was a focal concern (Figley, 1989). Secondary traumatization and burnout were experienced by spouses, not only in hearing about their loved one's past trauma but even more through ongoing interactions impacted by post-traumatic stress disorder (PTSD) symptoms involving emotional, behavioral, and substance abuse problems (Figley, 1998a). Ripple effects throughout the family network produced distress for children and other family members. Family involvement in treatment was deemed essential to address this family stress and, in turn, to enable the family to support the optimal recovery of the returned serviceperson. Currently, with the high rate of PTSD, suicide, traumatic brain injury, other severe injuries, and marital distress for deployed and returning combat troops, efforts to strengthen family resilience are a high priority in programs for US military families (MacDermid, 2010).

Family resilience-oriented services are also becoming a valuable approach in community recovery efforts in the wake of natural disasters, such as Hurricane Katrina, and in regions suffering ongoing conflict, political persecution, and/or terrorist attacks (Cohen *et al.*, 2002; Hernandez, 2002; Landau, 2007; Walsh, 2007; Girwitz *et al.*, 2008; Rowe & Liddle, 2008; Vigil & Geary, 2008; Knowles *et al.*, 2010).

Developmental perspective: family life cycle orientation

A family life cycle orientation views the family as a system moving forward over the life course of all members and across the generations (McGoldrick *et al.*, 2011). This developmental perspective is essential to understand and foster family resilience: (1) families navigate varied pathways in resilience with emerging challenges over time; (2) a pile-up of multiple stressors can overwhelm family resources; (3) the impact of a crisis may vary in relation to its timing in individual and family life cycle passage; and (4) a family's past experiences of adversity and response can generate catastrophic expectations or can serve as models of resilience.

Varied pathways in resilience

Most major stressors are not simply a short-term single event but rather a complex set of changing conditions with a past history and a future course (Rutter, 1987). Family resilience involves varied adaptational pathways over time, from the approach to a threatening event, through disruptive transitions, subsequent shockwaves in the immediate aftermath, and long-term reorganization. For example, in adaptation to loss, the immediate and long-term recovery for all members and their relationships will be influenced by how a family approaches the loss, facilitates emotional sharing and meaning-making, effectively reorganizes, and fosters reinvestment in life pursuits (Walsh & McGoldrick, 2004). Likewise, the experience of divorce proceeds from an escalation of pre-divorce tensions through disruption and reorganization of households and parent–child relationships; most experience transitional upheaval again with remarriage and stepfamily integration (Greene *et al.*, 2012). Given such complexity, no single coping response is invariably most successful; different strategies may prove useful in meeting emerging challenges. Some approaches that are functional in the short term may become rigid and dysfunctional over time. For example, with a sudden illness, a family must mobilize resources and pull together to meet the crisis, but later the family must shift gears with chronic disability and attend to the needs of other family members over a longer time (Rolland, 1994, 2012). Research on effective family processes for resilience over time in the context of loss, divorce, or illness can guide interventions. Brief modules can be timed to help families at various steps or transitions along their journey, helping them to integrate what has happened and meet anticipated challenges ahead.

Pile-up of stressors

Some families may do well with a short-term crisis but buckle under the cumulative strains of persistent or recurrent challenges, as with prolonged joblessness or ongoing complex trauma for those living in a conflict zone. A pile-up of internal and external stressors can overwhelm the family, heightening vulnerability and risk for subsequent problems. Multistressed, underresourced families, most often in impoverished minority communities, are often blamed for their difficulties. In contrast to problem-focused interventions, which too often increase parents' sense of deficit and despair, recent strengths-oriented family therapy approaches are intended to affirm and enhance family confidence and competencies (Combrinck-Graham, 2005; Minuchin *et al.*, 2006; Walsh, 2006). Intervention approaches using a strengths-oriented family system also treat complex problems of family violence and sexual abuse, often intertwined with substance abuse (e.g., Sheinberg & Fraenkel, 2001).

Stressful transitions

Functioning and symptoms of distress are assessed in the context of the multigenerational family system as it moves forward across the life cycle (McGoldrick *et al.*, 2011). Well-functioning families tend to have an evolutionary sense of time and a continual process of growth, change, and losses over the generations (Beavers & Hampson, 2003). This perspective helps members to see disruptive events and transitions also as milestones on their shared life passage.

A family resilience approach focuses on family functioning and adaptation around stressful life events and transitions (Lavee *et al.*, 1987; Walsh, 2009a). Some researchers have examined variables in risk and resilience around predictable, normative stressors, such as the transition to parenthood (Cowan & Cowan, 2012). More attention is directed to family processes for resilience associated with the disruptive impact of unanticipated, untimely events, such as the multiple transitions with divorce (Gorell Barnes, 1999; Greene *et al.*, 2012), the death of a child, or loss of a parent raising children (Greeff & Human, 2004; Greeff & van der Merwe, 2004; Walsh, 2009a). There is growing interest in family resilience with medical crises and adaptation to unfolding phases and transitions in chronic illness and disability (Campbell, 2003; Rolland, 2012).

Intergenerational legacies

The convergence of developmental and multigenerational strains heighten the risk for dysfunction. Distress increases exponentially when current stressors reactivate painful issues from the past (McGoldrick *et al.*, 2011). Unresolved conflicts and losses may surface when similar challenges are confronted. Family members may lose perspective, conflate immediate situations with past events, and either become overwhelmed by or cut off from painful feelings and contacts. Multigenerational anniversary patterns can be identified: many families function well until they reach a point in the life cycle passage that had been traumatic a generation earlier, particularly when a child reaches the same age that a parent experienced trauma. Family stories of past adversity and how they influence future expectations, from catastrophic fears to a hopeful outlook, can be illuminating. Legacies of resilience can also be found in adaptive response to adversity across the generations (Hauser, 1999).

Assessing family functioning and resilience

The assessment of family functioning is fraught with dilemmas (Walsh, 2012b). Views of normality and health are socially constructed. Clinicians and researchers bring their own assumptive maps into every evaluation and intervention, embedded in cultural norms, professional orientations, and personal experiences. Moreover, with recent social and economic transformations and a growing multiplicity of family kinship arrangements, no single model of family health or resilience fits all families and situations. Since the late 1980s, systems-oriented family process research has provided important empirical grounding for assessment of healthy family functioning (Beavers & Hampson, 2003; Epstein *et al.*, 2003; Olson & Gorall, 2003). Yet, family typologies tend to be static and acontextual; many offer a snapshot of interaction patterns within the family but lack multisystemic and developmental perspectives in relation to family challenges, resources, and constraints. Since families most often seek help in periods of crisis, clinicians must be cautious not to label their distress reflexively or to see differences from research norms as family pathology.

A family resilience framework offers several advantages. By definition, it focuses on family strengths under stress, in crisis, and facing adversity (Walsh, 2003). Second, it is assumed that no single model of healthy functioning fits all families or their situations. Functioning is assessed in context: relative to each family's values, structure, resources, and life challenges. Families forge varied pathways through adversity, fitting their cultural orientation, their emerging challenges, their life cycle passage, and their personal strengths and resources.

Use of genograms, timelines

Individual and family symptoms of distress are assessed in sociocultural and developmental contexts. A family genogram and timeline are essential tools for clinical assessment to schematize relationship information, track systems patterns over time, and guide intervention planning (McGoldrick *et al.*, 2008).

Particular attention should be paid to the timing of symptoms of distress: their co-occurrence with recent or threatening disruptive events in the family (Walsh & McGoldrick, 2004). For example, a son dropping out from school may be precipitated by his father's job loss and related family tensions, although family members may not initially note any connection. Frequently, individual symptoms coincide with stressful transitions, such as family separation or stepfamily formation, that require boundary shifts and re-definition of roles and relationships. It is important to attend to non-custodial parents and the extended kin network beyond the immediate household. The impact of stressful events should be explored in terms of (1) their impact on the family system, its members, and their relationships; and (2) how the family attempted to handle the problem situation, that is their proactive stance, immediate response, and long-term strategies.

Whereas genograms are most often used to focus on problematic family patterns, such as illness, conflict, or estrangement, a resilience-oriented approach also searches for positive influences, past, present, and potential. Inquiry is made about resourceful ways a family had dealt with past adversity and about models of resilience in the kin network that might be drawn on to inspire efforts to master current challenges. Families are also encouraged to make efforts to repair conflicts and reconnect with estranged loved ones who could contribute to child and family resilience.

The Walsh family resilience framework: key processes

The Walsh family resilience framework (Box 10.1) was developed as a conceptual map of key processes to guide assessment and intervention in clinical and community practice. This framework is informed by two decades of social science and clinical research on well-functioning family systems and on individual and family resilience. Synthesizing findings, nine processes for resilience are identified within three domains of family functioning: family belief systems, organization patterns, and communication processes. These processes can be assessed and targeted to strengthen family capacities to rebound from crises and master persistent life challenges (Walsh, 2003, 2006). Interventions aim to build family strengths as problems are addressed, thereby reducing risk and vulnerability. As the family becomes more resourceful, members gain ability to meet future challenges.

Family belief systems

Family resilience is fostered by shared beliefs that help members make meaning of their stressful situations, facilitate a positive, hopeful outlook, and provide transcendent or spiritual, values, practices, and purpose. Families can be helped to gain a sense of coherence (Antonovsky & Sourani, 1988; Antonovsky, 1998), recasting a crisis as a shared challenge that is comprehensible, manageable, and meaningful to tackle. Normalizing and contextualizing members' distress as natural or understandable in their crisis situation can depathologize their reactions and reduce blame, shame, and guilt. Drawing out and affirming family

Box 10.1 Key processes in family resilience

Belief systems

1. Make meaning of adversity:
   - view resilience as relationally based rather than "rugged individual"
   - normalize, contextualize adversity and distress
   - encourage sense of coherence: view crisis as a meaningful, comprehensible, manageable challenge
   - use causal/explanatory attributions: expectations.

2. Stimulate a positive outlook:
   - encourage hope, optimistic bias, confidence in overcoming odds
   - affirm strengths and build on potential
   - seize opportunities: active initiative and perseverance (can-do spirit)
   - master the possible, accept what cannot be changed, live with uncertainty.

3. Transcendence and spirituality:
   - larger values, purpose
   - spirituality: faith, practices, congregation; connectedness with nature
   - inspiration: envision new possibilities, creative expression, social action
   - transformation: learning, change, and growth from adversity.

Structural/organizational patterns

4. Flexibility:
   - open to change: rebound, reorganize, adapt to fit new challenges
   - find stability during disruption: continuity, dependability, follow-through
   - strong authoritative leadership: nurturance, protection, guidance.

5. Connectedness:
   - mutual support, collaboration, and commitment
   - respect individual needs, differences, and boundaries
   - reconnection, reconciliation of wounded relationships.

6. Social and economic resources:
   - mobilize kin, social, and community networks; use models and mentors
   - build financial security and balance work/family strains
   - use institutional supports (workplace, healthcare, family policy).

Communication/problem solving

7. Clarity:
   - clear, consistent messages (words and actions)
   - examine ambiguous information, truth seeking/truth speaking.

8. Open emotional expression:
   - share range of feelings (joy and pain; hopes and fears)
   - have mutual empathy; tolerance for differences
   - encourage pleasurable interactions, humor, respite.

9. Collaborative problem solving/preparedness:
   - creative brainstorming, resourcefulness
   - shared decision making, conflict management: negotiation, fairness
   - focus on goals, take concrete steps, build on success, learn from failure
   - proactive stance: prevent problems, avert crises, prepare for future challenges.

strengths in the midst of difficulties counters a sense of helplessness, failure, and despair as it reinforces shared pride, confidence, and a "can do" spirit. The en-*courage*ment of family members bolsters efforts to take initiative and persevere in efforts to overcome barriers. For resilience, family members focus efforts on mastering the possible, accepting that which is beyond their control. Spiritual resources, such as shared faith, practices of prayer or meditation, and religious/congregational involvement strengthen family bonds and resilience (Walsh, 2009b, 2010).

Family structure/organization

Family resilience is fostered by flexible structure, connectedness, mutual support, and teamwork in facing life challenges. In navigating disruptive changes and structural reorganization, families need to counterbalance flexibility with stability, particularly reassuring children and other vulnerable family members by providing security, continuities, and dependability.

Mutual support and teamwork facilitate resilience. Extended kin and social networks can be lifelines for support. Institutional policies (e.g., workplace, healthcare) that support family functioning are vital for distressed families to thrive.

Family communication processes

Family resilience is facilitated through clear information about their adverse situation and options, open emotional expression and pleasurable interactions for renewal, and collaborative problem solving. Families become more resourceful when interventions shift from a crisis-reactive mode to a proactive stance, anticipating and preparing to meet future challenges. Most important, interventions help families in problem-saturated situations to envision a better future and take concrete steps toward achieving their goals.

Practice applications of a family resilience orientation approach

A family resilience orientation can be applied usefully with a wide range of crisis situations, disruptive transitions, and persistent life challenges. Interventions utilize principles and techniques common among many strength-based family systems practice approaches, but attend more centrally to the impact of significant stressors and aim to strengthen the family resources and potential for positive adaptation. This approach also recognizes that families may forge varied pathways for resilience over time, depending on their adverse situation and their values, resources, and challenges. Principles guiding this approach are outlined in Box 10.2.

Family resilience-oriented practitioners serve as compassionate witnesses and facilitators, helping family members to share with each other their experience of adversity; to overcome silence, secrecy, shame, or blame; and to build mutual empathy and support. Respect for family strengths in the midst of suffering readily engages so-called "resistant" families, who are often reluctant to come for mental health services out of concerns that they will be judged as disturbed or deficient and blamed for their problems. Instead, family members are respectfully regarded as essential members of the healing team for recovery and resilience. Where they may have faltered, they are viewed as struggling with an overwhelming set of challenges and their best intentions are affirmed. Intervention efforts are directed to master those challenges through their shared efforts. (Box 10.3 gives practice guidelines.)

Box 10.2 Family resilience orientation: principles for practice

- Relational view:
  - a deficit view of families shifted to one of strengths
  - families seen as challenged by adversity, with potential for repair and growth.
- Systemic orientation:
  - interaction of biological, psychological, social, and spiritual influences
  - crisis/stress impacts family system: family response influences recovery of all members, relationships, and family unit
  - contextual view of crisis, symptoms of distress, and adaptation.
- Developmental perspective:
  - timing of symptoms and disruptive family challenges
  - pile-up of stressors, persistent adversity
  - varying adaptational challenges over time, varied pathways in resilience
  - fit with individual and family developmental phases/transitions
  - multigenerational patterns.

Box 10.3 Practice guidelines to strengthen family resilience

- Convey conviction in potential to overcome adversity through shared efforts.
- Use respectful language, framing to humanize and contextualize distress:
  - view as understandable, common in adverse situation (normal response to abnormal conditions)
  - decrease shame, blame, and pathologizing of family and individual members.
- Provide safe haven for family members to share pain, fears, challenges:
  - compassionate witness for suffering and struggle
  - facilitate their communication, mutual empathy, support, collaboration.
- Identify and affirm strengths, courage alongside vulnerabilities, constraints.
- Draw out potential for mastery, healing, and growth.
- Tap into kin, community, and spiritual resources to master challenges.

> **Box 10.3 (*cont.*)**
>
> - View crisis as opportunity for learning, change, and growth.
> - Shift focus from problems to possibilities:
>   - gain mastery, healing, and transformation out of adversity
>   - reorient future hopes and dreams.
> - Integrate adverse experience – and resilient response – into fabric of individual and relational life passage.

A family resilience orientation can be valuable in guiding clinical training, research, and community projects. A systemic assessment may lead to a variety of interventions or it may combine individual, couple, family, and multifamily group modalities depending on the relevance of different system levels to intervention aims. Putting an ecological view into practice, interventions may involve collaborative efforts of families with community agencies, the workplace, schools, healthcare providers, and other larger systems. Resilience-based family interventions can be adapted to a variety of formats including periodic family consultations or more intensive family therapy. Psychoeducational multifamily groups emphasize the importance of social support and practical information, offering concrete guidelines for crisis management, problem solving, and stress reduction as families navigate through stressful periods and face future challenges. Therapists or group leaders may help families to clarify specific stresses they are dealing with and to develop effective coping strategies, measuring success in small increments and maintaining family morale. Brief, cost-effective psychoeducational "modules" timed for critical phases of an illness or life challenge encourage families to accept and digest manageable portions of a long-term coping process (Rolland, 1994).

Examples of family resilience-based programs

Since the early 1990s, this family resilience metaframework has guided the development of clinical and community-based professional training, consultation, and services at the Chicago Center for Family Health (www.ccfhchicago.org). Collaborative programs have been designed to address a wide range of family challenges (Walsh, 2002, 2006, 2007; Rolland & Walsh, 2006):

- serious illness, disability, end-of-life issues, and caregiving challenges (e.g., "resilient partners" couples groups for couples living with multiple sclerosis)
- complicated and traumatic loss, healing, and resilience
- major disasters: family and community recovery and resilience
- refugee trauma and resilience
- complex trauma and family resilience in war-torn regions
- positive adaptation with divorce and stepfamily integration
- job loss and economic hardship: family resilience workshops for displaced workers in partnership with transition services
- family–school partnership programs: for at-risk youth
- gay and lesbian couples and families: overcoming challenges of stigma.

A few brief programmatic descriptions are offered here from our Center and from the work of colleagues elsewhere, to illustrate the potential utility of this approach. These illustrate working with families and communities.

Transitional stresses of job loss

One family resilience-based program addressed transitional adjustment of displaced workers when jobs were lost through factory closure or company downsizing. The Chicago Center designed family resilience-based psychoeducational workshops and counseling services in partnership with a community-based agency that specialized in job retraining and placement services. Rebounding from job loss involves dealing with prolonged transitional stresses of retraining and job search, and then gaining and retaining new employment. Job and income loss, as well as anxiety and uncertainty about re-employment success, often fuel depression, substance abuse, and marital/family conflict. Parental roles have to be realigned and the value of the displaced worker to the family has to be broadened from "breadwinner," particularly for men whose self-esteem is linked to that role. This pile-up of stress over many months, in turn, reduces the ability of spouses and family members to support workers' efforts. In one case, with the closing and relocation of a large clothing manufacturing plant, over 1800 workers lost their jobs. Most were African-American or Latino breadwinners for their families; many were single parents, with limited education or skills for employment in the changing job market. Resilience-focused workshops addressed the personal and familial impact of losses and transitional stresses and rallied family members as a resource team to support the best efforts of the displaced worker. Group topics focused on worker/family challenges and keys to resilience, such as identifying constraining beliefs and negative self-appraisals; identifying and affirming strengths, such as pride in doing a job well and qualities of dependability and loyalty. New competencies and benefits were generated by realigning household and childrearing tasks, developing mutually supportive bonds, and mobilizing extended family and community resources.

Multifamily groups for refugees

The value of a community-based family resilience approach with refugees and in war-torn communities was demonstrated in projects developed by the Chicago Center in collaboration with the Center on Genocide, Psychiatry, and Witnessing at the University of Illinois (Weine *et al.*, 2004; Walsh, 2006). In 1998–1999, multifamily groups were designed for Bosnian and Kosovar refugees who had suffered atrocities and traumatic loss of loved ones, homes, and communities in the Serbian "ethnic cleansing" campaign. The family resilience approach was sought out because many refugees were suffering symptoms of PTSD but were not utilizing mental health services because of feelings of shame and stigmatization they associated with psychiatric diagnoses of PTSD and mental disorders, and because of the narrow focus on individual symptoms of pathology. The community responded enthusiastically to the family-centered resilience orientation to foster recovery and positive adaptation.

This program, called CAFES for Bosnians and TAFES for Kosovars (Coffee/Tea and Family Education and Support), utilized a nine-week multifamily group format. Families readily participated because it tapped into the strong family-centered cultural values and was located in an accessible neighborhood storefront, where they felt comfortable. Offering a safe and compassionate setting to share stories of suffering and struggle, it also affirmed family strengths and resources, such as their courage, endurance, and faith; strong kinship networks; deep concern for loved ones; and determination to rise above their tragedies to forge a new life. Their efforts were encouraged to bridge cultures and, to the extent possible, to sustain kinship ties and gain a sense of belonging in both old and new

worlds (Falicov, 2007). To foster collaboration and to develop local resources, facilitators from their community were trained to co-lead groups and to be available as urgent needs might arise. This approach was experienced as respectful and empowering.

Kosovar Family Professional Educational Collaborative

The success of the CAFES and TAFES initiative led to development of the Kosovar Family Professional Educational Collaborative (KFPEC), an ongoing partnership in Kosovo between local mental health professionals and several teams of American family therapists. The aim of this project was to enhance the capacities of mental health professionals and paraprofessionals to address the overwhelming service needs in their war-torn region by strengthening family coping and recovery in the wake of widespread trauma and loss. In describing the value of this approach, Rolland and Weine (2000, p. 35) noted,

> The family, with its strengths, is central to Kosovar life, but health and mental health services are generally not oriented to families. Although "family" is a professed part of the value system of international organizations, most programs do not define, conceptualize, or operationalize a family approach to mental health services in any substantial or meaningful ways. Recognizing that the psychosocial needs of refugees, other trauma survivors, and vulnerable persons in societies in transition far exceed the individual and psychopathological focus that conventional trauma mental health approaches provide, this project aims to begin a collaborative program of family focused education and training that is resilience-based and emphasizes family strengths.

The consultants, sharing a multisystemic, resilience-oriented approach to address family challenges, encouraged Kosovar professionals to adapt the framework and develop their own practice methods to best fit local culture and service needs. The approach emphasized the importance of meeting with families to hear their stories, bearing witness to atrocities suffered, and eliciting the strengths and resources in family belief systems, organization, and communication processes. Interviews revealed that their Islamic teachings and the inspiration of family models and mentors were powerful wellsprings in resilience. One family drew strength from the mother's faith in Allah and her courage in carrying on after witnessing the murder of her husband and sons. An uncle shared stories with his nephews of the strong leadership and bravery of their deceased father and grandfather to inspire their best efforts for the future. In many families, strong cohesiveness and adaptive role flexibility enabled members to assume new responsibilities to fill in missing functions. Although their grief was immense, their resilience was remarkable. As one family member related, "Everyone belongs to the family and to the family's homeland, alive or dead, here or abroad. Everyone matters and everyone is counted upon" (Becker *et al.*, 2000, p. 29).

Traumatic loss and major disaster

There is increasing recognition among trauma and bereavement specialists of the intertwining of trauma, loss, grief, and resilience (Figley, 1998b; Bonanno, 2004; Litz, 2004; Malkinson *et al.*, 2005). In contrast to treatment programs focusing on individuals, multisystemic resilience-oriented approaches build healing networks that facilitate child, family, and community resilience (Walsh, 2007). These types of program create a safe haven for family and community members to share both deep pain and positive strivings. They can help families and communities to expand their vision of what is possible through collaboration, not only to survive trauma and loss, but to regain their spirit to thrive.

Lower Manhattan Community Recovery Project

Following the September 11 2001 (9/11) terrorist attacks, neighborhood schools closed and families were displaced for several months; parents and children were distressed on re-entry to homes and schools where they had experienced the trauma. Saul and colleagues (Landau & Saul, 2004) organized multifamily groups and parent–teacher networks in lower Manhattan neighborhoods directly affected. Later, they included local agencies, shopkeepers, and other residents. The process of family and community connectedness provided a matrix of healing and support. A neighborhood resource center and ongoing forums evolved to share experiences of trauma and resilience, mobilizing concerted action in recovery efforts. They formed a disaster preparedness initiative and developed such projects as a video narrative archive, a theater of witness project, a community website, a computer education program for seniors, and art and music projects, with long-lasting positive impact.

Family meetings as a community intervention for ambiguous loss

Another team of family systems-oriented therapists, co-led by Boss (Boss *et al.*, 2003), worked with families

of workers who were missing after the 9/11 attacks in concert with their labor unions. Multifamily group meetings were held in their union hall. Multilingual, multiracial intervention teams were attuned to the cultural diversity of families. Group leaders helped families to share anguishing experiences and communicated their basic premise: when a loved one remains missing, it is the situation of ambiguous loss that is abnormal, not distressed family members. The group interactions and mutual support were empowering, with several widows taking on leadership roles over time.

Research challenges and opportunities

The very flexibility of the concept of resilience, the complexity of systemic assessment, and the varied applications and intervention formats do pose daunting challenges for family assessment and intervention research. Given cultural and family diversity, and the probability that some processes may be more useful than others in dealing with varied challenges, findings from a particular study may not be generalizable to diverse populations and life challenges. That said, a number of recent and ongoing qualitative studies in many parts of the world are making progress in applying this family resilience framework to clarify which variables matter most for family resilience in a range of adverse situations, such as immigration, living with cancer, and death of a child, and in interventions to strengthen poor, fragile families to prevent child abandonment to the streets.

Conclusions

A family resilience orientation involves a crucial shift in emphasis from family deficits to family challenges, with conviction in the potential inherent in family systems for recovery and growth out of adversity. By targeting interventions to strengthen key processes for resilience, families become more resourceful in dealing with crises, weathering persistent stresses, and meeting future challenges. This conceptual framework can usefully be integrated with many strengths-based practice models and applied with a range of crisis situations, with respect for family and cultural diversity. Resilience-oriented services foster family empowerment as they bring forth shared hope, develop new and renewed competencies, and strengthen family bonds.

References

Antonovsky, A. (1998). The sense of coherence: An historical and future perspective. In H. McCubbin, E. Thompson, A. Thompson, & J. Fromer (eds.), *Stress, coping and health in families: Sense of coherence and resiliency* (pp. 3–20). Thousand Oaks, CA: Sage.

Antonovsky, A. & Sourani, T. (1988). Family sense of coherence and family adaptation. *Journal of Marriage and the Family*, **50**, 79–92.

Beavers, W. R. & Hampson, R. B. (2003). Measuring family competence. In F. Walsh (ed.), *Normal family processes: Growing diversity and complexity*, 3rd edn (pp. 549–580). New York: Guilford Press.

Becker, C., Sargent, J., & Rolland, J. S. (2000). Kosovar Family Professional Education Collaborative. *AFTA Newsletter*, **80**, 26–30.

Bonanno, G. A. (2004). Loss, trauma, and human resilience. *American Psychologist*, **59**, 20–28.

Boss, P. (2001). *Family stress management: A contextual approach*, 2nd edn. Thousand Oaks, CA: Sage.

Boss, P., Beaulieu, L., Wieling, E., & Turner, W. (2003). Healing loss, ambiguity, and trauma: A community-based intervention with families of union workers missing after the 9/11 attack in New York City. *Journal of Marital and Family Therapy*, **29**, 455–467.

Campbell, T. (2003). The effectiveness of family interventions for physical disorders. *Journal of Marital and Family Therapy*, **29**, 263–281.

Cohen, O., Slonim, I., Finzi, R., & Leichtentritt, R. (2002). Family resilience: Israeli mothers' perspectives. *American Journal of Family Therapy*, **30**, 173–187.

Combrinck-Graham, L. (2005). *Children in families at risk: Maintaining the connections*, 2nd edn. New York: Guilford Press.

Cowan, P. A. & Cowan, C. P. (2012). Normative family transitions, couple relationship quality and and healthy child development. In F. Walsh (ed.), *Normal family processes: Growing diversity and complexity*, 4th edn. New York: Guilford Press, in press.

Epstein, N., Ryan, C., Bishop, D., Miller, I., & Keitner, G. (2003). The McMaster model: A view of healthy family functioning. In F. Walsh (ed.), *Normal family processes: Growing diversity and complexity*, 3rd edn (pp. 581–607). New York: Guilford Press.

Falicov, C. (2007). Working with transnational immigrants: expanding meanings of family, community and culture. *Family Process*, **46**, 157–172.

Figley, C. R. (1989). *Helping traumatized families*. San Francisco, CA: Jossey-Bass.

Figley, C. R. (1998a) *Burnout in families: The systemic cost of caring*. San Francisco, CA: Jossey-Bass.

Figley, C. (ed.) (1998b). *The traumatology of grieving*. San Francisco, CA: Jossey-Bass.

Girwitz, A., Forgatch, M., & Wieling, E. (2008). Parenting practices as potential mechanisms for child adjustment following mass trauma. *Journal of Marital and Family Therapy*, **34**, 177–192.

Gorell Barnes, G. (1999). Divorce transitions: Identifying risk and promoting resilience for children and their parental relationships. *Journal of Marital and Family Therapy*, **25**, 425–441.

Greeff, A. P. & Human, B. (2004). Resilience in families in which a parent has died. *American Journal of Family Therapy*, **32**, 27–42.

Greeff, A. P. & van der Merwe, S. (2004). Variables associated with resilience in divorced families. *Social Indicators Research*, **68**, 59–75.

Green, R.-J. (2004). Risk and resilience in lesbian and gay couples. *Journal of Family Psychology*, **18**, 290–292.

Greene, S., Anderson, E., Forgatch, M. S., DeGarmo, D. S., & Hetherington, E. M. (2012). Risk and resilience after divorce. In F. Walsh (ed.), *Normal family processes: Growing diversity and complexity*, 4th edn. New York: Guilford Press, in press.

Hauser, S. T. (1999). Understanding resilient outcomes: Adolescent lives across time and generations. *Journal of Research on Adolescence*, **9**, 1–24.

Hernandez, P. (2002). Resilience in families and communities: Latin American contributions from the psychology of liberation. *Journal of Counseling and Therapy for Couples and Families*, **10**, 334–343.

Johnson-Garner, M. Y. & Meyers, S. A. (2003). What factors contribute to the resilience of African-American children within kinship care? *Child and Youth Care Forum*, **32**, 255–269.

Knowles, R., Sasser, D., & Garrison, M. E. B. (2010). Family resilience and resiliency following Hurricane Katrina. In R. Kilmer, V. Gil-Rivas, R. Tedeschi, & L. Calhoun (eds.), *Helping families and communities recover from disaster*. Washington, DC: American Psychological Association Press.

Landau, J. (2007). Enhancing resilience: Families and communities as agents for change. *Family Process*, **46**, 351–365.

Landau, J. & Saul, J. (2004). Facilitating family and community resilience in response to major disasters. In F. Walsh & M. McGoldrick (eds.), *Living beyond loss: Death in the family*, 2nd edn (pp. 285–309). New York: Norton.

Lansford, J. E., Ceballo, R., Abby, A., & Stewart, A. J. (2001). Does family structure matter? A comparison of adoptive, two-parent biological, single-mother, stepfather, and stepmother households. *Journal of Marriage and the Family*, **63**, 840–851.

Lavee, Y., McCubbin, H. I., & Olson, D. H. (1987). The effect of stressful life events and transitions on family functioning and well-being. *Journal of Marriage and the Family*, **49**, 857–873.

Litz, B. (2004). *Early intervention for trauma and traumatic loss*. New York: Guilford Press.

Luthar, S. S., Cicchetti, D., & Becker, B. (2000). The construct of resilience: A critical evaluation and guidelines for future work. *Child Development*, **71**, 543–562.

MacDermid, S. M. (2010). Family risk and resilience in the context of war and terrorism. *Journal of Marriage and Family*, **72**, 537–556.

Malkinson, R., Rubin, S., & Witztum, E. (2005). Terror, trauma, and bereavement: Implications for theory and therapy. In Y. Danieli, D. Brom, & J. Sills (eds.), *The trauma of terrorism: Sharing knowledge and shared care – An international handbook* (pp. 467–481). New York: Haworth.

McCubbin, H. & Patterson, J. M. (1983). The family stress process: The double ABCX model of adjustment and adaptation. *Marriage and Family Review*, **6**(Suppl.), 7–37.

McCubbin, H., McCubbin, M., McCubbin, A., & Futrell, J. (eds.) (1998). *Resiliency in ethnic minority families*: Vol. 1 *Native and immigrant families,* Vol. 2 *African-American families*. Thousand Oaks, CA: Sage.

McGoldrick, M., Gerson, R., & Petry, S. (2008). *Genograms: Assessment and intervention,* 3rd edn. New York: Norton.

McGoldrick, M., Carter, B., & Garcia Preto, N. (2011). *The expanded family life cycle: Individual, family, and social perspectives,* 4th edn. Needham Heights: Allyn & Bacon.

Minuchin, P., Colapinto, J., & Minuchin, S. (2006). *Working with families of the poor,* 2nd edn. New York: Guilford Press.

Olson, D. H. & Gorell, D. (2003). Circumplex model of marital and family systems. In F. Walsh (ed.), *Normal family processes: Growing diversity and complexity,* 3rd edn (pp. 514–544). New York: Guilford Press.

Oswald, R. F. (2002). Resilience within the family networks of lesbians and gay men: Intentionality and redefinition. *Journal of Marriage and the Family*, **64**, 374–383.

Patterson, J. (2002). Integrating family resilience and family stress theory. *Journal of Marriage and the Family*, **64**, 349–373.

Rolland, J. S. (1994). *Families, illness and disability: An integrative treatment model*. New York: Basic.

Rolland, J. S. (2012). Mastering family challenges in serious illness and disability. In F. Walsh (ed.), *Normal family processes: Growing diversity and complexity,* 4th edn. New York: Guilford Press, in press.

Rolland, J. S., & Walsh, F. (2006). Facilitating family resilience with childhood illness and disability. [Special issue on the family.] *Pediatric Opinion*, **18**, 1–11.

Rolland, J. S. & Weine, S. (2000). Kosovar Family Professional Educational Collaborative. *American Family Therapy Newsletter*, **79**, 34–35.

Rowe, C. L. & Liddle, H. A. (2008). When the levee breaks: Treating adolescents and families in the aftermath of Hurricane Katrina. *Journal of Marital and Family Therapy*, **34**, 132–148.

Rutter, M. (1987). Psychosocial resilience and protective mechanisms. *American Journal of Orthopsychiatry*, **57**, 316–331.

Sheinberg, M. & Fraenkel, P. (2001). *The relational trauma of incest: A family-based approach to treatment*. New York: Guilford Press.

Stinnett, N. & DeFrain, J. (1985). *Secrets of strong families*. Boston, MA: Little, Brown.

Ungar, M. (2004). The importance of parents and other caregivers to the resilience of high-risk adolescents. *Family Process*, **43**, 23–41.

Vigil, A. M. & Geary, D. C. (2008). A preliminary investigation of family coping styles and psychological well being among adolescent survivors of Hurricane Katrina. *Journal of Family Psychology*, **22**, 176–180.

Walsh, F. (1996). The concept of family resilience: Crisis and challenge. *Family Process*, **35**, 261–281.

Walsh, F. (2002). A family resilience framework: Innovative practice applications. *Family Relations*, **51**, 130–137.

Walsh, F. (2003). Family resilience: A framework for clinical practice. *Family Process*, **42**, 1–18.

Walsh, F. (2006). *Strengthening family resilience,* 2nd edn. New York: Guilford Press.

Walsh, F. (2007). Traumatic loss and major disaster: Strengthening family and community resilience. *Family Process*, **46**, 207–227.

Walsh, F. (2009a). Family transitions: Challenges and transitions. In M. Dulcan (ed.), *Textbook of child and adolescent psychiatry*. Washington, DC: American Psychiatric Press.

Walsh, F. (ed.) (2009b). *Spiritual resources in family therapy*. New York: Guilford Press.

Walsh, F. (2010). Spiritual diversity: Multifaith perspectives in family therapy. *Family Process*, **49**, 330–348.

Walsh, F. (2011). Families in later life: Challenges, opportunities, and resilience. In B. Carter & M. McGoldrick (eds.), *The expanded family life cycle,* 4th edn (pp. 261–277). Needham Heights, MA: Allyn & Bacon.

Walsh, F. (2012a). The "new normal family": Diversity and complexity. In F. Walsh (ed.), *Normal family processes: Growing diversity and complexity,* 4th edn. New York: Guilford Press, in press.

Walsh, F. (2012b). Clinical views of family normality, health, and dysfunction. In F. Walsh (ed.), *Normal family processes: Growing diversity and complexity,* 4th edn. New York: Guilford Press, in press.

Walsh, F. & McGoldrick, M. (2004). Loss and the family: A systemic perspective. In F. Walsh & M. McGoldrick (eds.), *Living beyond loss: Death in the family,* 2nd edn (pp. 3–26). New York: Norton.

Weine, S., Muzuravic, N., Kulauzovic, Y., *et al.* (2004). Family consequences of refugee trauma. *Family Process,* **43**, 147–160.

Community resilience: concepts, assessment, and implications for intervention

Fran H. Norris, Kathleen Sherrieb, and Betty Pfefferbaum

Introduction

Although stress research has emphasized individual well-being, many types of stress are experienced collectively: the events bring harm, pain, and loss to large numbers of people simultaneously. Natural disasters, terrorist attacks, war, political oppression, epidemics, and economic recessions happen to whole communities and, sometimes, whole societies. This is not to say that all exposed individuals experience the event identically; in a disaster, one person may lose a loved one, while another loses a home, and another only a few possessions. Nor is this to say that all exposed individuals respond identically; a person's psychological, social, and material resources powerfully shape his or her capacity to cope and function effectively. When stress pervades the community, however, these factors tell only part of the story. To have an ecologically valid understanding of mass trauma, we must recognize that survivors are connected and dependent upon one another's coping strategies. Their attributions and actions reflect a host of social influences, social comparisons, and emergent norms. They help each other but also compete for scarce resources. Household preparedness is vital, but one household can no more prepare for disaster than it could, on its own, protect itself from crime or disease, educate its children, or keep the roads safe. Consequently, an individual's resilience is inextricably linked to the community's ability to prepare for, respond to, and adapt to adverse conditions. Simply put, when problems are shared, so must be solutions.

In recognition of such interdependencies, "community resilience" has emerged as a key concept for disaster readiness, although by no means limited to this one goal (Norris *et al.*, 2008). This chapter will explore the concept of community resilience in some depth. Broadly, the chapter is organized into four

sections. The first section provides our perspective on the meaning of resilience, including definitions that work across levels of analysis (individual, family, organization, community, society). The second section describes the adaptive capacities theorized to yield community resilience. This is followed by an outline of measurement strategies and challenges in assessing capacities, including some of our own pilot work. The concluding section makes recommendations for intervention and raises issues that need to be addressed in future research.

Resilience as a process

Our perspective on the broader meaning of resilience has shaped our thinking about its specific application to communities. The concept of resilience appears in a variety of disciplines, including physics and engineering (Gordon, 1978; Bodin & Wiman, 2004), biology and ecology (e.g., Holling, 1973), sociology (e.g., Adger, 2000; Godschalk, 2003), and psychology (Werner & Smith, 1982; Rutter, 1993; Bonanno, 2004). Across domains of concern, most definitions of resilience emphasize a capacity for successful adaptation in the face of a disturbance, stress, or adversity. Attempting to integrate various definitions across levels of analysis, Norris and colleagues (2008, p. 130) defined resilience as "a process linking a set of adaptive capacities to a positive trajectory of functioning and adaptation after a disturbance." This definition of resilience encompasses two primary conceptions that are important for our discussion here.

First, in this definition, resilience *emerges from* adaptive capacities, but it is not synonymous with those capacities. Resilience is not a trait that an individual or community invariably has or does not have. Post-event trajectories are contingent upon both the capacities and the stressor. Resilience occurs when

Resilience and Mental Health: Challenges Across the Lifespan, ed. Steven M. Southwick, Brett T. Litz, Dennis Charney, and Matthew J. Friedman. Published by Cambridge University Press. © Cambridge University Press 2011.

resources are sufficiently strong to buffer or counteract the effects of a stressor such that a return to functioning, adapted to the altered environment, occurs. The more severe the stressor, the stronger the resources must be to create resilience. There is perhaps no person or community that would always exhibit resilience nor a person or community that would never exhibit resilience. The current emphasis on resilience is essentially a reframing or evolution of stress theory, now decades old, in which stress outcomes are viewed as the product of stressors interacting with risk and protective factors. Importantly, however, the contemporary frame of resilience directs attention to the potential of individuals and communities to adjust and stay well in the face of threats, losses, and challenges.

Second, resilience *is manifest in outcomes* of interest, but it is not synonymous with those outcomes. The definition of resilience as a process implies that it is not observed or measured directly, but it is evident in the patterns of change observed after significant stress. Norris *et al.* (2009) outlined six possible trajectories for post-traumatic stress symptoms, of which resilience was just one, the others being resistance, recovery, relapsing/remitting, delayed dysfunction, and chronic dysfunction. In analyses of two four-wave datasets collected from population-based samples after the 1999 floods/mudslides in Mexico and the 2001 terrorist attacks in New York, all of the hypothesized trajectories except one (relapsing/remitting) occurred with measurable frequency in one or both of the samples.

While the analyses conducted by Norris *et al.* (2009) focused on one particular outcome (post-traumatic stress), "wellness" provides a more complete criterion for assessing human adaptation (Cowen, 1983, 1994, 2000; Norris *et al.*, 2008), Wellness goes beyond the mere absence of psychopathology to include healthy patterns of behavior, adequate role functioning, and high quality of life. Community-level adaptation can be understood as "population wellness," defined as high and non-disparate levels of mental and behavioral health, role functioning, and quality of life in constituent populations. However, it is important not to confuse resilience, the process, with wellness, the outcome. A resilient trajectory could be observed for one outcome (e.g., post-traumatic stress) but not for another (e.g., quality of life). The outcomes of interest vary across levels of analysis, as do the specific resources that influence the patterns of change, but the basic nomenclature of adaptive capacities, observed trajectories, and adequate functioning applies to all.

Capacities for resilience

What we primarily seek to discover in resilience research is the capacity for resilience – those resources that increase the likelihood of adaptation as manifest in psychological or population wellness. Resilience rests on both the resources themselves and the dynamic attributes of those resources; we use the term "adaptive capacities" to capture this combination. Drawing upon the earlier work of Bruneau *et al.* (2003), we define adaptive capacities as resources with one or more dynamic attributes: *robustness*, the ability of the resource to withstand stress without suffering degradation; *redundancy*, the extent to which elements are substitutable in the event of disruption or degradation; and *rapidity*, the speed with which the resource can be accessed and used. By posing this definition, we aimed to integrate resilience perspectives with evidence showing that resources are not static – they evolve, strengthen, weaken, and rebound – and these trajectories are of interest in their own right (Hobfoll, 1988). Reaching a better understanding of the impact of critical incidents on community resources is one of the most critical and complex challenges for future research.

On the basis of their review of the literature, Norris *et al.* (2008) identified four primary sets of resources thought to yield community resilience: economic development, social capital, information and communication, and community competence. These sets are far from orthogonal, but they are also far from synonymous. Much has been written about these concepts, which are introduced here only briefly. There are innumerable possible linkages between elements in these sets (and between these elements and population wellness) that could be researched empirically across communities.

Economic development

Economic development encompasses three key elements relating to the level of economic resources, the diversity of those resources, and the equity of their distribution. Land and raw materials, physical capital, accessible housing, health services, schools, and employment opportunities create the essential resource base of a resilient community (Godschalk, 2003; Pfefferbaum *et al.*, 2007). Because of extensive interdependencies at the macroeconomic level, economic resilience depends not only on the capacities of individual businesses but also on the capacities of all the entities that depend on them and on which they depend (Rose, 2004, 2005).

Community resilience depends on both the volume of economic resources and their diversity. Communities that are dependent on a narrow range of resources are less able to cope with change that involves the depletion of that resource, a state that is sometimes referred to as "resource dependency" (Adger, 2000). Extreme events, such as droughts, floods, or infestations, increase the risk of being dependent on particular resources and, therefore, decrease resilience. Cutter *et al.* (2006) described one community that was particularly devastated by Hurricane Katrina in August 2005 because residents were almost totally reliant on the shrimping industry, on which the storm had a tremendous impact.

Societies do not allocate environmental risk equally, often making the poorest communities the weakest links in hazard mitigation (Tobin & Whiteford, 2002; Cutter *et al.*, 2003; Godschalk, 2003). Wisner (2001, p. 251) argued that mitigation plans in developing countries often fail to address the "root causes of disaster vulnerability, namely, the economic and political marginality of much of the population and environmental degradation." Poor communities not only are at greater risk for death and severe damage but are also often less successful in mobilizing support after disasters (Bolin & Bolton, 1986; Tobin & Whiteford, 2002). Ideally, the distribution or mobilization of support follows the "rule of relative needs," wherein the most support goes to those who need it the most. Often, however, the distribution of support follows the "rule of relative advantage," because one's embeddedness in the community, political connections, and social class determine the availability and accessibility of resources (Kaniasty & Norris, 1995). The capacity to distribute post-disaster resources to those who most need them seems vitally important for community resilience.

Social capital

The basic idea of social capital is that individuals invest, access, and use resources embedded in social networks to gain returns (Bourdieu, 1985; Lin, 2001). Social capital theorists debate the roles of self-interest and status attainment and whether social capital should be conceived as an individual, collective, or multilevel asset (Wellman & Frank, 2001). Theorists have also debated the extent to which people actively aim to increase their social capital (through investment) or whether, conversely, it arises from structural positions, families, and friendships (Kadushin, 2004).

For crisis response, an important dimension of social capital is the presence of interorganizational networks that are characterized by reciprocal links, frequent supportive interactions, overlap with other networks, the ability to form new associations, and cooperative decision-making processes (Goodman *et al.*, 1998). Comfort (2005, p. 347) noted that uncertainty often leads to efforts to broaden the "scope of actors, agents, and knowledge that can be marshaled." More generally, this trend necessitates networked as opposed to hierarchical systems for disaster response. Longstaff (2005) highlighted the importance of "keystones" or "hubs": "super-connected" network members who link one network to another (see also Fullilove & Saul, 2006). Despite the many values of dense networks, they are also more complex and, therefore, more uncertain. The efficiency of hubs may actually decrease resilience because the entire system fails if the hub is compromised (Allenby & Fink, 2005). Systems will be highly vulnerable if there is little redundancy for these connective functions.

Longstaff (2005) also noted the tendency to want individuals, groups, and organizations to come together tightly to resist danger. "Tight coupling" occurs when change in one component engenders a response from other components. This is not always bad, but tight coupling can also increase danger in some circumstances and can lead to premature convergence on solutions. "Loosely coupled" systems may be better at responding to local changes since any change they make does not require the whole system to respond (Longstaff, 2005). The happy medium may be loosely coupled organizations (to better respond to local needs) that are able to coordinate or collaborate (to facilitate access to their resources). The failure of relief organizations to work together results in "cracks" in the post-disaster service delivery network, whereas an effective service delivery system provides a complete set of services and linkages in which such cracks do not appear (Gillespie & Murty, 1994).

Social capital also encompasses the more familiar concept of social support, which refers to social interactions that provide individuals with actual assistance and embed them into a web of social relationships perceived to be loving, caring, and readily available in times of need (Barrera, 1986). Strong social support is vital for community resilience following crises (Goodman *et al.*, 1998; Ganor & Ben-Lavy, 2003; Tse & Liew, 2004; Pfefferbaum *et al.*, 2005). The overall pattern of help utilization resembles a pyramid with its broad foundation being the family, followed by other primary support groups, such as friends, neighbors, and co-workers, followed by formal agencies and other persons outside of the recipient's immediate circle (Kaniasty & Norris, 2000). Received support typically shows a mobilization pattern by increasing in the aftermath of disasters and correlating positively with severity of exposure. It protects against erosion of perceived support, which is a powerful protective factor for mental health (Norris & Kaniasty, 1996).

Another critical function of social networks is social influence. In emergencies, people look to similar others to help them to make decisions about appropriate behaviors. This idea, often characterized as "emergent norms," is among the oldest to be found in the sociology of disasters (Fritz & Williams, 1957). For example, the greater one's social ties, the more likely one is to receive information about recommendations to evacuate. Evacuation is often the only available strategy to save lives and reduce personal injuries. In an analysis of evacuation decisions before Hurricanes Hugo and Andrew, Riad et al. (1999) found that residents with stronger social support were twice as likely to evacuate as were residents with weaker social support. The important dimension was perceived support (e.g., ability to borrow money, get a ride, have a place to stay), not merely the number of ties.

For the most part, social support captures helping behaviors within family and friendship networks, but social capital also encompasses relationships between individuals and their larger neighborhoods and communities (Perkins et al., 2002). Three key social psychological dimensions of social capital are, therefore, sense of community, place attachment, and citizen participation. Sense of community is an attitude of bonding (trust and belonging) with other members of one's group or locale (Perkins et al., 2002), including mutual concerns and shared values. It is reliably believed to be an attribute of resilient communities (Ahmed et al., 2004; Landau & Saul, 2004; Tse & Liew, 2004; Pfefferbaum et al., 2007). Place attachment is closely related to one's sense of community. It implies an emotional connection to one's neighborhood or city, somewhat apart from connections to the specific people who live there (Altman & Low, 1992; Manzo & Perkins, 2006). Place attachment often underlies citizens' efforts to revitalize a community (Perkins et al., 2002) and, therefore, may be essential for community resilience. Place attachment may be of special note for disaster recovery, as these events have spatial parameters and will harm built and natural environments. In the worst of cases, people are displaced from neighborhoods and communities in which they are deeply rooted. The impact of displacement after disasters has often been profoundly adverse (e.g., Erikson, 1976; Oliver-Smith, 1986; Norris et al., 2005a), raising the possibility that place attachment could, in some circumstances, impair rather than facilitate individual resilience. However, place attachments increase the likelihood that the community as a whole has the will to rebuild (Manzo & Perkins, 2006).

Citizen participation is the engagement of community members in formal organizations, including religious congregations, school and resident associations, neighborhood watches, and self-help groups (Perkins et al., 2002). It is widely believed to be a fundamental element for community resilience (Goodman et al., 1998; Ganor & Ben-Lavy, 2003; Pfefferbaum et al., 2007). Empowering community settings are characterized by inspired, committed leadership and by opportunities for members to play meaningful roles (Maton & Salem, 1995). Quarantelli (1989) summarized the results of a series of observational studies of citizen groups that emerge with respect to hazardous waste sites, noting that they tend to have a small active core, a larger supporting circle that can be mobilized for specific tasks, and a greater number of nominal members. Most groups exist in conflict. Their goals are often vague and lofty at the outset but become more specific and achievable over time. Edelstein (1988) observed that leaders of citizen groups are usually those who have strongest attachments to place.

Information and communication

Information may be the primary resource in technical and organizational systems that enable adaptive performance (Comfort, 2005). By communication, we refer to the creation of common meanings and understandings and the provision of opportunities for members to articulate needs, views, and attitudes. Pfefferbaum et al. (2007), Goodman et al. (1998), and Ganor and Ben-Lavy (2003) have all argued that good communication is essential for community resilience or capacity.

Information and communication become vital in emergencies. People need accurate information about the danger and behavioral options, and they need it quickly. Public adherence to recommendations cannot be taken for granted, particularly when there is marked uncertainty about exposure, consequences of exposure, or the risks involved with following the recommendations (Reissman *et al.*, 2005). On the basis of her review, Longstaff (2005) argued that information increases survival only if it is "correct and correctly transmitted." In emergencies, when there is little time to check information, it is also important that the sender of the information be trusted. Closer, local sources of information are more likely to be relied upon than unfamiliar, distant sources. In fact, Longstaff concluded (2005, p. 62), "*A trusted source of information is the most important resilience asset that any individual or group can have*" (emphasis in original). Similarly, the Working Group on Governance Dilemmas in Bioterrorism Response (2004) concluded that trusted communication treats the public as a capable ally, invests in public outreach, and reflects the values and priorities of local populations.

Communication infrastructure is also a valuable resource. On the basis of their experiences in New York City after the September 11 2001 (9/11) terrorist attacks, Draper *et al.* (2006) maintained that it is advantageous for a lifeline (or hotline) system to be in place beforehand. These communication systems can be ramped up after the disaster to coordinate and deploy volunteers, and later they provide a central means for the public to learn about and access services (see also Norris *et al.*, 2006). The media also can be engaged to publicize available services and educate the public about typical reactions to disaster (e.g., Gist & Stolz, 1982; Norris *et al.*, 2006).

The remaining element in this set, less structural than the others, is the presence of communal narratives that give the experience shared meaning and purpose (Sonn & Fisher, 1998). Couto (1989) described how "group formulations" (narratives and symbols) became a mechanism for empowerment in Aberfan, South Wales, after a horrific environmental disaster took the lives of 104 school children and 20 adults. Writing about their own experiences in the aftermath of the 9/11 terrorist attacks in lower Manhattan, Landau and Saul (2004) concluded that community recovery depends partly on collectively telling the story of the community's experience and response. In an extraordinary anthropological study of six Guinean communities attacked by Sierra Leonean and Liberian forces (Abramowitz, 2005), symptoms of post-traumatic stress were much higher in three of the communities than in the others. In the three more distressed communities, respondents shared the feeling that government and non-governmental organizations had neglected them. Social rituals and practices, including

reciprocity and charity, were abandoned. There were widespread beliefs that some community members had prospered at the expense of others. In the three less distressed communities, residents shared a belief that customs and social practices would return to normal as soon as economic conditions improved. Most importantly, they had created a collective story that emphasized their resistance to the violence.

Community competence

Community competence is the capacity for meaningful, intentional action (Brown & Kulig, 1996/97). There appears to be high consensus that critical reflection and problem solving are fundamental prerequisites for community resilience (Goodman *et al.*, 1998; Bruneau *et al.*, 2003; Ganor & Ben-Lavy, 2003; Pfefferbaum *et al.*, 2007). Endangered communities must be able to learn about their risks and options and work together flexibly and creatively to solve problems. Longstaff (2005) argued that the capacity to acquire trusted and accurate information, to reflect on that information critically, and to solve emerging problems is far more important for community resilience than is a detailed security plan, which rarely foresees all contingencies (see also Comfort, 2005; Handmer & Dovers, 1996).

Cottrell (1976, p. 197) described a competent community as one in which "the various component parts of the community: (1) are able to collaborate effectively in identifying the problems and needs of the community; (2) can achieve a working consensus on goals and priorities; (3) can agree on ways and means to implement the agreed upon goals; and (4) can collaborate effectively in the required actions." Cottrell proposed that these competencies arose from commitment to the community as a relationship worthy of substantial effort, articulateness, communication, participation, and means for debate, discussion, and decision making. Many of these conditions were previously considered as aspects of social capital or information and communication, so it might be said that social capital and communication are prerequisites for community competence.

Collective action may depend heavily on the presence of "collective efficacy": community members' trust in the effectiveness of organized community action (Perkins & Long, 2002). Sampson *et al.* (1997) defined collective efficacy as a composite of mutual trust and shared willingness to work for the common good of a neighborhood. Paton and Johnston (2001) proposed that an initial focus on promoting collective efficacy would increase the likelihood of achieving success in working with a community to adopt mitigation strategies. Collective efficacy is highly related to empowerment (Perkins *et al.*, 2002), a process through which people lacking an equal share of valued resources gain greater access to and control over those resources (Rappaport, 1995). A particular relevant discussion of empowerment for our purposes was presented by Rich *et al.* (1995), who examined the dynamics of community empowerment after discovery of environmental hazards. The authors reasoned that meaningful participation in environmental action groups can be empowering and, conversely, that lack of opportunity for such participation can be disempowering. According to Rich and colleagues, the effectiveness of a community's response to a hazard is shaped by a combination of resources (such as sufficient education to understand the technical issues, money to hire lawyers or scientific advisors), a culture that permits challenges to authority, institutions that provide a basis for coordinating a response, and political mechanisms that involve citizens in decision making. In their model, empowerment progresses through a sequence of formal empowerment (mechanisms for citizen input), intrapersonal empowerment (feelings of personal competence and confidence), instrumental empowerment (ability to participate in and influence decision, as determined by knowledge, material resources, and persuasiveness), and substantive empowerment (ability to reach decisions that solve problems). The last of these stages is virtually synonymous with our broader meaning of community competence.

Assessment of capacities

Broadly, there are three approaches to the assessment of capacities for community resilience. Population-based surveys that are designed to allow responses from individual respondents to be aggregated to meaningful social units (neighborhoods, counties) have high potential but are considerably expensive. Existing national surveys are representative at the state level but cannot be used to describe smaller units of analysis. Consequently, in our work, we have focused on two very different, but perhaps complementary, approaches: community-based participatory methods and secondary analysis of social indicator data. The appropriate strategy may depend upon the scope of the analysis. At the local level, when the goal is to assess a single community or a small set of communities, participatory self-assessments may be most appropriate. When the goal is to assess multiple communities using a standardized metric, secondary analysis of social indicator and other publicly available data appears to be a promising approach. Each of these approaches is described in more detail below.

Participatory approaches

The Community Assessment of Resilience tool (CART) developed by Pfefferbaum and colleagues (2006) constitutes a community-based participatory approach to community resilience assessment and intervention. Community-based participatory research promotes collaboration between investigators and those being studied. These approaches can be used to investigate complex health, public health, or social concerns that occur disproportionately in communities marginalized with respect to health education and resources or to address challenging issues such as disparities in access to healthcare and outcomes (Meyer, 2000; Israel *et al.*, 2006; Cargo & Mercer, 2008; Flicker *et al.*, 2008). Inspired by the desire to stimulate community-based problem solving, CART not only builds on the principles of community-based participatory research it also promotes these principles by involving community representatives in both assessment and community-resilience building exercises.

The CART process begins by surveying community representatives about community resilience domains tested in community assessment studies and about additional specific concerns identified and refined in conjunction with community partners. The CART survey instrument incorporates four overlapping interrelated domains that characterize communities. Three of the domains are common to all of CART efforts: *connection and caring*, which includes relatedness, shared values, participation, support systems, equity, justice, hope, and diversity; *resources*, which includes natural, physical, financial, human, and social resources; and *transformative potential*, which includes data collection, analysis of community assets and shortcomings, and skill building that create the potential for community change. A fourth domain relates to the specific condition or adversity that concerns the community such as terrorism and disaster management, community violence, or poverty.

Community-based participatory approaches emphasize relationships to promote trust and mutual understanding, improve interactions, and foster collective problem solving between researchers and participants (Israel *et al.*, 1998; Cargo & Mercer, 2008; Cashman *et al.*, 2008; Christopher *et al.*, 2008). The CART approach relies on community partners to convene either a homogeneous or a heterogeneous mix of community leaders, neighborhood groups, selected professionals, residents, or other stakeholders to complete the community assessment and CART group activities. Rather than traditional methodology in which investigators study individuals whose sole input is to provide data (Israel *et al.*, 1998; Meyer, 2000; Macaulay & Nutting, 2006), community-based participatory approaches strive to improve the process and results by engaging the community in virtually all aspects of the work (Israel *et al.*, 1998; Macaulay & Nutting, 2006; Westfall *et al.*, 2006; Cargo & Mercer, 2008; Flicker *et al.*, 2008). Relying on the community's collective social experience and cultural perspective, community representatives can help to generate and refine theory, frame questions that address the community's concerns, and enhance the validity of research constructs (Israel *et al.*, 1998; Cargo & Mercer, 2008). Community partners help to design recruitment strategies and assessment and intervention processes that consider the needs and values of those involved, and they can assist in data collection by identifying and reaching out to potential participants (Macaulay & Nutting, 2006; Cashman *et al.*, 2008). They can advance the translation of research into practice; and they can promote the adoption and dissemination of results (Macaulay & Nutting, 2006; Cargo & Mercer, 2008; Cashman *et al.*, 2008). The community can benefit from this approach directly if newly generated knowledge is used to expand or enrich existing practices, services, programs, or policies (Israel *et al.*, 1998; Kemmis & McTaggart, 2005; Cargo & Mercer, 2008; Flicker *et al.*, 2008). Our CART community partners are engaged across many of these activities.

Designed to stimulate communication, analysis, and action, and to foster community participation and collaboration, community self-awareness, critical analysis, and skill development, the CART assessment and intervention reflect the principles of community-based participatory methodology. To initiate the process, CART community participants (e.g., a mix of community leaders, neighborhood members, selected professionals, and/or representatives of community organizations) complete the CART survey. The results provide information to generate a community profile incorporating findings by and across the CART domains (connection and caring, resources, transformative potential, and disaster management or other community concern). The initial survey is followed by a series of meetings in which the community participants review and interpret survey findings within the context of their community and concerns. Upon completion of the community resilience assessment phase, participants work together through group processes to explore the meaning of community, perceptions of the community resilience domains in application to specific community concerns, and potential resilience-enhancing actions. Based on survey results and knowledge of their community, group members identify community strengths and weaknesses, opportunities for improvement, external factors that might facilitate or impede change, and areas of disagreement. Group members then establish goals related to issues they choose to address, and they engage in strategic planning to prepare strategies and an action plan to enhance community resilience in support of the goals they have established. Strategies are then fielded, evaluated, and refined. Plans may be disseminated among community members and organizations, which may require training and other support to implement the strategies.

Several considerations arise in using community-based participatory research approaches. Colleagues, potential partners, and funders may need to be convinced of the value, validity, and reliability of this approach (Israel *et al.*, 1998). Community-based participatory approaches do require a long-term commitment of time and human capital to establish and nurture relationships with community partners, to conduct community assessments, and to incorporate stakeholder input throughout the process (Israel *et al.*, 1998; Macaulay & Nutting, 2006; Westfall *et al.*, 2006; Cashman *et al.*, 2008; Christopher *et al.*, 2008). We have been fortunate to identify partners who endorse the approach and appreciate the work we are promoting. While this approach is time and labor intensive, our experience has been positive and appears to support our ultimate goal of fostering community resilience building.

Social indicator research

The second potential approach to assessing community resilience relies on publicly available data to create a metric that can be applied across communities. In the disaster field, an excellent example is the Social Vulnerability Index (SOVI; Cutter *et al.*, 2003). Cutter and colleagues conducted factor analyses with data from all US counties to create the SOVI. It contains 11 factors representing income, age, race/ethnicity, occupation, commercial establishment density, single-sector industry, housing, and infrastructure dependence; these factors are used to depict community vulnerability. Although social vulnerability should be related (inversely) to community resilience, it is conceptually distinct, suggesting that new measures were needed.

The social indicator approach has been explored using the State of Mississippi as the pilot case, with county as the unit of analysis (Sherrieb *et al.*, 2010). In reviewing the literature related to the measurement of the capacities included in the Norris *et al.* (2008) model, it became apparent that "economic development" and "social capital" had structural characteristics that were possible to measure with secondary data, but the same was not true for "information and communication" and "community competence." Sherrieb *et al.* (2010) described previous measures of economic development and social capital in some detail, noting both their strengths and limitations with regard to utility for inclusion in a measure of community resilience. There has been considerable prior work on measurement of economic development. Well-known indices of economic development include (1) the gross domestic product, which provides the total value in national currency (dollars here) of all economic production in a given area in a year; (2) the Human Development Index, which has been used by the United Nations Development Programme (launched in 1990) as the marker for comparison of economic development across nations since 1990; and (3) the Social Health Index, which is derived from five potential indicators of social disadvantage: in the USA, rates of unemployment, poverty, high school drop out, violent crime, and Medicaid recipients (for further discussion of these measures, see Anderson, 1991; Horn, 1993; Shaw-Taylor, 1999; McGillivray, 2007).

Likewise, the literature defining, measuring, and modeling social capital is vast. Several measurements of social capital use an aggregate measurement derived from survey data. For example, Putnam (2000) and Kawachi *et al.* (1997) used measures from the General Social Survey conducted by the US National Opinion Research Center to determine social trust and organizational participation at the state level. Structural social capital indicators used by Kawachi *et al.* included per capita number of groups and associations such as churches, sports groups, political groups, and labor unions. Putnam (2000) included additional structural indicators measuring volunteerism, voting participation, service and participation in clubs, local organizations and community projects, and number of non-profit organizations per population size. Rupasingha *et al.* (2006) proposed a county-level model to measure social capital based on their definition of social capital as participation in associational activities. Their indicators included associational densities, presidential voter rates, census response rates, and per capita non-profit organizations. They argued that the degree of participation and density provides a good measure of social capital differences between regions.

Through a multistep process beginning with a "wish list" of measures and continuing through searching for and selecting indicators and validating indices, Sherrieb *et al.* (2010) selected 10 indicators to form an index of economic development: (1) employment rate, (2) median household income, (3) number of medical doctors per 10 000, (4) corporate tax revenues per 1000 population, and (5) percentage creative class occupations (measuring *resource level*); (6) income equity (inverse of the Gini coefficient), (7) racial differences in percentage with less than a high school education (measuring *resource equity*); and (8) net gain/loss rate in businesses over a year, (9) occupational diversity (percentage of occupations in the non-dominant industry for the area), and (10) urban influence (measuring *resource diversity*). Likewise, they selected seven indicators to form an index of social capital: (1) ratio of households with married parents with children to households with single female parents with children (measuring *social support*); (2) density of sports/arts organizations per 10 000, (3) density of civic organizations per 10 000, (4) voter percentage in 2004 presidential election, (5) religious adherents per 1000 (measuring *social participation*); and (6) net migration rate per 1000 in a three-year period, and (7) the inverse of the property crime rate (measuring *community bonds*).

In their initial research, Sherrieb *et al.* (2010) validated their measures against the SOVI and aggregated survey data from 21 Mississippi counties. (The availability of these survey data was their primary reason for using Mississippi as the pilot case.) Economic development and social capital were moderately correlated with each other ($r = 0.37$), but only 14% of the variance was shared by the three concepts, social capital, economic development, and SOVI. More than 50% of the variance in each measure was unique. These data support the premise that the three attributes share some common characteristics yet are distinct concepts. The Mississippi survey had included measures of collective efficacy, which were aggregated to the county level. Social capital was highly correlated with the aggregated collective efficacy measures (r values of 0.62 to 0.77), but the economic development and SOVI measures were not.

The distributions of scores were also consistent with what is known about different regions of Mississippi. For example, the rural region bordering the Mississippi River, known as the Delta historically, has been notable for its high rates of poverty. This area has some of the highest rates for infant, adolescent, and adult mortality in the USA (Woods, 1998). The region is also in the top highest 20% for social vulnerability when comparing the counties within the state and within the nation with SOVI (Hazards and Vulnerability Research Institute, 2008). The new community resilience measures provided comparable results as that region was in the lowest 20% for social capital, economic development, and community resilience.

Ultimately, the utility of measures of community resilience (or more correctly, capacity for community resilience) depends upon the ability of these measures to identify areas in need of strengthening. Areas low in community resilience and high in risk for disasters, terrorist attacks, or other collective threats are particularly important for efforts to build capacity. For example, Harrison County (Biloxi/Gulfport) was identified by Sherrieb et al. (2010) as being at high risk for disasters but low in social capital. Consequently, knowledge about the distribution of capacities and disaster risk can help to target specific interventions to facilitate resilience.

Despite their potential utility and feasibility, there are inherent limitations of archival data. Indicators that might be good measures of a concept are not always available, and there is a lag in the availability of data. Not only did Sherrieb et al. (2010) omit entire constructs, they were unable to measure the cognitive characteristics of social capital such as trust, reciprocity, norms, and values although the literature indicates that these are fundamental aspects of social capital. Despite this limitation, their indices of social capital and community resilience correlated with survey measures of collective efficacy, which addressed some of those cognitive aspects. We believe the study of Sherrieb et al. (2010) points to a useful method for future research that could be conducted with a larger, more geographically diverse sample of counties and a set of survey measures (such as the CART survey) developed specifically to capture the capacities thought to underlie community resilience.

Conclusions and implications

"Community preparedness" was recently legislated as one of four cross-cutting "target capabilities" required for federal emergency management (Post-Katrina Emergency Management Reform Act of 2006 [P.L. 109–295]). Representing a paradigm shift from earlier disaster mitigation approaches, community preparedness calls for the use and integration of all the community's resources into disaster planning, including those that exist outside of government as well as inside. Our work in identifying the adaptive capacities that underlie community resilience is consistent with this approach. While the distinction between community resilience and community preparedness is not completely clear, a resilience perspective takes us beyond making plans for a disaster toward building strengths in a community that will facilitate the process of resilience regardless of the nature of the shared adversity. Consequently, translation of our findings into policy recommendations involves a discussion of changes in the socioeconomic structure of at-risk communities.

The four sets of adaptive capacities provide a guide for enhancing community resilience. We repeat here the recommendations described in more detail by Norris et al. (2008).

First, to increase their resilience to disaster, communities must develop economic resources, reduce risk and resource inequities, and attend to their areas of greatest social vulnerability. Godschalk (2003) recommended that urban hazard mitigation activities be integrated with activities related to economic development and social justice, thereby "achieving the multiple objectives needed for a resilient system." Efforts to create economic diversity increase the probability that the community can withstand adversity or surprise. After a disaster, residents and grass-roots leaders should be vigilant to the equity of resource distribution. Competent communities may influence these dynamics through creative problem solving and political action.

Second, to access social capital, one of the primary resources of any community, local people must be engaged meaningfully in every step of the mitigation process. Enabled by professional practitioners, as necessary, community members must assess and address their own vulnerabilities to hazards, identify and invest in their own networks of assistance and information, and enhance their own capacities to solve problems created by "known or unknown unknowns" (e.g., Brown & Kulig, 1996/97; Coles & Buckle, 2004; Longstaff, 2005; Pfefferbaum *et al.*, 2007). As we reviewed here, the CART process is one structured approach that engages communities in this process. Non-indigenous practitioners best foster recovery by providing settings and resources that allow the community to take charge of the direction of change (van den Eynde & Veno, 1999; Landau & Saul, 2004; Perez-Sales *et al.*, 2005; Fullilove & Saul, 2006).

Third, pre-existing organizational networks and relationships are the key to rapidly mobilizing emergency and ongoing support services for disaster survivors. Loosely coupled but cooperative systems appear to provide the best combination of linkages and flexibility (Gillespie & Murty, 1994; Longstaff, 2005). A series of case studies of mental health system responses to major disasters, including the Oklahoma City bombing (Norris *et al.*, 2005b), the 9/11 terrorist attacks (Norris *et al.*, 2006), and many others (Elrod *et al.*, 2006) repeatedly revealed that developing organizational networks, coalitions, and cooperative agreements ahead of time is crucial, and that organizational plans should indicate how key constituencies will be involved. Program directors relied upon pre-existing relationships perhaps more than any other single resource to implement programs quickly. To work together after a disaster, systems must understand and trust each other, which is challenging if they have not worked together before.

Fourth, interventions are needed that boost and protect naturally occurring social supports in the aftermath of disasters. Fostering natural supports helps to ensure that communities and families retain the capacity to exchange emotional and instrumental support (Landau & Saul, 2004). Social support interventions are most effective when they build social skills and mutual support (Hogan *et al.*, 2002). Ideally, post-disaster support interventions furnish participants with knowledge, attitudes, and skills that can be used to recruit their own supports (Layne *et al.*, 2001).

Fifth, communities must plan for the unexpected; this means that communities must exercise flexibility and focus on building effective and trusted information and communication resources that function in the face of unknowns. Uncertainty is almost certain to exist after disasters. The most adaptive disaster management strategy is one that acknowledges complexity and uncertainty and relies on timely and trusted sources of information for rapid decision making as opposed to rigid plans (Longstaff, 2005). In contrast to command and control styles, problem-solving approaches allow for innovation and localized variations in response. Similarly, Godschalk (2003, p. 139) envisioned that "the public and private organization of a resilient city would both plan ahead and act spontaneously ...They would eschew simple command and control leadership, preferring to develop networks of leadership and initiative. They would set goals and objectives, but be prepared to adapt these in light of new information and learning."

Our primary hope is to foster creative thinking about how various pathways between economic development, social capital, information and communication, and community competence shape disaster readiness and recovery. Of course, there is then the question of how strongly the various adaptive capacities in this network contribute to the wellness of constituent populations. To date, research on the outcomes of community resilience is meager. Some studies have examined how individual-level perceptions of community resilience (Kimhi & Shamai, 2004; Pooley *et al.*, 2006), sense of community (Paton *et al.*, 2001), or collective efficacy (Benight, 2004) correlate with individual-level outcomes, but no study, to our knowledge, has truly examined how independently assessed community resources influence the post-disaster wellness of constituent populations.

The "prevention paradox" (Rose, 1981, 2001) is extremely important for future judgments regarding the relative influence (and significance for policy) of individual and community resilience resources. Effects that seem small in analyses of individuals may be quite large when extrapolated to populations. Traditional risk (or protective) factor research is almost assured to find that individual-level resilience resources (e.g., self-efficacy) have stronger effects within a study population than do community-level resilience resources (e.g., collective efficacy). This makes perfect sense from an ecological perspective, which distinguishes between proximal and distal influences on individual resilience and wellness, in turn. But proximal determinants protect only certain individuals, whereas distal effects protect everyone. If the underlying cause of an illness can be removed from the population, susceptibility of individuals within the population ceases to matter (Rose, 2001). Moreover, when the community itself is endangered, it does not merely function in the background as the context in which individuals flourish or do not. To paraphrase Trickett (1995), in this case, the community must become the figure, not the ground.

Acknowledgements

This research was supported by the US Department of Homeland Security through the National Consortium for the Study of Terrorism and Responses to Terrorism (grant N00140510629). However, any opinions, findings, and conclusions or recommendations in this document are those of the authors and do not necessarily reflect views of the US Department of Homeland Security.

References

Abramowitz, S. (2005). The poor have become rich, and the rich have become poor: Collective trauma in the Guinean Languette. *Social Science and Medicine*, **61**, 2106–2118.

Adger, W. (2000). Social and ecological resilience: Are they related? *Progress in Human Geography*, **24**, 347–364.

Ahmed, R., Seedat, M., van Niekerk, A., & Bulbulia, S. (2004). Discerning community resilience in disadvantaged communities in the context of violence and injury prevention. *South African Journal of Psychology*, **34**, 386–408.

Allenby, B. & Fink, J. (2005). Toward inherently secure and resilient societies. *Science*, **309**, 1034–1036.

Altman, I. & Low, S. (eds.) (1992). *Place attachment*. New York: Plenum Press.

Anderson, V. (1991). *Alternative economic indicators*. New York: Routledge.

Barrera, M. (1986). Distinctions between social support concepts, measures, and models. *American Journal of Community Psychology*, **14**, 413–445.

Benight, C. (2004). Collective efficacy following a series of natural disasters. *Anxiety, Stress, and Coping*, **17**, 401–420.

Bodin, P. & Wiman, B. (2004). Resilience and other stability concepts in ecology: Notes on their origin, validity, and usefulness. *ESS Bulletin*, **2**, 33–43.

Bolin, R. & Bolton, P. (1986). *Race, religion, and ethnicity in disaster recovery*. Boulder, CO: University of Colorado.

Bonanno, G. (2004). Loss, trauma, and human resilience: Have we underestimated the human capacity to thrive after extremely aversive events? *American Psychologist*, **59**, 20–28.

Bourdieu, P. (1985). The forms of capital. In J. Richardson (ed.), *Handbook of theory and research for the sociology of education* (p. 248). New York: Greenwood.

Brown, D. & Kulig, J. (1996/97). The concept of resiliency: Theoretical lessons from community research. *Health and Canadian Society*, **4**, 29–52.

Bruneau, M., Chang, S., Eguchi, R., *et al.* (2003). A framework to quantitatively assess and enhance the seismic resilience of communities. *Earthquake Spectra*, **19**, 733–752.

Cargo, M. & Mercer, S. L. (2008). The value and challenges of participatory research: Strengthening its practice. *Annual Review of Public Health*, **29**, 325–350.

Cashman, S. B., Adeky, S., Allen, A. J. 3rd, *et al.* (2008). The power and the promise: Working with communities to analyze data, interpret findings, and get to outcomes. *American Journal of Public Health*, **98**, 1407–1417.

Christopher, S., Watts, V., McCormick, A. K. H. G., & Young, S. (2008). Building and maintaining trust in a community-based participatory research partnership. *American Journal of Public Health*, **98**, 1398–1406.

Coles, E. & Buckle, P. (2004). Developing community resilience as a foundation for effective disaster recovery. *Australian Journal of Emergency Management*, **19**, 6–15.

Comfort, L. (2005). Risk, security, and disaster management. *Annual Review of Political Science*, **8**, 335–356.

Cottrell, L. Jr. (1976). The competent community. In B. Kaplan, R. Wilson, & A. Leighton (eds.), *Further explorations in social psychiatry* (pp. 195–209). New York: Basic Books, Inc.

Couto, R. (1989). Catastrophe and community empowerment: The group formulations of Aberfan's survivors. *Journal of Community Psychology*, **17**, 236–248.

Cowen, E. (1983). Primary prevention in mental health: Past, present, and future. In R. Felner, L. Jason, J. Moritsugu, & S. Farber (eds.), *Preventive psychology: Theory, research, and practice in community intervention* (pp. 11–25). New York: Pergamon Press.

Cowen, E. (1994). The enhancement of psychological wellness: Challenges and opportunities. *American Journal of Community Psychology*, **22**, 149–179.

Cowen, E. (2000). Community psychology and routes to psychological wellness. In J. Rappaport & E. Seidman (eds.), *Handbook of community psychology* (pp. 79–99). Dordrecht: Kluwer Academic.

Cutter, S., Boruff, B., & Shirley, W. L. (2003). Social vulnerability to environmental hazards. *Social Science Quarterly*, **84**, 242–261.

Cutter, S., Emrich, C., Mitchell, J., *et al.* (2006). The long road home: Race, class, and recovery from Hurricane Katrina. *Environment*, **48**, 10–20.

Draper, J., McCleery, G., & Schaedle, R. (2006). Mental health services support in response to September 11: The central role of the Mental Health Association of New York City. In Y. Neria, R. Gross, R. Marshall, & E. Susser (eds.), *9/11: Mental health in the wake of terrorist attacks* (pp. 282–310). New York: Cambridge University Press.

Edelstein, M. (1988). *Contaminated communities: The social and psychological impacts of residential toxic exposure.* Boulder, CO; Westview Press.

Elrod, C., Hamblen, J., & Norris, F. (2006). Challenges in implementing disaster mental health programs: State program directors' perspectives. *Annals of the American Academy of Political and Social Science*, **604**, 152–170.

Erikson, K. (1976). Loss of communality at Buffalo Creek. *American Journal of Psychiatry*, **133**, 302–305.

Flicker, S., Savan, B., Kolenda, B., & Mildenberger, M. (2008). A snapshot of community-based research in Canada: Who? what? why? how? *Health Education Research*, **23**, 106–114.

Fritz, C. & Williams, H. (1957). The human being in disasters: A research perspective. *Annals of the American Academy of Political and Social Science*, **309**, 42–51.

Fullilove, M. & Saul, J. (2006). Rebuilding communities post-disaster in New York. In Y. Neria, R. Gross, R. Marshall, & E. Susser (eds.), *9/11: Mental health in the wake of terrorist attacks* (pp. 164–177) New York: Cambridge University Press.

Ganor, M. & Ben-Lavy, Y. (2003). Community resilience: Lessons derived from Gilo under fire. *Journal of Jewish Communal Service*, Winter/Spring, 105–108.

Gillespie, D. & Murty, S. (1994). Cracks in a postdisaster service delivery network. *American Journal of Community Psychology*, **22**, 639–660.

Gist, R. & Stolz, S. (1982). Mental health promotion and the media: Community response to the Kansas City hotel disaster. *American Psychologist*, **37**, 1136–1139.

Godschalk, D. (2003). Urban hazard mitigation: Creating resilient cities. *Natural Hazards Review*, **4**, 136–143.

Goodman, R., Speers, M., McLeroy, K., *et al.* (1998). Identifying and defining the dimensions of community capacity to provide a basis for measurement. *Health Education and Behavior*, **25**, 258–278.

Gordon, J. (1978). *Structures.* Harmondsworth, UK: Penguin.

Handmer, J. & Dovers, S. (1996). A typology of resilience: Rethinking institutions for sustainable development. *Industrial and Environmental Crisis Quarterly*, **9**, 482–511.

Hazards and Vulnerability Research Institute (2008). *Social vulnerability maps and data.* Columbia, SC: Hazards & Vulnerability Research Institute, University of South Carolina, http://webra.cas.sc.edu/hvriapps/SOVI_Access/SOVI_search.aspx?Region =state&State=Missi ssippi&Search=Submit+Query (accessed February 18, 2011).

Hobfoll, S. (1988). *The ecology of stress.* New York: Hemisphere.

Hogan, B., Linden, W., & Najarian, B. (2002). Social support interventions: Do they work? *Clinical Psychology Review*, **22**, 381–440.

Holling, C. (1973). Resilience and stability of ecological systems. *Annual Review of Ecology and Systematics*, **4**, 1–23.

Horn, R. V. (1993). *Statistical indicators for the economic and social sciences.* Cambridge, UK: Cambridge University Press.

Israel, B. A., Schulz, A. J., Parker, E. A., & Becker, A. B. (1998). Review of community-based research: Assessing partnership approaches to improve public health. *Annual Review of Public Health*, **19**, 173–202.

Kadushin, C. (2004). Too much investment in social capital? *Social Networks*, **26**, 75–90.

Israel, B. A., Kreiger, J. W., Viahov, D., *et al.* (2006). Challenges and facilitating factors in sustaining community-based participatory research partnerships: Lessons learned from the Detroit, New York City, and Seattle Urban Research Centers. *Journal of Urban Health*, **83**, 1022–1040.

Kaniasty, K. & Norris, F. (1995). In search of altruistic community: Patterns of social support mobilization following Hurricane Hugo. *American Journal of Community Psychology*, **23**, 447–477.

Kaniasty, K. & Norris, F. (2000). Help-seeking comfort and receiving social support: The role of ethnicity and context of need. *American Journal of Community Psychology*, **28**, 545–582.

Kawachi, I., Kennedy, B. P., Lochner, K., & Prothrow-Stith, D. (1997). Social capital, income inequality, and mortality. *American Journal of Public Health*, **87**, 1491–1498.

Kemmis, S. & McTaggart, R. (2005). Participatory action research: Communicative action and the public sphere. In N. K. Denzin & Y. S. Lincoln (eds.), *The SAGE handbook of qualitative research* (pp. 559–603). Thousand Oaks, CA: Sage.

Kimhi, S. & Shamai, M. (2004). Community resilience and the impact of stress: Adult response to Israel's withdrawal from Lebanon. *Journal of Community Psychology*, **32**, 439–451.

Landau, J. & Saul, J. (2004). Facilitating family and community resilience in response to major disaster. In F. Walsh & M. McGoldrick (eds.), *Living beyond loss: Death in the family* (pp. 285–309). New York: Norton.

Layne, C., Pynoos, R., Saltzman, W., *et al.* (2001). Trauma/grief-focused group psychotherapy: School-based postwar intervention with traumatized Bosnian adolescents. *Group Dynamics: Theory, Research, and Practice*, **5**, 277–290.

Lin, N. (2001). *Social capital: A theory of social structure and action*. New York: Cambridge University Press.

Longstaff, P. (2005). *Security, resilience, and communication in unpredictable environments such as terrorism, natural disasters, and complex technology*. Cambridge, MA: Program for Information Resources Policy, Harvard University.

Macaulay, A. C. & Nutting, P. A. (2006). Moving the frontiers forward: Incorporating community-based participatory research into practice-based research networks. *Annals of Family Medicine*, **4**, 4–7.

McGillivray, M. (2007). Human well-being: Issues, concepts and measures. In M. McGillivray (ed.), *Human well-being: Concept and measurement* (pp. 1–22). New York: Palgrave MacMillan.

Manzo, L. & Perkins, D. (2006). Finding common ground: The importance of place attachment to community participation and planning. *Journal of Planning Literature*, **20**, 335–350.

Maton, K. & Salem, D. (1995). Organizational characteristics of empowering community settings: A multiple case study approach. *American Journal of Community Psychology*, **23**, 631–656.

Meyer, J. (2000). Qualitative research in health care: Using qualitative methods in health related action research. *British Medical Journal*, **320**, 178–181.

Norris, F. & Kaniasty, K. (1996). Received and perceived social support in times of stress: A test of the social support deterioration deterrence model. *Journal of Personality and Social Psychology*, **71**, 498–511.

Norris, F., Baker, C., Murphy, A., & Kaniasty, K. (2005a). Social support mobilization and deterioration after Mexico's 1999 flood: Effects of context, gender, and time. *American Journal of Community Psychology*, **36**, 15–28.

Norris, F., Watson, P., Hamblen, J., & Pfefferbaum, B. (2005b). Provider perspectives on disaster mental health services in Oklahoma City. *Journal of Aggression, Maltreatment, and Trauma*, **10**, 649–661.

Norris, F., Hamblen, J., Watson, P., *et al.* (2006). Toward understanding and creating systems of postdisaster care: A case study of New York's response to the World Trade Center disaster. In E. C. Ritchie, P. Watson, & M. Friedman (eds.), *Interventions following mass violence and disasters: Strategies for mental health practices* (pp. 343–364). New York: Guilford Press.

Norris, F., Stevens, S., Pfefferbaum, B., Wyche, K., & Pfefferbaum, R. (2008). Community resilience as a metaphor, theory, set of capacities, and strategy for disaster readiness. *American Journal of Community Psychology*, **41**, 127–150.

Norris, F., Tracy, M., & Galea, S. (2009). Looking for resilience: Understanding the longitudinal trajectories of responses to stress after major disasters. *Social Science and Medicine*, **68**, 2190–2198.

Oliver-Smith, A. (1986). *The martyred city*. Albuquerque, NM: University of New Mexico Press.

Paton, D. & Johnston, D. (2001). Disasters and communities: Vulnerability, resilience, and preparedness. *Disaster Prevention and Management*, **10**, 270–277.

Paton, D., Millar, M., & Johnston, D. (2001). Community resilience to volcanic hazard consequences. *Natural Hazards*, **24**, 157–169.

Perez-Sales, P., Cervellon, P., Vazquez, C., Vidales, D., & Gaborit, M. (2005). Post-traumatic factors and resilience: The role of shelter management and survivors' attitudes after the earthquakes in El Salvador 2001. *Journal of Community and Applied Social Psychology*, **15**, 368–382.

Perkins, D. & Long, D. (2002). Neighborhood sense of community and social capital: A multi-level analysis. In A. Fisher, C. Sonn, & B. Bishop (eds.), *Psychological sense of community: Research, applications, and implications* (pp. 291–318). New York: Plenum Press.

Perkins, D., Hughey, J., & Speer, P. (2002). Community psychology perspectives on social capital theory and community development practice. *Journal of the Community Development Society*, **33**, 33–52.

Pfefferbaum, R. L., Pfefferbaum, B., Wyche, K., Norris, F., & Reissman, D. (2006). *Community Assessment of Resilience Tool*. Oklahoma City, OA: Terrorism and Disaster Center of the National Child Traumatic Stress Network, http://www.oumedicine.com/Workfiles/College%20of%20Medicine/AD-Psychiatry/CART_description_060509.pdf (accessed March 2, 2011).

Pfefferbaum, B., Reissman, D., Pfefferbaum, R. L., Klomp, R. W., & Gurwitch, R. H. (2007). Building resilience to mass trauma events. In L. Doll, S. Bonzo, J. Mercy, & D. Sleet (eds.), *Handbook on injury and violence prevention interventions* (pp. 347–358). New York: Kluwer Academic.

Pooley, J., Cohen, L., & O' Connor, M. (2006). Links between community and individual resilience: evidence from cyclone affected communities in north west Australia. In D. Paton & D. Johnston (eds.), *Disaster resilience: An integrated approach* (pp. 161–173). Springfield, IL: Charles C. Thomas.

Putnam, R. (2000). *Bowling alone*. New York: Simon & Schuster.

Quarantelli, E. (1989). Characteristics of citizen groups which emerge with respect to hazardous waste sites. In D. Peck (ed.), *Psychosocial effects of hazardous toxic waste disposal on communities* (pp. 177–195). Springfield, IL: Charles C. Thomas.

Rappaport, J. (1995). Empowerment meets narrative: Listening to stories and creating settings. *American Journal of Community Psychology*, **23**, 795–807.

Reissman, D., Spencer, S., Tanielian, T., & Stein, B. (2005). Integrating behavioral aspects into community preparedness and response systems. In Y. Danieli, D. Brom, & J. Sills (eds.), *The trauma of terror: Sharing knowledge and shared care* (pp. 707–720). Binghamton, NY: Haworth Press.

Riad, J., Norris, F., & Ruback, R. B. (1999). Predicting evacuation in two major disasters: Risk perceptions, social influence, and access to resources. *Journal of Applied Social Psychology*, **29**, 918–934.

Rich, R., Edelstein, M., Hallman, W., & Wandersman, A. (1995). Citizen participation and empowerment: The case of local environmental hazards. *American Journal of Community Psychology*, **23**, 657–676.

Rose, A. (2004). Defining and measuring economic resilience to disasters. *Disaster Prevention and Management*, **13**, 307–314.

Rose, A. (2005). Analyzing terrorist threats to the economy: A computable general equilibrium approach. In P. Gordon, J. Moore, & H. Richardson (eds.), *Economic impacts of terrorist attacks* (pp. 196–217). Cheltenham, UK: Edward Elgar.

Rose, G. (1981). Strategy of prevention: Lessons from cardiovascular disease. *British Medical Journal*, **282**, 1847–1951.

Rose, G. (2001). Sick individuals and sick populations. *International Journal of Epidemiology*, **30**, 427–432.

Rupasingha, A., Goetz, S. J., & Freshwater, D. (2006). The production of social capital in US counties. *Journal of Socio-Economics*, **35**, 83–101.

Rutter, M. (1993). Resilience: some conceptual considerations. *Journal of Adolescent Health*, **14**, 626–631.

Sampson, R., Raudenbush, S., & Earls, F. (1997). Neighborhoods and violent crime: A multilevel study of collective efficacy. *Science*, **277**, 918–924.

Shaw-Taylor, Y. (1999). *Measurement of community health: The Social Health Index*. New York: University Press of America.

Sherrieb, K., Norris, F., & Galea, S. (2010). Measuring capacities for community resilience. *Social Indicators Research*, **99**, 227–247.

Sonn, C. & Fisher, A. (1998). Sense of community: Community resilient responses to oppression and change. *Journal of Community Psychology*, **26**, 457–472.

Tse, S. & Liew, T. (2004). New Zealand experiences: How is community resilience manifested in Asian communities? *International Journal of Mental Health and Addiction*, **2**, 1–8.

Tobin, G. & Whiteford, L. (2002). Community resilience and volcano hazard: The eruption of Tungurahua and evacuation of the *Faldas* in Ecuador. *Disasters*, **26**, 28–48.

Trickett, E. (1995). The community context of disaster and traumatic stress: An ecological perspective from community psychology. In S. Hobfoll & M. DeVries (eds.), *Extreme stress and communities: Impact and intervention* (pp. 11–25). Dordrecht: Kluwer Academic.

van den Eynde, J. & Veno, A. (1999). Coping with disastrous events: An empowerment model of community healing. In R. Gist & B. Lubin (eds.), *Response to disaster: Psychosocial, community, and ecological approaches* (pp. 167–192). Philadelphia, PA: Bruner/Mazel.

Wellman, B. & Frank, K. (2001). Network capital in a multilevel world: Getting support from personal communities. In N. Lin, K. Cook, & R. Burt (eds.), *Social capital: Theory and research* (pp. 233–273). New York: Aldine de Gruyter.

Werner, E. E. & Smith, R. S. (1982). *Vulnerable but invincible: A longitudinal study of resilient children and youth*. New York: McGraw-Hill.

Westfall, J. M., Van Vorst, R. F., Main, D. S., & Herbert, C. (2006). Community-based participatory research in practice-based research networks. *Annals of Family Medicine*, **4**, 8–14.

Wisner, B. (2001). Risk and the neoliberal state: Why post-Mitch lessons didn't reduce El Salvador's earthquake losses. *Disasters*, **25**, 251–268.

Woods, C. (1998). *Development arrested: The blues and plantation power in the Mississippi Delta*. New York: Verso.

Working Group on Governance Dilemmas in Bioterrorism Response (2004). Leading during bioattacks and epidemics with the public's trust and help. *Biosecurity and Bioterrorism: Biodefense Stategy, Practice, and Science*, **2**, 25–39.

Chapter

12

Trauma, culture, and resiliency

Carl C. Bell

Introduction

The generic principles for recovery from trauma and loss involve the reconstruction of meaning, the rebuilding of hope, and the sense of empowerment necessary to regain control over one's being and life (Herman, 1992). Constructs of meaning are inseparable from culture. Furthermore, genetic influences that put individuals at risk for developing traumatic symptoms cannot be adequately understood without taking into consideration their interdependence with environmental factors (Binder *et al.*, 2008), such as culture. This chapter highlights the interface between trauma, culture, and resiliency.

Apfel and Simon (1996), Masten and Coatsworth (1998), and Wolin and Wolin (1996) outlined the characteristics of resiliency as (1) resourcefulness; (2) ability to attract and use support; (3) curiosity and intellectual mastery; (4) compassion, with detachment; (5) conviction of one's right to survive; (6) ability to remember and invoke images of good and sustaining figures; (7) ability to be in touch with affects, not denying or suppressing major affects as they arise; (8) goal to live for; (9) vision of the possibility and desirability of restoration of civilized moral order; (10) the need and ability to help others; (11) ability to conceptualize; (12) an affective repertory; (13) altruism toward others; and (14) turning "traumatic helplessness" into "learned helpfulness." In addition to these characteristics of resiliency, there are more culturally bound characteristics of resiliency (Bell, 2001) such as (1) having a sense of "Atman" (true self); (2) developing *kokoro* (heart), also known as "indomitable fighting spirit" (Bell & Suggs, 1998); (3) having a totem, an animal spirit that lives inside; and (4) being able to cultivate *chi*, Chinese for internal energy (Cohen, 1997; Bell, 2000, 2008a).

Protective factors that cultivate resiliency and protect against trauma fall in to several categories (Bell *et al.*, 2005). Protective factors are biological (genetic such as intellectual ability, personality/temperamental traits, and toughness), psychological (intrapsychic attributes: adaptive mechanisms such as ego resiliency, motivation, humor and hardiness, and perceptions of self; emotional attributes: emotional well-being, life satisfaction, optimism, happiness, trust, dispositional optimism, dispositional hope, and life satisfaction; cognitive attributes: cognitive styles and processing, causal attribution such as an internal locus of control and blame, worldview or philosophy of life, change in philosophy of life, assumptive world, and wisdom; and spiritual attributes: spiritual well-being, spiritual development, existential issues, and attributes of post-traumatic growth), social (interpersonal skills, interpersonal relationships, connectedness, and social support), and environmental (such as positive life events and socioeconomic status). Culture intersects with these protective factors by facilitating practices that cultivate toughness, motivation, humor, hardiness, perceptions of self, optimism, trust, dispositional hope, dispositional optimism, life satisfaction, cognitive styles and processing, causal atribution (e.g., internal locus of control and blame), worldview or philosophy of life, change in life philosophy, assumptive world perspectives, wisdom, spiritual well-being, spiritual development, existential equipoise, interpersonal skills, interpersonal relationships, connectedness, and affinity for social support.

Cultural considerations for understanding resiliency

Culture is a complex, shared system of meaning consisting of learned behavior and meanings that are

---

Resilience and Mental Health: Challenges Across the Lifespan, ed. Steven M. Southwick, Brett T. Litz, Dennis Charney, and Matthew J. Friedman. Published by Cambridge University Press. © Cambridge University Press 2011.

socially transferred in various life-activity settings for purposes of individual and collective adjustment and adaptation (Marsella *et al.*, 2008). Accordingly, culture shapes and constructs our realities by contributing to our worldviews, perceptions, and orientations with ideas, morals, and preferences (Marsella, 2005). Further, culture changes and, as it is transmitted generation to generation, it is shaped by various inside and outside contexts and dynamics. This system of meaning consists of norms, beliefs, and values that proscribe behavior. As recovery from trauma intimately involves reconstruction of meaning, consideration of resiliency must take into account a person's specific cultural norms, beliefs, and values, and cultural dynamics (e.g., the subject's culture of origin and the extent of the subject's acculturation or level of ethnic identification). Further, "factors associated with ethnicity and culture strongly influence individuals' vulnerability and resilience; determine their coping styles, cognitive response to stress, and the nature of social support; shape their psychopathology, their experiencing of distress, and their clustering of symptoms; and influence the course and outcome of psychiatric conditions" (Charney *et al.*, 2002, p. 69). When evaluating another's status, Hansen (2002) suggested consideration of multicultural competencies such as knowing the person's history of victimization and manifestations of such issues as oppression, prejudice, marginalization, and their psychological sequelae; certainly these dynamics can influence resilience in negative and positive ways. Further, as family structures, gender roles, values, and beliefs differ across cultures and yet affect personality formation, developmental outcomes, and manifestations of mental illness and wellness, it is important to consider these dynamics of resilience or vulnerability as well.

Unfortunately, in an American culture highly charged with individualism, one of the most important, yet neglected, aspect in the field of stress and coping (Lazarus & Folkman, 1984) is the context of culture (Chun *et al.*, 2006). Currently, the cultural elements of individualism and collectivism are the most widely studied (Triandis, 1995). Individualism and collectivism consist of a set of values, attitudes, and behaviors that vary based on the value placed on the individual versus the individual's group (Hofstede, 1980). In individualistic cultures, the individual is the hub of attention and emphasis. Accordingly, individual freedoms, rights, and privileges are of utmost importance: "I think, therefore I am" is the key philosophy. In collectivistic cultures, by comparison an emphasis is placed on the group as a collective: "I am, because we are" is the key philosophy (Chun *et al.*, 2006). Locus of control is a very pertinent personality dimension to coping. Cross-cultural studies have revealed that individuals from individualistic cultures, such as European-Americans and New Zealanders, tend to have a stronger sense of internal locus of control than individuals from collectivistic cultures, such as the Japanese (Bond & Tornatzky, 1973; Mahler, 1974), the Chinese (Hamid, 1994), Asian Indians (Chandler *et al.*, 1982), and individuals from Zambia and Zimbabwe (Munro, 1979).

Some authors have noted that cultural, racial, and ethnic people of color are more adversely effected by various traumas (Bell, 2008b; Norris & Alegria, 2008). For example, Latinos and non-Hispanic blacks were more adversely affected by Hurricaine Andrew than were non-Hispanic whites (Perilla *et al.*, 2002). Following the September 11, 2001 terrorist attacks, Galea *et al.* (2005) found cultural, racial, and ethnic people of color were more likely to met criteria for post-traumatic stress disorder (PTSD) than non-Latino white respondents. Additionally, cultural, racial, and ethnic people of color within the USA are less likely than whites to seek mental health treatment until their symptoms are more severe. Further, they are less likely to seek treatment from mental health specialists as they are more inclined to use primary care or to use informal sources of support (Department of Health and Human Services, 2001). Also, it is less clear whether acculturation is a benefit (Marshall & Orlando, 2002) or detriment (Vega *et al.*, 1998) to resiliency. Issues of acculturative stress have been identified as strategies of non-dominant groups, such as integration, assimilation, separation, or marginalization; and of dominant groups, such as multiculturalism, melting pot, segregation, or exclusion (Berry, 2006).

Some researchers suggest that ethnic, racial, and cultural people of color seem to be more resilient than whites. For example, Ryff *et al.* (2003) reported that blacks report higher levels of psychological well-being than whites, and, after controlling for education, income, perceived discrimination, and other demographic variables, blacks would have an even better level of psychological well-being than whites if it were not for the finding that blacks experienced more discrimination than whites. Keyes (2007) found similar results and these observations are consistent with the observation that African-American women (despite their status in contemporary society resulting from sexism and discrimination) have the lowest suicide rates in the

USA (Goldsmith *et al.*, 2002). Unfortunately, there is a dearth of research on cultural, racial, and ethnic people of color (Department of Health and Human Services, 2001), so it is difficult to achieve clarity in issues of acculturation and resiliency.

Other authors have studied issues of hardiness (Maddi & Harvey, 2006). "Hardy attitudes" are commitment, control, and challenge, and "hardy skills" involve interacting with significant others in a fashion that enhances one's sense of social support. Hardiness involves self-care aimed at maintaining a level of arousal that is optimal for "hardy coping" and social interaction efforts. Self-efficacy, ego strength, optimism, resilience, post-traumatic growth, religiousness, endurance, patience, humility, and flexibility are aspects of hardiness. The notion of hardiness appears to be present in all cultural, racial, and ethnic groups; consequently, it can be considered a generic aspect of human nature (Maddi & Harvey, 2006).

Religious and spiritual coping are imbued with various aspects of culture. Culture shapes how people seek significance, how events are interpreted to have meaning for people, how familiar people are with the coping process, how they use specific modes of coping, and what vehicles they use for transformation of trauma (Pargament, 1997). Culture determines how people find meaning and gain control, comfort, intimacy, and closeness to God (regardless of how God is defined) so they can transform their traumatized lives (with the inherent sense of helplessness that accompanies trauma) into helpfulness and purpose (Klaassen *et al.*, 2006). Further, in order successfully to achieve a communal aspect to suffering and coping, cultural guidelines are necessary to shape community behavior. Culture shapes how people engage in active coping: planning, seeking instrumental social support, seeking emotional support, suppressing competing activities, practicing religion, reinterpreting events as positive and growth producing, accepting the trauma, focusing on and venting emotions, seeking calmness, denying psychologically and behaviorally avoiding, using alcohol/drugs, and engaging in humor (Carver *et al.*, 1989).

Monocultural ethnocentrism

Monocultural ethnocentrism is defined as the belief in one "right" culture and valuing that culture over others (Taylor, 2006). Monocultural ethnocentrism (usually European-centrism) makes it difficult to appreciate cultural differences between the cultural, racial,

and ethnic groups (Sue & Sue, 1999). This aspect of European and European-American culture also makes it difficult to appreciate diversity within racial groups. Achenbach (2008, p. 25) underscored this observation by noting

> Multicultural encounters can spawn both benefits and risks. For the study and treatment of psychopathology, the increasing salience of cultural variations forces us to question the generalizability of our mainly Western concepts. Until recently, much of the professional literature related to psychopathology was written primarily by Westerners from a handful of societies. These Westerners have written mainly about Westerners and for Westerners.

Unfortunately, monocultural ethnocentrism often precludes the appropriate use of exposure to multiple cultures as a creative source of possible coping responses.

Genetic/environmental interactions

Major depressive disorders have been linked to levels of serotonin in the brain, and many antidepressant drugs act by blocking reuptake of serotonin by acting directly on the brain serotonin transporter (5-HTT). Caspi and colleagues (2002) have examined gene–environmental interactions in the development of depression by looking at genetic variants of this transporter. One variant, *5HTTLPR*, moderated the influence of early childhood maltreatment and stressful life events on the development of depression. Kaufman and Henrich (2000) noted clinical studies of individuals with a history of abuse which suggested that the availability of a caring and stable parent or alternative guardian is one of the most important factors that distinguishes abused individuals with good developmental outcomes from those with more deleterious outcomes. Kaufman and colleagues (2006) also looked at the effect of social supports in moderating for genetic risk of depression in maltreated children, showing that maltreated children with positive social supports had depression scores that were only slightly greater than control subjects regardless of genotype. This indicates that the quality and availability of social supports is an extremely potent factor in determining risk for depression in maltreated children – with the effect greatest for those maltreated children with the most vulnerable genotypes (Kaufman *et al.*, 2006). Clearly, cultural context has the potential to influence parenting styles and the quality of social supports in a maltreated child's life.

The interaction between the parents and offspring (Thomas & Chess, 1977; Rettew *et al.*, 2006) can either be protective or a risk factor for illness. Therefore, taking a developmental psychopathology, family-based, gene–environment approach should better equip researchers and clinicians alike to understand etiopathology and ultimately treatment. The key is to prevent risk factors from becoming predictive factors by understanding protective factors (Bell, 2007). We should aim to devise strategies to keep children well, try particularly hard to prevent at-risk children from getting ill, and intervene with those who are already ill. Unfortunately, the major focus in mental health has been those who are already ill.

Religiosity as an environmental influence that can impact genetic expression

The concept that being raised in a religious household is protective has long been a core belief of religious disciplines. High levels of religious involvement predicts a reduce risk of substance misuse (Larson & Wilson, 1980; Payne *et al.*, 1991; Koenig *et al.*, 1994; Gorsuch, 1995), and Heath *et al.* (1999) found a protective effect of religious involvement and values against adolescent alcohol use. Spirituality has also been conceptualized by some as a genetic component of personality (Luby *et al.*, 1999; Cloninger, 2004). In a population-based adult twin sample, Kendler *et al.* (2003) found that general religiosity was inversely and significantly linked to nicotine dependence, alcohol dependence, drug misuse and dependence, and adult antisocial behavior. However, general religiosity was significantly related to panic disorder.

Maes *et al.* (1999) found that genetic factors could explain the association between church attendance and alcohol use in males, but in females, the association is primarily linked to shared environmental factors and genotype–environment covariance. In the Netherlands Twin Register adult twin sample, Koopmans *et al.* (1999) examined gene–environment interactions in the influence of religiosity on initiation of drinking in females and found a variance of 0% between high religiosity and initiation of drinking and 40% between low religiosity and initiation. Subjects with a religious upbringing and who participate in church activities scored lower on Sensation Seeking Questionnaire scales, with religiosity being associated with reduced genetic influence on disinhibition, particularly in males (Boomsma *et al.*, 1999).

Further, there is a wealth of psychiatric research indicating a relationship between degree of obsessive–compulsive disorder, culture, and religious identity and practice (Greenberg & Witztum, 1994; Chia, 1996; Raphael *et al.*, 1996; Texcan & Millet, 1997; Shooka *et al.*, 1998; Tek & Ulug, 2001; Abramowitz *et al.*, 2002; Greenberg & Shefler, 2002; Sica *et al.*, 2002; Rassin & Koster, 2003).

Our group and others have been struck by what appears to be the protective qualities of family-based activities and wonder whether the data are already strong enough to support a greater role for family-based approaches aimed at increasing family cohesion as a strategy for health and resilience promotion (Bell *et al.*, 2008; National Research Council & Institute of Medicine, 2009).

Specific cultural, racial, and ethnic considerations for cultivating resiliency

African-American resiliency systems

African-Americans have a number of characteristics that cultivate resiliency: historical experiences, cultural traits such as family characteristics, cultural values, ethnic orientation, strong kinship bonds, communal orientation, strong religious orientation, importance of tradition, strong work ethic, individual and academic achievement, respect for elders, harmony with nature, holistic thinking, adherence to mainstream American cultural norms and values, religion, communication styles, food, holidays, and health considerations (Billingsley, 1992; Jagers & Mock, 1995; Hill, 1997; Sue & Sue, 2003; Carswell & Carswell, 2008).

Racial socialization is a protective factor in African-American families (Klonoff & Landrine, 1999; Brook *et al.*, 2007; Corneille & Belgrave, 2007; Nasim *et al.*, 2007). Resiliency in African-American families is strongly associated with facilitating self-efficacy, parental supervision that is protective (Donenberg *et al.*, 2002), being future oriented, and spirituality (McCreary *et al.*, 2006). Nobles (1986) suggested that black families give their children a sense of history, sense of family, and sense of spirituality, and Staples (1976) noted the unique characteristic of the black family as being the non-kinship extended family: both of which are protective. Research finds the most common racial socialization message given to African-American youth was the importance of the work ethic and achievement. Racial and ethnic pride messages were next, and the third was race-related lessons about black heritage and historical traditions (Thornton *et al.*, 1990). Racial socialization messages are generally shown to have a protective effect (Stevenson *et al.*, 1997; Fischer & Shaw, 1999). Miller and MacIntosh (1999) have asserted that racial identity can create resilience by enhancing collective self-esteem. However, more research needs to be carried out on how African-American racial socialization processes are protective, as research results are mixed. For example, Arroyo and Zigler (1995) found that the more students endorsed racelessness, the more anxiety and depression they reported. However, these same students showed a greater sense of self-efficacy on achievement attitudes. Similarly, Anglin and Wade (2007) found that racial socialization positively contributes to academic adjustment, while internalized Afrocentric racial identity was negatively related to overall college adjustment.

American-Indian/Alaska Native resiliency systems

Like African-Americans, American-Indian/Alaska Natives have a great many challenges that cultivate their resiliency, for example the genocide and terrorism perpetrated against American-Indians in the eighteenth and nineteenth centuries (Johnson *et al.*, 2008). Similar to African-Americans, but to a greater extent, death rates from crime and disease are high in American-Indians. Further, substance abuse is a huge problem, with suicide rates being a close second to European-American rates (Goldsmith *et al.*, 2002). Native-American key values that foster resilience involve an emphasis on spirituality; sacredness of all living things and respect for nature, realized by cooperation and harmony with nature; cyclical thinking; interdependence between people; sharing and social responsibility; extended family; and respect for elders. Humor is a major part of many American-Indian cultures and these cultures gravitate toward approaches that emphasize values and strengths (Lafromboise *et al.*, 1990). A major strength for American-Indians is that their medicine is oriented toward healing through restoring the balance and harmony with the body and world using strategies involving spirituality, such as ritual purification in sweat lodges.

Arab-American resiliency systems

Arab, Muslim, and Middle Eastern people are very family oriented, with religious involvement and piety, including faith, prayer, and spiritual practices, being highly valued (Abi-Hashem, 2008). In addition, community, hospitality, truthfulness, thankfulness and gratitude, respect, esteem, contentment and satisfaction, generosity, dignity and honor, clear gender roles for the male and female, saving face and avoiding public shame, working hard and providing for your family, social obligations and relational duties, patience, and endurance are all very highly valued (Abi-Hashem, 2008). These cultural, racial, and ethnic groups use many metaphors, proverbs, and sayings containing cultural and spiritual wisdom (Abi-Hashem, 2008). Traditional therapies such as religious oaths, shrine visitation, purposeful prayers, evil eye protection, script writings, psychic activities, and natural therapies are common resiliency-cultivating approaches to life.

Asian cultural resiliency systems

Religion and philosophy vary across cultures, and religious and philosophical beliefs profoundly influence how people cope (Tweed & Conway, 2006). Further, people within the same culture have different approaches to suffering, adaptation, and the environment, resulting in different coping strategies. There is a vast array of cultural subgroups within the general Asian culture, and these subgroups are influenced to varying degrees by the three major religious and philosophies of Asian culture: Taoism, Confucianism, and Buddhism.

The ubiquity of change in Chinese culture was explored by Ji (2001), who found that Chinese participants in her study were more likely to affirm that change was ubiquitous in the world than were the European-American participants. This high expectation of change and of change in the direction of change (reversal of trends) coheres with the Taoist tradition of China (Chen, 2006a, 2006b). Taoism teaches a philosophy of life in terms of how, regardless of the circumstances, to live a contented, serene life with equipoise. In addition, in the tradition of sophisticated Asian culture, Taoism also proscribes mind/body practices that encourage breathing exercises that cultivate physical and mental well-being. Lao-tzu was clear that yin and yang rule nature thus "Fortune owes its existence to misfortune, and misfortune is hidden in fortune" (Chen, 2006b).

Individuals wise in Taoism know it is not either/or, but rather both/and.

Confucian tradition teaches the value of perseverance in response to difficulty; hence people from Asian cultures tend to believe in the utility of effort. Confucianism also emphasized family piety, a moral duty to respect and serve elders, ancestor worship, dignified expression, reserved manner of speaking, chaste temperament, and industriousness (Kaplan & Huynh, 2008); consequently, the tendency to catastrophize is minimized. (Research has shown clear links between catastrophizing and a lack of self-efficacy and risk of developing PTSD [Bryant & Guthrie, 2005].)

Buddhism, a multifaceted religion originating in India, has been an influential cultural force in Asia for more than 2500 years (Chen, 2006a). The conservative Theravada (southern Buddhism) – prevalent in Thailand, Sri Lanka, Burma, and Laos – adheres to the early scriptures believed to embody the authentic teachings of the Buddha. This form of Buddhism is called Hinayana ("lesser vehicle") by its critics because it mainly focuses on enlightenment of its practitioners. By comparison, the reportedly more evolved and adaptive Mahayana Buddhism ("great vehicle"), dominant in China, Taiwan, Japan, Korea, and Vietnam, stresses the ideal of Bodhisattvas: enlightened beings who vow to save all sentient beings from suffering. The Lotus Sutra, a central feature of Mahayana Buddhism, delves into the nature of the mind, and "ultimate reality," suggesting emptiness, is the highest possible stage in the evolution of human consciousness, because the mind is pure and "empty" of thoughts and feelings, thus allowing transcendence of dualistic consciousness (Chen, 2006a). From this expanded state of consciousness (Bell, 1980) comes wisdom, unconditional love, compassion, and a loss of the fear of death. Zen (Chan) developed out of Mahayana Buddhism and practices enlightenment through "direct seeing" of the true nature of the mind. Reportedly, Zen was introduced to China in the sixth century by an Indian monk named Bodhidharma (Oyama, 1966) or Ta Mo (Smith, 1964), who sought enlightenment through intuitive insights into the "self-nature" (true self). Bodhidharma was also extremely influential in the development of Asian martial arts.

Buddhist practices provide more than stress reduction, they provide a pathway that is free from life's troubles and sorrows. Like Christianity, effective coping in Buddhism requires spiritual/personal transformation, which is cultivated by mental and physical discipline leading to enlightenment to provide inner serenity and compassion. Buddhism is based on *catvāri āryasatyāni* ("four noble truths") (Byrom, 1976; Chen, 2006a). (1) *Dukkha*, the truth of suffering: – life has suffering (craving or greed; and aversion or hatred; ignorance or delusion). (2) *Tanha*, the truth of arising of suffering: suffering comes from craving and aversion. (3) *Nirvana*, the truth of liberation from suffering: freedom from suffering is possible by transforming craving or greed, aversion or hatred, ignorance or delusion by following the right path. (4) *Magga*, the truth of the eightfold path: right speech, right action, right living, right effort, right mindfulness, right meditation, right thought, and right understanding These eight paths can be classed as "morality," "meditation" (requiring regular efforts to practice mindfulness or bare attention in both formal meditation and in day to day life), and "wisdom" (the capacity to be non-attached to craving or greed, aversion or hatred, ignorance or delusion) (Chen, 2006a). These attributes are exemplified by various aphorisms: "Those who know themselves are enlightened" "Those who conquer themselves are strong" "The greatest woes comes from not knowing contentment; the greatest of faults comes from craving for gains" "A sage is free from excessive pursuit, extravagance and arrogance" (Ajaya, 1997).

Caribbean black resiliency system

The 10 key values of Eastern Caribbean people that help to cultivate resiliency are the extended family, a strong work ethic, multiculturalism and blacks' experience with racism, the value of education, spirituality, respect (as the culture is very authoritarian), veneration of elders and ancestors, communalism, creativity, and disaster as a result of negative actions (Dudley-Grant & Etheridge, 2008).

Asian Indian cultural resiliency system

There is a great deal of diversity within the Indian community that is complicated by differing levels of acculturation to Western society. Although Hinduism is most widely practiced, there are five other major religions, and most emphasize transcendence, holistic values, collectivism, self-realization, and transformation of the self (Prashantham, 2008). Developing a sense of "Atman" or "true self" is one way in which many Asian Indians cultivate their resiliency (Bell, 2001). Asian Indian cultural values that cultivate resilience include humility, respect, responsibility, politeness, morality, tolerance, spirituality, holistic perception, hospitality, and non-violence (Prashantham, 2008). Folk religions that emphasize *karma* are a large factor in encouraging people to take the "high road," and displays of anger (behind anger is hurt) are frowned upon because it disrupts harmony. Metaphors are very important forms of communication in India, and allegories are frequently used to convey truth. As in other cultures, Asian Indians have their own healing and strength-based strategies such as yoga, ayurveda, naturopathy, siddha treatment, homeopathy, unani treatment, tantra, shamans, reiki, pranic healing, kalari, and marma (Prashantham, 2008). Family is very important to Asian Indians and resiliency-cultivating practices that emphasize mind/body/sprit fit exactly into their cosmology. The capacity to take on responsibility for relatives outside of the nuclear family is another feature of the culture that assists in resiliency. Finally, beliefs in *karma* may lead to quicker acceptance of the inevitable, thus the catastrophizing resulting in increased risk for developing PTSD can be avoided (Bryant & Guthrie, 2005).

Latino/Native cultural resiliency systems

Like other cultural, racial, and ethnic groups, there is a great deal of diversity among Latin-Americans and, as with other groups, the generalizations presented may have exceptions. Most Latinos have a strong value for *familia* and extended kinship systems, suggesting strong regards for collectivism and interdependence. In addition, there is a strong Catholic influence within Latino cultures. Values that cultivate resiliency include *familismo* (family ties), *compadrazco* (friendship), and *personalismo* (warm personal relationships); other relationship values such as *respecto* (respect), *confianza* (trust), *caridad* (caring), *tener valor* (courage), and *fortaleza* (fortitude); and spiritual values such as *esperanza* (hope) and *fe* (faith) (Padilla & Borrero, 2006; Arredondo *et al.*, 2008). Working with such cultures requires awareness of the role of the family, the recognition of religion, and use of indigenous resources.

Don Miguel Ángel Ruiz (1997) provides an example of a Latino/Native cultural resiliency system in his outline of the four agreements from his tradition of the southern Mexican Toltec people: aggreement one, "be impeccable with your word"; aggreement two, "don't take anything personally"; aggreement three, "don't make assumptions"; and aggreement four, "always do your best."

Native Hawaiian resiliency systems

Native Hawaiian values that cultivate resiliency include *aloha* (affectionate, compassionate, and loving sentiments), *aina* (the environment nourishing the body, mental health, and relationships with the spiritual world), *ha'aha'a* (modesty or humility, interconnectedness, respect, and caring), *kokua* (helping other), *lokahi* (harmony), *mana* (divine or spiritual power), *ohana* (family), *alaka'i* (leadership), *pono* (justice), and *kela* (excellence) (McCubbin *et al.*, 2008). Social relationships are very important to Hawaiians and their values support these relationships. *Ho'oponopono*, aimed at restoring harmony, is another culturally specific resiliency-cultivating strategy of Hawaiian people (Rezentes, 1996). Native Hawaiians have three patterns of resilience: coherence or the family's capacity of developing a sense of trust, predictability, and manageability; problem-solving communication; and the family's shared ethnic identity (Thompson *et al.*, 1995).

General issues

Rather than simply approaching trauma from a diagnostic perspective, it is important to consider cultural aspects of salutogenesis as seeking to cope with trauma worldwide. Essential considerations in understanding the interface between trauma, culture, and resiliency include traditional healing practices, therapeutic contexts, culturally based medical practices, shamanic practices, assumptive belief systems about illness and health, perspectives on psychobiology of traumatic stress (e.g., mind–body relationships), a culture's implicit psychological and behavioral principles, the range of healer roles and practices, individual verses collective practices, and religious and spiritual involvement in healing and recovery (Wilson, 2008). Marsella (2005) outlined the generic salutogenic aspects of all cultures as beliefs, catharsis, confession, cultural re-embeddedness or separation, re-definition of problems or self, empathy, expression and verbalization of problems, faith, forgiveness, hope, identity development and awareness, information exchange, insight, interpretation of events, locus of control alterations, mobilization of endorphin and immune system, social supports, and so on. Throughout history, civilizations have experienced trauma and, accordingly, have developed practices, techniques, wisdom, and other skill sets to address this issue and to cultivate resiliency in preparation for the inevitable. In an insightful article, Wilson (2004) described the "abyss experience," which he defines as being confrontation with evil and death (i.e., the traumatic experience), experience with soul death and with non-being (i.e., absence of self/identity), a sense of abandonment by humanity (i.e., loss of connectedness), ultimate aloneness and despairing (i.e., separation and isolation), and cosmic challenge of meaning (i.e., spirituality and a sense of the mystical). Kohut (1966, p. 264) stated "Man's capacity to acknowledge the finiteness of his existence and to act in accordance with this painful discovery may well be his greatest psychological achievement…."

Marsella (2005) noted that all healing subcultures have (1) a set of assumptions about the nature of the problems that matches their worldview and construction of reality; (2) a set of assumptions about the context, settings, and requirements for healing to occur; (3) a set of assumptions and procedures to elicit particular expectations, emotions, and behaviors; (4) a set of requirements for activity and participation levels and/or roles for patient, family, and therapist; and (5) specific requirements for therapist training and skills expertise criteria. Unfortunately, as Satcher's report *Mental health: culture, race, and ethnicity* highlighted (Department of Health and Human Services, 2001), there is a dearth of research on mental health issues for various cultural, racial, and ethnic minority groups in the USA, and even less on resiliency and protective factors in these groups (Bell & Williamson, 2002).

Conclusions

In the West, in order fully to understand how trauma interfaces with culture and resiliency we need to overcome our monocultural ethnocentrism. We need to learn how to respect other cultures' resiliency-cultivating strategies and stop being critical of other cultures. To achieve this goal, we must develop a higher tolerance for what we do not understand because it is not familiar and become comfortable with diversity. We need a higher awareness that our culture is just one of many, and that there are similarities and commonalities among cultures, not solely differences. In order to understand how different cultures cultivate resiliency, we must seek to study and research different cultural strategies to create protective factors, strength, and resiliency in their groups. "Wisdom is achieved largely through man's ability to overcome his unmodified narcissism and it rests on his acceptance of the limitations of his physical, intellectual, and emotional powers" (Kohut, 1966, p. 268).

References

Abi-Hashem, N. (2008). Arab Americans: Understanding their challenges, needs, and struggles. In A. J. Marsella, J. L. Johnson, P. Watson, & J. Gryczynski (eds.), *Ethnocultural perspectives on disaster and trauma: Foundations, issues and applications* (pp. 115–173). New York: Springer.

Abramowitz, J. S., Huppert, J. D., Cohen, A. B., *et al.* (2002). Religious obsessions and compulsions in a non-clinical sample: The Penn Inventory of Scrupulosity (PIOS). *Behaviour Research and Therapy*, **40,** 825–838.

Achenbach, T. M. (2008). Multicultural perspectives on developmental psychopathology. In J. J. Hudziak (ed.), *Developmental psychopathology and wellness* (pp. 23–47). Washington, DC: American Psychiatric Press.

Ajaya, S. (1997). *Psychotherapy east and west: A unifying paradigm*. Honesdale, PA: Himalayan International Institute.

Anglin, D. M. & Wade, J. C. (2007). Racial socialization, racial identity, and Black students' adjustment to college. *Cultural Diversity and Ethnic Minority Psychology*, **13,** 207–215.

Apfel, R. J. & Simon, B. (eds.) (1996). *Minefields in their hearts* (pp. 9–11). New Haven, CT: Yale University Press.

Arredondo, P., Bordes, V., & Paniagua, F. A. (2008). Mexicans, Mexican Americans, Caribbean, and other Latin Americans. In A. J. Marsella, J. L. Johnson, P. Watson, & J. Gryczynski (eds.), *Ethnocultural perspectives on disaster and trauma: Foundations, issues and applications* (pp. 299–320). New York: Springer.

Arroyo, C. G. & Zigler, E. (1995). Racial identity, academic achievement, and the psychological well-being of economically disadvantaged adolescents. *Journal of Personality and Social Psychology*, **69,** 903–914.

Bell, C. C. (1980). States of consciousness. *Journal of the National Medical Association*, **72,** 331–334.

Bell, C. C. (2000). *Eight pieces of brocade*. Chicago, IL: Community Mental Health Council.

Bell, C. C. (2001). Cultivating resiliency in youth. *Journal of Adolescent Health*, **29,** 375–381.

Bell, C. C. (2007). Keeping promises: Ethics and principles in psychiatric practice. In Aspatore Books Staff (ed.), *The art and science of psychiatry* (pp. 7–38). Boston, MA: Aspatore Books.

Bell, C. C. (2008a). Asian martial arts and resiliency. *Ethnicity and Inequities in Health and Social Care*, **1**: 11–17.

Bell, C. C. (2008b). Should culture considerations influence early intervention? In R. Ursano & M. Blumenfield (eds.), *Early psychological intervention following mass trauma: Present and future directions* (pp. 127–148). Cambridge, UK: Cambridge University Press.

Bell, C. C. & Suggs, H. (1998). Using sports to strengthen resiliency in children – training "heart": Using sports to create resiliency. *Child and Adolescent Psychiatric Clinics of North America*, 7, 859–865.

Bell, C. C. & Williamson, J. (2002). Psychiatric services across the millennium: A celebration of 50 years of *Psychiatric Services* journal–special populations. *Psychiatric Services*, 53, 419–424.

Bell, C. C., Richardson, J., & Blount, M. A. (2005). Suicide prevention. In J. R. Lutzker (ed.), *Preventing violence: Research and evidence-based intervention strategies* (pp. 217–237). Washington, DC: American Psychological Press.

Bell, C. C., Bhana, A., Petersen, I., *et al.* (2008). Building protective factors to offset sexually risky behaviors among black South African youth: a randomized control trial. *Journal of the National Medical Association*, 100, 936–944.

Berry, J. W. (2006). Acculturative stress. In P. T. P. Wong & L. C. J. Wong (eds.), *Handbook of multicultural perspectives on stress and coping* (pp. 287–298). New York: Springer.

Billingsley, A. (1992). *Climbing Jacob's ladder: The enduring legacy of African-American families.* New York: Simon & Shuster.

Binder, E. B., Bradley, R. G., Liu, W., *et al.* (2008). Association of *FKBP5* polymorphisms and childhood abuse with risk of posttraumatic stress disorder symptoms in adults. *Journal of the American Medical Association*, 299, 1291–1305.

Bond, M. H. & Tornatzky, L. G. (1973). Locus of control in students in Japan and the United States: Dimensions and levels of response. *Psychologia: An International Journal of Psychology in the Orient*, 16, 209–213.

Boomsma, D. I., deGeus, E. J., van Baal, G. C., *et al.* (1999). A religious upbringing reduces the influence of genetic factors on disinhibition: Evidence for interaction between genotype and environment in personality. *Twin Research*, 2, 115–125.

Brook, J. S., Duan, T., Brook, D. W., & Ning, Y. (2007). Pathways to nicotine dependence in African American and Puerto Rican young adults. *American Journal of Addictions.* 16, 450–456.

Bryant, R. & Guthrie, R. M. (2005). Factor for posttraumatic stress: A study of trainee firefighters. *Psychological Science*, 16, 749–752.

Byrom, T. (trans.) (1976). *The Dhammapada: The sayings of the Buddha.* New York: Vintage Books.

Carswell, S. B. & Carswell, M. A. (2008). Meeting the physical, psychological, and social needs of African Americans following disaster. In A. J. Marsella, J. L. Johnson, P. Watson, & J. Gryczynski (eds.), *Ethnocultural perspectives on disaster and trauma: Foundations, issues and applications* (pp. 39–71). New York: Springer.

Carver, C. S., Scheier, M. & Weintraub, J. (1989). Assessing coping strategies: A theoretically based approach. *Journal of Personality and Social Psychology*, 56, 267–283.

Caspi, A., McClay, J., Moffitt, T. E., *et al.* (2002). Role of genotype in the cycle of violence in maltreated children. *Science*, 297, 851–854.

Chandler, T. A., Shama, D. D., Wolf, F. M., & Planchard, S. K. (1982). Multiattributional causality: A five cross-national samples study. *Journal of Cross-Cultural Psychology*, 12, 207–221.

Charney, D. S., Barlow, D. H., Botteron, K., *et al.* (2002). Neuroscience research agenda to guide development of a pathophysiologically based classification system. In D. A. Regier, D. J. Kupfer, & M. B. First (eds.), *Research agenda for DSM V* (pp. 31–84). Washington DC: American Psychiatric Press.

Chen, Y. H. (2006a). Coping with suffering: The Buddhist perspective. In P. T. P. Wong & L. C. J. Wong (eds.), *Handbook of multicultural perspectives on stress and coping* (pp. 73–90) New York: Springer.

Chen, Y. H. (2006b). The way of nature as a healing power. In P. T. P. Wong & L. C. J. Wong (eds.), *Handbook of multicultural perspectives on stress and coping* (pp. 91–103). New York: Springer.

Chia, B. H. (1996). A Singapore study of obsessive-compulsive disorder. *Sinagapore Medical Journal*, 37, 402–406.

Chun, C. A., Moos, R. H., & Cronkite, R. C. (2006). Culture: A fundamental concept for the stress and coping paradigm. In P. T. P. Wong & L. C. J. Wong (eds.), *Handbook of multicultural perspectives on stress and coping* (pp. 29–53). New York: Springer.

Cloninger, C. R. (2004). *Feeling good: The science of well-being.* New York: Oxford University Press.

Cohen, K. S. (1997). *The way of qigong.* New York: Ballantine Books.

Corneille, M. A. & Belgrave, F. Z. (2007). Ethnic identity, neighborhood risk, and adolescent drug and sex attitudes and refusal efficacy: The urban African American girls' experience. *Journal of Drug Education*, 37, 177–190.

Department of Health and Human Services (2001). *Mental health: Culture, race, and ethnicity. A supplement to "Mental Health: A Report of the Surgeon General".* Rockville, MD: US Department of Mental Health and Human Services, Substance Abuse and Mental Health Services Administration.

Donenberg, G., Wilson, H. W., Emerson, E., & Bryant, F. B. (2002). Holding the line with a watchful eye: The impact of perceived parental permissiveness and parental monitoring on risky sexual behavior among adolescents in psychiatric care. *AIDS Education and Prevention*, 14, 138–157.

Dudley-Grant, G. R. & Etheridge, W. (2008). Caribbean Blacks (Haitians, Jamaicans, Virgin Islanders, Eastern Caribbean): Responses to disasters in cultural context. In A. J. Marsella, J. L. Johnson, P. Watson, & J. Gryczynski (eds.), *Ethnocultural perspectives on disaster and trauma: Foundations, issues and applications* (pp. 209–240). New York: Springer.

Fischer, A. R. & Shaw, C. M. (1999). African Americans' mental health and perception of racist discrimination: Moderating effects of racial socialization experiences and self-esteem. *Journal of Counseling Psychology*, **46,** 395–407.

Galea, S., Vlahov, D., Tracy, M., *et al.* (2005). Hispanic ethnicity and post-traumatic stress disorders after a disaster: evidence from a general population survey after September 11, 2001. *Annals of Epidemiology*, **14,** 520–531.

Goldsmith, S. K., Pellman, T. C., Kleinman, A. M., *et al.* for the Committee on Psychopathology and Prevention of Adolescent and Adult Suicide and the Board on Neuroscience and Behavioral Health, National Institute of Medicine (2002). *Reducing suicide: A national imperative.* Washington, DC: National Academies Press.

Gorsuch, R. L. (1995). Religious aspects of substance abuse and recovery. *Journal of Social Issues*, **5,** 65–83.

Greenberg, D. & Shefler, G. (2002). Obsessive-compulsive disorder in ultra-orthodox Jewish patients: A comparison of religious and non-religious symptoms. *Psychological Psychotherapy*, **75,** 123–130.

Greenberg, D. & Witztum, E. (1994). Influence of cultural factors on OCD: Religious symptoms in a religious society. *Israel Journal of Psychiatry and Relations Science*, **31,** 211–220.

Hamid, P. N. (1994). Self-monitoring, locus of control, and social encounters of Chinese and New Zealand students. *Journal of Cross-Cultural Psychology*, **25,** 353–368.

Hansen, N. D. (2002). Teaching cultural sensitivity in psychological assessment: a modular approach used in a distance education program. *Journal of Personality Assessment*, **79,** 200–206.

Heath, A. C., Madden P. A. F., Grant, J. D., *et al.* (1999). Resiliency factors protecting against teenage alcohol use and smoking: Influences of religion, religious involvement and values, and ethnicity in the Missouri Adolescent Female Twin Study. *Twin Research*, **2,** 145–155.

Herman, J. (1992). *Trauma and recovery*. New York: Harper Collins.

Hill, R. B. (1997). *The strengths of African American families: Twenty-five years later*. Washington, DC: RB Books.

Hofstede, G. (1980). *Culture's consequences: Comparing values, behaviors, institutions, and organizations across nations*. Beverly Hills, CA: Sage.

Jagers, R. J. & Mock, L. O. (1995). The Communalism Scale and collectivistic–individualistic tendencies: Some preliminary findings. *Journal of Black Psychology*, **21,** 153–167.

Ji, L. J. (2001). Culture, change, and prediction. *Psychological Science*, **12,** 450–456.

Johnson, J. L., Baldwin J., Haring, R. C., *et al.* (2008). Essential information for disaster management and trauma specialists working with American Indians. In A. J. Marsella, J. L. Johnson, P. Watson, & J. Gryczynski (eds.), *Ethnocultural perspectives on disaster and trauma: Foundations, issues and applications* (pp. 73–113). New York: Springer.

Kaplan, A. S. & Huynh, U. K. (2008). Working with Vietnamese Americans in disasters. In A. J. Marsella, J. L. Johnson, P. Watson, & J. Gryczynski (eds.), *Ethnocultural perspectives on disaster and trauma: Foundations, issues and applications* (pp. 321–349). New York: Springer.

Kaufman, J. & Henrich, C. (2000). Exposure to violence and early childhood trauma. In C. Zeanah Jr. (ed.), *Handbook of infant mental health* (pp. 195–207). New York: Guilford Press.

Kaufman, J., Yang, B. Z., Douglas-Palumberi, H., *et al.* (2006). Brain derived neurotrophic factors–5-HTTLPR gene interactions and environmental modifiers of depression in children. *Biological Psychiatry*, **59,** 673–680.

Kendler, K. S., Aggen, S. H., Jacobson, K. C., *et al.* (2003). Does the level of family dysfunction moderate the impact of genetic factors on the personality trait of neuroticism? *Psychological Medicine*, **33,** 817–825.

Keyes, C. L. M. (2007). Promoting and protective mental health as flourishing: A complementary strategy for improving national mental health. *American Psychologist* **62,** 95–108.

Klaassen, D. W., McDonald, M. J., & James, S. (2006). Advance in the study of religious and spiritual coping. In P. T. P. Wong & L. C. J. Wong (eds.), *Handbook of multicultural perspectives on stress and coping* (pp. 105–132). New York: Springer.

Klonoff, E. A. & Landrine, H. (1999). Acculturation and alcohol use among Blacks: The benefits of remaining culturally traditional. *Western Journal of Black Studies*, **23,** 211–216.

Koenig, H., George, L., Meador, K., *et al.* (1994). Religious practices and alcoholism in a southern adult population. *Hospital and Community Psychiatry*, **45,** 225–231.

Kohut, H. (1966). Forms and transformations of narcissism. *Journal of American Psychoanalysis Association*, **14,** 243–272.

Koopmans, J. R., Slutske, W. S., van Baal, G. C. M., *et al.* (1999). The influence of religion on alcohol initiation: Evidence for genotype X environment interaction. *Behavioral Genetics*, **29,** 445–453.

Lafromboise, T. D., Trimble, J. E., & Mohatt, G. V. (1990). Counseling intervention and American Indian tradition: An integrative approach. *Counseling Psychologist*, **18**, 628–654.

Larson, D. & Wilson, W. P. (1980). Religious life of alcoholics. *Southern Medical Journal*, **73**, 723–727.

Lazarus, R. S. & Folkman, S. (1984). *Stress, appraisal, and coping*. New York: Springer.

Luby, J. L., Svrakic, D. M., McCallum, K., *et al.* (1999). The Junior Temperament and Character Inventory: Preliminary validation of a child self-report measure. *Psychological Reports*, **83**, 1127–1138.

Maddi, S. R. & Harvey, R. H. (2006). Hardiness considered across cultures. In P. T. P. Wong & L. C. J. Wong (eds.), *Handbook of multicultural perspectives on stress and coping* (pp. 409–426). New York: Springer.

Maes, H. H., Neale, M. C., Martin, N. G., *et al.* (1999). Religious attendance and frequency of alcohol use – same genes or same environment: A bivariate extended twin kinship model. *Twin Research*, **2**, 169–179.

Mahler, I. (1974). A comparative study of locus of control. *Psychologia: An International Journal of Psychology in the Orient*, **17**, 135–139.

Marsella, A. J. (2005). Culture and conflict: Understanding and negotiating different cultural constructions of reality. *International Journal of Intercultural Relations*, **29**, 651–673.

Marsella, A. J., Johnson, J. L., Watson, P., & Gryczynski, J. (2008). Essential concepts and foundations. In A. J. Marsella, J. L. Johnson, P. Watson, & J. Gryczynski (eds.), *Ethnocultural perspectives on disaster and trauma: Foundations, issues and applications* (pp. 3–14). New York: Springer.

Marshall, G. N. & Orlando, M. (2002). Acculturation and peritraumatic dissociation in youth adult Latino survivors of community violence. *Journal of Abnormal Psychology*, **111**, 166–174.

Masten, A. S. & Coatsworth, J. D. (1998). The development of competence in favorable and unfavorable environments. *American Psychologist*, **52**, 205–220.

McCreary, M. L., Cunningham, J. N., Ingram, K. M., & Fife, J. E. (2006). Stress, culture, and racial socialization. In P. T. P. Wong & L. C. J. Wong (eds.), *Handbook of multicultural perspectives on stress and coping* (pp. 487–513). New York: Springer.

McCubbin, L. D., Ishikawa, M. E., & McCubbin, H. I. (2008). The Kanaka Maoli: Native Hawaiians and their testimony of trauma and resilience. In A. J. Marsella, J. L. Johnson, P. Watson, & J. Gryczynski (eds.), *Ethnocultural perspectives on disaster and trauma: Foundations, issues and applications* (pp. 271–298). New York: Springer.

Miller, D. B. & MacIntosh, R. (1999). Promoting resilience in urban African American adolescents: Racial socialization and identity as protective factors. *Social Work Research*, **23**, 159–169.

Munro, D. (1979). Locus-of-control attribution: Factors among Blacks and Whites in Africa. *Journal of Cross-Cultural Psychology*, **10**, 157–172.

Nasim, A., Belgrave, F. Z., Jagers, R. J., Wilson, K. D., & Owens, K. (2007). The moderating effects of culture on peer deviance and alcohol use among high-risk African-American adolescents. *Journal of Drug Education*, **37**, 335–363.

National Research Council & Institute of Medicine (2009). *Preventing mental, emotional, and behavioral disorders among young people: Progress and possibilities*. Washington, DC: National Academies Press.

Nobles, W. (1986). *African psychology: Toward its reclamation, reascension, and revitalization*. Oaland, CA: Institute for the Advanced Study of Black Family Life and Culture.

Norris, F. H. & Alegria, M. (2008). Promoting disaster recovery in ethnic-minority individuals and communities. In A. J. Marsella, J. L. Johnson, P. Watson, & J. Gryczynski (eds.), *Ethnocultural perspectives on disaster and trauma: Foundations, issues and applications* (pp. 15–35). New York: Springer.

Oyama, M. (1966). *This is karate*. San Francisco: Japan Publications.

Padilla, A. M. & Borrero, N. E. (2006). The effects of acculturative stress on the Hispanic family. In P. T. P. Wong & L. C. J. Wong (eds.), *Handbook of multicultural perspectives on stress and coping* (pp. 299–317). New York: Springer.

Pargament, K. I. (1997). *The psychology of religion and coping*. New York: Guilford Press.

Payne, I., Bergin, A., Bielema, K., *et al.* (1991). Review of religion and mental health: Prevention and enhancement of psychological functioning. *Prevention Human Services*, **9**, 11–40.

Perilla, J. L., Norris, F. H., & Lavizzo, E. A. (2002). Ethnicity, culture, and disaster response: Identifying and explaining ethnic differences in PTSD six months after Hurricane Andrew. *Journal of Social and Clinical Psychology*, **21**, 20–45.

Prashantham, B. J. (2008). Asian Indians: Cultural considerations for disaster workers. In A. J. Marsella, J. L. Johnson, P. Watson, & J. Gryczynski (eds.), *Ethnocultural perspectives on disaster and trauma: Foundations, issues and applications* (pp. 175–207). New York: Springer.

Raphael, F. J., Rani, S., Bale, R., *et al.* (1996). Religion, ethnicity and obsessive-compulsive disorder. *International Journal of Social Psychiatry*, **42**, 38–44.

Rassin, E. & Koster, E. (2003). The correlation between thought-action fusion and religiosity in a normal sample. *Behaviour Research and Therapy*, **41**, 361–368.

Rettew, D. C., Stanger, C., McKee, L., *et al.* (2006). Interactions between child and parent temperament and child behavior problems. *Comprehensive Psychiatry*, **47**, 412–420.

Rezentes, W. C. (1996). *Ka lama kukui (Hawaiian psychology): An introduction.* Honolulu, HI: A'ali'I Books.

Ruiz, D. M. A. (1997). *The four agreements: A practical guide to personal freedom.* San Rafael, CA: Amber-Allen.

Ryff, C. D., Keyes, C. L. M., & Hughes, D. (2003). Status inequalities, perceived discrimination, and eudaimonic well-being: Do the challenges of minority life hone purpose and growth? *Journal of Health and Social Behavior*, **44**, 275–291.

Shooka, A., al-Haddad, M. K., & Raees, A. (1998). OCD in Bahrain: a phenomenological profile. *International Journal of Social Psychiatry*, **44**, 147–154.

Sica, C., Novara, C., & Sanavio, E. (2002). Religiousness and obsessive–compulsive cognitions and symptoms in an Italian population. *Behaviour Research and Therapy*, **40**, 813–823.

Smith, R. (ed). (1964). *Secrets of Shaolin Temple boxing.* Rutland, VT: Charles E. Tuttle.

Staples, R. (1976). *Introduction to black sociology.* New York: McGraw-Hill.

Stevenson, H. C., Reed, J., Bodison, P., & Bishop, A. (1997). Racism stress management: Racial socialization beliefs and the experience of depression and anger in African American Youth. *Youth and Society*, **29**, 197–222.

Sue, D. W. & Sue, D. (1999). *Counseling the culturally different: Theory and practice*, 3rd edn. New York: Wiley.

Sue, D. W. & Sue D. (2003). *Counseling the culturally diverse: Theory and practice*, 4th edn. New York: Wiley.

Taylor, J. F. (2006). Ethnocentric monocuturalism In Y. Jackson (ed.), *Encyclopedia of multicultural psychology* (p. 203). Thousand Oaks, CA: Sage.

Tek, C. & Ulug, B. (2001). Religiosity and religious obsessions in obsessive compulsive disorder. *Psychiatry Research*, **104**, 99–108.

Texcan, E. & Millet, B. (1997). Phenomenology of obsessive-compulsive disorders. Forms and characteristics of obsessions and compulsions in East Turkey. [In French.] *Encephale*, **23**, 342–350.

Thomas, A. & Chess, S. (1977). *Temperament and development.* New York: Brunner/Mazel.

Thompson, E. A., McCubbin, H. I., Thompson, H. I., & Elver, K. M. (1995). Vulnerability and resiliency in Native Hawaiian families under stress. In H. I. McCubbin, E. A. Thompson, H. I. Thompson, & J. E. Fromer (eds.), *Resiliency in ethnic minority families: Native and immigrant American families* (pp. 115–132). Madison, WI: University of Wisconsin System Center for Excellence in Family Studies.

Thornton, M. C., Chatters, L. M., Taylor, R. J., & Allen, W. R. (1990). Sociodemographic and environmental correlates of racial socialization by Black parents. *Child Development*, **61**, 401–409.

Triandis, H. C. (1995). *Individualism and collectivism.* Boulder, CO: Westbiew Press.

Tweed, R. G. & Conway, L. G. (2006). Coping strategies and culturally influenced beliefs about the world. In P. T. P. Wong & L. C. J. Wong (eds.), *Handbook of multicultural perspectives on stress and coping* (pp. 133–153). New York: Springer.

Vega, W. A., Kolody, B., Aguilar-Gaxiola, S., *et al.* (1998). Lifetime prevalence of DSM–III–R psychiatric disorders among urban and rural Mexican Americans in California. *Archives of General Psychiatry*, **55**, 771–778.

Wilson, J. P. (2004). The abyss experience and traumatic complex: A Jungian perspective of PTSD and dissociation. *Journal of Trauma in Dissociation*, **5**, 43–68.

Wilson, J. P. (2008). Culture, trauma, and the treatment of post-traumatic syndromes: A global perspective. In A. J. Marsella, J. L. Johnson, P. Watson, & J. Gryczynski (eds.), *Ethnocultural perspectives on disaster and trauma: Foundations, issues and applications* (pp. 351–375). New York: Springer.

Wolin, S. & Wolin, S. J. (1996). The challenge model: Working with strengths in children of substance-abusing parents. *Child and Adolescent Psychiatric Clinics of North America*, **5**, 243–256.

13

Loss and grief: the role of individual differences

Anthony D. Mancini and George A. Bonanno

Introduction

It is an unfortunate but inevitable fact of life that virtually all of us must face: people we are close to die. Despite this universality, researchers and theorists have long assumed that bereavement almost always results in significant, and sometimes incapacitating, distress. Curiously, the absence of distress after loss has itself been considered pathological and a likely harbinger of future difficulties (Middleton *et al.*, 1993). When bereaved persons fail to display the expected distress reaction, some have maintained that they are suppressing their grief (Middleton *et al.*, 1993) or lack an attachment to their spouse (Fraley & Shaver, 1999). Indeed, emotional expression following loss – particularly negative emotions – has long been considered cathartic, a necessary ingredient of healthy adjustment (Freud, 1957). Perhaps for this reason, bereaved people who appear outwardly resilient and who resume their lives with minimal disruptions have often been thought to possess extraordinary coping abilities.

However, this idea has increasingly come under fire (Bonanno, 2004). In fact, most bereaved people experience relatively transient disruptions in their ability to function effectively. Furthermore, research increasingly shows that there is a marked diversity in how people respond to loss. Indeed, it appears that three primary patterns or trajectories adequately describe most people's response to interpersonal loss. The largest category, usually from 50% to 60%, is characterized by stable, healthy levels of psychological and physical functioning relatively soon after a loss, or "resilience" (Bonanno, 2004; Mancini & Bonanno, 2006). A second category of bereaved persons (20–25%) displays more acute and persistent levels of distress but gradually they too recover their bearings and return to their former

level of functioning. The most problematic reaction is found among those with a persistent syndrome of a sometimes incapacitating distress that may take years to resolve. This pattern, often described as "complicated grief" (Bonanno *et al.*, 2007), is relatively rare, typically occurring in 10–15% of grievers (Bonanno & Kaltman, 2001). Two other types of bereavement response have also emerged recently, although they typically characterize only a small proportion of grievers. These include a chronic form of distress that *predated the loss and is exacerbated in its aftermath* (Bonanno *et al.*, 2002; Mancini *et al.*, 2011) and *dramatic improvement following loss* (A.D. Mancini, I. Galatzer-Levy, & G.A. Bonanno, unpublished data). Although each is quite uncommon (5–10%), these patterns have been confirmed using different methods and samples, suggesting that they are veridical.

This chapter considers the implications of these different patterns of grief response for how we understand the grieving process. To address this issue, we first review grief's varying manifestations. We then describe empirical findings on grieving across the three primary trajectories, focusing on qualitative differences. We conclude by considering the therapeutic implications of these differences in grieving and potential cultural variations.

The phenomenology of grief

How does the experience of grief manifest itself? Evidence increasingly suggests that four broad categories of disrupted functioning characterize the normative experience of loss (Bonanno & Kaltman, 2001): (1) cognitive disorganization, (2) dysphoric emotions, (3) health deficits, and (4) disruptions in social and occupational functioning.

Resilience and Mental Health: Challenges Across the Lifespan, ed. Steven M. Southwick, Brett T. Litz, Dennis Charney, and Matthew J. Friedman. Published by Cambridge University Press. © Cambridge University Press 2011.

Cognitive disorganization

In the initial aftermath of loss, some cognitive disorganization in adjusting to altered life circumstances has been widely noted, although this disorganization is by no means characteristic of all bereaved persons. Among the components of this disorganization are a sense of confusion and preoccupation with the loss, as well as having difficulty accepting the reality of their loss, a sense of derealization and disorganization, and preoccupation with memories of the deceased (Parkes & Weiss, 1983; Shuchter & Zisook, 1993). For example, a study of 350 conjugally bereaved individuals found that even two months after the loss up to 70% of the sample still found it "hard to believe" that their spouses had actually died, and approximately half (49%) continued to have this difficulty into the second year of bereavement (Zisook & Shuchter, 1993). Despite these continuing preoccupations, only a small proportion of the bereaved showed more extreme cognitive difficulties, such as difficulties concentrating (20%) or making decisions (17%).

Not surprisingly, bereaved persons are also commonly preoccupied with the memory of the deceased, especially soon after the loss. Particularly within the first year after the loss, it is common for bereaved persons to experience sudden recollections of the deceased that are not prompted by external events. These memories are often described as "unbidden," and, when they persist over a long period of time, they can be a source of considerable distress. In the study of Horowitz and colleagues (1997), for example, most bereaved persons (72%) reported such experiences even at six months after the loss. A more potentially problematic aspect of this continued engagement with the memory of the deceased is reflected in changes in identity after loss. For example, a substantial proportion of bereaved persons reported (87%) experiencing that "a piece of me is missing" (Zisook & Shuchter, 1993). Moreover, many of the bereaved (55%) found themselves doing things more like their deceased spouses, or even becoming more like their deceased spouses (39%). In another report, some bereaved individuals (14%) even experienced recurrent thoughts that their own death would follow, or mirror, their spouse's death (Horowitz et al., 1997). Given that these findings were observed in samples of middle-aged, and presumably healthy, individuals, they offer particularly compelling evidence of the potential impact of loss on cognitions about the self.

Some research also suggests that bereavement is associated with a concerted and enduring search to place the loss in a meaningful context. In a study of individuals who lost a child or a spouse in a car crash, for example, the search for meaning after a loss was found to unfold over the course of years (Lehman et al., 1987). As late as four to seven years after the sudden loss of a spouse or child, the vast majority of bereaved individuals continued to talk about the loss; to review memories, thoughts, or mental pictures of the deceased; or to ask themselves the questions "Why me?" or "Why my spouse/child?". Disconcertingly, 68% of the bereaved spouses and 59% of the bereaved parents reported that they had not found any meaning or made any sense at all of the loss. Indeed, a number of studies suggest that the search for meaning is usually associated with distress and may not help the person to resolve their grief. However, a recent study examining cancer survivors suggested that adaptation may be facilitated by making meaning out of the experience, as opposed to only searching for meaning. In other words, a persistent search for meaning in the aftermath of an acute stressor will only serve adaptive ends when it eventuates in a "meaning made" (Park et al., 2008).

Dysphoric emotions

Although bereavement obviously results in sadness, a variety of dysphoric emotions have also been linked to loss, most often centering around anger, irritability, hostility, sadness, fear, and guilt (Bowlby, 1980; Raphael, 1983; Osterweis et al., 1984). However, the frequency of these emotions is somewhat in doubt. Shuchter and Zisook (1993) used self-report measures to assay emotional experiences in the first year after the loss, finding that only a small portion of participants (less than 15%) endorsed emotions commonly linked to grieving, such as anger, guilt, and fear. This may be accounted for by the insufficiency of retrospective self-report measures to record ephemeral emotional experiences accurately. Indeed, a greater prevalence of dysphoric emotion during conjugal bereavement was observed in a subsequent study that measured facial expressions of emotion as they occurred during an interview six months after the loss (Bonanno & Keltner, 1997). Using this immediate, non-verbal assessment, anger and sadness were exhibited by almost two thirds of the bereaved participants, and contempt and disgust by approximately one third.

A more complex and mixed syndrome of dysphoric emotion is found in the common experience of yearning for the deceased. Unsurprisingly, yearning is a basic component of grief. Parkes (1970, p. 451) concluded that "the central and pathognomonic feature of grief" is an intense "pining" for the deceased, such that "without it grief cannot truly be said to have occurred and when present it is a sure sign of a person grieving." However, it is worth noting that yearning is a complex state, consisting of mixed positive and negative thoughts and feelings related to the lost loved one. Indeed, a critical point here is that although grief may evoke a range of emotional responses, grief is not synonymous with emotion. Whereas emotions are ephemeral responses to internal and environmental stimuli that condition certain action tendencies, grief is distinguished by its relatively enduring nature and by its recruitment of more long-term coping efforts to manage distress.

A similar dysphoric feature commonly associated with grieving is intense loneliness. Shuchter and Zisook (1993) reported that 59% of the widows and widowers they questioned during the first two months of bereavement experienced loneliness, while 37% felt lonely even when around other people. By the second year of bereavement, these proportions dropped to 39% and 23%, respectively; in contrast, only 3% of a match married sample endorsed experiencing any form of loneliness. Horowitz and colleagues (1997) reported similar findings, with 59% of their sample experiencing loneliness at six months after loss, and 38% experiencing loneliness at 14 months after loss.

Health deficits

There is considerable evidence that the stress of interpersonal loss also can carry a significant health cost. This has been observed most commonly in the form of increased doctor visits and complaints about general health, but more serious health problems have also been identified. A number of studies have suggested that interpersonal loss is associated with increased health difficulties, including shortness of breath, palpitations, digestive difficulties, loss of appetite, restlessness, and insomnia (Lindemann, 1944; Horowitz, 1986). One well-designed study compared health outcomes in elderly bereaved two months after loss and a comparison group matched for socioeconomic and demographic variables (Thompson et al., 1984). Compared with the matched control participants, the bereaved participants still reported worsened or new illnesses, more severe illnesses, increased use of medications, poorer perceived health, and poorer health relative to others of the same age.

In addition to these potential sequelae of loss, several studies have also examined the possible role of neuroendocrine activity, such as changes in cortisol or serum growth hormone levels, during bereavement. Although there is no evidence that neuroendocrine activity is altered significantly during bereavement or that it influences the course of grieving (Kim & Jacobs, 1993), evidence does suggest a link between grief and a relatively short-lived compromise in immune functioning (Irwin et al., 1987). This linkage, however, may be mediated by symptomatology in response to the loss. For example, Zisook and colleagues (1994) examined immune functioning variables in a sample of middle-aged conjugally bereaved women and in a sample of matched controls. There were no significant differences between the bereaved women at two months after loss and their married counterparts on any of the immune variables. However, when the bereaved sample was separated into depressed and non-depressed widows, depressed widows had a lower concentration of T-cells, lower natural killer cell activity, and a trend toward lower lymphocyte stimulation responses compared with the non-depressed widows. As compelling as the link between grief-related depression and a short-term suppression of immune functioning may be, it has not yet been demonstrated that the depressive aspects of grief exert a longer-term influence on immune functioning, or that the short-term suppression effects produce any lasting health consequences (Irwin & Pike, 1993). Additional research will be necessary to address this question further.

One dramatic and unfortunate consequence of bereavement is its impact on mortality, an association that appears to be particularly robust in the early months after a loss. In a striking demonstrations of the bereavement–mortality effect, researchers in Finland examined longitudinal data on 95 647 conjugally bereaved individuals in Finland during their first four years of bereavement (Kaprio et al., 1987). Compared with the average expected mortality rate in Finland, the conjugally bereaved individuals showed an overall 6.5% higher likelihood of dying. This increase was smaller (3.2% increase) for deaths by natural causes (e.g., cardiovascular disease). However, deaths by natural causes were almost twice as high as the normal expectancy rate in the first week of bereavement. Deaths by violent causes (e.g., traffic accidents) were even more likely (93% increase) among the bereaved individuals.

Finally, bereaved individuals showed considerably more deaths (242% increase) by suicide. Indeed, it is widely thought that bereavement increases the risk of dying, and this increased risk of mortality extends to all types of bereavement, particularly in the early months after the loss and particularly among younger bereaved individuals (Stroebe & Stroebe, 1993).

Disrupted social and occupational functioning

In addition to its cognitive, emotional, and somatic manifestations, grief has also been associated with disruptions in social and occupational functioning. These difficulties have been observed most commonly in the form of social withdrawal and isolation, and a concomitant difficulty in assuming or maintaining ordinary social and occupational roles. As with the other features of grief, disruptions in social and occupational functioning are common for most but not all bereaved individuals in the initial aftermath of a loss (Lindemann, 1944; Parkes & Weiss, 1983).

Bereaved individuals also may struggle in their roles as parents or in their careers (Parkes & Weiss, 1983). Several studies have shown that widowers report greater difficulties in their work roles both outside and inside the home, greater difficulties in managing spare time, and greater difficulties with their family roles (Tudiver et al., 1991). Similar findings were observed in a study conducted four to seven years after the sudden death of a spouse or child. The conjugally bereaved portion of the sample was still less likely to look forward to doing things with others, less confident that they could handle or cope with a serious problem or major change in their life, and rated the general state of their lives more negatively, compared with a matched married group. However, the bereaved parents in this study showed similar but non-significant trends toward the same results.

Bereavement also affects work performance and initiating and maintaining relationships. One study found that over a third (36%) of bereaved persons reported dissatisfaction in their work performance at seven months, and that 28% still endorsed this problem at 13 months (Shuchter & Zisook, 1993). Although these percentages show that dissatisfaction with work may not be as widespread as other grief-related difficulties, it was still more common among bereaved individuals relative to the 10% of the married comparison sample who reported such difficulties. A substantial proportion of bereaved persons still reported difficulties in developing new intimate relationships even six months after a loss (Horowitz et al., 1997). However, by 14 months, only about a third of the sample (32%) reported such difficulties.

Trajectories of loss and grief

Given that the experience of loss and grief takes on such varying manifestations, what are the implications of a trajectory approach for our understanding of individual differences in grieving? As discussed above, empirical evidence increasingly supports three primary or prototypical patterns of grief reaction: resilience, recovery, and chronic or complicated grief. Beyond the straightforward difference in the duration of grief symptoms across time, what does a trajectory approach suggest for our understanding of the qualitative aspects of grief? In other words, is the grief experience across the trajectories different in kind or just in duration and intensity? This question is taken up by first describing each trajectory pattern and briefly reviewing evidence for their prevalence before moving on to consider available empirical evidence for how the manifestations of grief described above would likely differ qualitatively across grief trajectories.

Resilience

The most prevalent response to loss is characterized by relatively stable psychological and physical functioning as well as the capacity for generative experiences and positive emotions. Elsewhere, we have described this capacity as *resilience*, and increasing evidence supports its distinctiveness as a trajectory in response to acute stress (Mancini & Bonanno, 2006; Bonanno & Mancini, 2008). In addition to bereavement, resilience has been observed in response to a wide variety of acute stressors, including the September 11 2001 terrorist attack (Bonanno et al., 2006), traumatic injury (DeRoon-Cassini et al., 2010), divorce (Mancini et al., 2011), and disease epidemic (Bonanno et al., 2008).

In the bereavement literature, an initial study focused on how people coped with the premature death of a spouse at midlife (Bonanno et al., 1995). Although using relatively small samples, this study demonstrated that a stable pattern of low distress over time, or resilience, could be clearly distinguished from the more conventionally understood pattern of recovery. More recent studies have provided additional evidence for the resilience trajectory. In an unusual study that followed a large sample of older married persons over the course of many years, the subset of persons who experienced the loss of their spouse showed surprisingly low levels of clinical depression, with approximately half reporting minimal to no symptoms at any point in the study (Bonanno et al., 2002). In another sample that included bereaved parents, bereaved spouses, and bereaved gay men, more than half reported minimal to no symptoms across time (Bonanno et al., 2005a). We found further confirmation for resilience as a distinct and common trajectory in response to loss in a recent study using a latent growth mixture modeling framework, a sophisticated statistical approach that permits the modeling of divergent trajectories of response across time (Muthén, 2004). In an analysis of over 16 000 German citizens who were followed over 20 years, 60% of persons who lost their spouse reported only a slight dip in life satisfaction and returned to baseline levels a year after the loss (Mancini et al., 2011).

What does the resilient trajectory suggest for our understanding of the grief response? It has long been assumed that the failure to grieve is indicative of an underlying but unseen psychopathology (Freud, 1957; Bowlby, 1980). Indeed, some have gone so far as to suggest that the appearance of mental health, when associated with a defensive disavowal of unpleasant aspects of the self, can be illusory (Shedler et al., 1993). Consistent with the illusion of mental health paradigm, there is a long history of associating resilience to loss with negative characteristics, including defensive denial, a lack of attachment to the spouse, and a delayed and more severe reaction to the loss.

Contrary to these speculations, an ample literature now suggests that the grief of resilient people is not marked by an absence of feeling. For example, when asked about their experiences soon after the loss, about 75% of those showing a resilient outcome trajectory reported experiencing intense yearning (painful waves of missing spouse) as well as pangs of intense grief at some point in the earliest months of bereavement (Bonanno et al., 2002). What is more, all but one of the bereaved people showing the resilient trajectory reported having experienced intrusive and unbidden thoughts about the loss that they could not get out of their mind, and that they found themselves ruminating, or going over and over what happened when the spouse died, in the earliest months of bereavement.

However, it appears that these aspects of grief are simply less debilitating and less persistent, in part because the loss is more quickly transmogrified into

memory and assumes a more benign and even comforting presence in the person's life. Bonanno et al. (2002) found that resilient people are particularly likely to experience positive emotions in tandem with memories of the deceased. Specifically, resilient people were better able than other bereaved participants to gain comfort from talking about or thinking about the spouse. For example, they were more likely than other bereaved people to report that thinking about and talking about their deceased spouse made them feel happy or at peace (Bonanno et al., 2004a). Moreover, this capacity remained stable over time but only for those in the resilient trajectory.

Although the resilient bereaved may experienced some cognitive disorganization related to the loss, recent evidence suggests that they largely maintain their equilibrium. For example, one characteristic of resilient people is a remarkable continuity in their identities. We found evidence for this continuity in a recent study in which we compared resilient and more symptomatic bereaved persons with a matched sample of married persons (A.D. Mancini, I. Galatzer-Levy, & G.A. Bonanno, unpublished data). Participants completed a task in which they identified traits associated with their identity (e.g., "kind" or "thoughtful"). Once the list was finalized, the researcher then asked the participant to indicate the extent that each trait had changed since the loss. When compared with bereaved persons with higher levels of symptoms, resilient individuals reported relatively little identity change at both 4 and 18 months after loss, and the degree of change did not differ from that reported by non-bereaved participants. Likewise, in qualitative examinations of the bereavement experience, the resilient bereaved reported a stable and continuous sense of who they are, a resource that appears to buffer them from the many changes entailed by the loss of a loved one (Bauer & Bonanno, 2001; Mancini & Bonanno, 2006).

In terms of health functioning, preliminary evidence suggests that the resilient bereaved also experience less-marked physiological consequences. To explore individual differences in somatic complaints over time, for example, Bonanno and colleagues (1999) categorized individuals according to their level of somatic symptoms across three time points, extending to 25 months after the loss. Two thirds of participants had either low levels of somatic complaints at each assessment or reported initial elevations of symptoms that dropped to normal levels between the first and second year. In a more recent analysis, self-reported health dysfunction strongly differentiated the resilient from trajectories of chronic grief and chronic high distress that predated the loss (Mancini *et al.*, 2011), further suggesting that the resilient bereaved experience fewer health problems following loss. Although it is likely that resilience would also attenuate or even nullify the mortality–bereavement link, this question has not been directly investigated and is thus an important topic of future research.

A hallmark of resilient bereaved people is their ability to continue to express and experience positive emotions even soon after a loss. For example, resilient individuals tend to exhibit more genuine laughs and smiles when speaking about the loss (Bonanno & Keltner, 1997), and also evoke more favorable responses in observers (Keltner, 1997). Moreover, resilient bereaved people also have fewest regrets about their behavior with the spouse, or about things they may have done or failed to do when he or she was still alive. Perhaps as a result, resilient individuals are less likely to search to make sense of or find meaning in the spouse's death, suggesting that they are less likely to engage in rumination, which is strongly associated with negative affective states (Nolen-Hoeksema *et al.*, 1997).

In sum, the resilient bereaved appear to experience a grief course marked by initial experiences of yearning and sadness but few disruptions in their ability to meet everyday obligations at work and in social relationships. In addition to experiencing relatively few health problems after the loss, the resilient bereaved also appear to retain a sense of a continuous self in spite of the loss and to experience a sense of comfort from memories of the deceased that remains stable across time.

Recovery

The term *recovery* connotes a trajectory in which normal functioning temporarily gives way to threshold or subthreshold psychopathology (e.g., symptoms of depression or post-traumatic stress disorder [PTSD]), usually for a period of at least several months, and then gradually returns to pre-event levels. This recovery pattern has long been considered the modal response to loss and other acute stressors (Brickman & Campbell, 1971). However, the empirical evidence has overwhelmingly shown that recovery typically characterizes only a minority of bereaved persons, at most 20% (Bonanno *et al.*, 2002; Mancini *et al.*, 2011).

According to a more traditional perspective, recovery might be seen as the healthiest response to bereavement, because it would appear to reflect an appropriate expression of the negative feelings associated with the loss. Such expression is often presumed to facilitate grief's resolution. As discussed above, however, evidence suggests that resilience is most characteristic of psychological health. Indeed, there is no evidence that grief-related symptoms early on in the bereavement experience are prognostic of better outcomes (Bonanno *et al.*, 2002, 2004b).

What is the bereavement experience like for people exhibiting this trajectory? At this point, there have been only a few direct examinations of recovery (Bonanno *et al.*, 2002, 2004b), making it somewhat difficult to characterize the grief experiences of such persons. Nevertheless, some aspects of their experience can be deduced from extant research. Bereaved persons who show the recovery pattern typically struggle with moderate levels of symptoms and experience difficulties carrying out their normal tasks at work or in the care of loved ones, but they somehow manage to struggle through these tasks and slowly but gradually begin to return to their pre-loss or baseline level of functioning, usually over a period of one or two years. Symptoms are relatively acute in the early stages of the loss. When compared with resilient persons, those in the recovery trajectory usually have more feelings of depression, difficulty enjoying activities, and sleeping symptoms early on, as well as experiencing more yearning and feelings of shock and despair about the loss. Although these symptoms typically resolve by 18 months, persons in the recovery trajectory do struggle to a greater extent than, for example, resilient persons. They also appear to experience fewer positive emotions in their experience of grief (Bonanno *et al.*, 2004a). For example, persons who demonstrate the recovery pattern see a decline over time in their capacity to derive comfort from positive memories of the deceased (Bonanno *et al.*, 2004a). This decline stands in sharp contrast to the resilient, whose memories of the deceased continue to provide undiminished comfort across time.

Chronic grief

The most problematic reaction to loss is characterized by a persistent syndrome of grief-related distress that can last for years after the loss. Although this type of reaction generally characterizes a small proportion of grievers, it can have profound effects on people's ability to function (Prigerson *et al.*, 1995, 1996). Theorists have long argued that chronic grief should be viewed as a separate form of psychopathology (Lichtenthal *et al.*, 2004), independent of diagnoses for major depression and PTSD. Until recently, evidence in support of a diagnostic category for chronic or "complicated" grief had been equivocal. One critical question that had not been adequately addressed is whether chronic grief has incremental validity in predicting functional outcomes over and above the predictive capacity of depression and PTSD symptoms. We recently investigated this question and confirmed that grief symptoms, when entered simultaneously into a regression equation with depression and PTSD symptoms, were associated with unique variance across different outcome measures (heart rate change and global functioning) and in two separate samples (Bonanno *et al.*, 2007). Therefore, chronic grief seems to be an independent form of psychopathology.

How does chronic grief differ from the recovery pattern? An obvious but perhaps principal difference between the conventional recovery pattern and chronic grief reactions is the duration of symptoms and their impact on functioning. However, duration of symptomatology does not appear to be the only factor to distinguish chronic reactions; severity of symptoms even in the initial months of bereavement also appears to inform such reactions. Recent research has shown, for example, that bereaved individuals who ultimately developed chronic reactions struggle with acute symptom levels in the early months of bereavement. These can include a dramatically reduced ability to perform well at work, to maintain relationships with friends or intimates, and to meet parenting obligations. These difficulties may persist for years after the loss, but at a minimum should endure for at least one year after bereavement to warrant the label "chronic grief."

Qualitative aspects of grief also differentiate chronic grief from the other trajectories

Although yearning typically characterizes all mourners, chronic grievers appear to experience a particularly acute form of it, one that has debilitating effects on their functioning. Parkes and Weiss (1983) identified a "high yearning" group of conjugally bereaved individuals who appeared to yearn for their deceased spouses "constantly," "frequently," or "whenever inactive." Pining like this is often a dominant feature of the day to day experience of chronic grievers. Indeed, the slightest peripheral cue – passing a restaurant associated with the deceased, for example – can activate the memory of the deceased, even when this cue has not entered

conscious awareness (Ehlers, 2006). The persistent and often distressing nature of the deceased's felt presence in the griever's life, along with the yearning that it occasions, appears to set in train a variety of consequences for adjustment, which mark chronic grief as distinct from other types of grieving.

Although most grievers experience some intrusive memories of the deceased or cognitive disorganization soon after a loss (for example, confusing someone on the street with the deceased), these experiences typically rapidly diminish in their intensity and frequency. For chronic grievers, however, the intrusive memories continue and may be accompanied by marked distress and autonomic arousal (Zisook *et al.*, 1998). In this way, chronic grief can resemble a syndrome with strong parallels to PTSD (Ehlers, 2006). In accord with this, a cardinal feature of chronic grief is avoidance. Chronic grievers are particularly likely, for example, to deploy avoidant strategies to manage feelings and reminders associated with the loss (Boelen *et al.*, 2006a). They may, for example, not talk to old friends or avoid places associated with the deceased. They may try to inoculate themselves against feelings related to the loss, try to push them out of awareness, or redirect their thoughts to mitigate their preoccupation with the deceased. These avoidant strategies for regulating the thoughts and feelings associated with the loss are typically ineffective, however, because they often reinforce the link between the memory of the deceased and the cognitive–affective structures with which it is associated (Boelen *et al.*, 2006b).

One avoidant strategy with particularly negative implications for bereavement is suppression, or inhibiting emotional–expressive behavior while feeling emotional arousal. Although research has yet to uncover a direct link between the use of suppression and chronic grief, it would appear likely, based on the central role of avoidance in chronic grievers' repertoire of coping behaviors, that suppression is often enacted in managing troubling feelings. Because of the cognitive resources required, the use of suppression inhibits the person's ability to absorb new information and, in this way, can impair interpersonal functioning (Gross & John, 2003), depriving the person of helpful resources. Consider, for example, a chronic griever who is preparing to attend a memorial for his or her loved one. To avoid being overwhelmed, the person may try to suppress the behavioral manifestations of his or her feelings, a coping strategy that entails significant cognitive resources and that is more likely to enhance autonomic arousal (Gross & John, 2003). As a consequence, the person would not only experience the event as more stressful but would also be deprived of some of the beneficial aspects of social interaction, including more cognitive integration of the loss.

Somewhat surprisingly, suppression and avoidance of the loss may also co-occur with an anxious preoccupation with the negative feelings related to the loss. One unfortunate consequence of this preoccupation is that chronic grievers' continuous expressions of pain may drive away potential avenues of social support (Coyne *et al.*, 1988; Kelly & McKillop, 1996; Keltner & Bonanno, 1997). This possibility received preliminary support in a recent study in which untrained observers were asked to rate their subjective reactions to videotapes of conjugally bereaved individuals as they described their loss to an interviewer (Keltner & Bonanno, 1997). Those bereaved participants who were perceived by the observers as less well adjusted also evoked in the observers greater frustration and less compassion. In a subsequent study (Capps & Bonanno, 2000), another group of untrained judges were shown narrative transcripts of these interviews. The more the bereaved participants described negative thoughts and emotions during the interview, the more the judges reported they would be inclined to avoid the participant. As can be seen, chronic grievers are in something of a double bind. If they suppress behaviors associated with their emotions, the benefits they derive from social interaction are sharply curtailed. Conversely, if they express their feelings of pain too much to their social network, they may erode the very relationships they are counting on for support.

Conclusions and clinical implications

This chapter has focused on individual differences in grieving, describing the widely varying manifestations of grief in response to loss. Based on a growing body of research, three primary trajectories of loss (resilience, recovery, and chronic grief) and two secondary trajectories (improvement and chronic distress) were identified that appear to characterize the experiences of most grievers. The empirical evidence for qualitative differences in the grief experience of persons in the different grief trajectories was then considered.

What are the implications of the heterogeneous nature of grief for clinical interventions? One obvious implication is that a one-size fits all approach for grief interventions, once commonly endorsed by grief theorists, is no longer tenable. Indeed, it has become increasingly clear that grief interventions are only appropriate for a minority of grievers, primarily those in the chronic grief trajectory. This position was recently underscored in an authoritative meta-analysis of grief interventions (Currier *et al.*, 2008). Perhaps the central finding of this meta-analysis is that studies that screen for more serious forms of grief show substantially stronger effects. In fact, in the absence of such screening, grief interventions show small effect sizes, substantially less than are observed in traditional therapies, and these effects are not retained at follow-up. Moreover, given the heterogeneity of grief, it would appear that it is necessary to employ a variety of clinical techniques tailored to the specific experiences of the griever, as opposed to generic therapeutic procedures that would be presumed to help all grievers. It is worth noting that this mandate stands in sharp contrast to traditional notions that grief is "work" and requires emotional expression or that grief proceeds in preordained stages (Wortman & Silver, 2001).

Although resilient persons are not appropriate candidates for intervention, their coping strategies may offer some intriguing avenues for clinical intervention (for a longer treatment of this issue, see Mancini & Bonanno [2006]). For example, one characteristic of resilient people is their ability to regulate emotion flexibility in response to situational demands. This capacity gives them a distinct coping advantage when faced with acute adversity (Bonanno *et al.*, 2004b). We are currently exploring how such skills might inform our understanding and treatment of chronic grief. Although no formal treatment approach exists to teach these kinds of skill directly, we suspect that coping flexibility might be learned or with practice improved among individuals who lack such abilities. Another clinical implication of the present review concerns the techniques used to regulate aversive emotions associated with loss. As discussed, the use of suppression, particularly for chronic grievers, carries with it a number of untoward complications (Gross & John, 2003). An alternative technique is cognitive reappraisal, which is antecedent focused (designed to anticipate the emotion) and involves construing a potentially stressful event in benign or growth-oriented terms in order to blunt its emotional impact (Gross & John, 2003). This may be a particularly important skill for chronic grievers, who are more vulnerable to distress under circumstances that activate their associations to the deceased. Although such techniques are standard components of clinical intervention, given the findings on individual differences in resilience, it seems worth emphasizing their potentially important role in interventions with bereaved persons.

One additional question is the role of contextual factors, such as the nature of the loss, caregiving strain, or material resources, and their impact on the grief experience. For example, although it might appear intuitive that sudden losses would be associated with more chronic grief, data have largely been equivocal on this question. However, one well-designed study, using a representative sample, appropriate control variables, and prospective data, found that the sudden loss of a loved one is not, by itself, associated with worse adjustment (Carr *et al.*, 2001). However, there is evidence that losses from violent causes (suicide, homicide, or violent accident) are associated with more symptomatology and lower levels of resilience (Kaltman & Bonanno, 2003). When the analysis controls for the violent nature of a loss, the impact of sudden losses is no longer significant. Caregiving strain, by contrast, appears not to be related to resilience per se, but it does predict an unusual trajectory of improved functioning following loss (Bonanno *et al.* 2002). Additional evidence for the crucial role of contextual factors was found in a recent analysis of a large panel dataset. Using a latent class framework, we not only validated the resilient trajectory empirically but we also found that one of the factors associated with resilience was less reduction in income following loss (Mancini *et al.*, 2011).

A final important question is the role of ethnic and cultural variations in resilience during bereavement. Western, independence-oriented countries tend to focus more heavily than collectivist countries on the personal experience of grief. Cushman (1990) has described a pervasive assumption in the West of a "bounded, interior self" in which autonomy and self-reliance are primary values and which stands in opposition to Eastern notions of a collectivist self. What are the implications of such cultural beliefs for coping with extreme adversity? Although we cannot take up this issue in detail, preliminary evidence suggests that coping strategies do hold different consequences for adjustment in different cultures. For example, bereaved people in China recover more quickly from loss than do bereaved Americans, and for the Chinese, coping is enhanced by a continuing psychological bond with the deceased (Bonanno *et al.*, 2005b), perhaps because the self is construed in connection to the broader community. By contrast, Americans bereaved persons who report a continuing bond to the deceased tend to do quite poorly (Bonanno *et al.*, 2005a), underlining the cultural imperative of a more individualistic society. These findings are consistent with the notion that adaptation may be linked to normative cultural values regarding appropriate grieving and views of the self. Moreover, these data raise the intriguing question of whether resilience has different meanings in different cultural contexts or, perhaps even more intriguing, whether different cultures may learn from each other about effective and not so effective ways of coping with extreme adversity.

References

Bauer, J. J. & Bonanno, G. A. (2001). I can, I do, I am: The narrative differentiation of self-efficacy and other self-evaluations while adapting to bereavement. *Journal of Research in Personality*, **35**, 424–448.

Boelen, P. A., van den Hout, M. A., & van den Bout, J. (2006a). A cognitive-behavioral conceptualization of complicated grief. *Clinical Psychology: Science and Practice*, **13**, 109–128.

Boelen, P. A., van den Bout, J., & van den Hout, M. A. (2006b). Negative cognitions and avoidance in emotional problems after bereavement: A prospective study. *Behaviour Research and Therapy*, **44**, 1657–1672.

Bonanno, G. A. (2004). Loss, trauma, and human resilience: Have we underestimated the human capacity to thrive after extremely aversive events? *American Psychologist*, **59**, 20–28.

Bonanno, G. A. & Kaltman, S. (2001). The varieties of grief experience. *Clinical Psychology Review*, **21**, 705–734.

Bonanno, G. A. & Keltner, D. (1997). Facial expressions of emotion and the course of conjugal bereavement. *Journal of Abnormal Psychology*, **106**, 126–137.

Bonanno, G. A. & Mancini, A. D. (2008). The human capacity to thrive in the face of potential trauma. *Pediatrics*, **121**, 369–375.

Bonanno, G. A., Keltner, D., Holen, A., & Horowitz, M. J. (1995). When avoiding unpleasant emotions might not be such a bad thing: Verbal–autonomic response dissociation and midlife conjugal bereavement. *Journal of Personality and Social Psychology*, **69**, 975–989.

Bonanno, G. A., Znoj, H., Siddique, H. I., & Horowitz, M. J. (1999). Verbal–autonomic dissociation and adaptation to midlife conjugal loss: A follow-up at 25 months. *Cognitive Therapy & Research*, **23**, 605–624.

Bonanno, G. A., Wortman, C. B., Lehman, D. R., *et al.* (2002). Resilience to loss and chronic grief: A prospective study from preloss to 18-months postloss. *Journal of Personality and Social Psychology*, **83**, 1150–1164.

Bonanno, G. A., Wortman, C. B., & Nesse, R. M. (2004a). Prospective patterns of resilience and maladjustment during widowhood. *Psychology and Aging*, **19**, 260–271.

Bonanno, G. A., Papa, A., Lalande, K., Westphal, M., & Coifman, K. (2004b). The importance of being flexible: The ability to both enhance and suppress emotional expression predicts long-term adjustment. *Psychological Science*, **15**, 482–487.

Bonanno, G. A., Moskowitz, J. T., Papa, A., & Folkman, S. (2005a). Resilience to loss in bereaved spouses, bereaved parents, and bereaved gay men. *Journal of Personality and Social Psychology*, **88**, 827–843.

Bonanno, G. A., Papa, A., Lalande, K., Nanping, Z., & Noll, J. G. (2005b). Grief processing and deliberate grief avoidance: A prospective comparison of bereaved spouses and parents in the United States and the People's Republic of China. *Journal of Consulting and Clinical Psychology*, **73**, 86–98.

Bonanno, G. A., Galea, S., Bucciarelli, A., & Vlahov, D. (2006). Psychological resilience after disaster: New York City in the aftermath of the September 11th terrorist attack. *Psychological Science*, **17**, 181–186.

Bonanno, G. A., Neria, Y., Mancini, A., *et al.* (2007). Is there more to complicated grief than depression and posttraumatic stress disorder? A test of incremental validity. *Journal of Abnormal Psychology*, **116**, 342–351.

Bonanno, G. A., Ho, S. M. Y., Chan, J. C., *et al.* (2008). Psychological resilience and dysfunction among hospitalized survivors of the SARS epidemic in Hong Kong: A latent class approach. *Health Psychology*, **27**, 659–667.

Bowlby, J. (1980). *Attachment and loss.* New York: Basic Books.

Brickman, P. & Campbell, D. T. (1971). Hedonic relativism and planning the good society. In M. H. Appley (ed.), *Adaptation level theory: A symposium* (pp. 287–302). New York: Academic Press.

Capps, L. & Bonanno, G. A. (2000). Narrating bereavement: Thematic and grammatical predictors of adjustment to loss. *Discourse Processes*, **30**, 1–25.

Carr, D., House, J. S., Wortman, C., Neese, R., & Kessler, R. C. (2001). Psychological adjustment to sudden and anticipated spousal loss among older widowed persons. *Journals of Gerontology* **56B**, S237–S248.

Coyne, J. C., Wortman, C. B., & Lehman, D. R. (1988). The other side of support: Emotional overinvolvement and miscarried helping. In B. H. Gottlieb (ed.), *Marshaling social support: Formats, processes, and effects* (pp. 305–330). Thousand Oaks, CA: Sage.

Currier, J. M., Neimeyer, R. A., & Berman, J. S. (2008). The effectiveness of psychotherapeutic interventions for bereaved persons: A comprehensive quantitative review. *Psychological Bulletin*, **134**, 648–661.

Cushman, P. (1990). Why the self is empty: Toward a historically situated psychology. *American Psychologist*, **45**, 599–611.

DeRoon-Cassini, T., Mancini, A. D., Bonanno, G. A., & Rusch, M. (2010). Psychopathology and resilience following traumatic injury: a latent growth mixture model analysis. *Rehabilitation Psychology*, **55**, 1–11.

Ehlers, A. (2006). Understanding and treating complicated grief: What can we learn from posttraumatic stress disorder? *Clinical Psychology: Science and Practice*, **13**, 135–140.

Fraley, R. C. & Shaver, P. R. (1999). Loss and bereavement: Attachment theory and recent controversies concerning "grief work" and the nature of detachment. In J. Cassidy & P. R. Shaver (eds.), *Handbook of attachment: Theory, research, and clinical applications* (pp. 735–759). New York: Guilford Press.

Freud, S. (1957). Mourning and melancholia. In J. Strachey (ed.), *The standard edition of the complete psychological works of Sigmund Freud,* Vol. 14 (pp. 152–170). London: Hogarth Press.

Gross, J. J. & John, O. P. (2003). Individual differences in two emotion regulation processes: Implications for affect, relationships, and well-being. *Journal of Personality and Social Psychology*, **85**, 348–362.

Horowitz, M. J. (1986). *Stress response syndromes,* 2nd edn. Northvale, NJ: Jason Aronson.

Horowitz, M. J., Siegel, B., Holen, A., *et al.* (1997). Diagnostic criteria for complicated grief disorder. *American Journal of Psychiatry*, **154**, 904–910.

Irwin, M. R. & Pike, J. (1993). Bereavement, depressive symptoms, and immune function. In M. S. Stroebe, W. Stroebe, & R. O. Hansson (eds.), *Handbook of bereavement: Theory, research, and intervention* (pp. 160–171). Cambridge, UK: Cambridge University Press.

Irwin, M. R., Daniels, M., Weiner, H., *et al.* (1987). Immune and neuroendocrine changes during bereavement. *Psychiatric Clinics of North America*, **10**, 449–465.

Kaltman, S. & Bonanno, G. A. (2003). Trauma and bereavement: Examining the impact of sudden and violent deaths. *Journal of Anxiety Disorders*, **17**, 131–147.

Kaprio, J., Koskenvuo, M., & Rita, H. (1987). Mortality after bereavement: A prospective study of 95 647 bereaved persons. *American Journal of Public Health*, **77**, 283–287.

Kelly, A. E. & McKillop, K. J. (1996). Consequences of revealing personal secrets. *Psychological Bulletin*, **120**, 450–465.

Keltner, D. (1997). Signs of appeasement: Evidence for the distinct displays of embarrassment, amusement, and shame. In P. Ekman & E. L. Rosenberg (eds.), *What the face reveals: Basic and applied studies of spontaneous expression using the Facial Action Coding System (FACS)* (pp. 133–160). London: Oxford University Press.

Keltner, D. & Bonanno, G. A. (1997). A study of laughter and dissociation: Distinct correlates of laughter and smiling during bereavement. *Journal of Personality and Social Psychology*, **73**, 687–702.

Kim, K. & Jacobs, S. C. (1993). Neuroendocrine changes in bereavement. In M. S. Stroebe, W. Stroebe, & R. O. Hansson (eds.), *Handbook of bereavement: Theory, research, and intervention* (pp. 143–159). Cambridge, UK: Cambridge University Press.

Lehman, D. R., Wortman, C. B., & Williams, A. F. (1987). Long-term effects of losing a spouse or child in a motor vehicle crash. *Journal of Personality and Social Psychology*, **52**, 218–231.

Lichtenthal, W. G., Cruess, D. G., & Prigerson, H. G. (2004). A case for establishing complicated grief as a distinct mental disorder in DSM-V. *Clinical Psychology Review*, **24**, 637–662.

Lindemann, E. (1944). Symptomatology and management of acute grief. *American Journal of Psychiatry*, **101**, 141–149.

Mancini, A. D. & Bonanno, G. A. (2006). Resilience in the face of potential trauma: Clinical practices and illustrations. *Journal of Clinical Psychology*, **62**, 971–985.

Mancini, A. D., Bonanno, G. A., & Clark, A. (2011). Stepping off the hedonic treadmill: latent class analyses of individual differences in response to major life events. *Journal of Individual Differences*, in press.

Middleton, W., Moylan, A., Raphael, B., Burnett, P., & Martinek, N. (1993). An international perspective on bereavement related concepts. *Australian and New Zealand Journal of Psychiatry*, **27**, 457–463.

Muthén, B. (2004). Latent variable analysis: Growth mixture modeling and related techniques for longitudinal data. In D. Kaplan (ed.), *Handbook of quantitative methodology for the social sciences* (pp. 345–368). Newbury Park, CA: Sage.

Nolen-Hoeksema, S., McBride, A., & Larson, J. (1997). Rumination and psychological distress among bereaved partners. *Journal of Personality and Social Psychology*, **72**, 855–862.

Osterweis, M., Solomon, F., & Green, F. (1984). *Bereavement: Reactions, consequences, and care*. Washington, DC: National Academy Press.

Park, C. L., Edmondson, D., Fenster, J. R., & Blank, T. O. (2008). Meaning making and psychological adjustment following cancer: The mediating roles of growth, life meaning, and restored just-world beliefs. *Journal of Consulting and Clinical Psychology*, **76**, 863–875.

Parkes, C. M. (1970). The first year of bereavement: a longitudinal study of the reaction of London widows to the death of their husbands. *Psychiatry*, **33**, 444–467.

Parkes, C. M. & Weiss, R. S. (1983). *Recovery from bereavement*. New York: Basic Books.

Prigerson, H. G., Maciejewski, P. K., Reynolds, C. F. 3rd, *et al.* (1995). Inventory of Complicated Grief: A scale to measure maladaptive symptoms of loss. *Psychiatry Research*, **59**, 65–79.

Prigerson, H. G., Bierhals, A. J., Kasl, S. V., *et al.* (1996). Complicated grief as a disorder distinct from bereavement-related depression and anxiety: A replication study. *American Journal of Psychiatry,* **153**, 1484–1486.

Raphael, B. (1983). *Recovery from bereavement*. New York: Basic Books.

Shedler, J., Mayman, M., & Manis, M. (1993). The illusion of mental health. *American Psychologist*, **48**, 1117–1131.

Shuchter, S. R. & Zisook, S. (1993). The course of normal grief. In M. S. Stroebe, W. Stroebe, & R. O. Hansson (eds.), *Handbook of bereavement: Theory, research, and intervention* (pp. 23–43). Cambridge, UK: Cambridge University Press.

Stroebe, M. S. & Stroebe, W. (1993). The mortality of bereavement: A review. In M. S. Stroebe, W. Stroebe, & R. O. Hansson (eds.), *Handbook of bereavement: Theory, research, and intervention* (pp. 175–195). Cambridge, UK: Cambridge University Press.

Thompson, L. W., Breckenridge, J. N., Gallagher, D., *et al.* (1984). Effects of bereavement on self-perceptions of physical health in elderly widows and widowers. *Journal of Gerontology*, **39**, 309–314.

Tudiver, F., Hilditch, J., Permaul, J. A., *et al.* (1991). A comparison of psychosocial characteristics of new widowers and married men. *Family Medicine*, **23**, 501–505.

Wortman, C. B. & Silver, R. C. (2001). The myths of coping with loss revisited. In M. S. Stroebe, R. O. Hansson, W. Stroebe & H. Schut (eds.), *Handbook of bereavement research: Consequences, coping, and care* (pp. 405–429). Washington, DC: American Psychological Press.

Zisook, S. & Shuchter, S. R. (1993). Major depression associated with widowhood. *American Journal of Geriatric Psychiatry*, **1**, 316–326.

Zisook, S., Shuchter, S. R., Irwin, M., & Darko, D. F. (1994). Bereavement, depression, and immune function. *Psychiatry Research*, **52**, 1–10.

Zisook, S., Chentsova-Dutton, Y., & Shuchter, S. R. (1998). PTSD following bereavement. *Annals of Clinical Psychiatry*, **10**, 157–163.

Chapter

14

Reorienting resilience: adapting resilience for post-disaster research

Jennifer Johnson and Sandro Galea

Introduction

The past few years have seen an increase in research interest about resilience after specific traumatic events. One of the more interesting developments in the peer-reviewed literature about the topic is a broadening of the term "resilience," extending it from its original formulation pertaining to individual experiences and individual reactions (Bonanno, 2004; Butler *et al.*, 2007; de Mel *et al.*, 2008; Ganzel *et al.*, 2008) to considerations of populations or groups who collectively experience traumatic events (Bruneau *et al.*, 2003; Kendra & Wachtendorf, 2003; Vale & Campanella, 2005; Norris *et al.*, 2008). This chapter focuses on the particular challenges that arise when considering resilience of communities in the context of collectively experienced traumatic events, typically called disasters. This extension is referred to as a "multilevel" conception of resilience, recognizing that in this formulation resilience is both an "individual level" and a "community level" phenomenon.

Although the term disaster represents a broad range of human experiences, disasters have in common their disruption of collectively experienced normal life. This chapter first briefly introduces disaster public health research before going on to discuss the origins and application of resilience as a multilevel concept. A perspective is offered on the meaning and uses of resilience in disaster research and the challenges of applying the concept of multilevel resilience to disaster settings. This is followed by a brief review of the special challenges disasters pose across the multiple levels of human organization – from the molecular to the ecological. Finally, resilience is reoriented in terms of disasters and future research directions are suggested within this rapidly evolving and dynamic concept.

Disaster research

This section introduces and orients readers who are not familiar with the disaster literature. Disasters are quite common occurrences worldwide. It is estimated that nearly 500 disasters occur every year (excluding droughts and war) in which around 50 000 people die, 74 000 are injured, 5 million are displaced, and 80 million are affected (Norris *et al.*, 2005). Norris (2005, p. 141) aptly describes the challenges that disasters pose: "For the survivors, disasters may engender an array of stressors, including threat to one's life and physical integrity, exposure to the dead and dying, bereavement, profound loss, social and community disruption, and ongoing hardship."

Disasters are costly – both in terms of human life (Figure 14.1) and financial loss (Figure 14.2). This is illustrated with two examples of the financial and life losses in two very different disasters. The Indian Ocean tsunami of 2004 caused around 230 000 deaths and material loss in excess of US$10 billion, not counting the indirect costs, clean-up, or the cost of morbidity and mortality (Smolka, 2006). The tsunami had an impact on countries more than 5 000 km away from its source (United Nations Office for the Coordination of Humanitarian Affairs, 2005). Less than one year after the tsunami, Hurricane Katrina struck the US Gulf Coast, resulting in an estimated 1800 known fatalities (Knabb *et al.*, 2005) and an estimated total economic loss of $125 billion (Risk Management Solutions, 2005). The damages from this disaster were far reaching, including impaired oil-refining capacity through destroyed oil rigs, destruction of transportation arteries through damaged bridges and roads, and displacement for thousands of residents into shelter or temporary housing (Knabb *et al.*, 2005). Although these two settings and disasters are very different, the

Resilience and Mental Health: Challenges Across the Lifespan, ed. Steven M. Southwick, Brett T. Litz, Dennis Charney, and Matthew J. Friedman. Published by Cambridge University Press. © Cambridge University Press 2011.

loss experienced in each will impact affected individuals and the communities for generations to come.

Of particular concern, the rate and cost of disasters have increased in the last half-century. The Center for Research on the Epidemiology of Disasters reports an increase in the number of natural disasters since the early 1980s, particularly for hydrological and meteorological disaster types (Scheuren *et al.*, 2008). Figure 14.1 shows a breakdown of the number of natural disasters by number of victims from 1987 to 2006; the number of disasters increases for each category over this period (Hoyois *et al.*, 2007). Smolka (2006) showed an increase in economic and insured losses from natural disasters from 1950 to 2005, even after adjusting for inflation (Figure 14.2).

The increases in occurrence and cost of natural disasters are likely caused by a combination of factors: concentration of populations in urban areas (Klein *et al.*, 2003; Smolka, 2006; James *et al.*, 2008), development of risky coastal/valley regions (Smolka, 2006; James *et al.*, 2008), increasing complexity of modern societies and technology (Smolka, 2006), and global warming/climate change (Klein *et al.*, 2003; Smolka, 2006; James *et al.*, 2008). Human settlement in hazardous areas often destroys local ecosystems that act as protection against natural disasters (Mileti, 1999). Moreover, some hazard mitigation efforts only postpone the inevitable and often put more life and property at risk when the eventual event occurs (Mileti, 1999). In addition, the increasing reliance on and interconnectedness of

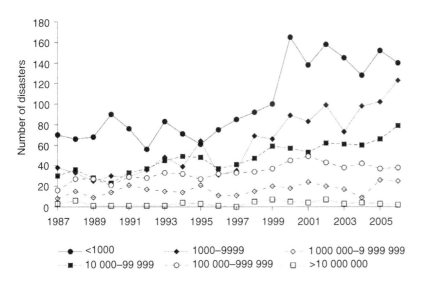

Figure 14.1 Number of natural disasters by number of victims. (Based on Figure 10 in Hoyois *et al.*, 2007. Reproduced with permission from EM-DAT: The OFDA/CRED International Disaster Database – Université catholique de Louvain – Brussels (www.emdat.be).)

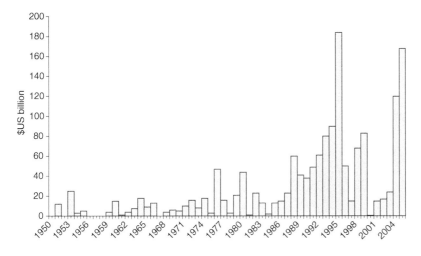

Figure 14.2 Economic losses from large-scale natural disasters 1950–2005, adjusted for inflation. (Reproduced, with permission, from figure 1, Smolka, 2006.)

technology puts the world at far greater risk of severe damage from technological disasters (Mitchell & Townsend, 2005). For example, the Nimda computer virus, which struck 85 000 servers worldwide about one week after the September 11, 2001 (9/11) terrorist attack, led to far more Internet congestion, outages, and economic damage than the infrastructure damage from the 9/11 terrorist attacks (Mitchell & Townsend, 2005).

The incidence and consequences of disasters are far from equally distributed across regions of the world. Asian nations, particularly population-dense India and China, were the hardest hit by natural disasters in 2007, representing 37% of reported natural disasters, 90% of reported victims, and 46% of economic damages from natural disasters (Scheuren et al., 2008). India and China both ranked in the highest 10 countries for number of disasters, number of disaster deaths, and economic damages from disaster in 2006 as well (Hoyois et al., 2007). In addition to death and financial cost, disasters are often associated with psychopathology for exposed individuals. The severity of psychological impairment following natural disasters is higher in less wealthy nations than in more wealthy ones, while the pattern of impairment severity following technological disasters is the opposite (Norris et al., 2002).

Disaster research in public health aims to identify the short- and long-term outcomes of disasters as well as the distribution of those outcomes in populations. Disaster research is heavily informed by disasters occurring in more wealthy nations. A recent meta-analysis on behavioral health outcomes following terrorist events found 88 of 111 published articles on this topic were in North American populations, while only 5 of 227 worldwide terrorist incidents were located in North America (DiMaggio & Galea, 2006). Of 160 articles on psychosocial consequences of disasters reviewed by Norris and colleagues (2002), 91 (57%) were from the USA and territories, 46 (29%) from other wealthy countries, and 23 (14%) were from less wealthy nations. Disaster research is also unequally distributed by disaster type. In the Norris review, over 55% of the published literature was on the consequences of natural disasters, 34% on technological disasters, and 11% on mass violence (Norris et al., 2002). This is likely a reflection of the frequency of disaster occurrence, the severity of consequences, and the media attention and public awareness of each type of event (e.g., a drought versus a bombing).

For a number of reasons, disaster research is less empirically informed than many other fields of research today. Abramson and colleagues (2007) conducted an assessment of medical and public health literature on disasters, finding 32% of articles to be reviews or commentary, 24% case studies, 12.2% surveys, 8.3% program or policy evaluation, 6.6% quasi-experimental/observational, 6.6% secondary data analysis, and less than 10% key informant interview, clinical trial, epidemiological investigation, operational research, or focus group. In summary, these authors found about as much review and commentary on the subject as original research. Disasters are particularly difficult to study for a number of reasons. Most disasters are unanticipated, yet study planning, institutional review board approvals, and funding all take time to obtain. In addition, existing records may be damaged in the disaster and records taken just after the disaster may be of far lower quality owing to confusion and lack of coordination in an overwhelmed system. Lastly, research in less wealthy nations may be challenged by lack of ongoing surveillance and lack of existing health infrastructure.

Resilience: origins of a multilevel concept

The concept of resilience has gained much momentum since the late 1990s. With roots in the engineering field, the term has come to represent individual psychological, family, social, and ecological processes. Below, we briefly review the origins of resilience and highlight its importance as a multilevel concept in disaster research.

Resilience began as a technical engineering concept meaning the speed of return to equilibrium after displacement (Bodin & Wiman, 2004) or the "ability to store strain energy and deflect elastically under a load without breaking or being deformed" (Gordon, 1978, p 129). While this definition is specific and easily defined and measured, it has limited applicability to human systems, which are both proactive and reactive, have multiple possible equilibrium states, and evolve over time.

Ecological definitions of resilience vary. Holling defined resilience as the persistence of a system and its ability to absorb disturbance without damaging or altering the relationships within it (Holling, 1973). Klein and colleagues (2003, p. 40) defined resilience by two components: "the amount of disturbance a system can absorb and still remain within the same state or domain of attraction and the degree to which the system is capable of self-organization." These definitions are applicable to human systems in that they allow for multiple stable states and for a dynamic, evolving system. In addition, they define the system's resilience through its relationships, rather than physical properties, further increasing applicability and relevance to human populations.

In medicine, the term resilience was originally co-opted by developmental psychologists and used to describe children who, despite adverse genetic or environmental conditions, exceeded expectations of psychological adaptation and wellness (Butler et al., 2007). At its most extreme, resilience has been suggested to be synonymous with invulnerability (Rutter, 1993). Applied to broader psychology, resilience has been defined as the ability to endure temporary upheaval with no apparent disruption in ability to function at work or in relationships (Bonanno, 2004). Bonanno articulated a trajectory of resilience that is distinct from recovery, where temporary psychopathology follows trauma and is gradually overcome. Egeland and colleagues (1993) defined resilience as a process: "the development of competence despite severe or pervasive adversity." These definitions of resilience are specific to human psychology and easily measured by various pre-ordained levels of functioning or competence (e.g., hours worked, quality of life). However, this definition does not allow for the multiple possible equilibrium states in community or group systems. Nor does it adequately capture community factors or feedback between multiple actors.

Community resilience, a relatively new concept, is gaining in importance in disaster research today. Like Egeland, Norris and colleagues (2008, p. 131) defined community resilience as a process rather than an outcome: "a process of linking a set of adaptive capacities to a positive trajectory of functioning and adaptation in constituent populations after disturbance." Mileti (1999, p. 4) described a similar concept, "Sustainability means that a locality can tolerate – and overcome – damage, diminished productivity, and reduced quality of life from an extreme event without significant outside assistance." This conceptualization of resilience examines the function of systemic features, rather than individual features, making it a potentially very useful concept for the purposes of identifying potential avenues for community-level intervention. However, the expansion of resilience to consider disaster-affected populations faces a number of challenges that we will return to below.

The use and meaning of the concept of resilience in disaster research

The concept of resilience is important in disaster research for a number of reasons. First, a return to normalcy is appropriate and unambiguously desirable in many post-disaster contexts. The infrastructure and institutions of a community, including such things as electricity, clean water, gas, sewage, and health services, are often easily objectified and measured in both pre- and post-disaster setting. They are also related to an issue that individual members of the community are most concerned with: is it safe to go home? Return to normalcy has profound importance in terms of individuals' outlooks on life (de Mel et al., 2008), daily functioning (Jordan et al., 2004), and work performance (Boscarino et al., 2006).

The concept of resilience may also serve a functional purpose. As Vale and Campanella (2005, p. 340), noted, "In a sense, the notion of a resilient city is a societally and economically productive form of denial." The denial of pathology following disaster may pave the way for the return of investment in a community on all levels. Former Federal Emergency Management Agency administrator James Lee Witt is quoted as saying, "all disasters are political" (Abramson et al., 2007). Demonstration of resilience may be an end in and of itself, particularly where administrators need to prove their worth.

When the salience of the resilience concept in both social and political terms is recognized, it is then not surprising that resilience has tremendous utility in both disaster research and disaster planning. Two key works in the area are those of Norris and colleagues (2008) and Bruneau and colleagues (2003). Norris et al. (2008) discusses how disasters, in addition to shocking the system often simultaneously damage the very resources necessary for a resilient response. Bruneau and colleagues (2003, pp. 737–738) outlined four characteristics thought to predict community resilience: "ability to withstand a given level of stress or demand without suffering degradation or loss of function" (robustness), "the extent to which elements, systems, or other units of analysis exist that are substitutable" (redundancy), "the capacity to identify problems, establish priorities, and mobilize resources when conditions exist that threaten to disrupt some element" (resourcefulness), and "the capacity to meet priorities and achieve goals in a timely manner in order to contain losses and avoid future disruption" (rapidity). Although the utility of a resourcefulness factor has recently been challenged in the prediction of community resilience, the other three have become generally accepted in recent literature on the subject (Norris *et al.*, 2008).

Bruneau *et al.* (2003) continued to specify examples of these measures, such as partial power restored to households within one hour, for social performance of rapidity. Other factors are more challenging to evaluate (operationalize, quantify, and judge) in the post-disaster setting. Moreover, disaster planners are ideally interested in the effectiveness of pre-disaster community characteristics to predict post-disaster resilience. To continue the example above, what pre-disaster aspects of a community's social infrastructure make power restoration within one hour post-disaster possible? While more empiric evidence is needed to inform disaster planning efforts, these are clearly very good places to start.

Disasters as a special challenge to multiple levels of functioning

Unlike many traumatic events, disasters act all at once on individuals, families, and communities. This section of the chapter provides a brief overview of the multilevel consequences of disasters that challenge our multilevel concept of resilience. Disaster threats to the individual include direct threat of injury and death, physiological changes, mental health consequences, and indirect and ongoing risk of injury. Threats to the family include property loss and financial/employment concerns. Threats to the community include cultural/identity conceptualization, economic, and political concerns.

Physical health

Disasters are often characterized by their capacity for causing mass injury and death. For those who have perished, resilience is moot. Direct threat of death and injury depends on disaster type (Llewellyn, 2006), timing, and severity (Peleg *et al.*, 2002), as well as individual circumstances such as proximity, location, and quality of infrastructure (Peleg *et al.*, 2002). Risk of injury or death also depend on demographic characteristics, where those with lower power and resources are generally at highest risk of an adverse event, for example

women, children, and the elderly (Nishikiori *et al.*, 2006), and people with mental disorders, physical disabilities, recent hospitalization, or low income (Chou *et al.*, 2004). Because of the unexpected nature of many disasters, individuals are unable to control their exposure to many of these risk factors for death and injury. Survivors with permanent injuries may have ongoing medical needs (Rathore *et al.*, 2007; Tauqir *et al.*, 2007) and resilience means moving on in the face of disability, where a "return to normalcy" may not be possible.

Disaster-related stress is associated with physiological and anatomical changes in survivors. Exposure to the Oklahoma City bombing was associated with neurological reactivity six to seven years later (Tucker *et al.*, 2007). Three to four years after the 9/11 terrorist attacks, proximity to the attacks was associated with gray matter volume changes in brain areas related to mental disorders (Ganzel *et al.*, 2008). Animal models support the role of stress-induced brain changes (Helmreich *et al.*, 1999). Disaster exposure is also associated with short-term death from cardiac conditions (Leor *et al.*, 1996; Gold *et al.*, 2007); higher resting heart rate, serum cholesterol, and triglycerides (Trevisan *et al.*, 1992); and long-term higher resting heart rate (Bland *et al.*, 2000) and serum uric acid levels (Trevisan *et al.*, 1997), particularly for individuals who have lost financial or social resources in the disaster (Trevisan *et al.*, 1997; Bland *et al.*, 2000). Exposure to disasters in utero is associated with changes to the adult physiological profile, including cortisol and testosterone levels (Huizink *et al.*, 2008), glucose tolerance, atherogenic lipid profile, and fibrinogen concentrations (Roseboom *et al.*, 2001). In these ways, disaster-associated stress may have long-term or lifelong impacts, even generations later.

Psychological health

The psychological impacts of disasters are often more heterogeneous, widespread, and longer lasting than their physical impact. Vicarious grief after disasters is disproportionate to their burden, compared with more chronic problems of disease or malnutrition (Chochinov, 2005). Mental health problems following disasters have been reported by those directly affected (e.g., injured [Hoven *et al.*, 2003] or relocated [Soeteman *et al.*, 2007]), those indirectly affected (e.g., witnessing burial of corpses [Ghaffari-Nejad *et al.*, 2007]), and those unaffected or vicariously affected by disaster (e.g., living in the same country [Silver *et al.*,

2002] or exposed to the media [Wayment, 2004]). Specific mental health outcomes following disaster include post-traumatic stress disorder (Galea *et al.*, 2005), depression (Armenian *et al.*, 2002; Bromet & Havenaar, 2007), anxiety (Grievink *et al.*, 2007), sleep problems (Dirkzwager *et al.*, 2006; Grievink *et al.*, 2007), behavioral problems (Reijneveld *et al.*, 2003; Chemtob *et al.*, 2008), suicidality (Chou *et al.*, 2003; Loganovsky *et al.*, 2008), and decreased quality of life (Wang *et al.*, 2000; Slottje *et al.*, 2007).

The trajectory of mental illness following disasters is tremendously heterogeneous and may last years to decades (Thomas, 2006; Chou *et al.*, 2007; Tucker *et al.*, 2007; Loganovsky *et al.*, 2008). Mental health trajectory following a disaster may be influenced by other forms of recovery (e.g., financial [Nandi *et al.*, 2004]); perceived support (Tang, 2007); demographic factors such as age, race, gender, or education level (Bonanno *et al.*, 2007); recent or past life stressors (Bonanno *et al.*, 2007); genetic background (Kilpatrick *et al.*, 2007); or time alone (de Mel *et al.*, 2008). As with risk for physical harm, the probability of a resilient trajectory of mental health is influenced by many factors outside individual control.

Environmental health

In addition to the direct risk of physical injury and death, disasters may also produce environmental conditions with protracted or even delayed health impact. Reduced air quality is associated with worsening or new respiratory complaints following volcanic eruptions (Michaud *et al.*, 2004; Shimizu *et al.*, 2007), forest fires (Moore *et al.*, 2006), haze disasters (Kunii *et al.*, 2002), and bombing incidents (Lioy *et al.*, 2002). Mold following hurricanes and flood disasters may result in infections and allergic or hypersensitivity reactions (Metts, 2008). Reduced water quality following storms and flooding may be associated with an increased incidence of infectious disease (Kondo *et al.*, 2002). Industrial disasters may cause soil contamination and bioaccumulation (Meharga *et al.*, 1999). Agricultural contamination with radioactive substances may find its way into milk and foodstuffs, wood, mushrooms, berries, and game (Alexakhin *et al.*, 2007). After Chernobyl, consumption of agricultural foodstuffs from the affected region was a leading source of accidental irradiation (Alexakhin *et al.*, 2007). These few examples provide a brief glimpse of the environmental challenges to health resilience that disasters pose

through their persistence, lack of individual control over exposure, and their delayed or unanticipated impact. These indirect risks may also exact a toll on psychological well-being.

Rescue and clean-up operations

In order to respond adaptively to disaster, communities must mobilize rescue and clean-up personnel. Yet these same people that lead a community to a resilient response are, themselves, at a higher risk for persistent physical and psychological impairment. The impact on rescue and clean-up personnel is highlighted because they are part of a resilient response and, at the same time, prone to negative outcomes as individuals. Of the 2801 people killed in the 9/11 terrorist attacks, 343 were fire and 60 law enforcement personnel (14%) (Bradt, 2003). Time spent on the disaster scene has been associated with occupational exposure and symptomology, often in a dose–response manner (Feldman *et al.*, 2004). Rescue and clean-up personnel may also be exposed to unusual industrial chemicals (e.g., petrofluorochemicals used in fire-fighting foams [Tao *et al.*, 2008]). Disaster-associated exposures may lead to chronic health problems for rescue and clean-up personnel. For example, rescue and police officers responding to the Tokyo subway sarin attack showed chronic problems, with memory decline three to four years later in a dose–response manner with exposure level (Nishiwaki *et al.*, 2001). One year after the 9/11 terrorist attacks, workers showed lung function decline equivalent to 12 years of age-related decline (Banauch *et al.*, 2006). In addition to short- and long-term physical risks, rescue and clean-up workers have shown excess risk of suicide (Rahu *et al.*, 1997), chronic anxiety, depression, somatic symptoms, obsessive–compulsive symptoms, interpersonal sensitivity, hostility, and sleeping problems (Huizink *et al.*, 2006). While rescue and clean-up workers are essential to disaster response and recovery, they bear a great challenge to their individual health resilience in that their exposure far exceeds that of most bystanders and may continue for months or years after the disaster.

Displacement

Displacement is a far more common direct consequence of disasters than death or injury. Loss of shelter leaves people vulnerable to disease (Kondo *et al.*, 2002) and heat or cold (Llewellyn, 2006). Those in temporary living conditions may suffer from chronic undernutrition

(Jayatissa *et al.*, 2006), mental illness, the worsening of chronic diseases, and lack of access to medical care for years after disaster (Shehab *et al.*, 2008). Primary concerns for displaced populations include economic security; physical and economic access to food; relative freedom from disease and infection; access to clean water, air, and non-degraded land; security from violence and threats; security of cultural identity; and protection of their basic human rights (Kett, 2005). Displacement after disaster poses a major challenge to physical and mental well-being; displaced persons have often lost family members and economic resources and are vulnerable to physical and mental health assaults, sometimes over a protracted time period.

Disasters and the family

In addition to the hazards that disasters pose to individuals who come in contact with these events, families also suffer disaster losses that in many ways differ from the losses experienced by individuals. Families suffer property loss after disasters through severe direct damage (Madamala *et al.*, 2007), disaster sequelae (e.g., fires after the Kobe earthquake [Shaw & Goda, 2004]), and post-disaster involuntary resettlement programs (Badri *et al.*, 2006). For small business owners, damage to the workplace predicts non-return (Madamala *et al.*, 2007). Relocation may also be motivated by avoidance of traumatic reminders (Salcoglu *et al.*, 2008). In addition to property, loss of family "irreplaceables" (lost sentimental possessions) is common after disaster (Galea *et al.*, 2008). Family loss is associated with a number of mental health problems, including posttraumatic stress disorder (Armenian *et al.*, 2000; Chou *et al.*, 2007) and suicide (Chou *et al.*, 2003). Even threatened loss is predictive of distress (O'Neill *et al.*, 1999).

Displaced families often have to change their primary source of income, particularly those families originally employed in agriculture or commercial activities (Badri *et al.*, 2006). Families reliant on individuals suffering permanent disaster-related injury may require a substantial transition in employment to maintain their financial security (Gul *et al.*, 2008). Displaced families may be forced to spend more on their households in an unfamiliar environment (Badri *et al.*, 2006). This increased expenditure, combined with job transition and loss of savings, may result in increased borrowing for daily needs and debt. Because property and possessions may be a family's main source of income or form of investment, their loss in disasters often produces profound economic vulnerability.

Disasters and the community: relationships between people and place

In addition to destruction of the physical environment in which communities are situated, disasters pose several challenges to other elements of community, including concepts of identity and relationship with the environment. Disasters may shatter traditional assumptions of security, predictability, and trust (Walsh, 2007). The following quote from a focus group in Tamil Nadu, India following the Indian Ocean tsunami shows how cultural conceptualizations of the relationship between people and nature can be altered by disaster (Rajkumar *et al.*, 2008, p. 847): "We have been taught in our childhood how to survive during storms and cyclones. We would be alert only when we were sailing over the sea. On the shore, we would be relaxed like sleeping in our mother's lap. This is the first time we learned that the sea might hit us even when we are on the shore."

Individual self-assessments of a community's capacity to deal successfully with the ongoing challenge may have an impact on the relationship between disaster threat and mental health of its members (Kimhi & Shamai, 2004).

Post-disaster resettlement and changes in day to day living further disrupt the cultural relationship between people and place (Oliver-Smith, 1991; Dugan, 2007). Temporary living situations that separate disaster survivors from their communities are associated with adverse mental health consequences (Perez-Sales *et al.*, 2005). Interestingly, Perez-Sales and colleagues showed that when emergency shelters organized tent assignment by community of origin, survivors had fewer feelings of humiliation and emotional discomfort. While the preservation of community groups is ideal after disaster, it is not always possible. Challenges to the cultural relationship with place, nature, and people pose serious challenges to the cultural resilience of communities following disaster.

Economic and political impact

Disasters also pose a challenge to the economic and political well-being of communities. Loss of public infrastructure, utilities, and communications following disaster are common challenges to businesses and residents within and around disaster-affected communities (Centers for Disease Control and Prevention, 2006). Restoration of transportation methods, such as railways, roads, and harbors, after disasters is essential to economic restoration and may take years to accomplish (Shaw & Goda, 2004). Shared public resources such as hospitals, universities, and schools are often damaged and are sometimes permanently closed in the wake of disaster (Guidry & Margolis, 2005; Schultz *et al.*, 2007; Ayyala & Sacks, 2008) Lastly, disasters may have large-scale economic and political consequences for entire countries, particularly where they disrupt locations of centralized power (e.g., the Mexico City earthquake [Davis, 2005]).

Relocation caused by disasters disrupts the economic and political relationships between people and place in terms of resource availability, access to employment and labor resources, territoriality, leadership structures, and intergroup relations (Oliver-Smith, 1991). Resettlement also affects the political and economic environment of host communities where displaced persons settle (Badri *et al.*, 2006).

Where disasters are associated with mass demographic shift, they may result in the restructuring of class systems within communities. After the Indian Ocean tsunami, socioeconomic and cultural differences between fisherman and lower castes in India were reduced, because both groups suffered property loss and lived as neighbors in emergency shelters (Rajkumar *et al.*, 2008). In addition, because fishermen were at greater risk of death (Nishikiori *et al.*, 2006), the tsunami resulted in the opening of lucrative fisherman jobs to survivors of lower castes (Rajkumar *et al.*, 2008). After the Manjil earthquake, resettled communities saw an increase in women working outside the home because of a lack of home-related farm work and an overall decreased reliance on agriculture for household income (Badri *et al.*, 2006). Many of these examples showcase the power of disaster-affected communities to adapt through large-scale demographic and economic changes. Community adaptations to altered economic and political circumstances may be delayed, however, by prolonged uncertainty in the aftermath of disaster or reduced overall assets (De Silva & Yamao, 2007).

At other times, disasters may bring to light underlying vulnerability and result in more accurate future estimations of risk. After the 9/11 terrorist attacks, insurance premiums on prominent buildings in New York City increased by as much as 300% as the downtown area was seen as an area of concentrated risk (Vale & Campanella, 2005).

Some measures of economic resilience are fairly intuitive (e.g., return of power, restoration of railway travel), but these measures are by no means comprehensive. The next section reviews the limitations and challenges to applying resilience theory to disaster settings.

Challenges in applying resilience to disasters

The earlier part of this chapter provided a brief introduction to disaster research and looked at the history, uses, and meaning of the term resilience before giving an overview of the dimensions along which disaster disruption acts to challenge individual, family, and community well-being. Yet, adaptation and continued existence are far more common outcomes than extinction following disaster. Clearly, then, resilience is an apposite construct for disaster research. However, thinking of resilience as a multilevel construct poses particular challenges, especially where communities have actually changed shape through drastic demographic shift and physical change to the environment. The expansion of resilience to consider disaster-affected communities is associated with a number of challenges, including (1) the identification of the population of interest, (2) the quantification of "baseline" state, and (3) the measurement of adaptation in a meaningful way. Lastly, this form of resilience is concerned with population-level functioning and is, therefore, potentially insensitive to the heterogeneity of impact among subgroups within the system. These issues are discussed in more detail below.

Defining community

One of the principal challenges faced by the expansion of resilience to a multilevel construction is the definition of community. In social sciences, the community has been defined as a group of people bound by social, functional, cultural, or circumstantial connection (Chaskin, 1997). Communities are dynamic, negotiated, voluntary, and neither totally inclusive nor exclusive (Chaskin, 1997). Norris and colleagues (2008, p. 128) more broadly defined the term "community" to better suit the purposes of community resilience theory: "Communities are composed of built, natural, social, and economic environments that influence one another in complex ways." However, communities may span large geographic regions (e.g., the Jewish-American community). In addition, populations are not merely the sum of individuals, just as population health is not the sum of individual health (Reidpath,

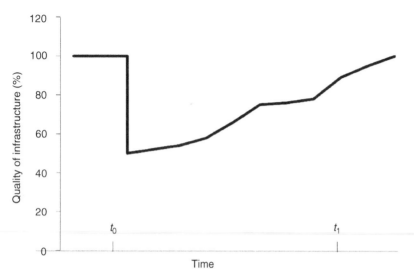

Figure 14.3 Defining baseline as "quality of infrastructure" after disaster. t_0, time of an earthquake when damage to community infrastructure results in a 50% fall; t_1, time at which the community returns to close to 100% quality of infrastructure. (Based on data in Bruneau et al., 2003.)

2005). Lastly, the boundaries that define community are likely to vary from observer to observer.

Compounding these challenges, disasters influence areas that do not necessarily match the boundaries observers may ascribe to communities. For example, injury and death in the Indian Ocean tsunami was multicontinental – including the Seychelles, Maldives, Somalia, India, Bangladesh, Myanmar, Thailand, Malaysia, and Indonesia (United Nations Office for the Coordination of Humanitarian Affairs, 2005). Even when destruction and death are isolated to a single city, the impact may be felt over an entire country. For example, students at Northern Arizona University who experienced no personal bereavement in the 9/11 terrorist attacks showed disaster-focused distress, including grief, survivor guilt, and intrusive thoughts of the disaster (Wayment, 2004). Exposure to media, mediated by perceived similarity to victims, was associated with disaster-focused distress nearly six months after the attacks (Wayment, 2004). Hurricane Katrina caused direct damage to numerous communities in the states of Louisiana and Mississippi, with hurricane-related deaths reported in the parishes of Orleans, St. Bernard, and Jefferson (Brunkard et al., 2008). The majority of deaths occurred in the Orleans parish, specifically in the lower ninth ward, in Lakeview and Gentilly, adjacent to Lake Pontchartrain (Brunkard et al., 2008). The multidimensional impact of Hurricane Katrina crossed state, city, and neighborhood boundaries. Researchers interested in community resilience following disasters are challenged to define their unit of analysis in a meaningful way.

Return to what baseline?

Another challenge in the extension of resilience to the community is the definition of a baseline level of functioning. Bruneau and colleagues (2003) provided a framework for assessing earthquake resilience (Figure 14.3). In this diagram, t_0 is the time of an earthquake when damage to community infrastructure results in a 50% drop. Over time, restoration projects repair the damage and the community returns to 100% quality of infrastructure by time t_1. The authors go on to describe several illustrative performance measures, such as percentage of homes with power immediately after an earthquake and time required to initiate and complete critical response tasks (e.g., fire-fighting, search and rescue).

However, measures of functionality are fundamentally set by an a-priori understanding of "normal" function that frequently are dependent on disciplinary perspectives. For example, economists measure loss to economic output (e.g., Rose, 2006), civil engineers assess transportation network coverage and accessibility (Chang & Nojima, 2001), and religious leaders measure the recovery of faith and spiritual life (Ford et al., 2003). Research on these different community traits may show differential recovery trajectories for the same community. This heterogeneity of recovery path is likely to occur across the multilevel conceptualizations of resilience. For example, recovery of livelihood for individual business owners may not reflect their mental health recovery (de Mel et al., 2008). It is possible that resilience of some types of functionality

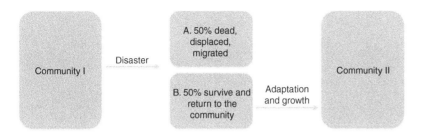

Figure 14.4 Hypothetical extreme flood disaster in Wayne County, MI.

may by asynchronous with, and may even be in contrast to, recovery in other areas.

Resilience for whom?

Further compounding these challenges, a return to a community-wide baseline may actually belie the true heterogeneity of disaster impact on subgroups within the same community. Because resilience relies on the pre-existing resources of a community, the rebound of that community may reflect, or even worsen, pre-existing disparities. Vale and Campanella (2005, pp. 12–13) posed some very difficult questions on this subject:

> What we call 'recovery' is also driven by value-laden questions about equity. Who sets the priorities for the recovering communities? How are the needs of low-income residents valued in relation to the pressing claims of disrupted businesses? Who decides what will be rebuilt where, and which voices carry forth the dominant narratives that interpret what transpires? Who gets displaced when new facilities are constructed in the name of recovery?

Community resilience is fundamentally concerned with the persistence of the system. The processes that lead to system persistence, however, are not universally aligned with resilience processes in individuals or within subgroups of communities. A simplistic, hypothetical example uses an extreme flood disaster in Wayne County, MI (Figure 14.4). After the disaster, 50% of pre-disaster residents have been killed, displaced, or migrated; while 50% of residents survive the disaster and return to the community, adapt, and grow. To what degree do researchers care about those who preserve the system (B) more than those who are no longer contributing to the system (A)? Does it matter what group A individuals are doing now (e.g., contributing to other communities, in temporary housing, dead)? To what degree were the two groups similar or different in the first place? What might determine whether a given individual falls into group A or B? How do we describe the resilience of this community?

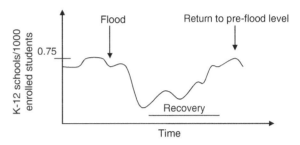

Figure 14.5 Educational system resilience (public schools, K-12) following hypothetical flood disaster in Wayne County, MI.

This example uses a hypothetical number of operational K-12 public schools per 1000 enrolled students in the county as a measure of system functioning (Figure 14.5), based on the Census American Factfinder and Wayne County Regional Educational Service Agency for construction of these data. From the system standpoint, it would appear that the community has responded resiliently, with a return to the pre-flood (baseline) level of education system functioning. When broken down by school district (Figure 14.6), however, we see that the demography of different districts has actually changed. While Detroit and Dearborn display a return to baseline school-to-student ratio after the disaster, many of the families living below poverty simply never moved back to Detroit after the disaster. The number of students decreased by 40 000, and yet the community shows resilience. How should we describe this community's response to disaster? Do those 40 000 students and their families enter our equation?

These questions are related to the more general question of how we wish to use the concept of resilience. If we want to use the term as a theoretical objective – a term used to motivate leaders to make their communities more equitable, diversify their economic base, and cultivate social networks and collective efficacy in the name of disaster preparedness – then its current definition may suffice. However, if we are tempted to use it in an evaluative way to assess how

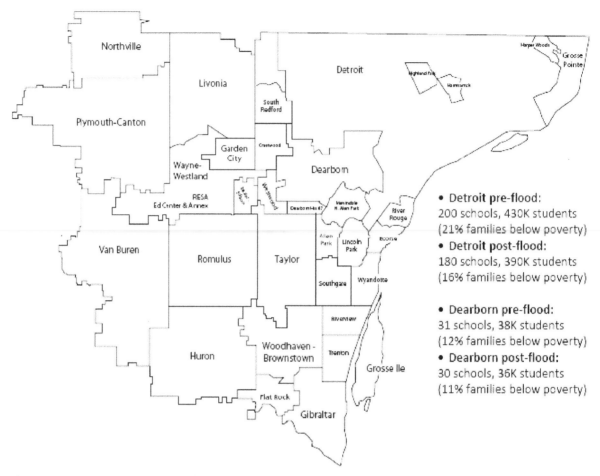

Figure 14.6 Educational system resilience following hypothetical flood disaster in Wayne County, MI by school system. K, indicates 1000.

communities respond to disasters based on measured quantities and qualities of functioning and to inform future responses based on generalizable conclusions, then the operationalization of this concept needs to incorporate a distributional perspective as well as one focused on system wellness.

Hurricane Katrina provides a well-documented example of the devastation disaster causes and the mass population shift that occurs as a result. After its first landfall in Louisiana, Hurricane Katrina moved northeast, making its second landfall in Hancock County, Mississippi, destroying more than a third of homes in the county (Centers for Disease Control and Prevention, 2006). The US Census shows that New Orleans residents who moved after Hurricane Katrina were very different from those who stayed (Figures 14.7 and 14.8; Koerber, 2006). Koerber shows that those who stayed in New Orleans were disproportionately

white, while those who moved were disproportionately black; likewise, the age distribution of residents who stayed and moved were different, with non-movers being older. In other situations, disasters may cause mass resettlement of entire populations. For example, after the Manjil earthquake, residents of two villages, Balklor and Jamal-Abad, were relocated and integrated into a larger village, Ab-Bar, causing dramatic and complex changes to all three groups (Badri *et al.*, 2006).

Just as individual outcomes after disasters are inequitably distributed, this pattern is replicated on a higher level of analysis: "There is never a single, monolithic vox populi that uniformly affirms the adopted resilience narrative in the wake of disaster… marginalized groups or peoples are generally ignored in the narrative construction process" (Vale & Campanella, 2005, p. 341). Just as subcommunities do not have equitably distributed pre-disaster resources, they do not equitably

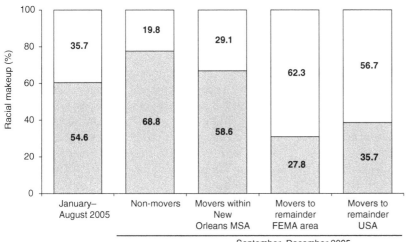

Figure 14.7 Racial makeup of residents in the New Orleans metropolitan statistical area (MSA) before Hurricane Katrina (January–August 2005) and after (September–December 2005). FEMA area, area covered by the Federal Emergency Management Agency. (Based on data in Koerber, 2006.)

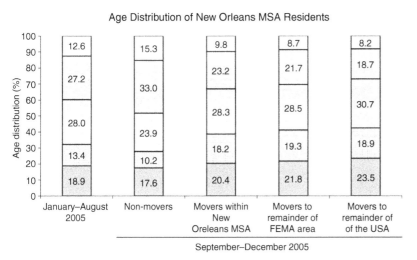

Figure 14.8 Age distribution of residents in the New Orleans metropolitan statistical area (MSA) before Hurricane Katrina (January–August 2005) and after (September–December 2005). FEMA area, area covered by the Federal Emergency Management Agency. (Based on data in Koerber, 2006.)

share disaster impact or resilience processes after disaster. For example, researchers found that a school's probability of being flooded one week after Hurricane Floyd depended on race and income level of students – schools in low-income areas with a majority of black students were twice as likely to be flooded as non-low-income schools with a majority of non-black students (Guidry & Margolis, 2005). In addition to the higher risk of flooding, schools in low-income areas will have fewer resources to deal with the health consequences of flooding, such as respiratory illness.

Defining value-neutral resilience and failure

It has been suggested that disasters are a catalyst for positive social change (Paton, 2006). Others assert that disasters are not usually accompanied by changes to the pre-disaster establishment (Vale & Campanella, 2005). Are there situations where resilience may actually worsen social problems or increase future vulnerability? Many researchers have denounced the utility of a universally positive conceptualization of resilience: "Are cities resilient because their recovery has followed some particular identifiable model, or are they resilient only because interpreters choose to define resilience in such fluid and malleable ways" (Vale & Campanella, 2005, p. 335). For evaluation purposes, we must be equipped with a value-neutral conceptualization of resilience.

Davis (2005) provides a compelling case study on the Mexico City 1985 earthquake: the bulk of damage was located in the city center, including death, injury, and damage to buildings; while disruption of power and telecommunications extended to businesses outside the city. While survivors inside the city had emergency shelter and medical needs, financial and large-scale manufacturers outside the city required phones and electricity to continue business. Davis argued that the city's response prioritized economic and political interests over efforts to provide emergency shelter and medical needs and, later, housing reconstruction for displaced residents. "Their 'resilience' – expressed as an insistence on continuing business as usual – may prevent them from acting in ways that most constructively promote recovery and reconstruction" (Davis, 2005, p. 275). Davis' recognition of a resilient process with both positive and negative consequences for individuals and subgroups is highly unusual in resilience literature. This approach should be encouraged in future research.

Lastly, we suggest that multilevel resilience must be defined in a way that allows for failure. The technical homologue of resilience failure would mean a material that breaks or deforms under strain. Examples of ecological resilience failure include the extinction of a species, a reduction in the diversity of a ecological system, or decreased stability of the system. A psychological homologue of resilience failure would be persistent disruption in quality of life or ability to function. A failure of community resilience would connote a negative trajectory of community functioning and adaptation or increased social vulnerability after disaster. If we want to evaluate the degree to which communities respond with resilience to disaster, we must identify levels of quantifiable characteristics that describe both a resilient and a non-resilient response in meaningful ways.

Reorienting resilience

This chapter has identified some of the major challenges in the application of resilience to disaster settings, particularly for the concept of community resilience. These challenges have led some to question the usefulness of the concept of resilience in context of disasters (Klein *et al.*, 2003). We suggest, however, that disasters expose pre-existing vulnerabilities and capacities of individuals and communities that indeed provide insight about positive trajectories following disruption. The abandonment of disaster resilience as an evaluative construct would result in a missed opportunity for the assessment of disaster preparedness and response. The challenge today is to define resilience as a unified concept that can be used to compare experiences across contexts, despite the heterogeneity of disasters. We propose three main ways forward that may address some of the challenges identified here. We intend these to inform future work in the area and to encourage discussion and debate about ways forward.

First, the community level of analysis is both meaningful and practical in resilience research. However, both communities and disasters are geographically diffuse. In addition, disaster exposure is more dimensional than it is dichotomous. Disaster researchers are challenged to define the boundaries of communities in ways that reflect identity and shared environment, rather than convenience. Research that quantifies individuals as either "affected" or "unaffected" by disaster, usually based on some threshold level of exposure, may contradict the true gradient nature of disasters on populations. Research in this area should aim to identify a simple way to assess disaster impact on individuals and communities across multiple dimensions.

Second, aggregate measures of system performance (e.g., return of water or power) are truly useful qualities for assessing community functioning. A return to aggregate baseline functioning after the disruption of disaster may be an appropriate measure for some dimensions of system resilience. However, aggregate values often belie the differential impact of disasters on subgroups within the community. The concept of community resilience must be sensitive to the heterogeneity of disaster impacts, resilience processes, and outcomes among subgroups within a community while maintaining the assessment of shared, systemic functioning.

Third, the common definition of resilience as a "return to normalcy" is appealing. However, a universally positive conceptualization of resilience is misleading. Where system resources after disaster are meager, different dimensions of system resilience may work in competition with one another. Where one dimension of the community functioning (e.g., economic) is prioritized over other important elements (e.g., temporary housing), demonstrated resilience in that prioritized dimension may belie an increase in overall system vulnerability. The concept of resilience, then, must be both multidimensional and value neutral. In addition, resilience must be defined in a way that allows for failure. If we wish to use resilience as a way to evaluate disaster response, disaster planners and researchers should negotiate concrete, measurable outcomes at each level of a system that indicate successful resilience and define what level of system performance indicates failed resilience.

Conclusions

This chapter has outlined the challenges that disasters pose to the resilience of individuals, families, and communities and discussed the ways in which disasters may transform the way researchers and theorists think about resilience. Three main ways forward were outlined in the hope of inspiring new discourse on this burgeoning topic. Resilience is both theoretically compelling and useful in the field of disaster planning and research. However, much development is needed to truly realize the potential of resilience as an evaluative tool in these fields.

References

Abramson, D. M., Morse, S. S., Garrett, A. L., & Redlener, I. (2007). Public health disaster research: Surveying the field, defining its future. *Disaster Medicine and Public Health Preparedness*, **1**, 57–62.

Alexakhin, R. M., Sanzharova, N. I., Fesenko, S. V., Spiridonov, S. I., & Panov, A. V. (2007). Chernobyl radionuclide distribution, migration, and environmental and agricultural impacts. *Health Physics*, **93**, 418–426.

Armenian, H. K., Morikawa, M., Melkonian, A. K., *et al.* (2000). Loss as a determinant of PTSD in a cohort of adult survivors of the 1988 earthquake in Armenia: Implications for policy. *Acta Psychiatrica Scandinavica*, **102**, 58–64.

Armenian, H. K., Morikawa, M., Melkonian, A. K., *et al.* (2002). Risk factors for depression in the survivors of the 1988 earthquake in Armenia. *Journal of Urban Health: Bulletin of the New York Academy of Medicine*, **79**, 373–382.

Ayyala, R. & Sacks, J. G. (2008). Tulane after Katrina. *Ophthalmology*, **115**, 922–923.

Badri, S. A., Asgary, A., Eftekhari, A. R., & Levy, J. (2006). Post-disaster resettlement, development and change: A case study of the 1990 Manjil earthquake in Iran. *Disasters*, **30**, 451–468.

Banauch, G. I., Hall, C., Weiden, M., *et al.* (2006). Pulmonary function after exposure to the World Trade Center collapse in the New York City fire department. *American Journal of Respiratory and Critical Care Medicine*, **174**, 312–319.

Bland, S. H., Farinaro, E., Krogh, V., *et al.* (2000). Long term relations between earthquake experiences and coronary heart disease risk factors. *American Journal of Epidemiology*, **151**, 1086–1090.

Bodin, P. & Wiman, B. L. B. (2004). Resilience and other stability concepts in ecology: Notes on their origin, validity, and usefulness. *ESS Bulletin*, **2**, 33–43.

Bonanno, G. A. (2004). Loss, trauma, and human resilience: Have we underestimated the human capacity to thrive after extremely aversive events? *American Psychologist*, **59**, 20–28.

Bonanno, G. A., Galea, S., Bucciarelli, A., & Vlahov, D. (2007). What predicts psychological resilience after disaster? The role of demographics, resources, and life stress. *Journal of Consulting and Clinical Psychology*, **75**, 671–682.

Boscarino, J. A., Adams, R. E., & Figley, C. R. (2006). Worker productivity and outpatient service use after the September 11th attacks: Results from the New York City terrorism outcome study. *American Journal of Industrial Medicine*, **49**, 670–682.

Bradt, D. A. (2003). Site management of health issues in the 2001 World Trade Center disaster. *Academic Emergency Medicine*, **10**, 650–660.

Bromet, E. J. & Havenaar, J. M. (2007). Psychological and perceived health effects of the Chernobyl disaster: A 20-year review. *Health Physics*, **93**, 516–521.

Bruneau, M., Chang, S. E., Eguchi, R. T., *et al.* (2003). A framework to quantitatively assess and enhance the seismic resilience of communities. *Earthquake Spectra*, **19**, 733–752.

Brunkard, J., Namulanda, G., & Ratard, R. (2008). Hurricane Katrina deaths, Louisiana, 2005. *Disaster Medicine and Public Health Preparedness*, **2**, 215–223.

Butler, L. D., Morland, L. A., & Leskin, G. A. (2007). Psychological resilience in the face of terrorism. In B. Bongar, L. Brown, L. Beutler, J. Breckenridge & P. Zimbardo (eds.), *Psychology of terrorism* (pp. 400–417). New York: Oxford University Press.

Centers for Disease Control and Prevention (2006). Rapid community needs assessment after Hurricane Katrina: Hancock county, Mississippi, September 14 – 15, 2005. *Morbidity and Mortality Weekly Report*, **55**, 234–236.

Chang, S. E. & Nojima, N. (2001). Measuring post-disaster transportation system performance: The 1995 Kobe earthquake in comparative perspective. *Transportation Research Part A: Policy and Practice*, **35**, 475–494.

Chaskin, R. J. (1997). Perspectives on neighborhood and community: A review of the literature. *Social Science Review*, **71**, 521–547.

Chemtob, C. M., Nomura, Y., & Abramovitz, R. A. (2008). Impact of conjoined exposure to the World Trade Center attacks and to other traumatic events on the behavioral problems of preschool children. *Archives of Pediatrics and Adolescent Medicine*, **162**, 126–133.

Chochinov, H. M. (2005). Vicarious grief and response to global disasters. *Lancet*, **366**, 697–698.

Chou, F. H., Wu, H. C., Chou, P., *et al.* (2007). Epidemiologic psychiatric studies on post-disaster impact among Chi-Chi earthquake survivors in Yu-Chi, Taiwan. *Psychiatry and Clinical Neurosciences*, **61**, 370–378.

Chou, Y. J., Huang, N., Lee, C. H., *et al.* (2003). Suicides after the 1999 Taiwan earthquake. *International Journal of Epidemiology*, **32**, 1007–1014.

Chou, Y. J., Huang, N., Lee, C. H., *et al.* (2004). Who is at risk of death in an earthquake? *American Journal of Epidemiology*, **160**, 688–695.

Davis, D. E. (2005). Reverberations: Mexico city's 1985 earthquake and the transformation of the capital. In L. J. Vale & T. J. Campanella (eds.), *The resilient city: How modern cities recover from disaster* (pp. 255–280). New York: Oxford University Press.

de Mel, S., McKenzie, D., & Woodruff, C. (2008). Mental health recovery and economic recovery after the tsunami: High-frequency longitudinal evidence from Sri Lankan small business owners. *Social Science and Medicine*, **66**, 582–595.

De Silva, D. A. & Yamao, M. (2007). Effects of the tsunami on fisheries and coastal livelihood: A case study of tsunami-ravaged southern Sri Lanka. *Disasters*, **31**, 386–404.

DiMaggio, C. & Galea, S. (2006). The behavioral consequences of terrorism: A meta-analysis. *Academic Emergency Medicine*, **13**, 559–566.

Dirkzwager, A. J., Kerssens, J. J., & Yzermans, C. J. (2006). Health problems in children and adolescents before and after a man-made disaster. *Journal of the American Academy of Child and Adolescent Psychiatry*, **45**, 94–103.

Dugan, B. (2007). Loss of identity in disaster: How do you say goodbye to home? *Perspectives in Psychiatric Care*, **43**, 41–46.

Egeland, B., Carlson, E., & Sroufe, L. A. (1993). Resilience as process. *Development and Psychopathology*, **5**, 517–528.

Feldman, D. M., Baron, S. L., Bernard, B. P., *et al.* (2004). Symptoms, respirator use, and pulmonary function changes among New York City firefighters responding to the World Trade Center disaster. *Chest*, **125**, 1256–1264.

Ford, C. A., Udry, J. R., Gleiter, K., & Chantala, K. (2003). Reactions of young adults to September 11, 2001.

Archives of Pediatrics and Adolescent Medicine, **157**, 572–578.

Galea, S., Nandi, A., & Vlahov, D. (2005). The epidemiology of post-traumatic stress disorder after disasters. *Epidemiologic Reviews*, **27**, 78–91.

Galea, S., Tracy, M., Norris, F., & Coffey, S. F. (2008). Financial and social circumstances and the incidence and course of PTSD in Mississippi during the first two years after Hurricane Katrina. *Journal of Traumatic Stress*, **21**, 357–368.

Ganzel, B. L., Kim, P., Glover, G. H., & Temple, E. (2008). Resilience after 9/11: Multimodal neuroimaging evidence for stress-related change in the healthy adult brain. *Neuroimage*, **40**, 788–795.

Ghaffari-Nejad, A., Ahmadi-Mousavi, M., Gandomkar, M., & Reihani-Kermani, H. (2007). The prevalence of complicated grief among Bam earthquake survivors in Iran. *Archives of Iranian Medicine*, **10**, 525–528.

Gold, L. S., Kane, L. B., Sotoodehnia, N., & Rea, T. (2007). Disaster events and the risk of sudden cardiac death: A Washington state investigation. *Prehospital and Disaster Medicine*, **22**, 313–317.

Gordon, J. (1978). *Structures*. Harmondsworth, UK: Penguin Books.

Grievink, L., van der Velden, P. G., Stellato, R. K., *et al.* (2007). A longitudinal comparative study of the physical and mental health problems of affected residents of the firework disaster Enschede, the Netherlands. *Public Health*, **121**, 367–374.

Guidry, V. T. & Margolis, L. H. (2005). Unequal respiratory health risk: Using GIS to explore hurricane-related flooding of schools in eastern North Carolina. *Environmental Research*, **98**, 383–389.

Gul, S., Ghaffar, H., Mirza, S., *et al.* (2008). Multitasking a telemedicine training unit in earthquake disaster response: Paraplegic rehabilitation assessment. *Telemedicine Journal and e-Health*, **14**, 280–283.

Helmreich, D. L., Watkins, L. R., Deak, T., *et al.* (1999). The effect of stressor controllability on stress-induced neuropeptide mRNA expression within the paraventricular nucleus of the hypothalamus. *Journal of Neuroendocrinology*, **11**, 121–128.

Holling, C. S. (1973). Resilience and stability of ecological systems. *Annual Review of Ecology and Systematics*, **4**, 1–23.

Hoven, C. W., Duarte, C. S., & Mandell, D. J. (2003). Children's mental health after disasters: The impact of the World Trade Center attack. *Current Psychiatry Reports*, **5**, 101–107.

Hoyois, P., Below, R., Scheuren, J., & Guha-Sapir, D. (2007). *Annual disaster statistical review: Numbers and trends 2006*. Brussels: Centre for Research on the Epidemiology of Disasters.

Huizink, A. C., Slottje, P., Witteveen, A. B., *et al.*
(2006). Long term health complaints following the
Amsterdam air disaster in police officers and firefighters. *Occupational and Environmental Medicine*, **63**,
657–662.

Huizink, A. C., Bartels, M., Rose, R. J., *et al.* (2008).
Chernobyl exposure as stressor during pregnancy
and hormone levels in adolescent offspring. *Journal of
Epidemiology and Community Health*, **62**, e5.

James, J. J., Subbarao, I., & Lanier, W. L. (2008). Improving
the art and science of disaster medicine and public
health preparedness. *Mayo Clinic Proceedings*, **83**,
559–562.

Jayatissa, R., Bekele, A., Piyasena, C. L., & Mahamithawa, S.
(2006). Assessment of nutritional status of children
under five years of age, pregnant women, and lactating
women living in relief camps after the tsunami in Sri
Lanka. *Food and Nutrition Bulletin*, **27**, 144–152.

Jordan, N. N., Hoge, C. W., Tobler, S. K., *et al.* (2004). Mental
health impact of 9/11 Pentagon attack: Validation of a
rapid assessment tool. *American Journal of Preventive
Medicine*, **26**, 284–293.

Kendra, J. M. & Wachtendorf, T. (2003). Elements of
resilience after the World Trade Center disaster:
Reconstituting New York City's emergency operations
centre. *Disasters*, **27**, 37–53.

Kett, M. (2005). Displaced populations and long term
humanitarian assistance. *British Medical Journal*, **331**,
98–100.

Kilpatrick, D. G., Koenen, K. C., Ruggiero, K. J., *et al.* (2007).
The serotonin transporter genotype and social support
and moderation of posttraumatic stress disorder and
depression in hurricane-exposed adults. *American
Journal of Psychiatry*, **164**, 1693–1699.

Kimhi, S. & Shamai, M. (2004). Community resilience and
the impact of stress: Adult response to Israel's withdrawal
from Lebanon. *Journal of Community Psychology*, **32**,
349–451.

Klein, R. J. T., Nicholls, R. J., & Thomalla, F. (2003).
Resilience to natural hazards: How useful is this concept?
Environmental Hazards, **5**, 35–45.

Knabb, R. D., Rhome, J. R., & Brown, D. P. (2005). *Tropical
cyclone report: Hurricane Katrina*. Miami, FL: National
Hurricane Center, http://www.nhc.noaa.gov/pdf/TCR-
AL122005_Katrina.pdf (accessed February 10, 2011).

Koerber, K. (2006). *Migration patterns and mover
characteristics from the 2005 ACS gulf coast area special
products: Detailed tables*. Washington, DC: Housing and
Economic Household Statistics Division, US Census
Bureau.

Kondo, H., Seo, N., Yasuda, T., *et al.* (2002). Post-flood:
infectious diseases in Mozambique. *Prehospital and
Disaster Medicine*, **17**, 126–133.

Kunii, O., Kanagawa, S., Yajima, I., *et al.* (2002). The 1997
haze disaster in Indonesia: Its air quality and health
effects. *Archives of Environmental Health*, **57**, 16–22.

Leor, J., Poole, W. K., & Kloner, R. A. (1996). Sudden cardiac
death triggered by an earthquake. *New England Journal of
Medicine*, **334**, 413–419.

Lioy, P. J., Weisel, C. P., Millette, J. R., *et al.* (2002).
Characterization of the dust/smoke aerosol that
settled east of the World Trade Center (WTC) in lower
Manhattan after the collapse of the WTC 11 September
2001. *Environmental Health Perspectives*, **110**, 703–714.

Llewellyn, M. (2006). Floods and tsunamis. *Surgical Clinics
of North America*, **86**, 557–578.

Loganovsky, K., Havenaar, J. M., Tintle, N. L., *et al.* (2008).
The mental health of clean-up workers 18 years after
the Chernobyl accident. *Psychological Medicine*, **38**,
481–488.

Madamala, K., Campbell, C. R., Hsu, E. B., Hsieh, Y. H., &
James, J. (2007). Characteristics of physician relocation
following Hurricane Katrina. *Disaster Medicine and
Public Health Preparedness*, **1**, 21–26.

Meharga, A. A., Osborna, D., Pain, D. J., Sanchez, A., &
Naveso, M. A. (1999). Contamination of Donana food-
chains after the Aznalcollar mine disaster. *Environmental
Pollution*, **105**, 387–390.

Metts, T. A. (2008). Addressing environmental health
implications of mold exposure after major flooding.
*American Association of Occupational Health Nurses
Journal*, **56**, 115–120; quiz 121–122.

Michaud, J. P., Grove, J. S., & Krupitsky, D. (2004). Emergency
department visits and "vog"-related air quality in Hilo,
Hawai'i. *Environmental Research*, **95**, 11–19.

Mileti, D. (1999). *Disasters by design: A reassessment of
natural hazards in the United States*. Washington, DC:
Joseph Henry Press.

Mitchell, W. J. & Townsend, A. M. (2005). Cyborg agonistes:
Disaster and reconstruction in the digital electronic era.
In W. J. Mitchell & A. M. Townsend (eds.), *The resilient
city: How modern cities recover from disaster* (pp. 313–
335). New York: Oxford University Press.

Moore, D., Copes, R., Fisk, R., *et al.* (2006). Population
health effects of air quality changes due to forest fires in
British Columbia in 2003: Estimates from physician-
visit billing data. *Canadian Journal of Public Health*, **97**,
105–108.

Nandi, A., Galea, S., Tracy, M., *et al.* (2004). Job loss,
unemployment, work stress, job satisfaction, and the
persistence of posttraumatic stress disorder one year
after the September 11 attacks. *Journal of Occupational
and Environmental Medicine*, **46**, 1057–1064.

Nishikiori, N., Abe, T., Costa, D. G., *et al.* (2006). Who
died as a result of the tsunami? Risk factors of mortality

among internally displaced persons in Sri Lanka: A retrospective cohort analysis. *BMC Public Health*, **6**, 73.

Nishiwaki, Y., Maekawa, K., Ogawa, Y., *et al.* (2001). Effects of Sarin on the nervous system in rescue team staff members and police officers 3 years after the Tokyo subway Sarin attack. *Environmental Health Perspectives*, **109**, 1169–1173.

Norris, F. H., Friedman, M. J., Watson, P. J., *et al.* (2002). 60 000 disaster victims speak: Part I. An empirical review of the empirical literature, 1981–2001. *Psychiatry*, **65**, 207–239.

Norris, F. H., Baker, C. K., Murphy, A. D., & Kaniasty, K. (2005). Social support mobilization and deterioration after Mexico's 1999 flood: Effects of context, gender, and time. *American Journal of Community Psychology*, **36**, 15–28.

Norris, F. H., Stevens, S. P., Pfefferbaum, B., Wyche, K. F., & Pfefferbaum, R. L. (2008). Community resilience as a metaphor, theory, set of capacities, and strategy for disaster readiness. *American Journal of Community Psychology*, **41**, 127–150.

Oliver-Smith, A. (1991). Successes and failures in post-disaster resettlement. *Disasters*, **15**, 12–23.

O'Neill, H. K., Evans, B. A., Bussman, M. D., & Strandberg, D. K. (1999). Psychological distress during the red river flood: Predictive utility of the conservation of resources model. *Applied Behavioral Science Review*, **7**, 159–169.

Paton, D. (2006). Disaster resilience: Building capacity to co-exist with natural hazards and their consequences. In D. Paton & D. Johnston (eds.), *Disaster resilience: An integrated approach* (pp. 3–10). Springfield, IL: Charles C. Thomas.

Peleg, K., Reuveni, H., & Stein, M. (2002). Earthquake disasters: Lessons to be learned. *Israel Medical Association Journal*, **4**, 361–365.

Perez-Sales, P., Cervellon, P., Vazquez, C., Vidales, D., & Gaborit, M. (2005). Post-traumatic factors and resilience: The role of shelter management and survivors' attitudes after the earthquakes in El Salvador (2001). *Journal of Community and Applied Social Psychology*, **15**, 368–382.

Rahu, M., Tekkel, M., Veidebaum, T., *et al.* (1997). The Estonian study of Chernobyl cleanup workers: II. incidence of cancer and mortality. *Radiation Research*, **147**, 653–657.

Rajkumar, A. P., Premkumar, T. S., & Tharyan, P. (2008). Coping with the Asian tsunami: Perspectives from Tamil Nadu, India on the determinants of resilience in the face of adversity. *Social Science and Medicine*, **67**, 844–853.

Rathore, M. F., Rashid, P., Butt, A. W., *et al.* (2007). Epidemiology of spinal cord injuries in the 2005 Pakistan earthquake. *Spinal Cord: The Official Journal of the International Medical Society of Paraplegia*, **45**, 658–663. doi:10.1038/sj.sc.3102023

Reidpath, D. D. (2005). Population health. More than the sum of the parts? *Journal of Epidemiology and Community Health*, **59**, 877–880.

Reijneveld, S. A., Crone, M. R., Verhulst, F. C., & Verloove-Vanhorick, S. P. (2003). The effect of a severe disaster on the mental health of adolescents: A controlled study. *Lancet*, **362**, 691–696.

Risk Management Solutions (2005). *RMS combines real-time reconnaissance with risk models to estimate Katrina losses*. Newark, CA: Risk Management Solutions, www.rms.com/newspress/pr_091905_hukatrina_lossmethodology.asp (accessed February 10, 2011).

Rose, A. (2006). Economic resilience to disasters: Toward a consistent and comprehensive formulation. In D. Paton, & D. Johnston (eds.), *Disaster resilience: An integrated approach* (pp. 226–248). Springfield, IL: Charles C. Thomas.

Roseboom, T. J., van der Meulen, J. H., Ravelli, A. C., *et al.* (2001). Effects of prenatal exposure to the Dutch famine on adult disease in later life: An overview. *Molecular and Cellular Endocrinology*, **185**, 93–98.

Rutter, M. (1993). Resilience: Some conceptual considerations. *Journal of Adolescent Health*, **14**, 626–631, 690–696.

Salcoglu, E., Basoglu, M., & Livanou, M. (2008). Psychosocial determinants of relocation in survivors of the 1999 earthquake in Turkey. *Journal of Nervous and Mental Disease*, **196**, 55–61.

Scheuren, J., le Polain de Waroux, O., Below, R., Guha-Sapir, D., & Ponserre, S. (2008). *Annual disaster statistical review: The numbers and trends 2007*. Melin, Belgium: Jacoffset.

Schultz, C. H., Koenig, K. L., & Lewis, R. J. (2007). Decision-making in hospital earthquake evacuation: Does distance from the epicenter matter? *Annals of Emergency Medicine*, **50**, 320–326.

Shaw, R. & Goda, K. (2004). From disaster to sustainable civil society: The Kobe experience. *Disasters*, **28**, 16–40.

Shehab, N., Anastario, M. P., & Lawry, L. (2008). Access to care among displaced Mississippi residents in FEMA travel trailer parks two years after Katrina. *Health Affairs*, **27**, w416–w429.

Shimizu, Y., Dobashi, K., Hisada, T., *et al.* (2007). Acute impact of volcanic ash on asthma symptoms and treatment. *International Journal of Immunopathology and Pharmacology*, **20**(Suppl. 2), 9–14.

Silver, R. C., Holman, E. A., McIntosh, D. N., Poulin, M., & Gil-Rivas, V. (2002). Nationwide longitudinal study of psychological responses to September 11. *Journal of the American Medical Association*, **288**, 1235–1244.

Slottje, P., Twisk, J. W., Smidt, N., *et al.* (2007). Health-related quality of life of firefighters and police officers 8.5 years after the air disaster in Amsterdam. *Quality of Life Research*, **16**, 239–252.

Smolka, A. (2006). Natural disasters and the challenge of extreme events: Risk management from an insurance perspective. *Philosophical Transactions. Series A, Mathematical, Physical, and Engineering Sciences*, **364**, 2147–2165.

Soeteman, R. J., Yzermans, C. J., Kerssens, J. J., *et al.* (2007). Health problems presented to family practices in the Netherlands 1 year before and 1 year after a disaster. *Journal of the American Board of Family Medicine*, **20**, 548–556.

Tang, C. S. (2007). Trajectory of traumatic stress symptoms in the aftermath of extreme natural disaster: A study of adult Thai survivors of the 2004 southeast Asian earthquake and tsunami. *Journal of Nervous and Mental Disease*, **195**, 54–59.

Tao, L., Kannan, K., Aldous, K. M., Mauer, M. P., & Eadon, G. A. (2008). Biomonitoring of perfluorochemicals in plasma of New York state personnel responding to the World Trade Center disaster. *Environmental Science and Technology*, **42**, 3472–3478.

Tauqir, S. F., Mirza, S., Gul, S., Ghaffar, H., & Zafar, A. (2007). Complications in patients with spinal cord injuries sustained in an earthquake in northern Pakistan. *Journal of Spinal Cord Medicine*, **30**, 373–377.

Thomas, C. R. (2006). Psychiatric sequelae of disasters. *Journal of Burn Care and Research*, **27**, 600–605.

Trevisan, M., Jossa, F., Farinaro, E., *et al.* (1992). Earthquake and coronary heart disease risk factors: A longitudinal study. *American Journal of Epidemiology*, **135**, 632–637.

Trevisan, M., O' Leary, E., Farinaro, E., *et al.* (1997). Short- and long-term association between uric acid and a natural disaster. *Psychosomatic Medicine*, **59**, 109–113.

Tucker, P. M., Pfefferbaum, B., North, C. S., *et al.* (2007). Physiologic reactivity despite emotional resilience several years after direct exposure to terrorism. *American Journal of Psychiatry*, **164**, 230–235.

United Nations Office for the Coordination of Humanitarian Affairs (2005). *Indian Ocean earthquake-tsunami 2005, flash appeal*. New York: United Nations.

Vale, L. J. & Campanella, T. J. (2005). *The resilient city: How modern cities recover from disaster*. New York: Oxford University Press.

Walsh, F. (2007). Traumatic loss and major disasters: Strengthening family and community resilience. *Family Process*, **46**, 207–227.

Wang, X., Gao, L., Zhang, H., *et al.* (2000). Post-earthquake quality of life and psychological well-being: Longitudinal evaluation in a rural community sample in northern China. *Psychiatry and Clinical Neurosciences*, **54**, 427–433.

Wayment, H. A. (2004). It could have been me: Vicarious victims and disaster-focused distress. *Personality and Social Psychology Bulletin*, **30**, 515–528.

Chapter 15

Rape and other sexual assault

Heidi S. Resnick, Constance Guille, Jenna L. McCauley, and
Dean G. Kilpatrick

Introduction

This chapter describes the prevalence of rape and the
risk of associated mental health problems, including
definition of key terms such as rape. The particular
focus of the chapter is on post-traumatic stress disorder
(PTSD) as a primary mental health problem associated with rape. Major methodological approaches to
the study of rape, related risk, resilience, and associated mental health problems are described, and advantages and disadvantages and implications of the major
approaches are discussed. Findings from the literature related to risk and protective factors for PTSD are
reviewed in general, as well as what is known specifically about risk and protective factors for PTSD given
exposure to rape. The discussion is concluded by considering the implications for future research related to
etiology and/or intervention in relation to the study of
resilience.

Prevalence of rape

Rape is a common problem in many countries, including America. Carefully conducted epidemiological
studies estimate the proportion of women who have
been raped is between 12.6% and 16.1% in the USA
(Kilpatrick et al., 1992, 2007a; Tjaden & Thoennes,
2000). Based on the most recent estimates and the 2005
US Census data, an estimated 20.2 million women have
been raped, with an estimated 1.1 million women who
have been raped within a given year (Kilpatrick et al.,
2007b). Furthermore, the incidence of rape is likely to
be increasing, with recent lifetime prevalence estimates
of rape being higher than those obtained in the early
1990s. There is substantial evidence to support significant untoward consequences of rape. Women who are
victims of rape are at a significantly increased risk for
mental health problems, substance abuse, and poor

physical health compared with non-victims (Steketee
& Foa, 1987; Resick, 1993; Resnick et al., 1993, 1997;
Kessler et al., 1995; Kilpatrick et al., 1997, 2003). In particular, findings from epidemiological studies indicate
that rape or completed sexual assault, compared with
other traumatic events, is associated with greatest risk
of PTSD (Kilpatrick et al., 1989; Norris, 1992; Resnick
et al., 1993; Kessler et al., 1995). While estimates vary,
approximately half of rape victims develop PTSD
(Breslau et al., 1998); so not all women who experience rape develop emotional problems, but, given
the high prevalence of rape and the substantial cost
associated with this adverse event, it is not surprising
that researchers have focused on predictors of PTSD
among rape victims. A significant consequence of this
focus is that little is understood about the characteristics of those who appear to endure rape with minimal
adverse sequelae. A better understanding of the human
capacity to maintain healthy, symptom-free functioning or resilience in the face of significant adversity is of
great importance to the study of PTSD. It is useful to
identify protective factors as well as risk factors for psychopathology, both to understand resilience in the face
of known risk factors and to identify potentially modifiable risk factors that might be targeted in interventions promoting resilience (e.g., providing secondary
prevention once a woman has been sexually assaulted).
For example, knowing characteristics of rape that elevate risk may help to identify those who are resilient
even under high-risk conditions and to identify individual, system response, or social response factors that
produce more positive outcomes under those conditions. Consequently, the major objective of this chapter is to review what is known about risk and protective
factors for PTSD after exposure to rape, with particular emphasis on factors related to resilience. Prior to
this review, important terms will be defined and key

Resilience and Mental Health: Challenges Across the Lifespan, ed. Steven M. Southwick, Brett T. Litz, Dennis Charney, and
Matthew J. Friedman. Published by Cambridge University Press. © Cambridge University Press 2011.

methodological issues identified that should be considered in a review of rape and resilience and how well extant research is capable of providing information on resilience. Our review will draw on what existing reviews of the literature tell us about risk and protective factors for PTSD in general, as well as what we know about risk and protective factors for PTSD given exposure to rape specifically.

Definition of terms

Rape

Rape is a form of sexual assault that is defined as a felony crime in the USA and many other nations. The crime of rape has several major elements. First, rape involves some type of sexual penetration of the victim's vagina, mouth, or anus. Second, the sexual activity must be unwanted by the victim. Third, the tactics used by the perpetrator must involve (1) use of force or threat of force or other harm to the victim, (2) using alcohol or drugs to render a victim too incapacitated to control his or her behavior or protect themself, or (3) taking advantage of a victim who is incapacitated or unconscious and who, therefore, is unable to protect themself. Although rape victims can be male or female, in this chapter they will be referred to as female.

Forcible rape. The tactic used by the perpetrator is force or threat of force or other harm to the victim or someone else (e.g., the perpetrator threatens to hurt the victim's children if the victim does not cooperate).

Drug- or alcohol-facilitated rape. The tactic used by the perpetrator is to deliberately give the victim drugs or alcohol without her permission in an attempt to get her high or drunk and then to commit an unwanted sexual act.

Incapacitated rape. The victim voluntarily uses alcohol or drugs and is passed out, or awake but too drunk or high to consent or control her behavior.

Statutory rape. The perpetrator has sexual penetration with someone who is defined by law as too young to be capable of giving consent.

Attempted rape. This is a type of sexual assault that occurs when no sexual penetration as defined above occurs but an unsuccessful attempt by the perpetrator to commit a rape as defined above has occurred.

Rape acknowledgement. Not all women who have experienced an event that meets the legal definition of rape define what happened as rape, and, therefore, they do not think of themselves as rape victims.

Unacknowledged rape. An event that has the legal elements of rape but that is not perceived by the victim to have been a rape. Unacknowledged rape victims are victims of rape who do not acknowledge that what happened to them was a rape.

Resilience

As described by Bonanno (2004), resilience is defined as the absence of an emotional disorder following exposure to a potentially traumatic event. In the context of this chapter, resilience is defined as either failure to develop PTSD after a rape occurs or rapid recovery from PTSD if PTSD does develop after a rape occurs. Although this definition of resilience will be used, it is important to note that true resilience is much more than the absence of psychopathology (e.g., post-traumatic growth). However, there is so little research on these other measures of resilience that this is the definition that will be used.

Methodological issues

Characteristics of an ideal study of post-rape resilience

Ideal studies do not exist, but if they did, here is what they would look like. First, the sample of rape victim studies would be representative of the population of rape victims of interest. This would ensure that both the victims and the rapes they experienced are representative of all rape victims and all rape cases. Second, there would be careful measurement of all pre-rape, rape, and post-rape variables that are thought to be risk or protective factors for PTSD or related problems. Third, PTSD and related problems would be measured before the rape as well as a sufficient number of times afterwards to permit assessment of the trajectory of PTSD and related problems before, immediately after the rape, and several time thereafter. Fourth, an appropriate comparison group of non-victims of rape would be included and assessed to make it possible to establish the extent to which PTSD and other problems are rape related (i.e., their prevalence is significantly higher among rape victims than among non-victims). Fifth, the longitudinal PTSD data would be used to identify the trajectories of changes in PTSD status after a rape to determine victims who are resilient versus those who are not resilient.

A research study with these elements would be ideally suited to address post-rape resilience for several reasons. First, because it would include a representative sample of all rape victims as opposed to a biased sample that excluded some important types of victim, any findings would be much more generalizable. Second, longitudinal assessment of PTSD status before and after rape would permit trajectories of change to be tracked, thereby establishing which rape victims are resilient. Third, comprehensive measurement of potential risk and protective factors would permit the examination of a wide range of biopsychosocial risk and protective factors related to resilience or lack of same.

Not surprisingly, no studies meet all these criteria. In general, extant studies fall into two groups. The first group of studies are epidemiological and involve screening for history of rape among representative, probability samples of female adolescents, young adults, or adult women living in households or colleges (Tjaden & Thoennes, 2000; Fisher *et al.*, 2003; Kilpatrick *et al.*, 2007b). Such studies are generally retrospective, not longitudinal, and they rarely involve collection of biological risk or protective factor measures. A major strength of these studies is that their samples of rape victims are much more likely to be representative of the population of all rape victims from which they are drawn. An additional strength is that such studies are more likely to capture the full range of changes in PTSD and other mental problems that occur as a result of a rape because they include victims who are having few problems as well as those who are having many problems. A final strength of these studies is that they are more likely to include a representative distribution of risk and protective factors.

The second group of studies involves obtaining data from the subset of rape victims who report crimes to police, seek services from rape crisis centers or other victim assistance agencies, or who respond to advertisements seeking rape victims to participate in research on rape. The last method for recruiting victims yields only a convenience sample, from which results cannot be generalized. Samples obtained from the subset of rape victims who report their crimes and/or who seek assistance can provide valuable information,

particularly because many such studies involve longitudinal assessments after the rape. However, it has long been known that the majority of women who are raped do not report the crime to police (e.g., Kilpatrick, 1983; Kilpatrick *et al.*, 1992) or seek services from rape crisis centers (Kilpatrick & Veronen, 1983). To the extent that there are major differences between samples including the types of victim (and their cases) participating in these studies and the population of all rape victims and cases, such studies might be expected to yield biased information about resilience following rape.

Unacknowledged rape and how it can bias participation in rape research

There is ample evidence that many victims of experiences that meet the legal definition of rape do not perceive what happened to them as a rape (Kilpatrick *et al.*, 2007b). These unacknowledged rape victims are unlikely to report cases to police, to seek services from rape crisis centers or other service agencies, or to participate in research projects that are recruiting for "rape victims," because they do not think what happened to them was a rape and they do not think of themselves as rape victims. As noted, even if the rape is acknowledged as such, the vast majority of rape victims do not report the assault to police or other authorities, particularly if drugs or alcohol were involved in the rape (Resnick *et al.* 2000). For example, in a recent study of a national household probability sample of 3001 adult women and a sample of 2000 women recruited nationwide from colleges, Kilpatrick and colleagues (2007b) found that 18% of women in the general population sample and 11.5% of women in the national college student sample reported a lifetime history of rape including forcible, incapacitated rape or drug- and alcohol-facilitated rape. Among those who experienced forcible rape, only 18% of women in the general population sample and 16% of the college women reported the incident to police or other authorities. An even smaller percentage of the general population sample (10%) and the college women sample (7%) reported rapes that occurred as a result of drug or alcohol facilitation or incapacitation. These data confirm the belief that most rape victims do not report their cases to police.

If there are differences in cases that are acknowledged as rapes or not, cases that are reported to police or not reported, and among rape victims who do and do not participate in rape research, this could have a substantial impact on the characteristics of the rape victims and rape cases that have been included in various studies. Likewise, if some of the same variables that predict whether a rape case is acknowledged, or reported, or that result in victims seeking services, also increase risk of PTSD and/or related disorders, then some of what we think we know about risk and resilience after rape may have been obtained from biased samples of rape victims that do not include the full range of rape cases and rape victims. For example, Rothbaum et al. (1992) found that 94% of a sample of rape victims who reported to police, sought medical care, or rape crisis center services met diagnostic criteria for PTSD at two weeks after the assault while 50% continued to meet criteria three months later. In contrast, Resnick et al. (1993) found that 32% of women who had ever been raped in a national household probability sample of US adult women met lifetime PTSD criteria. However, prevalence of lifetime PTSD was 45% among victims of either rape or physical assault when such incidents included both fear of death/injury or actual injury (Resnick et al., 1993). Consequently, Resnick and colleagues suggested that differences in PTSD prevalence across studies might relate to such differences in assault or other characteristics that distinguish rape victims or rape incidents that are or are not reported to authorities. Consistent with this notion regarding differences in PTSD or other outcomes among those reporting to police or other authorities, acknowledgement of rape has been found to be associated with greater symptoms of PTSD (Layman et al., 1996; Zinzow et al., 2010) and physical health complaints (Conoscenti & McNally, 2006).

To further investigate whether women who report rape to police or other authorities are more likely to also meet criteria for PTSD, we conducted analyses within the original National Women's Study sample of 4008 women. Women who had experienced at least one rape incident as an adult were asked in reference to a first or most recent rape assault whether they had reported the incident to police or other authorities. Occurrence of PTSD was assessed with the National Women's Study PTSD module (Resnick et al., 1993) using DSM-IV criteria (American Psychiatric Association, 1994). Of 218 women who had experienced an adult rape, 23.9% had reported one or more lifetime rape incident to police or other authorities. Those who reported an assault to police were significantly more likely to meet criteria for lifetime PTSD (44.2% and 28.9%, respectively) (chi square = 4.23 [df 1, n =218]; $p < 0.05$). These data are interesting and indicate a prevalence of PTSD

approaching that found by Rothbaum et al. (1992) at 12 weeks post-rape among those who had reported an assault to police, hospital, or rape crisis personnel. Most importantly, these data demonstrate that rape victims who report their cases to police were more likely to have PTSD than those who do not report.

As reviewed by Fisher et al. (2003), demographic characteristics such as older age at time of assault and assault characteristics such as injury or other indicators of severity are risk factors for reporting to police, self-acknowledgement of rape (Layman et al., 1996; Conoscenti & McNally, 2006), and seeking post-rape medical services (Resnick et al., 2000). Furthermore, as reported by Kilpatrick et al. (2007b), positive predictors of reporting of a most recent or only rape within the general population sample included verbal threat, injury, or fear of death or injury. Therefore, findings indicate that women who self-acknowledge rape, report rape, or are seen in medical settings are also more likely to have experienced the types of rape that greatly increase the risk of PTSD. Specifically, both injury and fear of death or injury have consistently been identified as risk factors for PTSD within studies that have evaluated outcomes associated with a range of traumatic events including rape (Kilpatrick et al., 1989; Resnick et al., 1993). These data demonstrate the biases inherent to convenience samples of rape victims and underscore the need to study all victims of rape among the general population.

Reviews of the extant literature: risk and protective factors for post-traumatic stress disorder in general

Although much is known concerning risk factors for PTSD, research examining protective factors is in its relative infancy. However, important information can be distilled from understanding which factors increase risk of psychopathology following a traumatic event. One of the first attempts to summarize factors that impact later development of PTSD was by Shalev and colleagues (1996). After reviewing 38 studies, they identified several risk factors for PTSD including pre-trauma vulnerability (e.g., psychiatric family history, sex, genes, neuroendocrine factors, personality traits, early trauma, negative parenting experiences, and lower education), peritraumatic events (e.g., magnitude of the trauma, preparation for the event, immediate reactions to the event including dissociation and coping responses), and post-trauma factors (e.g., symptom trajectory, social support, other life stress). The identification of these risk factors is laudable and served as a basis for subsequent explorations of individual vulnerability factors that have attempted to overcome some of the limitations of these initial data, including generalizability, heterogeneity of studies, and inconsistency in replication of risk factors (Brewin et al., 2000).

Simultaneously, Brewin et al. (2000) and Ozer et al. (2003), conducted independent meta-analyses of risk factors for PTSD in trauma-exposed adults. The first meta-analysis (Brewin et al., 2000) included studies of multiple types of trauma among military and civilian populations, with combined sample sizes of 1149 to 11 000 subjects. In addition to identifying the absolute and relative effect sizes of 14 risk factors for PTSD, including multiple pre-trauma variables (age, gender, socioeconomic status, education, race, family psychiatric history, intelligence, childhood adversity, and previous trauma), peritrauma and post-trauma variables (trauma severity, social support and life stress), they also examined the moderating effects of various sample and study characteristics. Overall Brewin et al. (2000) found that, when both military and civilian populations were combined, the risk of PTSD was enhanced to a small extent by pre-trauma characteristics (effect sizes ranging from 0.5 to 0.19) and to a somewhat larger extent by peritraumatic and post-traumatic experiences (effect sizes ranging from 0.23 to 0.40). However, the extent of effect for the majority of predictors differed by sample, with most of the pre-trauma variables predicting PTSD in military veterans compared with civilian samples. Very few of the pre-trauma predictors, with the exception of prior psychiatric history, childhood abuse and family psychiatric history, had effects of similar magnitude across studies, with the effect of some pre-trauma predictors, including gender, age at trauma, and race, disappearing in certain subsets of studies. These data suggest that attempts to identify a universal set of pre-trauma predictors of PTSD that is valid across different traumatized groups is premature and it underscores the complex interaction between the person exposed and the nature of exposure in predicting PTSD. As suggested by Brewin et al. (2000), these data serve as a springboard to begin to investigate the dynamic between pre-trauma characteristics and how these interact with peritrauma and post-trauma factors in the development of PTSD.

Independent of Brewin's conclusions, Ozer et al. (2003) began exploring this interaction and focused their meta-analysis on mainly two types of predictor: personal characteristics relevant for psychological processing of the trauma and outstanding features of the traumatic event or its effects. Specifically, seven risk factors were explored, including prior trauma, prior psychological adjustment, family history of psychopathology, perceived life threat during the trauma, post-trauma social support, peritraumatic emotional responses, and peritraumatic dissociation. The results revealed similar effect sizes among comparable predictors to those found by Brewin et al. (2000), and that, overall, peritraumatic psychological processes, not prior characteristics, were the strongest predictors of PTSD. Consistent with the findings of Brewin et al. (2000), Ozer et al. (2003) also found that predictors varied based on study sample and characteristics (i.e., type of traumatic event, time elapsed since the event, type of sample, and method of PTSD assessment). While each of these variables moderated at least two of the predictors, the most consistent and salient variable was type of event. Interpersonal violence, classified as civilian assault, rape, and domestic violence, compared with violence that occurred in the military, increased the effect sizes of almost all the predictors, including history of prior trauma, prior psychological adjustment, family history of psychopathology, and perceived life threat during the trauma. These findings suggest that the characteristics of the individual must be considered in combination with the nature of the traumatic event when attempting to determine who will become symptomatic following a traumatic event. Therefore, in order to understand the risk factors for the development of PTSD, it may be helpful to study traumatic events that are more homogeneous in nature.

Reviews of the extant literature: risk and protective factors for post-traumatic stress disorder specifically for exposure to rape

Steketee and Foa (1987) conducted an early review of the extant rape literature that addressed risk factors for short-term and longer-term reactions and that evaluated risk factors in terms of demographics, rape characteristics, initial acute responses, and post-rape stressors including interaction with the criminal justice system. As with the reviews discussed above, the information is organized in terms of pre-assault, peri-assault, and post-assault risk factors with a range of outcomes. As noted in the review by Steketee and Foa (1987) and subsequent reviews (Resnick *et al.*, 1991; Resick, 1993), rape has been associated with a range of problems including anxiety, depression, substance abuse, poor self-esteem, physical health complaints, and problems in social and sexual functioning – in addition to PTSD. Findings from early reviews are noted here and updated findings regarding risk factors are provided. There is a relatively greater emphasis in this review on predictors of PTSD, with resilience viewed as non-PTSD, given the primary focus of many reports on PTSD as an outcome.

Pre-trauma factors associated with post-rape functioning

A number of pre-assault characteristics have been shown to influence post-rape functioning. Although the majority of studies have focused on the relationship between pre-assault characteristics and post-assault dysfunction, valuable information can be gained from these studies that may increase our understanding of factors associated with post-trauma adjustment. Overall, the pre-assault characteristics most heavily investigated in post-rape functioning are (1) demographic information, (2) prior assault history, and (3) prior psychological functioning or prior psychiatric history. As noted above, these studies are often retrospective in nature and the populations studied likely do not accurately represent all rape victims. The limitations discussed above should be kept in mind when reviewing the extant literature that follows.

Demographics

Demographic characteristics are some of the most heavily investigated factors in the development of PTSD, but their role in predicting recovery from sexual assault is unclear. The extant literature investigating demographic factors as a predictor of PTSD among sexual assault survivors is inconsistent (Ullman *et al.*, 2007a), with some studies highlighting these factors as correlates and others not finding an association (Koss *et al.*, 2002). For example, two studies have found older age to be protective (Ullman *et al.*, 2007a), with less severe PTSD symptoms, but several earlier studies reviewed found no effect of age (Steketee & Foa, 1987). The findings reviewed by Steketee and Foa (1987) on effects of education and marital status and response to rape are also mixed. These contradictory results may reflect differences in sampling approach, because

some rape victims were recruited via epidemiological approaches while others were recruited from clinical or community-based populations and are subject to the aforementioned biases. In addition, certain demographic characteristics can have both positive and negative effects. For example, being married does not necessarily imply a positive and supportive relationship, and may, in fact, be an added stressor for some. Furthermore, education may be moderated by other demographic factors such as socioeconomic status and, therefore, account for some of these contradictory findings.

One demographic characteristic that appears to be a consistent predictor of poorer post-rape functioning is lower economic status (Kilpatrick *et al.*, 1985; Resnick *et al.*, 2007). Given that history of rape and physical assault may be prevalent among those with reduced economic resources and in fact may contribute to lower resources (Bassuk *et al.*, 1996; Byrne *et al.*, 1999), it may be important to develop strategies to increase economic resources among women at risk for victimization and in the post-assault period. Similar to social support (discussed below in reference to post-assault factors), baseline economic and social support may also be conceptualized as pre-assault risk factors related to either resilience or poor adjustment post-assault.

The impact of demographic characteristics, as well as assault and post-assault characteristics, on current PTSD symptoms were evaluated in a study of 600 female sexual assault survivors recruited from college, community, and mental health agencies (Ullman *et al.*, 2007b). All forms of sexual victimization were included, including completed rape, attempted rape, sexual coercion, and unwanted sexual contact occurring during adolescence or adulthood (age 14 years and over) and childhood (aged under 14 years). Among the demographic variables, race, education, and marital status were not related to PTSD symptoms, but older age at the time of the assault was related to less severity of PTSD symptoms. These findings may suggest that adults, compared with teenagers, are somehow more resilient when faced with sexual assault. It is possible that, with age, comes more experience in dealing with traumatic events. Also, adults are likely to have more resources and better-developed coping strategies to handle this experience compared with young adults. One caveat to these data, however, is that participants were a convenience sample of volunteers from the community who responded to advertisements and notices for women who had a history of unwanted sexual experiences. As noted above, such women are self-acknowledged victims, who may differ in terms of assault characteristics and other variables from those within more representative samples. Consequently, these demographic risk factors and other predictors of PTSD may not generalize to more representative samples.

In a longitudinal study of a nationally representative sample of 3006 women, Acierno et al. (1999) identified separate risk factors for PTSD after rape and after physical assault. Whereas demographic variables did not predict post-rape PTSD, lower education did predict post-assault PTSD among physical assault victims. These data highlight another important area of investigation in the study of PTSD, which is revictimization. Demographic variables such as young age and minority status increased the risk of being raped or physically assaulted, respectively (Acierno et al., 1999). Given that history of prior assault is a risk factor for PTSD, it is important to identify those at risk for revictimization in an effort to intervene to avoid further traumatic event exposure and its devastating consequences.

Prior assault history

One of the most consistent findings from epidemiological and clinical samples is that many survivors of rape also have histories of other traumatic events, and multiple traumatic events are associated with increased risk of PTSD (Kramer & Green, 1991; Resnick et al., 1995; Ozer et al., 2003; Ullman et al., 2007a; Cougle et al., 2009). For example, Resnick et al., (1995) found a PTSD prevalence of 67% three months after rape among women with a prior history of sexual or physical assault compared with 23% among women without that history. These findings are consistent with earlier studies suggesting that those with a history of multiple rapes, compared with a single incident rape, showed greater distress following a recent assault and reported more intense nightmares and fears one year after the assault (Resick, 1993). Resnick et al. (1995) found that women with a prior history of assault also had lower cortisol levels in the immediate hours following a rape compared with women without such histories. These data highlight important biological differences among women with a history of prior assault and women without such a history and are consistent with most studies, but not all, that found low cortisol levels among adults with chronic PTSD (reviewed by Pervanidou, 2008). Resnick et al. (1995) did not find associations between

cortisol levels and PTSD in this small sample of recent rape victims. However, as noted, women with prior assault histories had lower cortisol levels post-rape and were also subsequently found to have higher prevalence of PTSD. Although dysfunction of the hypothalamic–pituitary–adrenal (HPA) axis in the context of trauma is not completely understood, low cortisol levels may reflect an altered stress response as the result of prior trauma. It is also possible that an attenuated stress-response system may confer additional risk for PTSD following subsequent victimization, or it may correlate with other factors that increase risk of PTSD following a subsequent assault.

Altered HPA activity and glucocorticoid receptor sensitivity have been shown to be associated with PTSD (Yehuda, 2001; Yehuda et al., 2004) and there is increasing evidence that the interaction of biological (i.e., genetic) and environmental (i.e., childhood traumatic events) factors may predict adult PTSD. Binder et al. (2008) examined variants in the gene *FKBP5* (a regulator of glucocorticoid receptor sensitivity) in a sample of low-income, predominantly African-American subjects recruited from an inner city general medical clinic. These results showed that the variants in *FKBP5* were associated with higher levels of adult PTSD symptoms, but only among individuals exposed to two or more types of child abuse (including sexual abuse). There was no effect of genotype for individuals who experienced only one type of child abuse or no child abuse. While the topic of childhood abuse is beyond the scope of this chapter, these results demonstrate that the combination of genotype and exposure to traumatic events, in this case early life trauma, influences adult PTSD outcomes. These findings are important and highlight the need to consider childhood traumatic event exposure, severity of different types of traumatic event, and/or multiple exposures as potential risk factors for the development of PTSD in the aftermath of rape within studies of potential genetic risk factors. Such research may also shed light on the association between prior traumatic event exposure and PTSD.

Prior assault history is not only associated with PTSD but also with a number of other psychiatric conditions and treatment responses. Resnick et al. (2007) found that prior history of rape was a significant predictor of PTSD, depression, and other anxiety symptom frequency following a recent rape, and that prior history moderated the effects of a brief secondary preventive intervention designed to prevent or reduce PTSD, depression, and substance abuse. Specifically, frequency of PTSD and depressive symptoms were significantly lower among women with a prior history of rape who were exposed to a video intervention prior to the rape examination that contained information about the examination and modeling and information about post-rape coping strategies than in those who received standard care. Women without a prior history of rape appeared to be more resilient. In addition, among women without a prior history of rape, those in the video group reported somewhat higher frequency or intensity of PTSD and general anxiety symptoms at six weeks after rape assessment but not at six months after rape.

Prior psychological functioning (or mental health history)

The majority of early studies, but not all, have found prior psychological functioning to play an important role in the immediate, recent, and long-term post-rape adjustment periods (Resick, 1993). As reviewed by Resick, findings from most but not all early longitudinal studies of recent rape victims indicated that prior history of mental health problems was associated with greater distress within the first few days post-assault or increased distress or prevalence of post-rape criteria for a psychiatric condition at one month after rape or at longer-term follow-ups. These study samples included primarily rape victims who reported to police, rape crisis centers, or other authorities.

Other research has demonstrated high prevalence of rape and physical assault among those with serious mental illness, including mood disorders, schizophrenia, PTSD, and substance abuse (Goodman *et al.*, 2001; Cusack *et al.*, 2004). Findings indicate that the vast majority (87–91%) of patients in the US public mental health system report a history of exposure to one or more serious traumatic events (Cusack *et al.*, 2004) and more than one third may experience a past year incident of physical or sexual assault (Goodman *et al.* 2001). Data from these and other studies indicate that there may be a cyclical relationship between mental health problems and victimization by assault, such that history of assault increases risk of mental health problems, which may also increase risk of new victimization and associated worsening of mental health problems. Those with serious mental illness may be particularly vulnerable to assault victimization.

Findings from Resnick *et al.* (1992) indicated an interaction between retrospectively assessed pre-crime diagnosis of depression, crime severity characteristics,

and post-crime PTSD. Specifically, participants who met criteria for depression with age of onset before exposure to crime were significantly more likely to meet criteria for post-crime PTSD only among those whose attacks included fear of death, sustained injury, or rape. Prior mental health history was not related to crime exposure itself and did not appear to be a vulnerability factor for PTSD in the absence of these crime severity characteristics. These findings are partially consistent with Koss *et al.* (2002), who examined the psychological, physical, and social impact of rape among a large university-based sample of women. They found a negative influence on post-rape recovery with "psychological problem history," defined as self-reported behavioral problems (i.e., acting out, referral to juvenile services, substance abuse) as well as a history of psychiatric hospitalization, suicide attempts, and pharmacological and psychological treatment. However, psychological problem history had direct effects on social maladjustment, self-blame, and assault severity, which are all factors that have been shown to associate with poor post-rape adjustment and PTSD. These findings suggest that the negative impact of psychological problem history is possibly moderated by maladaptive coping strategies (i.e., self-blame), poor social skills, or assault characteristics (i.e., assault severity) and is not necessarily a predictor of poorer post-assault adjustment. In addition, the role of prior or complex assault history and its role in influencing adjustment prior to a subsequent rape needs to be considered and may have important treatment implications. Consequently, those with significant prior traumatic event history may also benefit from intervention addressing responses and problems associated with such events. Post-rape interventions aimed at improving social skills and addressing issues of self-blame may impart resilience among rape victims.

Peritraumatic factors associated with post-rape functioning

This section considers factors linked to the assault time frame, such as assault characteristics, peritraumatic reactions, rape acknowledgement, and post-assault concerns.

Assault characteristics

In their early review of the literature related to rape, Steketee and Foa (1987) stated that most extant studies reported no significant associations between rape characteristics or situational factors and PTSD. In addition, findings were mixed across the small number of studies that found associations between assault characteristics and post-rape indicators of functioning. Some studies found that the more violent or potentially injurious the assault the poorer the adjustment over time, in terms of mood, psychiatric problems, and physical health complaints, while another set of studies found that severity was related to better self-esteem and sexual functioning. As suggested by Steketee and Foa (1987), the mixed findings might be attributed to the possibility that increased severity may relate differentially to the varied outcomes studied. Consequently, they suggested that higher threat or more violent assaults might be associated with negative mental health outcomes in some studies but with less guilt and hence some positive functioning as observed in other studies. This could be seen as consistent with findings reported by Ullman et al. (2007a) that indicated that life threat during a sexual assault was significantly positively correlated with positive social reactions while also being positively correlated with PTSD.

A more complicated issue is that life threat was also positively correlated with negative social reactions. It is likely that this is a function of the fact that more severe assaults (in terms of injury or perceived life threat) are more likely to be self-acknowledged as rape and are also more likely to be reported, which increases the likelihood of others knowing about the incident and responding in negative as well as positive ways. In fact, in an earlier study, Ullman and Filipas (2001) found that injury and life threat were positively correlated with the number of support providers told about the assault and with the average number of negative social reactions. The numbers of support providers and the average number of negative social reactions were also significantly positively correlated with each other.

The lack of any reported differences in the majority of studies and/or inconsistent findings observed may also have related to the selective nature of samples studied. Early studies of functioning post-rape typically included women identified through rape crisis or hospital programs serving recent victims (e.g., Kilpatrick et al., 1979; Calhoun et al., 1982; Frank & Stewart, 1984). The more restricted range of characteristics of reported cases and/or an extremely high prevalence of PTSD may make it difficult to identify assault-related risk factors in these samples. In the Rothbaum et al. (1992) longitudinal study of recent rape victims, 94% met all but duration criteria for PTSD at two weeks after assault

and almost 50% met criteria at three months post-rape. As reviewed by Resick (1993), findings do not support the notion that stranger rape is more severe than rapes by known assailants in terms of negative mental health outcomes. In fact, rapes by known assailants including dating or marital partners appear to be similar in terms of negative mental health consequences (Kilpatrick et al., 1988; Koss et al., 1988). Data from more representative sample studies indicate that injury as a part of an assault increases risk of current PTSD among those with history of rape, controlling for other predictors (Acierno et al., 1999). Similarly, Kilpatrick et al. (1989) examined a large probability sample of community women who were assessed for a range of crime-exposure histories and found that the experiences of injury, fear of death or injury, and the crime type of rape were all significant predictors of PTSD. Kilpatrick et al. found that rape was the only type of crime studied that was a significant predictor of PTSD even after controlling for injury and threat characteristics. A majority (78%) of women reporting all three history characteristics met criteria for PTSD. Resnick et al. (1993), in a large national sample of women, found that both injury and fear of death or injury were predictors of lifetime PTSD among women with histories of rape or physical assault. Ullman and colleagues (Ullman & Filipas, 2001; Ullman et al., 2007a), using a range of strategies to recruit women with sexual assault histories from the community and various service agencies, also found that perceived life threat was a significant correlate of PTSD among victims of sexual assault. However, other assault characteristics studied, including offender violence (Ullman et al., 2007a) or injury (Ullman & Filipas, 2001), were not related to PTSD. Consequently, one of the more consistent assault time frame predictors of PTSD may in itself be a perception or response, albeit a response that is highly correlated with objective threat characteristics such as injury as a result of assault (e.g., Ullman & Filipas, 2001).

Peritraumatic reactions

Consistent with the finding that the subjective perception of fear of death or injury during assault is predictive of PTSD or other negative outcomes, results of numerous studies indicate that early distress responses post-rape are strong positive predictors of PTSD or other long-term patterns of anxiety or distress (Kilpatrick et al., 1985; Girelli et al., 1986; Rothbaum et al., 1992). The studies by Kilpatrick et al. (1985) and Rothbaum et al. (1992) indicated that distress at two weeks after rape positively predicted ongoing distress and PTSD at three months after rape. Other data indicate that anxiety or distress reported at the time of rape or immediately afterwards may be a risk factor for later anxiety and PTSD symptoms (Girelli *et al.*, 1986; Resnick *et al.*, 2005). However, possible emotional avoidance, or reduced acute reactions in the early aftermath of assault, has also been hypothesized as a risk factor for later problems in functioning (Gilboa-Schechtman & Foa, 2001). Dunmore *et al.* (2001) found that retrospectively reported cognitive reactions that included mental defeat, confusion, and detachment were predictive of PTSD severity at later assessments among victims of sexual or physical assault. Several studies have identified panic reactions as common responses in the aftermath of rape, or other assault, that are associated with later PTSD (Resnick *et al.*, 1994; Falsetti *et al.*, 1995; Bernat *et al.*, 1998; Kilpatrick *et al.*, 1998). The study of panic and other acute reactions and cognitions appears to be important given the finding that subjective factors, including perceived life threat, were more predictive of psychological distress than objective assault characteristics among victims of interpersonal violence (Weaver & Clum, 1995).

Understanding emotional and cognitive perception variables that commonly occur during sexual assault and that are predictive of PTSD or other problems post-assault should inform development of secondary and tertiary preventive interventions. For example, as part of the video intervention developed by Resnick and colleagues (2005), information about panic reactions during the assault was included in order to normalize such reactions and provide an explanation of the functional underpinnings of physical sensations that might occur during an extremely stressful event, and to address the possibility that conditioned responses might occur later with reminders. The rationale for including this component was that this might normalize such reactions and reduce fear of panic sensations in and of themselves. In addition, potential cognitions related to blame and concern about negative responses from others within the formal medical setting were addressed by providing positive models of both rape crisis and hospital personnel responding in a supportive way. Another major rationale for the development and use of a video intervention designed to reduce acute distress and later psychopathology post-rape was the hypothesis that many components of the forensic rape examination (e.g., pelvic examination) might serve as strong rape-related cues, potentially raising acute

distress. Modeling of successful coping with examination procedures was included to possibly help prepare women to deal with the upcoming potential stressor.

The pattern of symptoms over time among rape victims is also very important to think about in terms of resilience or recovery issues. Significant decreases in PTSD or anxiety by three months after rape have been reported based on longitudinal studies (Kilpatrick *et al.*, 1979; Rothbaum *et al.*, 1992). Kilpatrick and Calhoun (1988) suggested that it was critical to keep information about the naturalistic course of recovery in mind when evaluating the efficacy of treatment programs implemented soon after a rape, because a significant proportion of individuals would be likely to recover over time.

Rape acknowledgement

As noted above, self-acknowledgement of rape has been found to be associated with more stereotypic or violent assaults (Koss, 1985), greater symptoms of PTSD (Layman *et al.*, 1996), and physical health complaints (Conoscenti & McNally, 2006). More recently, Kilpatrick *et al.* (2007b) assessed how often forcible, drug- or alcohol-facilitated or incapacitated rapes were acknowledged as rape. Specifically, women were asked in reference to up to two separate rape incidents whether they perceived the incident as unpleasant but not a crime, a crime but not a rape, or rape. Results within the college sample indicated that forcible rape incidents were most likely (51%) to be perceived as rape. One third (32%) of such incidents were perceived as a crime but not a rape, and 15% were seen as unpleasant but not a crime. Within the college sample, only 25% of incidents that involved unwanted penetration but that involved incapacitation through either voluntary or administered substances were perceived as rape; 40% were seen as crime other than rape, and 31% were perceived as unpleasant but not a crime. Parallel data in the general population sample indicated that 71% of forcible incidents were perceived as rape, 18% were perceived as crime, and 7% were perceived as unpleasant incidents. Substance-related rapes were perceived as rape in 45% of the cases; 28% were perceived as crime, and 22% were perceived as unpleasant incidents.

Some previous studies have examined associations between rape acknowledgement and PTSD without controlling for assault factors such as perceived life threat or force, which relate to both acknowledgement and PTSD (e.g., Layman *et al.*, 1996). A recent study by Littleton and Henderson (2009) of 346 rape victims recruited from a large university sample found that 39% of rapes were acknowledged. Acknowledgement was associated with more violent assaults and more frequent PTSD symptoms; however, in a structural equation model controlling for assault severity, acknowledgement was not a significant predictor of PTSD. Further, the effects of assault characteristics on PTSD were not direct but rather were associated indirectly with PTSD via the association of more violent assaults with more maladaptive coping strategies, including wishful thinking, social withdrawal, and self-criticism; these, in turn, were predictive of PTSD. In a comparison of acknowledged and unacknowledged rape and non-rape victims in a volunteer community sample, Conoscenti and McNally (2006) found that acknowledged and unacknowledged rape victims did not differ from each other on a standardized measure of PTSD symptom frequency. Both unacknowledged and acknowledged rape victims reported more health complaints than non-victims, while acknowledged rape victims reported more health symptoms than unacknowledged victims.

Zinzow et al. (2010) reported findings within the general population sample of 3001 women participating in the aforementioned study of forcible and drug- and alcohol-facilitated rape. History of both forcible rape and drug/alcohol-facilitated rape was associated with increased prevalence of PTSD compared with prevalence among non-rape victims. Zinzow et al. also examined characteristics of a most recent or only rape incident in association with PTSD diagnosis within the subsample of 556 rape victims and found positive correlations between rape acknowledgement and peritraumatic fear, injury, memory of event, force, and forcible rape. Acknowledgement of an incident as rape and/or as a crime was inversely related to incapacitated or drug/alcohol-facilitated rapes. Acknowledgement of most recent rape as either a rape or as a crime was a risk factor for PTSD diagnosis, controlling for assault characteristics that had been associated with PTSD on a univariate level. Although, as noted by Littleton and Henderson (2009), there are some mixed findings regarding association between acknowledgement and mental health correlates of rape, controlling for characteristics of assault, it does appear that acknowledgement tends to be positively correlated with those characteristics of assault that increase risk of PTSD. Whether acknowledgement or perception of more severe victimization is a unique predictor of negative

mental health consequences after controlling for such assault characteristics is equivocal at this point, but it may be relevant to consider as a cognitive variable that could be addressed in a constructive way in the context of secondary prevention.

Concerns in the aftermath of assault

Data from household probability samples (Kilpatrick et al., 1992, 2007b) indicate that victims of rape report post-assault concerns about health that include fear of pregnancy, HIV/AIDS, or other sexually transmitted diseases. Such concerns were reported by at least 40% of women who had been raped in the previous five-year period in the National Women's Study (Kilpatrick et al., 1992) and by 50% or more of rape victims in the general household probability study of forcible and drug- and alcohol-facilitated or incapacitated rape (Kilpatrick et al., 2007b). Both studies also found that concerns about negative evaluation by family members or others were reported as or more frequently than concerns about health. In a more select sample of those reporting the assault to police or other authorities, Resnick and colleagues (2002) found that concerns about HIV infection from the assault were reported by a majority of women. Greater concern regarding health issues such as sexually transmitted diseases may relate to formal reporting and was associated with receipt of post-rape medical care (Resnick et al., 2000). Programs that facilitate women receiving basic healthcare needs and addressing their health and other concerns might promote resilience following assault. Outreach to those not seeking post-assault services might reduce barriers to those who do not currently report assault.

Post-rape factors associated with post-rape functioning

Several post-assault factors have been shown to have varying degrees of influence on post-rape resilience. In general, the factors receiving the most empirical attention include social support, victim coping strategies, experience of additional traumas/life stressors, and accessing post-rape resources such as crisis counseling or psychological treatment. As with the personal and rape characteristics considered in this chapter, the research on these post-rape factors has been conducted with a wide range of populations, in a wide range of settings; the limitations of the extant literature mentioned at the outset of this chapter should be kept in mind.

Social support

The literature on social support has several ways of defining the reactions received by rape victims from either formal of informal recipients of disclosures. *Positive social reactions* or *social support* reactions are those in which the rape survivor feels that the response to disclosure is positive or neutral, whereas *negative social reactions* have been defined as reactions in which the victim feels blamed, disbelieved, or unsupported (reviewed by Ullman, 1999). Positive and negative social reactions are distinguishable from lack of social support, which is most often considered to be a separate factor with respect to resilience and recovery. In general, negative social reactions to disclosure have been consistently associated with lower levels of resilience, greater use of unhealthy coping styles such as avoidance and self-blame, and more severe levels of PTSD symptoms (Andrews *et al.*, 2003; Ullman *et al.*, 2007a, 2007b; reviewed by Ullman, 1999). Further, measures of perceived lack of social support have been associated with poorer recovery (Brewin *et al.*, 2000), whereas perceived satisfaction with level of social support received has been shown to buffer against initial risk for the development of PTSD (Andrews *et al.*, 2003).

The data regarding the impact of positive social support are much less straightforward, and more mixed with respect to findings. Initial research on the role of social support found that victim-perceived supportive reactions were associated with fewer reported physical health symptoms and more positive overall physical health ratings (Kimmerling & Calhoun, 1994). Although Ullman (1999) noted that some of the extant literature found positive social support to be protective, a significant portion of the literature reported non-significant findings regarding the impact of positive social support on the recovery process. More recent research with self-identified survivors of adult rape has, surprisingly, found greater frequency of social contact, positive social support, and higher levels of global support were associated with higher levels of PTSD symptoms (Ullman *et al.*, 2007a, 2007b). While this might suggest that support somehow leads to PTSD symptoms, it may simply reflect the fact that more symptomatic women seek more help, as has been noted in other studies.

Finally, the literature suggests that person and rape characteristics not only influence to whom women disclose their rape experience but also from whom they are most likely to receive support (Ullman & Filipas,

2001). Borja and colleagues (2006) examined the role of formal positive, informal positive, formal negative, and informal negative social reactions in contributing to the post-rape adjustment of over 100 college women. Results of that study indicated that only informal negative reactions significantly increased women's report of PTSD symptoms, whereas positive social support from both formal and informal sources were correlated with better adjustment/post-traumatic growth. None of the various forms of social reactions were significantly associated with general psychological distress. This study highlights the complexities of the relation between social support and post-rape adjustment in suggesting that both valence (positive versus negative) and source (formal versus informal) of support are important considerations.

The literature on social support has several limitations worthy of note. First, it is limited by its reliance on data from non-representative (most often community, but at times college) women who self-identify as "rape victims." As previously discussed, sampling methodology can limit the populations to which research findings can be generalized and applied. Another limitation of this area of research is that it lacks standard operational definitions of the various types of support and often relies heavily (or exclusively) on subjective perceptions of supportive/unsupportive reactions. That is, similar reactions may be interpreted as positive by some and interpreted as negative reactions by others (Ullman, 1999). Since almost all studies of social support have relied on retrospective self-report, it is also possible that respondent's current evaluation of the social support they received post-rape has been influenced by their present level of adjustment. That is, women reporting higher levels of current symptoms may be more likely to remember and highlight the negative social reactions they received in the more immediate rape aftermath Even given these limitations, we may still cautiously draw two main conclusions from the social support literature: (1) perception of positive support and that the level of support meets the individual need of the rape survivor are associated with recovery and resilience; and (2) negative reactions are seldom, if ever, associated with resilience and are often associated with poorer general recovery.

Coping

When confronted with an adverse life experience such as rape, women may employ a wide array of coping strategies, and may use them to varying degrees either in tandem or succession. When reading the summary of research on post-rape coping and resilience presented below, it is important to keep in mind that various measures of coping strategies exist, some measuring dominant coping styles (e.g., Frazier & Burnett, 1994), while others measure relative frequency of use of an array of coping strategies (e.g., Gutner *et al.*, 2006). However, despite these nuances in measurement, several general conclusions may be drawn from the existing literature on coping strategies and post-rape resilience.

First, approach-oriented coping strategies have generally been found to be associated with fewer post-traumatic stress symptoms and recovery, include cognitive restructuring, expressed emotion, seeking social support, counseling, positive distancing, and keeping busy (Frazier & Burnett, 1994; Valentiner *et al.*, 1996; Gutner *et al.*, 2006). Frazier and colleagues (2005) longitudinally surveyed a sample of women reporting their rape experience to an emergency medical facility and found that perceptions of control over the recovery process were significantly associated with greater use of cognitive restructuring; this, in turn, was associated with less reported distress post-rape. Similar results were found in a volunteer community sample of female adult rape survivors, with greater perceptions of control being associated with fewer PTSD symptoms (Ullman *et al.*, 2007a).

Second, avoidance-oriented coping strategies have generally been found to be associated with greater PTSD symptom severity and lower levels of resilience (Cohen & Roth, 1987; Santello & Leitenberg, 1993; Ullman, 1999; Ullman *et al.*, 2007b). The term *avoidance coping* has been used in a litany of research to apply to a range of coping strategies with the common element of disengagement or withdrawal. For example, among a community-recruited sample of self-identifying rape victims, Frazier and Burnett (1994) found that the most unhelpful coping strategies (those associated with higher mental health symptom levels) include avoidance strategies such as staying home and withdrawing from others. Similarly, wishful thinking, which may be viewed as a form of cognitive withdrawal, was associated with higher levels of PTSD symptoms among an adult clinical sample of rape victims (Valentiner *et al.*, 1996). Research sampling college survivors of rape has contributed similar findings of poorer adjustment among women employing higher levels of disengagement coping strategies (Santello & Leitenberg, 1993).

Third, as mentioned above with respect to social reactions and social support, victims' self-blame has also been shown to have a positive correlation with higher levels of post-rape psychopathology. Self-blame (e.g., there is something wrong with me as a person that led to my victimization; it was my fault I was raped) has, with high level of consistency, been associated with greater levels of PTSD symptomology. Frazier and colleagues (Frazier, 2003; Frazier *et al.*, 2004, 2005) have specifically examined behavioral self-blame (which they refer to as *past control*, or the notion that the victim's actions were to blame for the assault), consistently finding that it was associated with higher levels of distress. In addition, the correlation between measures of self-blame and higher levels of psychological distress, in turn, have been shown to influence health outcomes when examined in a cross-sectional sample of women with rape experiences (Koss *et al.*, 2002).

Finally, there is an important conceptual issue that must be considered with respect to any potential relationships that are found to exist between coping or self-blame and PTSD. Although it is generally assumed that avoidant coping strategies and/or behavioral self-blame are causative risk factors for PTSD, one can also make the case that people who develop PTSD have a greater need than those who are resilient to use a variety of coping strategies (including avoidant ones) than their counterparts who are not coping with PTSD symptoms. Likewise, it could be argued that self-blame is a self-protective cognitive coping strategy that is more likely to occur among people who develop PTSD than among those who do not. Consequently, it is equally plausible to hypothesize that PTSD causes maladaptive coping and self-blame as it is to hypothesize that maladaptive coping and/or self-blame causes PTSD. Clearly, only well-designed longitudinal research can establish which of these hypotheses is correct.

Additional stress and trauma

Women's experience of rape does not occur in isolation from additional life stresses. In fact, some evidence suggests that women experiencing sexual assault victimization are at increased risk for the additional life stress produced by unemployment, divorce, and reduced income (Byrne *et al.*, 1999). It is likely that this notable resource loss has a bidirectional relationship with post-rape distress. Research supports post-rape distress as a contributor to women's loss of resources (Monnier *et al.*, 2002). In turn, general life stress has been shown to be one of most consistent predictors of

PTSD development in meta-analysis, with medium to large effect sizes (Brewin *et al.*, 2000). Among a group of rape survivors, Resnick *et al.* (2007) found that having lower economic resources was a risk factor for poorer functioning after rape. Given that history of rape and physical assault are prevalent among those with reduced economic resources and, in fact, may contribute to lower resources (Bassuk *et al.*, 1996; Byrne *et al.*, 1999), it may be important to develop strategies to increase economic resources among women at risk for victimization and in the post-assault period. Similar to social support (discussed below in reference to post-assault factors), baseline economic and social support may also be conceptualized as pre-assault risk factors related to either resilience or poor adjustment post-assault.

Subsequent exposure to another traumatic event may appear to decrease resilience among rape survivors. Much empirical evidence exists that many women have multiple experiences of rape (Messman & Long, 1996; Breitenbecher & Scarce, 1999; Rich *et al.*, 2004). Women with a history of prior rape are at 2 to 4.5 times greater risk for future victimization than women without a rape history, making prior rape history one of the strongest risk factors for subsequent assault (Gidycz *et al.*, 1995, Humphrey & White, 2000). Women with a history of multiple victimizations are at greater risk for lacking satisfying social relationships and utilizing escapism/avoidant coping techniques, both of which have been previously identified as risk factors for poorer adjustment (Ellis *et al.*, 1982; Proulx *et al.*, 1995).

Several factors should be considered when considering the role of additional life stress and trauma in women's resilience against rape. First, direct prospective examinations of the contribution of additional life stress and subsequent trauma exposure to the development of PTSD (or other relevant mental health problems) have yet to be conducted. Second, the literature on revictimization is somewhat confused by the fact that many studies define revictimization as at least one incident of childhood sexual victimization and subsequent victimization in adulthood, whereas other studies have defined revictimization more in line with the discussion of multiple victimizations presented in this chapter.

Conclusions and future directions

The majority of studies investigating risk and resilience factors among rape victims, although laudable, have the potential to yield potentially biased information because of the methodological approaches used (e.g., typically retrospective nature of epidemiological studies and non-generalizable results from convenience samples typically restricted to volunteer samples or those reporting the assault to police or other authorities). In order to fill in the gaps in our understanding of factors that promote resilience among rape victims, future studies need to address these limitations.

First, as described in the methodological section of this chapter, an ideal study of risk and resilience would include a large representative sample of women who would be assessed for "baseline" characteristics including both psychological and biological markers thought to be important for risk or protection against PTSD. This sample would then be followed over time to allow for assessment of traumatic events, including rape, as well as for PTSD and related problems in those who experienced rape compared with those who did not. This would allow for the identification of potential risk and protective factors related to resilience in a large representative sample of women. Ultimately, these results would be more generalizable than the convenience samples.

Second, despite employing an adequate study design to identify key risk and resilience factors among rape victims, these data may still be limited by rape victims' tendency to avoid acknowledging rape. As noted above, many victims who meet the legal definition of rape do not acknowledge what happened to them as a rape. Given the findings that rape acknowledgement is related to characteristics of assault that are predictive of PTSD or other negative mental health outcomes, studies that ask participants if they have been raped or sexually assaulted, rather than using behavioral definitions, and studies that gather volunteer respondents (all of whom will identify as having an unwanted sexual assault history) may include primarily or more predominantly sexual assault victims who have experienced higher rates of injury and perceived life threat and, in turn, may observe higher prevalence of PTSD. In order to avoid this potential bias, when researchers are inquiring about rape experiences among participants, it is important to employ behavioral definitions of rape as opposed to asking participants if they have been raped or sexually assaulted.

Also, as highlighted throughout this chapter, the majority of the literature has focused on factors that predict post-rape PTSD or other psychopathology. The identification of key risk factors for psychopathology can be used to study resilience in the face of known risk factors as well as to identify potentially modifiable risk factors that may be targeted in interventions to promote resilience or that constitute secondary prevention efforts once a woman has been sexually assaulted. A second line of investigation would be to identify protective factors among a cohort of those that have thrived in the face of adversity. In addition, more research should focus on risk factors and potential interventions for other problems such as substance abuse.

Using what we know to foster greater resilience and design early interventions to speed recovery

Little is known about strategies that might promote resilience after rape. Such approaches might include public education about realistic characteristics of rape and about functional coping strategies in the aftermath of rape. The latter type of information about how to report an incident or what to do in the immediate aftermath is often put forth by rape crisis centers but it is heavily focused on criminal justice system or evidence-gathering issues. Information designed to reduce blame or shame by addressing true characteristics of rape may also be disseminated by service agencies, but these are typically given to women who have already been victimized. Outreach to college campuses and community education events are also often conducted by rape crisis agencies, but the potential impact of such educational approaches in terms of resilience following rape has not been empirically studied to our knowledge. More widespread public education programs targeting potential social support providers or recipients of disclosure have also not been evaluated. Such approaches might promote resilience by reducing negative social reactions and increasing positive supportive responses. Rape crisis agencies often conduct education with formal service providers such as police, with the goal of reducing negative responses. Similarly, sexual assault response teams, including nurses and other criminal justice personnel, attempt to provide such education across disciplines in order to improve the quality of services provided and/or the investigation of rape cases. Empirical evaluation of the impact of such approaches on treatment of rape victims or perceived formal responses by rape victims is lacking. Additionally, minimal information is available about

the direct impact of rape crisis advocates who provide information and support to rape victims during the medical examination, through the criminal justice process, or in the period after rape. However, the limited information available suggests that such services are helpful to survivors (reviewed by Campbell et al., 2005; Martin et al., 2007; Decker & Naugle, 2009).

More information is available regarding secondary prevention or early intervention approaches (primarily targeting the individual and her cognitive or behavioral coping strategies) designed to be implemented soon after a rape with the goal of reducing acute distress and preventing or reducing longer-term problems such as PTSD. Treatment implemented after an individual already has PTSD would be considered tertiary intervention. Kilpatrick and colleagues (2007b) reviewed strategies and findings pertaining to rape-related secondary and tertiary interventions. They noted that propranolol is an example of a pharmacological early intervention that has been evaluated in small studies with victims of different traumatic events (e.g., Famularo et al., 1988; Pitman et al., 2002; Vaiva et al., 2003). They suggested that the initial promising findings showing relatively lower prevalence of PTSD or lower intensity of physiological responding need to be replicated within larger samples. Mixed findings have been observed related to psychosocial early interventions, which include cognitive-behavioral approaches delivered within hours, days, or weeks after a rape. For example, Kilpatrick and Veronen (1983) found symptom improvement among victims of rape who received four to six hours of an early cognitive-behavioral skills-based intervention between 6 and 21 days after an assault, but improvement was not greater than that seen in the control group. Foa and colleagues (1995) found that a brief multisession cognitive-behavioral intervention delivered within one month of an assault (including rape) was associated with reduced prevalence of PTSD at the end of treatment but not at a follow-up at 5.5 months after the assault. A subsequent study by Foa and colleagues (2006) comparing brief cognitive-behavioral therapy, assessment control, or supportive counseling implemented within one month after an assault found reduced symptoms of PTSD and general anxiety associated with the cognitive-behavioral treatment relative to the supportive counseling condition when assessed at three months after the assault. Differences between groups were not observed at longer-term follow-up. Findings from the study by Foa and colleagues were seen as consistent with the possibility that early cognitive-behavioral intervention might accelerate recovery post-assault.

As described above, Resnick and colleagues (1999, 2005) developed a psychoeducational cognitive-behavioral intervention delivered in a video format and designed to be shown prior to the rape examination that is routinely conducted whenever a rape victim reports the assault to police or seeks post-rape medical services. The video has two major components, the first of which provides information about the medical examination and modeling of a woman successfully going through procedures. In addition, hospital and rape crisis personnel are introduced and positive messages are conveyed by these individuals regarding the fact that the assault was not the individual's fault but that they have control over their recovery. This component was designed to reduce anxiety related to the medical examination and to provide a positive supportive context at the time of the exam. The second component of the video includes psychoeducation and modeling of coping strategies in the aftermath of assault, which include in vivo graduated exposure, behavioral activation, identification of cues or situations that may be associated with drug or alcohol use, and promotion of activities and contexts that do not involve substance use. Information about acute reactions of panic and a learning theory model of possible later reactions to reminders of assault is presented in order to try to prevent fear of physiological arousal sensations and to provide a model for understanding the rationale for in vivo exposure exercises.

A randomized clinical trial compared the video intervention with standard care among a group of rape victims who were seen for standard post-rape medical care. Data indicated that, among women with a prior history of rape, those in the video group reported significantly lower frequency of PTSD symptoms and severity of depression symptoms at assessment approximately six weeks after rape compared with women in the standard care sample. Women without a prior history of rape appeared to be more resilient in terms of reported symptom frequency and intensity over time. No differences in symptoms of psychopathology were observed related to intervention at longer-term follow-up assessment at approximately six months post-rape (Resnick *et al.*, 2007). Results of this study indicated a significant moderating effect of prior history of rape. It was hypothesized that women with a prior history of assault, who are also at risk of more severe problems following a new incident, might also

understand the content of the video intervention and it may have been more salient to them given their prior history of assault and/or subsequent reactions including PTSD.

The review of risk and resilience factors related to differential outcomes following rape may identify which approaches or components may be useful for integrating with other promising interventions to promote resilience or recovery. There are a number of such strategies that can be envisaged. Wider dissemination of information about characteristics of rape and helpful responses to others who have experienced assault could be evaluated to see if such information leads to attitude and/or behavior change, greater resilience, or more positive support/reduced negative support in the aftermath of rape. Strategies to enhance perceived control or efficacy would appear to be useful and could perhaps be taught as general ways of coping with stressors. Greater emphasis might be given to improving social support of victims in the aftermath of assault and such a strategy could then be evaluated empirically. Assistance with economic or other resources in the aftermath of rape could be instigated, similar to the components augmenting the treatment strategy used by Zatzick and colleagues (2004) for patients with traumatic injuries. Finally, additional attention should be given to developing and evaluating potentially effective early interventions and exploring possible individual differences in response to interventions to determine which approaches may be useful given identified risk or resilience factors.

Acknowledgements

Support for writing was provided by NIDA Grant R01 DA023099–02 (*Prevention of Postrape Drug Abuse: Replication Study and Training*) and Grant 5 *T32* MH018869–22 (*Traumatic Stress Across the Lifespan: A Biopsychosocial Training Program*) (principal investigator, Dean Kilpatrick).

References

Acierno, R., Resnick, H., Kilpatrick, D. G., Saunders, B., & Best, C. L. (1999). Risk factors for rape, physical assault, and posttraumatic stress disorder in women: examination of differential multivariate relationships. *Journal of Anxiety Disorders*, **13**, 541–563.

American Psychiatric Association (1994). *Diagnostic and statistical manual of mental disorders,* 4th edn. Washington, DC: American Psychiatric Press.

Andrews, B., Brewin, C., & Rose, S. (2003). Gender, social support, and PTSD in victims of violent crime. *Journal of Traumatic Stress*, **16**, 421–427.

Bassuk, E. L., Weinreb, L. F., Buckner, J. C., *et al.* (1996). The characteristics and needs of sheltered homeless and low income housed mothers. *Journal of the American Medical Association*, **276**, 640–646.

Bernat, J. A., Ronfeldt, H. M., Calhoun, K. S., & Arias, I. (1998). Prevalence of traumatic events and peritraumatic predictors of posttraumatic stress symptoms in a nonclinical sample of college students. *Journal of Traumatic Stress*, **11**, 645–664.

Binder, E. B., Bradley, R. G., Liu, W., *et al.* (2008). Association of *FKBP5* polymorphisms and childhood abuse with risk of posttraumatic stress disorder symptoms in adults. *Journal of the American Medical Association*, **299**, 1291–1305.

Bonanno, G. A. (2004). Loss, trauma, and human resilience: Have we underestimated the human capacity to thrive after extremely aversive events? *American Psychologist*, **59**, 20–28.

Borja, S., Callahan, J. L., & Long, P. J. (2006). Positive and negative adjustment and social support of sexual assault survivors. *Journal of Traumatic Stress*, **19**, 905–914.

Breitenbecher, K. H. & Scarce, M. (1999). A longitudinal evaluation of the effectiveness of a sexual assault education program. *Journal of Interpersonal Violence*, **14**, 459–478.

Breslau, N., Kessler, R. C., Chilcoat, H. D., *et al.* (1998). Trauma and posttraumatic stress disorder in the community: the 1996 Detroit Area Survey of Trauma. *Archives of General Psychiatry*, **55**, 626–632.

Brewin, C. R., Andrews, B., & Valentine, J. D. (2000). Meta-analysis of risk factors for posttraumatic stress disorder in trauma-exposed adults. *Journal of Consulting and Clinical Psychology*, **68**, 748–766.

Byrne, C. A., Resnick, H. S., Kilpatrick, D. G., Best, C. L., & Saunders, B. E. (1999). The socioeconomic impact of interpersonal violence on women. *Journal of Consulting and Clinical Psychology*, **67**, 362–366.

Calhoun, K. S., Atkeson, B. M., & Resick, P. A. (1982). A longitudinal examination of fear reactions in victims of rape. *Journal of Counseling Psychology*, **29**, 655–661.

Campbell, R., Patterson, D., & Lichty, L. F. (2005). The effectiveness of sexual assault nurse examiner (SANE) programs: A review of psychological, medical, legal, and community outcomes. *Trauma, Violence, and Abuse*, **6**, 313–329.

Cohen, L. J. & Roth, S. (1987). The psychological aftermath of rape: Long-term effects and individual differences in coping. *Journal of Social and Clinical Psychology*, **5**, 525–534.

Conoscenti, L. M. & McNally, R. J. (2006). Health complaints in acknowledged and unacknowledged rape victims. *Journal of Anxiety Disorders*, **20**, 372–379.

Cougle, J. R., Resnick, H., & Kilpatrick, D. G. (2009). Does prior exposure to interpersonal violence increase risk of PTSD following subsequent exposure? *Behaviour Research and Therapy*, **47**, 1012–1017.

Cusack, K. J., Frueh, B. C., & Brady, K. T. (2004). Trauma history screening in a community mental health center. *Psychiatric Services*, **55**, 157–162.

Decker, S. E. & Naugle, A. E. (2009). Immediate intervention for sexual assault: A review with recommendations and implications for practitioners. *Journal of Aggression, Maltreatment and Trauma*, **18**, 419–441.

Dunmore, E., Clark, D. M., & Ehlers, A. (2001). A prospective investigation of the role of cognitive factors in persistent posttraumatic stress disorder (PTSD) after physical or sexual assault. *Behaviour Research and Therapy*, **39**, 1063–1084.

Ellis, E., Atkeson, B., & Calhoun, K. (1982). An examination of differences between multiple-and single-incident victims of sexual assault. *Journal of Abnormal Psychology*, **91**, 221–224.

Falsetti, S. A., Resnick, H. S., Dansky, B. S., Lydiard, R. B., & Kilpatrick, D. G. (1995). The relationship of stress to panic disorder: Cause or effect? In C. M. Mazure (ed.), *Does stress cause psychiatric illness?* (pp. 111–147). Washington, DC: American Psychiatric Press.

Famularo, R., Kinscherff, R., & Fenton, T. (1988). Propranolol treatment for childhood posttraumatic stress disorder, acute type: a pilot study. *Archives of Pediatric Adolescent Medicine*, **142**, 1244–1247.

Fisher, B. S., Daigle, L. E., Cullen, F. T., & Turner, M. G. (2003). Reporting sexual victimization to the police and others: Results from a national-level study of college women. *Criminal Justice and Behavior*, **30**, 6–38.

Foa, E. B., Hearst-Ikeda, D., & Perry, K. J. (1995). Evaluation of a brief cognitive-behavioral program for the prevention of chronic PTSD in recent assault victims. *Journal of Consulting and Clinical Psychology*, **63**, 948–955.

Foa, E. B., Zoellner, L. A., & Feeny, N. C. (2006). An evaluation of three brief programs for facilitating recovery after assault. *Journal of Traumatic Stress*, **19**, 29–43.

Frank, E. & Stewart, B. D. (1984). Depressive symptoms in rape victims. *Journal of Affective Disorders*, **7**, 77–85.

Frazier, P. A. (2003). Perceived control and distress following sexual assault: A longitudinal test of a new model. *Journal of Personality and Social Psychology*, **84**, 1257–1269.

Frazier, P. & Burnett, J. (1994). Immediate coping strategies among rape victims. *Journal of Counseling and Development*, **72**, 633–639.

Frazier, P., Steward, J., & Mortensen, H. (2004). Perceived control and adjustment to trauma: A comparison across events. *Journal of Social and Clinical Psychology*, **23**, 303–324.

Frazier, P., Mortensen, H., & Steward, J. (2005). Coping strategies as mediators of the relations among perceived control and distress in sexual assault survivors. *Journal of Counseling Psychology*, **52**, 267–278.

Gidycz, C., Hanson, K., & Layman, M. (1995). A prospective analysis of the relationships among sexual assault experiences: An extension of previous findings. *Psychology of Women Quarterly*, **19**, 5–29.

Gilboa-Schechtman, E. & Foa, E. B. (2001). Patterns of recovery from trauma: the use of intraindividual analysis. *Journal of Abnormal Psychology*, **110**, 392–400.

Girelli, S. A., Resick, P. A., Marhoefer-Dvorak, S., & Hutter, C. K. (1986). Subjective distress and violence during rape: Their effects on long-term fear. *Violence and Victims*, **1**, 35–45.

Goodman, L., Salyers, M., & Mueser, K., *et al.* (2001). Recent victimization in women and men with severe mental illness: Prevalence and correlates. *Journal of Traumatic Stress*, **14**, 615–633.

Gutner, C., Rizvi, S., Monson, C., & Resick, P. (2006). Changes in coping strategies, relationship to the perpetrator, and posttraumatic distress in female crime victims. *Journal of Traumatic Stress*, **19**, 813–823.

Humphrey, J. A. & White, J. W. (2000). Women's vulnerability to sexual assault from adolescence to young adulthood. *Journal of Adolescent Health*, **27**, 419–424.

Kessler, R. C., Sonnega, A., Bromet, E., Hughes, M., & Nelson, C. B. (1995). Posttraumatic stress disorder in the National Comorbidity Survey. *Archives of General Psychiatry*, **52**, 1048–1060.

Kilpatrick, D. G. (1983). Rape victims: Detection, assessment, and treatment. *Clinical Psychologist*, **36**, 92–95.

Kilpatrick, D. G. & Calhoun, K. S. (1988). Early behavioral treatment for rape trauma: Efficacy or artifact. *Behavior Therapy*, **19**, 421–427.

Kilpatrick, D. G. & Veronen, L. J. (1983). Treatment for rape related problems: Crisis intervention is not enough. In L. H. Cohen, W. L. Claiborn, & C. A. Spector (eds.), *Crisis intervention* (pp. 165–185). New York: Human Sciences Press.

Kilpatrick, D. G., Veronen, L. J., & Resick, P. A. (1979). The aftermath of rape: Recent empirical findings. *American Journal of Orthopsychiatry*, **49**, 658–669.

Kilpatrick, D. G., Veronen, L. J., & Best, C. L. (1985). Factors predicting psychological distress among rape victims.

In C. R. Figley (ed.), *Trauma and its wake* (pp.113–141). New York: Brunner/Mazel.

Kilpatrick, D. G., Best, C. C., Saunders, B. E., & Vernon, L. J. (1988). Rape in marriage and in dating relationships: How bad is it for mental health? *Annals of the New York Academy of Sciences*, **528**, 335–344.

Kilpatrick, D. G., Saunders, B. E., Amick-McMullan, A., *et al.* (1989). Victim and crime factors associated with the development of crime-related post-traumatic stress disorder. *Behavior Therapy*, **20**, 199–214.

Kilpatrick, D. G., Edmunds, C. N., & Seymour, A. K. (1992). *Rape in America: A report to the nation.* Arlington, VA: National Victim Center and the Medical University of South Carolina.

Kilpatrick, D. G., Acierno, R., Resnick, H. S., Saunders, B., & Best, C. L. (1997). A 2-year longitudinal analysis of the relationship between violent assault and substance use in women. *Journal of Consulting and Clinical Psychology*, **65**, 834–847.

Kilpatrick, D. G., Resnick, H. S., Freedy, J. R., *et al.* (1998). The posttraumatic stress disorder field trial: Emphasis on criterion A and overall PTSD diagnosis. In T. Widiger, A. Frances, H. Pincus, *et al.* (eds.), *DSM-IV sourcebook*, Vol. 4 (pp. 303–344). Washington, DC: American Psychiatric Press.

Kilpatrick, D. G., Ruggiero, K. J., Acierno, R., *et al.* (2003). Violence and risk of PTSD, major depression, substance abuse/dependence, and comorbidity: Results from the national survey of adolescents. *Journal of Consulting and Clinical Psychology*, **71**, 692–700.

Kilpatrick, D. G., Resnick, H. S., Ruggiero, K. J., Conoscenti, L. M., & McCauley, J. (2007a). *Drug-facilitated, incapacitated, and forcible rape: A national study. Final report submitted to the National Institute of Justice, May 2007* [NCJ 219181]. Rockville, MD: National Institute of Justice.

Kilpatrick, D. G., Amstadter, A. B., Resnick, H. S., & Ruggiero, K. J. (2007b). Rape related PTSD: Issues and interventions. *Psychiatric Times*, **24**, 7.

Kimmerling, R. & Calhoun, K. S. (1994). Somatic symptoms, social support, and treatment seeking among sexual assault victims. *Journal of Consulting and Clinical Psychology*, **62**, 333–340.

Koss, M. P. (1985). The hidden rape victim. *Psychology of Women Quarterly*, **48**, 61–75.

Koss, M. P., Dinero, T. E., & Seibel, C. A. (1988). Stranger and acquaintance rape: Are there differences in victim's experience? *Psychology of Women Quarterly*, **12**, 1–24.

Koss, M. P., Figueredo, A. J., & Prince, R. J. (2002). Cognitive mediation of rape's mental, physical, and social health impact: Tests of four models in cross-sectional data. *Journal of Consulting and Clinical Psychology*, **70**, 926–941.

Kramer, T. L. & Green, B. L. (1991). Posttraumatic stress disorder as an early response to sexual assault. *Journal of Interpersonal Violence*, **6**, 160–173.

Layman, M. J., Gidycz, C. A., & Lynn, S. J. (1996). Unacknowledged versus acknowledged rape victims: situational factors and posttraumatic stress. *Journal of Abnormal Psychology*, **105**, 124–131.

Littleton, H., & Henderson, C. E. (2009). If she is not a victim, does that mean she was not traumatized? *Violence Against Women*, **15**, 148–167.

Martin, S. L., Young, S. K., Billings, D. L., & Bross, C. C. (2007). Health care-based interventions for women who have experienced sexual violence. *Trauma, Violence, and Abuse*, **8**, 3–18.

Messman, T. L. & Long, P. J. (1996). Child sexual abuse and its relationship to revictimization in adult women: A review. *Clinical Psychology Review*, **16**, 397–420.

Monnier, J., Resnick, H., Kilpatrick, D., & Seals, B. (2002). The relationship between distress and resource loss following rape. *Violence and Victims*, **17**, 85–92.

Norris, F. H. (1992). Epidemiology of trauma: Frequency and impact of different potentially traumatic events on different demographic groups. *Journal of Consulting and Clinical Psychology*, **60**, 409–418.

Ozer, E. J., Best, S. R., Lipsey, T. L., & Weiss, D. S. (2003). Predictors of posttraumatic stress disorder and symptoms in adults: A meta-analysis. *Psychological Bulletin*, **129**, 52–73.

Pervanidou, P. (2008). Biology of post-traumatic stress disorder in childhood and adolescence. *Journal of Neuroendocrinology*, **20**, 632–638.

Pitman, R. K., Sanders, K. M., Zusman, R. M., *et al*. (2002). Pilot study of secondary prevention of posttraumatic stress disorder with propranolol. *Biological Psychiatry*, **51**, 189–192.

Proulx, J., Koverola, C., Fedorowicz, A., & Kral, M. (1995). Coping strategies as predictors of distress in survivors of single and multiple sexual victimization and nonvictimized controls. *Journal of Applied Social Psychology*, **25**, 1464–1483.

Resick, P. A. (1993). The psychological impact of rape. *Journal of Interpersonal Violence*, **8**, 223–255.

Resnick, H. S., Kilpatrick, D. G., & Lipovsky, J. A. (1991). Assessment of rape-related posttraumatic stress disorder: stressor and symptom dimensions. *Journal of Consulting and Clinical Psychology*, **3** 561–572.

Resnick, H. S., Kilpatrick, D. G., Best, C. L., & Kramer, T. L. (1992). Vulnerability–stress factors in development of posttraumatic stress disorder. *Journal of Nervous and Mental Disease*, **180**, 424–430.

Resnick, H. S., Kilpatrick, D. G., Dansky, B. S., Saunders, B. E., & Best, C. L. (1993). Prevalence of civilian trauma and posttraumatic stress disorder in a representative national sample of women. *Journal of Consulting and Clinical Psychology*, **61**, 984–991.

Resnick, H. S., Falsetti, S. A., Kilpatrick, D. G., & Foy, D. W. (1994). Associations between panic attacks during rape assaults and follow-up PTSD or panic-attack outcomes. In *Proceedings of the 10th Annual Meeting of the International Society of Traumatic Stress Studies*, Chicago, November.

Resnick, H. S., Yehuda, R., Pitman, R. K., & Foy, D. W. (1995). Effect of previous trauma on acute plasma cortisol level following rape. *American Journal of Psychiatry*, **152**, 1675–1677.

Resnick, H. S., Acierno, R., & Kilpatrick, D. G. (1997). Health impact of interpersonal violence. Section II: Medical and mental health outcomes. *Behavioral Medicine*, **23**, 79–85.

Resnick, H. S., Acierno, R., Holmes, M., Kilpatrick, D., & Jager, N. (1999). Prevention of post-rape psychopathology: Preliminary findings of a controlled acute rape treatment. *Journal of Anxiety Disorders*, **13**, 359–370.

Resnick, H. S., Holmes, M. M., Kilpatrick, D. G., *et al*. (2000). Predictors of post-rape medical care in a national sample of women. *American Journal of Preventive Medicine*, **19**, 214–219.

Resnick, H. S., Monnier, J., Seals, B., *et al*. (2002). Rape-related HIV risk concerns among recent rape victims. *Journal of Interpersonal Violence*, **17**, 746–759.

Resnick, H. S., Acierno, R., Kilpatrick, D. G., Holmes, M. (2005). Description of an early intervention to prevent substance abuse and psychopathology in recent rape victims. *Behavior Modification*, **29**, 156–188.

Resnick, H. S., Acierno, R., Waldrop, A. E., *et al*. (2007). Randomized controlled evaluation of an early intervention to prevent post-rape psychopathology. *Behaviour Research and Therapy*, **45**, 2432–2447.

Rich, C. L., Combs-Lane, A. M., Resnick, H. S., & Kilpatrick, D. G. (2004). Child sexual abuse and adult sexual revictimization. In L. J. Koenig, L. S. Doll, A. O'Learey, & W. Pequegnat (eds.), *From child sexual abuse to adult sexual risk: Trauma, revictimization, and intervention* (pp. 49–68). Washington DC: American Psychiatric Press.

Rothbaum, B. O., Foa, E. B., Riggs, D. S., Murdock, T., & Walsh, W. (1992). A prospective examination of post-traumatic stress disorder in rape victims. *Journal of Traumatic Stress*, **5**, 455–475.

Santello, M. & Leitenberg, H. (1993). Sexual aggression by an acquaintance: Methods of coping and later psychological adjustment. *Violence and Victims*, **8**, 91–104.

Shalev, A. Y., Peri, T., Canetti, L., & Schreiber, S. (1996). Predictors of PTSD in injured trauma survivors: a prospective study. *American Journal of Psychiatry*, **153**, 219–225.

Steketee, G. & Foa, E. B. (1987). Rape victims: Post-traumatic stress responses and their treatment: A review of the literature. *Journal of Anxiety Disorders*, **1**, 69–86.

Tjaden, P. & Thoennes, N. (2000). Prevalence and consequences of male-to-female and female-to-male partner violence as measured by the National Violence Against Women Survey. *Violence Against Women*, **6**, 142–161.

Ullman, S. (1999). Social support and recovery from sexual assault: A review. *Aggression and Violent Behavior*, **4**, 343–358.

Ullman, S. E. & Filipas, H. H. (2001). Predictors of PTSD symptom severity and social reactions in sexual assault victims. *Journal of Traumatic Stress*, **14**, 369–389.

Ullman, S., Filipas, H. H., Townsend, S. M., & Starzynski, L. L. (2007a). Psychosocial correlates of PTSD symptom severity in sexual assault survivors. *Journal of Traumatic Stress*, **20**, 821–831.

Ullman, S., Townsend, S. M., Filipas, H. H., & Starzynski, L. L. (2007b). Structural models of the relations of assault severity, social support, avoidance coping, self-blame, and PTSD among sexual assault survivors. *Psychology of Women Quarterly*, **31**, 23–37.

Vaiva, G., Ducrocq, F., Jezequel, K., *et al.* (2003). Immediate treatment with propranolol decreases posttraumatic stress disorder two months after trauma. *Biological Psychiatry*, **54**, 947–949.

Valentiner, D., Foa, E., Riggs, D., & Gershuny, B. (1996). Coping strategies and posttraumatic stress disorder in female victims of sexual and nonsexual assault. *Journal of Abnormal Psychology*, **105**, 455–458.

Weaver, T. L. & Clum, G. A. (1995). Psychological distress associated with interpersonal violence: A meta-analysis. *Clinical Psychology Review*, **15**, 115–140.

Yehuda, R. (2001). Biology of posttraumatic stress disorder. *Journal of Clinical Psychiatry*, **62**, 41–46

Yehuda, R., Golier, J. A., Halligan, S. L., Meaney, M., & Bierer, L. M. (2004). The ACTH response to dexamethasone in PTSD. *American Journal of Psychiatry*, **161**, 1397–1403

Zatzick, D., Roy-Byrne, P., Russo, J., *et al.* (2004). A randomized effectiveness trial of stepped collaborative care for acutely injured trauma survivors. *Archives of General Psychiatry*, **61**, 498–506.

Zinzow, H., Resnick, H., Amstadter, A., *et al.* (2010). Drug and alcohol-facilitated, incapacitated, and forcible rape in relation to mental health in a national sample of women. *Journal of Interpersonal Violence*, **25**, 2217–2236.

Chapter

16

The stress continuum model: a military organizational approach to resilience and recovery

William P. Nash, Maria Steenkamp, Lauren Conoscenti, and Brett T. Litz

Introduction

Resilience in the face of adversity is vital for military service members to survive potential threats to their own lives and safety and to accomplish assigned missions, often for the sake of others' survival and welfare. The ability of service members to bounce back from operational stress may also determine how successfully they reintegrate with their families and communities after returning from deployment, whether they can continue to work in military professions, and whether they develop potentially disabling mental disorders or other serious behavioral problems. Military organizations have long traditions of selecting, training, and sustaining service members to endure intense and persistent operational stress without losing their abilities to function on the battlefield, but other indices of resilience have only recently attracted the sustained interest of the military. As military organizations develop programs to promote a broader spectrum of desired stress outcomes, they are faced with a choice between expecting traditional resilience-building methods to meet untraditional objectives and creating entirely novel approaches to resilience.

Academic interest in the psychological, biological, social, and personality-trait differences associated with successful adaptation to combat and operational experiences has increased rapidly since the late 1990s. Underlying recent studies in this area has been the assumption that the incidence of various mental health and functional problems associated with combat and operational experiences might be reduced if modifiable risk and resilience factors could be identified and then targeted in military prevention programs. Unfortunately, research and translational programs to enhance resilience in members of the armed services have, so far, been limited by the lack of a unified or paradigmatic approach to conceptualizing the military and extra-military processes and functions that may lead to resilient outcomes, and even by the lack of a consensus definition of resilience. Uniform methods of measuring resilience processes or outcomes also do not yet exist. The little empirical research that has been conducted in the military has significant internal and external validity problems, greatly limiting their power to inform prevention or intervention practices, which is the basic goal of resilience research.

To promote clarity about the concept of resilience in the military, and to foster future research, this chapter begins by considering the concept of resilience in the military as comprising of different classes of positive stress outcome. The chapter then considers potential metrics for each and briefly surveys existing evidence that the military has been successful at developing and sustaining each aspect of resilience in its service members. The goal is to identify the greatest ongoing challenges for military resilience program development. One recently developed, evidence-informed approach to promoting resilience and recovery is then described that specifically emphasizes military ecological validity: the Combat and Operational Stress Control (COSC) program in the US Marine Corps and its parallel in the US Navy, the Operational Stress Control (OSC) program. The rationale, conceptual framework, and intervention strategies common to both programs are outlined. The chapter concludes with a call for well-designed outcome studies of programs that attempt to fill the current gaps in military resilience programs.

Military resilience challenges

Almost any mission with which a military unit may be tasked – whether assaulting an opposing military force, countering a civilian insurgency, conducting

Resilience and Mental Health: Challenges Across the Lifespan, ed. Steven M. Southwick, Brett T. Litz, Dennis Charney, and Matthew J. Friedman. Published by Cambridge University Press. © Cambridge University Press 2011.

peacekeeping, or providing humanitarian assistance in the wake of a disaster – can expose service members to mortal danger, loss, and moral compromise with an intensity and relentlessness hard to imagine in most other settings (e.g., Litz, 2007; Nash, 2007a; Litz *et al.*, 2009). Returning from deployment exposes service members to an entirely different set of adaptive challenges, some of which may be just as overwhelming as those experienced during deployment. Examples include the stress of coming home to a broken family, a lost civilian job, or financial ruin. Both during and after deployment to an operational theater, service members face the challenge of mourning losses, finding meaning in experiences that seem senseless, and making peace with enduring memories of death and destruction. Resilience challenges for military service members and the organizations that support them, therefore, arguably encompass at least three broad forms: (1) *operational resilience*, which may be defined as the ability to maintain occupational role functioning and psychological performance during operational deployments despite stressor exposures, and perhaps despite internal distress and conflict (see Litz, 2005); (2) *post-deployment resilience*, which may be defined as the ability to reacquire and maintain effective role functioning in largely non-military settings after returning from deployment, and so again to be a productive member of a family and civilian society; and (3) *psychological resilience*, which may be defined as the ability to adapt physically, mentally, and spiritually to operational stressor exposures, and the sometimes lasting changes they engender, without developing a significant mental disorder or behavioral problem.

Though obviously interrelated, these three broad resilience challenges in the military have very different historical and scientific bases, and they depend on different methods for promotion and metrics for assessment. Each will now be briefly described in its historical and scientific context.

Operational resilience

Extreme stress is not an incidental byproduct of armed conflict but rather one of its central features and immediate objectives. Success in traditional warfare has often been determined by which side possesses the greater ability to endure and continue fighting despite the potentially overwhelming challenges and hardships each side intentionally inflicts upon the other (von Clausewitz, 1982 [orginally published 1832]).

Troops in battle who are disabled by stress, even briefly, or who lose their ability to remain calm and make rational decisions in the face of chaos lose operational effectiveness and may quickly become physical casualties. Some of the historically highest physical casualty rates have been experienced by ground combat units engaged in disorganized and panicked retreats. Similarly, the success of western nations and deployed military units to prevail in modern, asymmetrical warfare against non-governmental insurgencies or terrorist groups depends on their abilities to remain focused on constructively "winning the hearts and minds" of populations even while repeatedly enduring attacks from within the population's ranks – attacks that have great potential to provoke terror, horror, helplessness, rage, and a desire to seek vengeance rather than to build hospitals, schools, and sewage systems. The weapons of global terrorism, including the growing threat of rogue nuclear incidents, directly target the resilience of societies and their governments.

At the unit level, the desired outcomes of operational resilience include mission effectiveness, readiness, and force preservation. At the individual level, the simplest desired outcome is to avoid becoming a stress casualty (i.e., being incapacitated) by continuing to maintain at least the minimum required ability to function in assigned operational military roles. Stated more positively, the objectives of individual and unit-level operational resilience are performance enhancement despite hardships and losses, and the development and maintenance of the time-honored military traits of courage, fortitude, and valor (e.g., Moran, 1967 [originally published 1945]). Operational resilience has been so central to the effectiveness of fighting forces that methods for promoting it have been in existence since ancient times. In the Roman army (Phang, 2008), for example, the goal of all training and discipline was to develop *virtus* (courage in battle) without *ferocia* (madness), and *animus* (confidence) and *impetus* (enthusiasm) without excessive *ira* (anger). The same warrior ideal of controlled aggression, summoned by external authority but restrained by internal moral values, can be found in military cultures throughout history (French, 2003). Much the same tools are available to the military today as were in use in ancient times to promote operational resilience: pre-induction selection, tough and realistic training, the building of unit cohesion through shared successes in the face of shared hardships, and engaged leadership (Nash *et al.*, 2011).

239

At its most basic level, operational resilience is easy to measure in service members because the primary target outcome is simple and easy to quantify over the fixed period of observation of each deployment. Most simply, operational resilience may be quantified as the inverse of the incidence of disabling combat or operational stress casualties in a deployed force. A deployed unit that has suffered a 10% stress casualty rate may be said to be 90% operationally resilient. At the less basic level of optimum individual performance despite stress load, metrics for operational resilience are less clear and simple, and may not be easily collected.

How successful has the military been at promoting operational resilience in its service members and units? Using the simple metric of the rates of stress casualties requiring medical evacuation, the US military has enjoyed considerable and sustained success in promoting operational resilience. After World War II, when as many as 10% of all troops were disabled by "battle fatigue" or some mental health diagnosis, stress casualties rates fell to approximately 3.7% during the Korean War, and as low as 1.2% in Vietnam (Nash, 2007b). Shorter and more predictable tour lengths and generally lower physical casualty rates were credited for some of this apparent improvement in operational resilience over time. According to the 2005 report of the US Army Mental Health Advisory Team (MHAT; the MHAT-II report), the last annual MHAT report to include stress-casualty data, behavioral health diagnoses accounted for 7.1% of all medical evacuations from Iraq (527 of 7415) between March and September 2003 (the initial invasion), and 6.0% of all medical evacuations from Iraq during the same months the following year (Mental Health Advisory Team, 2005). Given that approximately 181 356 soldiers deployed to Iraq during 2003 (Hoge *et al.*, 2006), the stress casualty rate among the personel during the initial invasion of Iraq was only 527 (0.29%). By any standard, the modern US military may be considered highly successful at promoting and maintaining operational resilience.

Post-deployment resilience

It is likely that returning service members and veterans have always faced significant challenges readapting to civilian life, and that operational stress has always followed them home to their families and communities after they have participated in armed conflict. These challenges are clearly described in ancient Greek tragedies (Shay, 1994, 2002) and in the diaries and letters of American Civil War soldiers and veterans (Dean, 1997). The ancient Greeks understood that war – particularly the brutal, close-up variety they practiced – could darken the psyches of surviving veterans with a *miasma* (pollution) that was difficult, at best, to wash away, and that could result in illness, death, or the destruction of families long after the war had ended (Meagher, 2006). Like many other ancient Greek insights, however, this understanding of the post-deployment consequences of combat stress was somehow forgotten, only to be slowly and painfully rediscovered over the past century. The world was shocked by the murders over six weeks in 2002 of four military wives by their active duty husbands at Fort Bragg, North Carolina, home of the army's special operations command (Starr, 2002). Three of the four assailants had recently returned from combat operations in Afghanistan.

Unlike the military's approach to operational resilience, tools for promoting post-deployment resilience have changed considerably over the centuries. Public purification rites and rituals to remove the stain of war have long been used to promote reintegration into civil society after war. In ancient Greece, public performances of dramas of homecoming, written for audiences of veterans by playwrights who, like Sophocles and Euripides, were veterans themselves, may have been crucial for the socialization of returning warriors (Meagher, 2006). In the USA, organized programs to promote post-deployment resilience have only recently become a priority. Troops returning from the US Civil War, World War I, and the Vietnam War were notoriously left to fend for themselves to too great an extent unless they qualified for government-supplied financial or medical assistance. Despite the myriad of readjustment problems experienced by Vietnam combat veterans, US military services only first implemented ongoing programs to promote post-deployment resilience, such as "Warrior Transition" in the Marine Corps and "Battlemind" in the US Army, in the wake of the Fort Bragg murders in 2002. Both Warrior Transition and Battlemind, as initially conceived, are single-session psychoeducational classes delivered to service members immediately before or after they return from a theater of war (see Nash *et al.*, 2011). Another method in use by the military to promote post-deployment resilience is a brief "decompression" period in a location intermediate between war zone and home, such as the "Third Location Decompression" currently employed by Canadian forces (Marin, 2004), among others. Perhaps most important for post-deployment resilience is the provision by military organizations of ongoing support for their own service members and veterans by peers and leaders, as well as a full range of social and health programs. Notable in this regard is the US Marine Corps' Marine for Life program (http://www.m4l.usmc.mil).

Metrics suggesting a lack or deficiency of post-deployment resilience may be drawn from the rates of occurrence of a number of objective post-deployment behaviors. Examples include post-deployment vehicle accidents, substance misuse or abuse, family violence, divorce, and post-deployment suicide. How successful has the US military been at promoting post-deployment resilience indexed this way? A survey of recent news articles on the subject gives anecdotal evidence that a lot more work needs to be done in this area. For example, in an eerie echo of the 2002 Fort Bragg murders, three female soldiers were killed in 2008 by their military husbands or boyfriends, also at Fort Bragg (Burleigh, 2008). A series of homicides at Fort Carson, Colorado, between November 2008 and May 2009, triggered an epidemiological investigation (US Army Center for Health Promotion and Preventive Medicine, 2009). Less anecdotal evidence for a current gap in post-deployment resilience promotion also comes from the news media, often quoting government reports, regarding the rising rates in the military of suicide, substance abuse, domestic violence, and divorce (e.g., Anon, 2009; Stewart, 2009; Tyson, 2009). Unfortunately, data regarding the prevalence of these post-deployment problems in military populations are sparse in the current professional medical and psychological literature. Nevertheless, it is clear that current gaps exist in the promotion of post-deployment resilience in the military.

Psychological resilience

Psychological resilience, as defined here, is most closely related to the concept of resilience commonly found in the mental health literature – that is, the ability to maintain a stable, healthy level of psychological and physical functioning despite exposure to losses, potentially traumatic events, or other extreme stressors (e.g., Bonanno, 2004). Since levels of psychological and physical functioning must strongly influence behaviors and role performance both during and after deployment, psychological resilience is fundamental to the other two aspects of resilience discussed above. But psychological resilience deserves to be discussed separately from both operational and post-deployment resilience because the methods available for promoting it, and the possible metrics for assessing it, may be very different. Observable post-exposure behaviors, for example, may be very poor indicators of levels of psychological resilience because even extreme distress may be invisible to all but the most intimate of social contacts, and the impacts of physical, psychological, social, or spiritual changes resulting from stressor exposures may be long delayed. By definition, psychological resilience is more than merely meeting minimum standards of behavior during circumscribed periods of time. To a much greater extent than operational or post-deployment resilience, psychological resilience must be viewed as *a process* rather than a state or trait, and studied longitudinally rather than in cross-section.

The military has only recently focused its resilience-building efforts on the promotion of psychological resilience, at least in part because of its long tradition of viewing the qualities that contribute to operational resilience as sufficient to also ensure long-term psychological health and well-being in service members after they returned home. In the traditional warrior ethos, qualities like courage and fortitude have been seen as the primary, if not sole, determinants of psychological resilience as well as resilience on the battlefield. The logical flip-side of this belief has been that those who lacked psychological resilience after returning from a theater of war must also have been lacking in courage and fortitude (Nash, 2007b). Such attitudes might lead to the conclusion that stress disorders such as post-traumatic stress disorder (PTSD) are not legitimate illnesses or injuries, even among those who provide healthcare in the military. In a recent survey of a self-selected but large sample of convenience of 310 army healthcare providers at Fort Hood, Texas, 18% endorsed having little or no confidence that PTSD was a "real illness caused by military service" (Stahl, 2009).

Regardless of attitudes and traditional beliefs, the goal of psychological resilience programs must be to prevent long-term psychological distress or dysfunction and, instead, to encourage psychological health, strength, and well-being. These are the clear goals set for US military psychological health programs by the Department of Defense Task Force on Mental Health, chartered by Congress in 2006. In its report back to Congress in 2007, the Task Force established four overarching goals for military psychological health programs: (1) build a culture of support for psychological health in the military; (2) ensure the availability to service members and their families of a full continuum of excellent care; (3) provide sufficient resources to achieve these ends; and (4) empower line military leaders to plan and coordinate integrated prevention, identification, and treatment efforts (US Department of Defense Task Force on Mental Health, 2007).

How well has the military met the psychological resilience challenge? Does the low rate of battlefield combat stress casualties during the current conflicts in Iraq and Afghanistan signal a low rate of mental disorders among its veterans? According to recent epidemiological studies, psychological resilience remains a significant problem for the military. The rate of PTSD among service members and veterans who have served in the wars in Iraq and Afghanistan is in the range 10–18%, and the prevalence does not diminish over time (Litz & Schlenger, 2009). In addition, PTSD is but one of many adverse mental health outcomes possible in those exposed to combat; others include depressive, anxiety, and substance use disorders. Another source of data regarding psychological resilience in the military is the reports of the US Army's MHAT teams, chartered by the Army Surgeon General every year since 2003 to assess the mental health of soldiers currently deployed to Iraq and Afghanistan. The MHAT studies have reported that among US Army soldiers currently deployed to Iraq, the prevalence of significant mental disorder symptoms, whether of post-traumatic stress, depression, or anxiety, has varied from a low of 12.6% in 2005 to a high of 20% in 2007 (Mental Health Advisory Team, 2003, 2005, 2006a, 2006b, 2008, 2009). Year-to-year variations correlated well with recent levels of combat exposure and other risk factors rather than in response to institutional resilience building or other intervention programs .

The US Navy and Marine Corps approach to resilience and recovery

Every military service branch has responded to the resilience challenges described above by developing and fielding new programs designed to reduce the rates of adverse stress outcomes and, instead, to promote wellness and optimal performance. Rather than survey these myriad new programs, none of which has yet been proven effective by well-designed outcome or program-evaluation studies, we turn now to a description of one particular approach to resilience and recovery that was recently developed in the US Marine Corps as its COSC program, and subsequently adapted

for use in the US Navy as the OSC program (Marine Corps Combat Development Command & Navy Warfare Development Command, 2010). Although these two service-specific programs differ somewhat, they share common goals, guiding assumptions, core concepts, and tools for intervention. The presentation of the program is structured in a way that we feel can lead to measurement strategies, testable predictions, and empirical research, and can hopefully serve as a model for the field.

Program overview and goals

The COSC and OSC programs are comprehensive, system-wide occupational stress management programs whose primary goal is to *promote resilience* of all the three types described above, including operational resilience during deployments, post-deployment resilience after returning, and psychological resilience throughout military careers and beyond. Therefore, COSC and OSC target wellness and the prevention of mental disorders rather than the enhancement of performance. A secondary goal for these programs is to provide a common language and framework to integrate all resilience and recovery efforts within US Navy and Marine Corps units *under the leadership of military commanders* and their chains of command. The COSC and OSC have been developed and implemented stepwise, beginning approximately in 1999.

Guiding assumptions and rationale

The following are the key underlying assumptions and the rationales that guide the COSC and OSC programs, along with the rationale for each.

Assumption 1. The *stress states lie along a broad spectrum* for members of the military services, from wellness and thriving, at one end, to illness and disability, at the other, with important intermediate stress states signaling varying levels of risk for role impairment and long-term mental disorders. There are many more possible stress outcomes than the extreme states of affliction or resistance. Furthermore, stress states are not fixed over time but evolve as trajectories.

Rationale. Epidemiological research has often focused on dichotomous outcomes from stressor exposures, such as the presence or absence of PTSD, for example. However, when symptom burden among stress-exposed service members and veterans is assessed using continuous rather than dichotomous measures, it is clear that levels of clinical and subclinical distress and dysfunction are distributed broadly at any point in time (Shalev, 2002; Bonanno *et al.*, 2006), and that symptoms change along identifiable trajectories as time progresses (e.g., Bonanno, 2004; Dickstein *et al.*, 2010).

Assumption 2. Regardless of how strong, capable, and well prepared someone is prior to stressor exposure, *anyone can be stressed beyond their adaptive capacity*. Given sufficient exposure to stressors, many individuals will express at least subclinical distress and dysfunction, even though few will develop chronic mental disorders.

Rationale. Pre-exposure preparation programs have not yet been found to effectively prevent adverse stress outcomes such as PTSD in trauma-exposed individuals (Whealin *et al.*, 2008). In studies of risk and resilience factors for PTSD, among the greatest determinants of mental health outcomes have been the cumulative burden of stressor exposures (e.g., Bonanno *et al.*, 2007; King *et al.*, 2008) and peri-exposure psychological processes (Ozer *et al.*, 2003), rather than pre-exposure factors. The finding by army researchers in World War II that every soldier had a breaking point defined by duration of continuous exposure to combat (Appel & Beebe, 1946) has been echoed by the findings of recent researchers that the risk for mental disorder symptoms increases with each month of deployment (Mental Health Advisory Team, 2008).

Assumption 3. To be maximally effective, mental disorder prevention programs in the military must intervene *not only before service members are exposed* to potentially toxic stressors, but also *after they develop even subclinical levels of distress or dysfunction* in the context of trauma, loss, or other extreme stress. In order to provide targeted interventions for symptomatic individuals, prevention must also include effective methods for identifying who, at any given moment, is symptomatic. *Military psychological health programs must promote both resilience and recovery.*

Rationale. Using the nomenclature endorsed by the Institute of Medicine Committee on Prevention of Mental Disorders (Mrazek & Haggerty, 1994), the greatest evidence exists to support the effectiveness of *indicated* prevention interventions, which target individual subclinical distress and dysfunction, rather than *selective* or *universal* prevention interventions targeting high-risk groups or entire populations, respectively (Feldner *et al.*, 2007). Furthermore, since even so-called resilient individuals often experience at least brief periods of subclinical distress and dysfunction in the aftermath of trauma or loss (Bonanno, 2004), and early symptom burden is a marker of risk for future pathology (Shalev, 2002), recovery may be more relevant to prevention efforts than resilience.

Assumption 4. Whereas certain aspects of resilience are determined by pre-existing individual traits and capabilities, promoting resilience of all types throughout the lives and careers of service members and their families is only possible by *leveraging all available systemic resources*, including those in the physical, psychological, social, and spiritual domains. One of the resources that is most crucial for the promotion and maintenance of resilience in military units and families is their organic leadership. The responsibility for resilience and recovery programs in the military resides with line leaders at all levels; it cannot be delegated to medical, mental health, or religious ministry personnel.

Rationale. The early literature on resilience correlated the ability to bounce back quickly from adversity with individual risk and protective factors such as age, gender, ethnicity, and enduring personality traits such as hardiness (Kobasa *et al.*, 1982; Taft *et al.*, 1999). However, evidence has accrued that positive outcomes in the face of adversity depend on complex interactions between the individual and the environment, with significant roles played by availability of resources and social systems such as families, communities, and cultures (e.g., Taft *et al.*, 1999; Waller, 2001; Hobfoll *et al.*, 2009).

Core concept: the stress continuum model

A prerequisite for implementing an organization-wide effort in the military to promote resilience and recovery, and to prevent adverse stress outcomes, is a language and classification system for stress that can be employed equally by military leaders, service members, chaplains, family members, and medical and mental health professionals. Every member of the organization must hold a similar concept of the stress states to be promoted or prevented, and each must share a similar understanding of the words used to describe these states. Such commonalities of language and conception are not easily achieved among the many stakeholders of resilience and stress prevention in a military organization, given the many cultural, educational, and professional differences that divide them. To meet this challenge, the commanding generals of the US Marine Corps' three air–ground–logistics Marine Expeditionary Forces (MEFs) convened a working group in 2007 consisting of Marine leaders, chaplains, and medical and mental health professionals. The charter for this Tri-MEF COSC Working Group charged it with developing a multidisciplinary but leader-oriented, organization-wide, stigma-reducing approach to resilience, wellness, and prevention that was consistent with both the warrior ethos and current science. The result of the Working Group's deliberations was the combat and operational stress continuum model, a heuristic that divided the spectrum of possible stress states into four color-coded zones designated green (ready), yellow (reacting), orange (injured), and red (ill). Although the boundaries between these four stress zones are neither sharp nor easily defined by available metrics, the conceptual definition of each zone was believed by the multidisciplinary members of the Tri-MEF Working Group to have strong face validity and be consistent with current evidence and theory (Nash, 2011). Importantly, the line Marine leaders that commissioned the Tri-MEF Working Group saw the continuum model as a way to integrate and coordinate the resilience efforts of line commanders and caregivers throughout the organization, throughout unit deployment cycles and throughout the careers of individual service members. What follows is a brief description of the four zones of the model.

Ready: the green zone

The green zone is the zone of *adaptive coping, optimal functioning, and personal well-being*. The green zone is not the absence of stress, for the lives of marines, sailors, and their family members are seldom without stress, but rather its effective mastery without the experience of significant distress or impairment in physical, social, or occupational functioning. The ability to remain in the green zone under stress, and to return quickly to it once affected by stress, are two crucial aspects of resilience. Training and experiences of mastery that

increase individuals' resistance to hardship and adversity may be said to "grow the green zone" for them: that is, increase the range of stress challenges that they are able to endure without becoming distressed or dysfunctional in any significant way. Military training, social cohesion, and leadership are also engineered to enhance the ability of service members to bounce quickly back to the green zone once the source of perturbing stress has been removed.

Attributes and behaviors characteristic of the green zone include high levels of physical and cognitive performance, remaining calm and steady both physically and emotionally, sustained confidence in oneself and others, and behaving ethically and morally. Other green zone characteristics include receiving adequate and restful sleep, maintaining proper nutrition and physical fitness, retaining a sense of humor, and remaining engaged socially and spiritually.

The green zone is the zone of stress *resistance* rather than stress resilience, in that green zone stress, by definition, causes only minimal changes in perceived distress and functional abilities. Individuals in the green zone do not need to bounce back because they are not significantly bent. Therein lies the limitation of the green zone, and the reason that military training intentionally and repeatedly stresses service members well beyond their levels of green zone comfort. As with physical training in preparation for athletic competition, training must repeatedly and increasingly challenge individuals slightly beyond their current capacities in order to develop greater strength, power, and endurance.

Reacting: the yellow zone

The yellow zone is the zone of *mild and temporary distress or changes in functioning owing to stress*. By definition, yellow zone stress reactions are always temporary and reversible since yellow zone stress does not significantly exceed individuals' coping capacities. Each individual's yellow zone, therefore, is defined by their current level of resilience in body, mind, and spirit – their current ability to bounce back from hardship and adversity of various levels of intensity. It is crucial for service members to acquire and maintain broad yellow zone stress capacities because the yellow zone is where most operational challenges are met. Hence, military training repeatedly and intentionally pushes service members into their yellow zones. While preparing for a war zone deployment, entire military units are led through yellow zone training challenges of ever-increasing difficulty. Like athletes, warfighters seek to finish their training regimens at near-peak capacity.

As defined, yellow zone stress causes subjective distress, decrements in functioning, or both. Subjective distress in the yellow zone may include emotions of anxiety, fear, anger, or sadness. Yellow zone cognitions may include worrying or fantasies of either quitting or retaliating against those who are inflicting current stressors. Changes in physical functioning in the yellow zone may include high levels of physiological arousal, causing a rapid heart rate and breathing, sweating, and tremulousness. They may also include diarrhea, nausea, or other physical symptoms of strain. Cognitive changes in the yellow zone are those associated with very high and sustained levels of physiological arousal, such as distractibility, poorly sustained attention, slowed recall, and poor problem solving. Behaviors characteristic of the yellow zone may include irritability, difficulty falling asleep, or changes in appetite, levels of enjoyment, motivation, enthusiasm, or social connectedness.

The defining characteristics of yellow zone distress and changes in functioning are that they are always mild and temporary, and they always disappear completely once the source of stress is no longer present. Yellow zone stress is, by definition, a level of stress to which a particular individual is resilient and, therefore, able to rebound from without incurring lasting damage to body, mind, or spirit. Yellow zone stress does not leave a mental or emotional scar. Of course, as each individual endures repeated challenges over time, and as resources for resilience are depleted, yellow zone capacities may dwindle and resilience may be progressively lost.

Injured: the orange zone

The orange zone represents the first significant departure in the stress continuum model from more traditional views of combat and operational stress, which tended to conceive of any and all experiences of distress or dysfunction in the context of military operations as normal and transient, regardless of severity or persistence. For example, the COSC doctrinal publication FM4–02–51 defines "combat and operational stress reaction" (COSR) as follows (US Army, 2006, pp. 1–5):

> This term can be applied to any stress reaction in the military unit environment. Many reactions look like symptoms of mental illness (such as panic, extreme anxiety, depression, hallucinations), but they are only transient reactions to the traumatic stress of combat and the cumulative stresses of military operations. Some individuals may have behavioral disorders that existed prior to deployment or disorders that were first present during deployment, and need BH intervention beyond the interventions for COSR.

Implied in this definition of COSR is the conceptualization of combat stress, dating back to the early years of World War I, as not genuine expressions of injury or illness induced by stress but rather as always temporary and reversible, except in those individuals weakened by pre-existing disorders of character or mental functioning (see Lerner, 2003). The same symptoms of distress or dysfunction, if experienced somewhere other than in a theater of war, might be conceived very differently, and might receive very different treatment. In fact, the same symptoms as those considered a normal COSR during deployment might be diagnosed and treated as PTSD if they were still evident after the deployment ended.

The orange zone of "stress injury" was established to address some of the drawbacks of the traditional view of combat stress as essentially all yellow zone, no matter how disabling. In particular, a stress zone was needed that represented subclinical or pre-clinical levels of distress or dysfunction interposed between the yellow zone of normal, necessary, and transient stress reactions and the more severe and diagnosable mental disorders (the red zone). Without a stress zone between normal and disordered, there could be no target for the early indicated prevention interventions that might spell the difference between recovery and chronic disability. Also, the traditional view of psychological resilience as determined solely by the same qualities necessary for functional operational resilience, such as courage and fortitude, has increased the stigma associated with being damaged by the stress of military service, and erected barriers of shame and denial between injury and care (Nash et al., 2009).

Orange zone stress is defined as more persistent and severe distress or dysfunction resulting from stressors that exceed, in intensity or duration, the functional limits of individuals' biological, psychological, social, and spiritual coping machinery. Whereas yellow zone stress represents a bending under force, orange zone stress is conceived to represent a literal wound in the body, mind, or spirit caused by stress. If one conceives of an injury as a disruption in normal integrity that resulting in a decrement in normal functioning, then the evidence in support of the concept of literal, rather than figurative, injuries under stress comes from many sources. For example, a disruption of sustaining attachments caused by the death of someone or something cherished may result in at least short-term, if not enduring, changes in self-concept and relationship to the world (Papa *et al.*, 2008; Prigerson *et al.*, 2009). Similarly, to the extent internalized cognitive schemata form the structure of personality and other mental functioning, events that violate deeply held assumptions, beliefs, or values can cause enduring psychological, social, and spiritual dysfunction (Janoff-Bulman, 1992; Litz *et al.*, 2009). There is also accruing evidence from both pre-clinical and clinical studies that severe stress can cause a number of lasting changes in brain structure and function (e.g., Bremner, 2006; Heim & Nemeroff, 2009; Martin *et al.*, 2009). High levels of cortisol in the brain seen in stress have been implicated in the loss of glutamate neurons in the prefrontal cortex and hippocampus in circuits important for the control of physiological arousal, emotion, and cognition; these circuits act through metabolic pathways similar to those changed in head trauma, stroke, and a wide variety of degenerative brain diseases (Kruman & Mattson, 1999; McEwen, 2000, 2008; Giza & Hovda, 2001).

Although the clinical literature has not yet elucidated the causes and effects of orange zone stress, the lessons of history teach that there are at least four distinct yet overlapping sources of stress injury: (1) life threat, (2) loss, (3) moral compromise, and (4) cumulative wear and tear. The stress continuum model, as employed by the OSC and COSC programs, alerts leaders and caregivers to the possibility of orange zone stress in the wake of specific events that are potentially traumatic, potentially morally injurious, or involve the loss of cherished persons or things. It also draws attention to cumulative stress, from all sources over months or years, as a fourth possible source of stress injury.

Orange zone stress is a subclinical and pre-clinical state from which most individuals are expected to recover (e.g., Shalev, 2002). However, the orange zone is also a marker of risk, both for possible failure of role performance (loss of operational resilience) and future mental disorders or behavioral problems (loss of psychological resilience). The risk indexed by orange zone stress is conceived to persist for an indefinite period of time after acute distress and dysfunction fade.

III: the red zone

The red zone is the zone of diagnosable mental disorders arising in individuals exposed to combat or other operational stressors. Because red zone illnesses are mental disorders, they can only be diagnosed by health professionals. Nevertheless, commanders, unit leaders, peers, and family members can and should be aware of the characteristic symptoms of stress illnesses so that they can identify them and make appropriate referrals as soon as possible. The most widely recognized stress illness is PTSD, but well-recognized mental disorders arising from stressor exposures in vulnerable individuals include depressive and anxiety disorders, and substance abuse and dependence.

The five core leader functions for psychological health

The combat and operational stress continuum model described above is broad in its scope, encompassing all conceivable responses and outcomes to stress, both for service members and their families. Clearly, no one group of individuals can manage the entire stress continuum as defined. At left end of the continuum – the green and yellow zones – the activities of line leaders predominate to promote resiliency. Here, universal and selective prevention are paramount. At the far right of the continuum, the red zone is the purview of medical and mental health professionals, supported by chaplains and other social and spiritual support personnel. Individual service members and family members bear responsibility for maintaining their own psychological health across the stress continuum, including building their own resiliency, managing their own stress reactions, and recognizing and getting help for stress injuries and illnesses when needed. To promote resilience, recovery, and reintegration across the stress continuum, leaders in the US Marine Corps and Navy have developed and promulgated a set of five core leader functions for psychological health: (1) strengthen, (2) mitigate, (3) identify, (4) treat, and (5) reintegrate.

Strengthen

The first core function for leaders is to strengthen service members before they are exposed to operational stressors. Individuals enter military service with a set of pre-existing strengths and vulnerabilities based on genetics, prior life experiences, personality style, family supports, and a host of other factors that may be largely immutable. However, centuries of experience in military organizations, as well as a number of research studies, have demonstrated that commanders of military units can do much to enhance the resilience of unit members and their families through a number of universal prevention interventions. These interventions fall into the three broad categories of training, unit cohesion, and leadership.

Tough, realistic training develops physical and mental strength and endurance, enhances warfighters' confidence in their ability as individuals and as members of units to cope with the challenges they will face, and inoculates them to the stressors they will encounter. Exactly how pre-exposure to stress enhances resilience is not well understood, but emerging evidence suggests that both psychological and biological mechanisms are involved. Well-trained service members have lower heart rates and higher levels of neuropeptide Y, a neurotransmitter that promotes calmness in the face of severe stress (Morgan et al., 2000; Eaton et al., 2007). They also face familiar challenges with greater confidence and less anxiety-induced loss of mental focus or dissociation (Morgan et al., 2001).

Unit cohesion, defined broadly as mutual trust and support in a social group, is developed through sharing adversity over time in a group with a stable membership. Two-way communication, both horizontally among peers and vertically between leaders and subordinates, is essential to unit cohesion. Most leaders know how to build cohesive units given enough time and unit stability, but a too-common challenge is to try to maintain unit cohesion in the face of rotations into and out of the unit, including casualties and combat replacements. Certainly, the unit rotation policies currently practiced in the US military are more conducive to unit cohesion than the individual rotations common during the Vietnam era, but individual augmentees and members of reserve or National Guard units may still be disadvantaged regarding this important ingredient to strengthening.

Although complex and multifaceted, leadership is an essential factor for the strengthening of unit members and families. Leaders strengthen unit members by teaching and inspiring them, keeping them focused on mission essentials, instilling confidence, and providing a model of ethical and moral behavior. Another crucial way in which leaders enhance the resilience of their unit members is by providing a resource of courage and fortitude on which unit members can draw during times of challenge (Moran, 1967).

Military organizations in the USA are currently investing a great deal in new methods to augment pre-exposure strengthening through enhanced fitness, neurocognitive training, and stress inoculation using sensory immersion trainers. One challenge facing line leaders hoping to strengthen their unit members through training is to deliver training that is adequately tough and realistic without making it so tough that it inflicts orange zone injuries on the training field. Another challenge is to recognize the limits of pre-exposure universal prevention interventions. Military psychological health programs must also provide selective interventions for yellow zone stress reactions, and indicated interventions for orange zone stress injuries.

Mitigate

The second core function is to mitigate stressors throughout deployment cycles in order to reduce the stress burden placed on service members and their families. Optimal mitigation of stress requires balancing competing priorities. On the one hand is the need to intentionally subject service members to stress in order to train and toughen them, and to accomplish assigned missions while deployed. On the other hand are the imperatives to reduce or eliminate stressors that are not essential to training or mission accomplishment and to ensure adequate sleep, rest, and restoration to allow recovery between challenges. Resilience, courage, and fortitude can be likened to leaky buckets that are constantly being drained by stress. To keep them from running dry, these buckets must be frequently refilled through the provision of all necessary physical, psychological, social, and spiritual resources. Mitigation activities include physical interventions such as ensuring adequate sleep, rest, and nutrition, and maintaining physical health and fitness. They also can include social and spiritual replenishment activities such as shared successes, recreation, religious practices, and after-action reviews as a means by which leaders can reinforce ethical standards and give meaning to sacrifices and losses. Given the correlation between length of deployment and stress, the most important mitigation strategies may be simply limiting the duration of deployments and increasing the length of dwell time between deployments.

Identify

Since even the best pre- and peri-exposure prevention efforts cannot eliminate all significant post-exposure distress and dysfunction, effective psychological health promotion requires continuous monitoring of stressors and stress outcomes. Operational leaders must know the individuals in their units, including their specific strengths and weaknesses, and the nature of the challenges they face both in the unit and in their home lives. Leaders must recognize when individuals' confidence in themselves or their peers or leaders is shaken, or when units have lost cohesion because of casualties, changes in leadership, or challenges to the unit. Most importantly, every unit leader must know which stress zone each unit member is in at every moment, day to day. Service members cannot be depended upon to recognize their own stress reactions, injuries, and illnesses, particularly while deployed to operational settings. The external focus of their attention and their denial of discomfort, necessary to thrive in an arduous environment, make it difficult for them to recognize their own stress states. In addition, stigma can be an insurmountable barrier to admitting stress problems, once recognized, to someone else. Effective indicated prevention depends on leaders, caregivers, peers, and family members recognizing orange zone stress in others. For this reason, education and training on stress zone identification is afforded to all personnel groups in the US Navy and Marine Corps at various points in their careers, particularly before and after operational deployments.

Treat

The fourth leader function for psychological health promotion is to treat orange and red zone stress once identified. The operative verb, "treat," may imply clinical care provided by a licensed medical or mental health professional. But in the context of the OSC and COSC programs, what is meant is not clinical care but intervention of any kind, at any level. Viewed in this way, the treatment function is the responsibility of everyone in the organization, since effective interventions for subclinical states may be provided by almost anyone trained to provide such help.

To fill the gap in intervention strategies lying between routine leadership and clinical mental healthcare, the US Navy and Marine Corps developed a set of indicated prevention tools targeting orange zone stress in operational environments. This intervention is known as *combat and operational stress first aid* (COSFA) and provides evidence-informed strategies to promote recovery (see Hobfoll *et al.*, 2007) in the hands of line leaders, non-mental healthcaregivers, and others (Nash *et al.*, 2008). The COSFA intervention includes seven actions, divided into three levels of care: (1) continuous aid (check and coordinate), (2) primary aid (cover and calm), and (3) secondary aid (connect, competence, and confidence).

The first continuous aid action, *check*, is merely the imperative to assess and reassess individuals exposed to potential orange zone stressors, in order to recognize current stress zone, needs, and risks. The check action takes into account two critical components of the stress continuum model: the differential risks posed by the four zones of the stress continuum, and the trajectories over which symptoms change over time. There are few settings in which longitudinal assessment is as easy to perform by involved leaders, caregivers, and peers as in military units, given the closeness and involvement that characterizes such organizations. The second continuous aid action, *coordinate*, makes maximum use of the extended support system intrinsic to military organizations by connecting those in need with available resources.

The two primary aid actions, *cover and calm*, are tools for acute crisis response. Cover means to get to cover, or to make safe, whatever that may require. Calm actions target physiological arousal, emotional intensity, and cognitive disorganization. Primary aid is seldom required, but when it is needed, the need is acute. Therefore, everyone at every level of the organization should be trained in both verbal and non-verbal actions for primary aid.

Secondary aid actions are designed to promote recovery and healing from orange zone stress over a longer period of time, and they are intended to be performed mostly by senior leaders and caregivers, since they require the greatest communication skills, authority, and responsibility. The *connect* action of COSFA merely means to promote social support, especially from peers and family members, in the aftermath of orange zone stress. The *competence* action includes all mentoring, teaching, and counseling activities geared toward the recovery of functional skills in all important areas, including self-care, social interacting, and occupational performance. The final secondary aid action, *confidence*, targets obstacles to self-esteem and hope in the wake of orange zone stress, particularly high levels of guilt, shame, or blame. Restoration of confidence often depends on more realistic self-appraisal, but it also may require forgiveness of self and others for perceived failures.

The treatment function of the COSC and OSC programs also encompasses referral, consultation, and case management to ensure higher levels of care are obtained when they are needed. Finally, this treatment function challenges leaders at all levels to remove the obstacles to care posed by stigma in all its forms.

Reintegrate

The final leader function for psychological health, reintegrate, seeks to conserve precious personnel resources by returning individuals to duty as soon and as completely as possible as they recover and heal from stress. The reintegration imperative challenges military line leaders and medical support personnel to continuously monitor the functional capacities and self-confidence of service members as they recover, and to apply rational standards to decisions regarding fitness for duty and worldwide deployability. For stress-affected individuals to be effectively reintegrated into their units, stigma must be continuously addressed, and the confidence of both the stress-affected person and their peers and small unit leaders must be restored. This process may take months to bring to successful conclusion. In those cases in which substantial recovery and return to full duty is not anticipated, the challenge for operational commanders is to assist service members as they transition to civilian life and Veterans Affairs care.

Conclusions

The US Navy and Marine Corps have developed parallel programs (COSC and OSC) to promote resiliency and recovery in their members, not only to preserve operational functional capacities but also to promote post-deployment functioning and long-term health and well-being. The conceptual foundation for these programs is as the combat and operational stress continuum model, a heuristic that promotes communication and integration of resilience and recovery efforts throughout the organization. The model classifies stress states in four color-coded stress zones, each representing a different level of risk for failure of role performance and a future mental disorder. Leaders in the US Navy and Marine Corps bear responsibility for several core functions necessary to promote psychological health across the stress continuum. Unique to these programs and the stress continuum model on which they are based is a major focus on identifying subclinical or pre-clinical stress injuries in order to apply indicated prevention interventions when needed.

Although the COSC and OSC programs were devised based on available evidence, the programs have yet to be proven effective by well-designed outcome or program evaluation studies. Program evaluation studies are needed to validate the major components of these programs, including the stress continuum model, the core leader functions, and COSFA.

There is a broad need for program evaluation research across the spectrum of resilience training efforts in the military. We argue that useful research can only come from cogent and well-articulated conceptual frameworks. We urge decision makers, developers, and researchers to lay out the goals, assumptions, and rationale for each component of their respective models, as we have done in this chapter. This will help to address the big challenges in the field, which are to operationally define resilience; to gain a consensus about what "pre-clinical" states of distress or dysfunction entail, and how to measure these states; to agree on the key constructs of interest and to derive or cull measures of various predictor variables and outcomes; to conduct longitudinal research so that causal inferences can be generated about risk and resilience factors in the military; and to use this information to conduct ongoing program evaluation.

References

Anon. (2009). Divorces rising in military. *New York Times*, November 28, 2009, http://www.nytimes.com/2009/11/28/us/28brfs-DIVORCESRISI_BRF.html (accessed January 8, 2010).

Appel, J. W. & Beebe, G. W. (1946). Preventive psychiatry: an epidemiologic approach. *Journal of the American Medical Association*, **131**, 1469–1475.

Bonanno, G. A. (2004). Loss, trauma, and human resilience: Have we underestimated the human capacity to thrive after extremely aversive events? *American Psychologist*, **59**, 20–28.

Bonanno, G. A., Galea, S., Bucciarelli, A., & Vlahov, D. (2006). Psychological resilience after disaster: New York City in the aftermath of the September 11th terrorist attack. *Psychological Science*, **17**, 181–186.

Bonanno, G. A., Galea, S., Bucciarelli, A., & Vlahov, D. (2007). What predicts psychological resilience after disaster? The role of demographics, resources, and life stress. *Journal of Consulting and Clinical Psychology*, **75**, 671–682.

Bremner, J. D. (2006). Stress and brain atrophy. *CNS and Neurological Disorders*, **5**, 503–512.

Burleigh, N. (2008). The Fort Bragg murders. *People*, 70, December 15, 2008, http://www.people.com/people/archive/article/0,20245668,00.html (accessed January 8, 2010).

Dean, E. T. (1997). *Shook over hell: Post-traumatic stress, Vietnam, and the civil war*. Cambridge, MA: Harvard University Press.

Dickstein, B. D., Suvak, M., Stein, N., Adler, A. B., & Litz, B. T. (2010). Examining variability in the natural course of

PTSD: predictors of symptom trajectory. *Journal of Traumatic Stress*, **23**, 331–339.

Eaton, K., Sallee, F. R., & Sah, R. (2007). Relevance of neuropeptide Y (NPY) in psychiatry. *Current Topics in Medicinal Chemistry*, **7**, 1645–1659.

Feldner, M. T., Monson, C. M., & Friedman, M. J. (2007). A critical analysis of approaches to targeted PTSD prevention: Current status and theoretically derived future directions. *Behavior Modification*, **31**, 80–115.

French, S. E. (2003). *Code of the warrior: Exploring warrior values past and present*. Lanham, MD: Rowman & Littlefield.

Giza, C. C. & Hovda, D. A. (2001). The neurometabolic cascade of concussion. *Journal of Athletic Training*, **36**, 228–235.

Heim, C. & Nemeroff, C. B. (2009). Neurobiology of posttraumatic stress disorder. *CNS Spectrums*, **14**(Suppl. 1), 13–24.

Hobfoll, S. E., Watson, P., Bell, C. C., *et al.* (2007). Five essential elements of immediate and mid-term mass trauma intervention: Empirical evidence. *Psychiatry*, **70**, 283–315.

Hobfoll, S. E., Palmieri, P. A., Johnson, R. J., *et al.* (2009). Trajectories of resilience, resistance, and distress during ongoing terrorism: The case of Jews and Arabs in Israel. *Journal of Consulting and Clinical Psychology*, **77**, 138–148.

Hoge, C. W., Auchterlonie, J. L., & Milliken, C. S. (2006). Mental health problems, use of mental health services, and attrition from military service after returning from deployment to Iraq or Afghanistan. *Journal of the American Medical Association*, **2295**, 1023–1032.

Janoff-Bulman, R. (1992). *Shattered assumptions: Towards a new psychology of trauma*. New York: Free Press.

King, L. A., King, D. W., Bolton, E. E., Knight, J. A., & Vogt, D. S. (2008). Risk factors for mental, physical, and functional health in Gulf War veterans. *Journal of Rehabilitation Research and Development*, **45**, 395–408.

Kobasa, S. C., Maddi, S. R., & Kahn, S. (1982). Hardiness and health: a prospective study. *Journal of Personality and Social Psychology*, **42**, 168–177.

Kruman, I. I. & Mattson, M. P. (1999). Pivotal role of mitochondrial calcium uptake in neural cell apoptosis and necrosis. *Journal of Neurochemistry*, **72**, 529–540.

Lerner, P. (2003). *Hysterical men: War, psychiatry, and the politics of trauma in Germany, 1890–1930*. Ithaca, NY: Cornell University Press.

Litz, B. T. (2005). Has resilience to severe trauma been underestimated? *American Psychologist*, **60**, 262.

Litz, B. T. (2007). Research on the impact of military trauma: Current status and future directions. *Military Psychology*, **19**, 217–238.

Litz, B. T. & Schlenger, W. E. (2009). PTSD in service members and new veterans of the Iraq and Afghanistan wars: a bibliography and critique. *PTSD Research Quarterly*, **20**, 1–7.

Litz, B. T., Stein, N., Delaney, E., *et al.* (2009). Moral injury and moral repair in war veterans: A preliminary model and intervention strategy. *Clinical Psychology Review*, **29**, 695–706.

Marin, A. (2004). *From tents to sheets: an analysis of the, C.F. experience with third location decompression after deployment*. [Report from the Ombudsman, Canadian Forces, July 29, 2004.] Ottawa: Ombudsman for the Canadian Forces, http://www.ombudsman.forces.gc.ca/rep-rap/sr-rs/tld-dtl/app-ann-01-eng.asp (accessed January 18, 2010).

Marine Corps Combat Development Command & Navy Warfare Development Command (2010). *Combat and operational stress control*. [MCRP 6–11C/NTTP 1–15M.] Quantico, VA: Marine Corps Combat Development Command.

Martin, E. I., Ressler, K. J., Binder, E., & Nemeroff, C. B. (2009). The neurobiology of anxiety disorders: brain imaging, genetics, and psychoneuroendocrinology. *Psychiatric Clinics of North America*, **32**, 549–575.

McEwen, B. S. (2000). The neurobiology of stress: from serendipity to clinical relevance. *Brain Research*, **886**, 172–189.

McEwen, B. S. (2008). Central effects of stress hormones in health and disease: Understanding the protective and damaging effects of stress and stress mediators. *European Journal of Pharmacology*, **583**, 174–185.

Meagher, R. E. (2006). *Herakles gone mad: Rethinking heroism in an age of endless war*. Northampton, MA: Olive Branch Press.

Mental Health Advisory Team (2003). *Operation Iraqi Freedom (OIF)*. [Report, December 16, 2003.] Washington, DC: US Army Medical Department, http://www.armymedicine.army.mil/reports/mhat/mhat.html (accessed August 30, 2009).

Mental Health Advisory Team (2005). *Operation Iraqi Freedom (MHAT-II)*. [Report, January 30, 2005.] Washington, DC: US Army Medical Department, http://www.armymedicine.army.mil/reports/mhat/mhat.html (accessed August 30, 2009).

Mental Health Advisory Team (2006a). *Operation Iraqi Freedom 04–06 (MHAT-III)*. [Report, May 29, 2006.] Washington, DC: US Army Medical Department, http://www.armymedicine.army.mil/reports/mhat/mhat.html (accessed January 18, 2010).

Mental Health Advisory Team (2006b). *Operation Iraqi Freedom 05–07 (MHAT-IV)*. [Final Report, December 17, 2006.] Washington, DC: US Army Medical Department, http://www.armymedicine.army.mil/reports/mhat/mhat.html (accessed January 18, 2010).

Mental Health Advisory Team (2008). *Operation Iraqi Freedom 06–08: Iraq, Operation Enduring Freedom 8.* [Afghanistan Report February 14, 2008.] Washington, DC: US Army Medical Department, http://www.armymedicine.army.mil/reports/mhat/mhat.html (accessed August 30, 2009).

Mental Health Advisory Team (2009). *Operation Iraqi Freedom 07–09 (MHAT-VI).* [Report, May 8, 2009.] Washington, DC: US Army Medical Department, http://www.armymedicine.army.mil/reports/mhat/mhat.html (accessed August 30, 2009).

Moran, C. M. W. (1967). *The anatomy of courage.* Boston: Houghton Mifflin. [Original published in 1945.]

Morgan, C. A., Wang, S., Mason, J., *et al.* (2000). Hormone profiles in humans experiencing military survival training. *Biological Psychiatry*, **47**, 891–901.

Morgan, C. A., Hazlett, G., Wang, S., *et al.* (2001). Symptoms of dissociation in humans experiencing acute, uncontrollable stress: a prospective investigation. *American Journal of Psychiatry*, **158**, 1239–1247.

Mrazek, P. J. & Haggerty, R. J. (eds.) (1994). *Reducing risks for mental disorders: Frontiers for preventive intervention research.* Washington, DC: National Academies Press for the Committee on Prevention of Mental Disorders, Institute of Medicine.

Nash, W. P. (2007a). The stressors of war. In C. R. Figley & W. P. Nash (eds.), *Combat stress injuries: Theory, research, and management* (pp. 11–31). New York: Routledge.

Nash, W. P. (2007b). Combat/operational stress adaptations and injuries. In C. R. Figley & W. P. Nash (eds.), *Combat stress injuries: Theory, research, and management* (pp. 33–63). New York: Routledge.

Nash, W. P. (2011). US Marine Corps and Navy combat and operational stress continuum model: A tool for leaders. In E. C. Ritchie (ed.), *Operational behavioral health* (pp. 193–204). Washington, DC: Borden Institute.

Nash, W. P., Westphal, R. J., Watson, P., & Litz, B. T. (2008). Combat and operational stress first aid (COSFA): A toolset for military leaders. In *Proceedings of the Psychological Health and Traumatic Brain Injury Warrior Resilience Conference of the Defense Centers of Excellence*, Fairfax, VA, November 2008.

Nash, W. P., Silva, C., & Litz, B. T. (2009). The historical origins of military and veteran mental health stigma, and the stress injury model as a means to reduce it. *Psychiatric Annals*, **39**, 789–794.

Nash, W. P., Krantz, L., Stein, N., Westphal, R. J., & Litz, B. (2011). Two approaches to meeting the challenges of mental health prevention in the military: Army Battlemind and the Navy–Marine Corps Stress Continuum. In J. Ruzek, J. Vasterling, P. Schnurr,

& M. Friedman (eds.), *Posttraumatic stress reactions: Caring for the veterans of the global war on terror* (pp. 193–214). New York: Guilford Press.

Ozer, E. J., Best, S. R., Lipsey, T. L., & Weiss, D. S. (2003). Predictors of posttraumatic stress disorder and symptoms in adults: a meta-analysis. *Psychological Bulletin*, **129**, 52–73.

Papa, A., Neria, Y., & Litz, B. T. (2008). Traumatic bereavement in war veterans. *Psychiatric Annals*, **38**, 686–691.

Phang, S. E. (2008). *Roman military service: Ideologies of discipline in the late republic and early principate.* New York: Cambridge University Press.

Prigerson, H. G., Horowitz, M. J., Jacobs, S. C., *et al.* (2009). Prolonged grief disorder: Psychometric validation of criteria proposed for DSM-V and ICD-11. *PLoS Medicine*, **6**, e1000121.

Shalev, A. Y. (2002). Acute stress reactions in adults. *Biological Psychiatry*, **51**, 532–543.

Shay, J. (1994). *Achilles in Vietnam: Combat trauma and the undoing of character.* New York: Scribner.

Shay, J. (2002). *Odysseus in America: Combat trauma and the trials of homecoming.* New York: Scribner.

Stahl, S. M. (2009). Crisis in army psychopharmacology and mental health care at Fort Hood. *CNS Spectrums*, **14**, 677–684.

Starr, B. (2002). Fort Bragg killings raise alarm about stress: No connection established to assailant's Afghanistan duty. *CNN.com*, July 27, 2002, http://archives.cnn.com/2002/US/07/26/army.wives (accessed January 8, 2010).

Stewart, P. (2009). US Army suicides set to hit new high in 2009. *Reuters*, November 17, 2009, http://www.reuters.com/article/idUSN1752246 (accessed January 8, 2010).

Taft, C. T., Stern, A. S., King, L. A., & King, D. A. (1999). Modeling physical health and functional health status: the role of combat exposure, posttraumatic stress disorder, and personal resource attributes. *Journal of Traumatic Stress*, **12**, 3–23.

Tyson, A. S. (2009). Army's suicide rate "horrible," general says. *Washington Post*, November 18, 2009, http://www.washingtonpost.com/wp-dyn/content/article/2009/11/17/AR2009111703426.html (accessed January 8, 2010).

US Army (2006). *Combat and operational stress control.* [FM 4-02.51.] Washington, DC: Department of the Army, http://www.fas.org/irp/doddir/army/fm4-02-51.pdf (accessed February 17, 2011).

US Army Center for Health Promotion and Preventive Medicine (2009). *Epidemiologic consultation 14-HK-OB1U-09: Investigation of homicides at Fort Carson, Colorado, November 2008–May 2009.* Washington, DC: US Army Center for Health Promotion and Preventive Medicine, http://www.armymedicine.army.mil/reports/

FinalRedactedEpiconReport14July2009.pdf (accessed January 18, 2010).

US Department of Defense Task Force on Mental Health (2007). *An achievable vision: Report of the Department of Defense Task Force on Mental Health*. Falls Church, VA: Defense Health Board.

von Clausewitz, C. (1982). *On war*. New York: Penquin Books. [Original published in 1832.]

Waller, M. A. (2001). Resilience in ecosystemic context: evolution of the concept. *American Journal of Orthopsychiatry*, **71**, 290–297.

Whealin, J. M., Ruzek, J. I., & Southwick, S. (2008). Cognitive behavioral theory and preparation for professionals at risk for trauma exposure. *Trauma, Violence, and Abuse*, **9**, 100–113.

Chapter 17

Resilience in the face of terrorism: linking resource investment with engagement

Stevan E. Hobfoll, Brian Hall, Katie J. Horsey, and Brittain E. Lamoureux

Introduction

Since the terrorist attacks in Washington and New York on September 11, 2001 (9/11), there have been a flurry of studies on the impact of terrorism and war. Not surprisingly, research has focused on the negative health and mental health impact of these events. In particular, research has focused on how direct and indirect exposure to terrorism and war relate to increased post-traumatic stress disorder (PTSD) and depression (Galea *et al.*, 2002; Bleich *et al.*, 2003; Panamaki *et al.*, 2005; Hobfoll *et al.*, 2006a, 2006b; Agronick *et al.*, 2007). The major goal of terrorism in particular, and in many senses the purpose of war, is to impact the enemy's civilian population psychologically to motivate them to capitulate to demands, or to make them psychologically suffer for perceived wrongs they have done. Indeed, this second goal of terrorism, to inflict harm without a clear political goal, is increasingly the stance taken by terrorists. Whether it is Hamas, Hezbollah, Al Qa'ida or the Tamil Tigers, it is not always clear what they are actually asking for, or if there is agreement among them as to what "victory" would even look like. Rather, they often strike out to cause the "enemy" to suffer in exchange for their suffering.

The study of traumatic psychological injury has continued value. In particular, we know little about how people react to ongoing terrorism (Bleich *et al.*, 2003; Hobfoll *et al.*, 2006a), circumstances where populations must quickly evacuate (Palmieri *et al.*, 2008), or to different kinds of attack (shootings, stabbings, bioterrorism, etc.). Nor do we know much about instances where attacks are of large scale, even though in places like Iraq terrorist attacks have often been of major, repeated scale. Studies of national samples in regions of ongoing terrorism and war are particularly important to study because both direct and indirect exposure takes a heavy toll on such populations (Stein *et al.*, 2004; Somer *et al.*, 2005; Shalev *et al.*, 2006).

At the same time, there is new interest in how people may respond resiliently in the face of terrorism and war. Bonanno and colleagues (Bonanno, 2005; Bonanno *et al.*, 2005, 2006, 2007) noted that following the attacks on the World Trade Center the majority of individuals did not develop significant symptoms, and even those who initially showed signs of disorder recovered fairly quickly. Likewise, Norris *et al.* (2007) and Layne *et al.* (2007) have encouraged the discussion and study of what resiliency might look like and how it might better be studied following mass casualty. Such interest is not new as the study of resiliency has long interested psychology and psychiatry. Several seminal theorists who witnessed the events of World War II, including concentration camps, and the following period noted the importance of salutogenic processes (Frankl, 1963; Caplan, 1964), but their work was seldom matched with empirical study, even if their ideas were rich and potentially heuristic.

Several recent studies have examined resilience in the face of terrorism and war. Galea *et al.* (2002), in their examination of Manhattan residents following the 9/11 terrorist attacks, found that over 40% did not report any PTSD symptoms. Examining the same sample, Bonanno *et al.* (2006) noted that 65.1% of their sample reported no or one symptom of PTSD in the six months following the World Trade Center attacks. Even among those highly exposed in this sample, around one third remained resilient using these strict criteria.

This chapter will map out two theoretical frameworks that have been employed in different areas of stress research and apply them to an understanding of resiliency in the face of mass casualty and terrorism in

Resilience and Mental Health: Challenges Across the Lifespan, ed. Steven M. Southwick, Brett T. Litz, Dennis Charney, and Matthew J. Friedman. Published by Cambridge University Press. © Cambridge University Press 2011.

particular. One, *conservation of resources (COR) theory* (Hobfoll, 1988, 1989, 2001) has been used across the continuum of levels of stress. This theory has been particularly applied to traumatic stress (Hobfoll, 1991) and has been used to aid an understanding of disaster (Freedy *et al.*, 1994; Norris & Kaniasty, 1996; Benight *et al.*, 1999) and terrorism (Hobfoll *et al.*, 2006a, 2007; Hall *et al.*, 2008; Palmieri *et al.*, 2008). *Engagement theory*, in contrast, has been most successfully applied to work-related stress (Schaufeli *et al.*, 2002), and is a major emerging theory within the positive psychology movement (Seligman & Csikszentmihalyi, 2000). The two theories fit extremely well, in part, because engagement thinking was informed by COR theory, but also because COR theory speaks to how stress operates on individuals, groups, and communities and engagement theory speaks to outcomes that are related to human resiliency in the face of challenge. This differs greatly from how resiliency has generally been examined, which is most often in terms of the lack of the psychopathology or resiliency-related resources that help to prevent or limit psychopathology. Instead, engagement theory speaks to positive outcomes that are true markers of resilient, positive responding.

Conservation of resources theory and resiliency

Conservation of resources theory is based on several principles and corollaries that must be delineated to understand the theory and move forward in applying it to mass casualty responding and terrorism and war responding in particular. Unlike other stress theories, COR theory emphasizes the centrality of both loss and gain cycles, and an understanding of both is critical to understanding potential resiliency.

The theory begins with the tenet that individuals strive to obtain, retain, foster, and protect those things they centrally value. They employ key resources in order to conduct this self, social, and societal regulation. This tenet places COR theory in the context of a motivational theory that goes beyond stress and challenge, suggesting instead that this is the normal course of human responding. It needs also be stated that what is centrally valued is universal and includes health, well-being, peace, family, self-preservation, and a positive sense of self, even if the core elements of sense of self differ culturally. This also means that humans will exist in, build, foster, and protect social and societal systems that enable these same valued ends.

Conservation of resources theory next states several key principles that have been supported today in literally hundreds of studies of stress and trauma (Hobfoll & Lilly, 1993; Hobfoll, 2001):

principle 1: the primacy of resource loss
principle 2: resource investment
principle 3: the salience of gain under situations of resource loss.

These principles give rise to three corollaries, which will be described as they arise.

Principle 1: the primacy of resource loss

The first principle of COR theory is that resource loss is disproportionately more salient than resource gain. Resources include object resources (e.g., car, house), condition resources (e.g., employment, marriage), personal resources (e.g., key skills and personal traits such as self-efficacy and self-esteem), and energy resources (e.g., credit, knowledge, money). The disproportionate impact of resource loss is seen in both the degree and the speed of impact, as losses have large impact and typically also have rapid impact. It might appear at odds to again emphasize resource loss when this chapter focuses on resiliency. However, stating the primacy of loss emphasizes the main task of resilient responding, that is to offset the powerful, usually rapid, and often long-term impact of resource loss.

Resource loss is primary across all stress levels. However, there are both quantitative and qualitative differences under conditions of traumatic stress, and more specifically when trauma occurs communally in situations of mass trauma (Hobfoll, 1991, 1998). First, the process of resource loss following terrorism and war occurs with even greater rapidity, as people's world can literally be altered fundamentally and at core levels of life, family, and society. Further, as terrorism and war occur on the level of community, the extent of resource breakdown affects the full continuum of society, resulting in decrements of reserves for both individuals and individual families, and across families and organizations. Indeed, if great enough or chronic, the breakdown may deplete the reserves established for treatment and intervention, which can become quickly overwhelmed.

Principle 2: resource investment

The second principle of COR theory is that people must invest resources in order to protect against resource loss, recover from losses, and gain resources. The first corollary of COR theory relates to this:

corollary 1: those with greater resources are less vulnerable to resource loss and more capable of orchestrating resource gain; conversely, those with fewer resources are more vulnerable to resource loss and less capable of resource gain.

The principle and the corollary related to resource investment and gain are central to any understanding of resiliency. They posit that resiliency is an active process and one that demands personal, social, and societal resources. It is a balancing act and demands hard work in the service of coping, particularly in situations such as terrorism and war, where there are often significant and rapid losses and often no clear end to threat.

Given that terrorism and war can result in profound resource loss, the means of protection of resources or their reinstatement in the aid of resiliency is particularly challenging. Indeed, it may often be beyond individuals' self-capacity, at least initially, and require major influx of social support or formal therapeutic and resource intervention from government and non-governmental organizations that respond to disaster, war, and terrorism. This means that the reconstitution of resources to stabilize individuals and families often demands resources that are part of functional community processes: what Iscoe (1974) called *competent communities*. The therapist, intervention apparatus, and aid agencies are major resources that can provide a variety of support that is outside the armamentarium of individuals, families, or organizations, and that may act directly or as advocates.

Gain cycles that follow large disasters or mass casualties and foster resiliency are potentially deceptive. Kaniasty and Norris (1995) have noted that, following a brief period of altruistic sharing of resources, people and social systems may become more neutral about sharing resources, or even become competitive for resources. Moreover, for those who are most disenfranchised in a society, the altruistic period of resource sharing may not reach them. Families and care agencies may attempt to take care of their own and their communities, but if they are cut off from the major bank of community resources, their efforts may be insufficient to sustain resiliency processes.

The processes of resource gain to aid resiliency are also challenged by the nature of resource conservation. Specifically, COR theory states that individuals, families, and organizations have a strong motivation to withhold resource reserves, and consequently tend to be conservative in their resource investment. Even in instances of massive loss, there is motivation and logic in withholding resources for the unknown challenges that are yet to come. For those who are resource rich, the threat to their reserves will require a greater degree of loss or more long-standing loss. Yet, terrorism and war, if directly impacting even those who are resource rich, can result in depletion of the resources that might have contributed to gain cycles. For those who lack basic resource reserves on social, economic, or emotional levels, this situation will be more immediate and may even occur on note of the threat of terrorism or disaster, before losses actually occur.

This suggests that one of the major challenges of resiliency processes will be to respond with resource investment at major levels, which implies having the resources and the willingness to spend or invest resources. A consequence of this is that those with major resource reservoirs will be more likely to be resilient and that those who are willing to, or are directed to, effectively spend and invest resources will do best. Implied in this is a level of strategy of resource investment, and to the extent that terrorism and war cause a challenge at unpracticed ways of coping, the successful pattern of resiliency responding may have a large creative element.

Principle 3: the salience of gain

Principle 3 is paradoxical. Although resource loss is more potent than resource gain, the salience of gain increases under situations of resource loss (Hobfoll *et al.*, 1999). The paradoxical increase in saliency of resource gain is accentuated during traumatic situations and is a critical insight as to the substance and even the counterintuitive strength of resiliency efforts. This follows because, under conditions of high loss, even efforts that result in small gains may elicit positive expectancy and hope, and lead to further goal-directed efforts. In this manner, resource gains that under less-stressful circumstances would be appraised as trivial may objectively offer a lifeline to survival (e.g., "I am not alone," "Rescuers are on there way," "I now see what I need to do, even if it will be difficult") or may be imbued with meaning (e.g., "People still care," "God is with me").

When turning to engagement theory, below, it will be increasingly clear the processes of investing resources can result in positive outcomes that can counterbalance and even at times offset the negative impact of traumatic events such as war and terrorism.

This is not to romanticize these processes, as resiliency may come in tandem with or interlaced with troubling emotions and thoughts.

Resource loss and gain spirals

The first two principles of COR theory concerning loss primacy and investment of resources, in turn, lead to two key further corollaries, which pertain to resource loss and gain spirals (Hobfoll, 1988, 1998):

corollary 2: those who lack resources are not only more vulnerable to resource loss, but initial loss begets future loss

corollary 3: while those who possess resources are more capable of gain and initial resource gain begets further gain, because loss is more potent than gain, loss cycles will be more impactful and more accelerated than gain cycles.

Understanding these changes the approach to trauma from one that might be more static to a more dynamic moving target of challenges that require ongoing efforts in the service of coping and resiliency efforts.

In the context of major stress and traumatic community stress, corollary 2 is paramount (Norris & Kaniasty, 1996) as loss cycles are central to mass casualty and occur with both force and increasing momentum. Particularly where people are broadly impacted beyond individual loss, where many families are affected and social structures become overburdened or even lost amidst attacks, resource loss cycles can become overwhelming. For resiliency, this means that efforts to halt loss cycles will require great energy, significant resources, and will be ongoing. In a mass casualty disaster or terrorist attack, individuals may lose the very social, personal, and societal resources that are key to their normal coping processes, now required with accelerating need (Klingman & Cohen, 2004). For example, if a family already under financial strain loses the primary breadwinner, or where the general economy has collapsed as in Palestine, trauma results in loss cycles that undermine the structure and availability of even primary resources such as food, shelter, and, in the case of a highly unsafe area, lives. Perhaps even more fundamental in such cycles is the realistic understanding that one cannot even protect one's family given the randomness of attack.

Recent research has illustrated the critical nature of resource loss spirals subsequent to natural disasters or terrorist attacks that have led to many casualties. In the aftermath of the Northridge earthquake, Sattler (2006) reported how individuals subject to secondary stressors, such as living in shelters, continued to experience resource loss and loss spirals that were difficult to break. Secondary resource strain and loss will continue to impact psychological outcomes, such as PTSD, and challenge recovery (Pynoos *et al.*, 2004). Psychosocial resource losses, as well as material losses and losses to the community on service and structural levels, follow in the wake of initial losses and mediate the relationship between disaster (e.g., flood) exposure and psychological distress (Smith & Freedy, 2000). Because secondary stressors can lead to a taxing of personal resources beyond that of the original trauma, the demand on resources continues until resources can be gained and loss halted. Seen this way, resiliency is not a single state but a trajectory, which must be followed for individuals.

In war zones and where terrorism is ongoing, the potency of resource loss over resource gain is clear, illustrating the great challenge to resiliency. At the same time as individuals, families, organizations, and the society itself make efforts to cope with the changing reality, the losses may continue to mount and prior avenues for coping and gaining resources may be interrupted or lost (Klingman, 2006). War presents a unique situation in which resources are lost both as a consequence of attacks and also through their withdrawal for redirection to fighting the enemy. This can impact healthcare, transportation, food, medication, social support networks, jobs, finances, and basic access to services.

Corollary 3 suggests that resiliency processes will be stretched as losses occur. However, at the same time, efforts to strive for resiliency will continue and be fostered if resources are available or can be fostered through informal or formal support efforts.

Resiliency resources are important in understanding resource gain in the face of trauma. Resiliency resources again must be considered on the level of individuals, families, and community. Key resiliency resources that function to offset psychological distress and aid well-being include self-efficacy, deeply imbued sense of optimism, self-esteem, social support, and higher socioeconomic status and social status in the community. As we turn to engagement theory, below, these will become clearer as they are integral to the process of engagement, both as a process and in being engaged as an outcome.

Defensive responding under conditions of resource lack

The fourth corollary of COR theory is fundamental for an understanding of mass casualty trauma:

corollary 4: those who lack resources are likely to adopt a defensive posture to conserve their resources.

Following terrorism and during periods of war and the consequent onslaught of resource loss, individuals, families, and organizations will often adopt a defensive posture. Under such circumstances a new "logic" occurs – the logic of defense. This has been understood on the individual level where denial, projection, sublimation, and rationalization take place, but it is less well understood under situations of mass casualties. However, we can be guided by some understanding of underlying processes. People tend to follow a defensive course in a logical sequence when there are known, practiced, accepted avenues of response. This means that people are practiced when they are addressing circumstances that they have gone through before. However, people are generally not prepared on individual, family, and organizational levels (including government) for situations of war and terrorism. Even in regions such as Israel, where practiced coping might be expected, many circumstances are so new and different as to trap people into using strategies that have poor fit.

Defensive coping is probably more integral to resiliency than might first be assumed. We tend to place defensive coping in a negative light and active, proactive coping in a positive light. As Breznitz (1983) indicated, there are many levels of defensive coping and they are fundamental to successful adaptation to extreme circumstances. People need to titrate the full weight of their losses and the challenges that await them, and some degree of optimistic bias can aid these efforts (Carver & Scheier, 1998). It is possible, however, that those who are more resilient will be less destructive in their defensive patterns and remain more prosocial; however, this premise, like much in this chapter, is largely speculative.

Engagement theory and resiliency

The positive psychology revival has led to interest in engagement as the counterbalance to the burnout and other distress-indicative processes (Schaufeli *et al.*, 2002). This work on engagement is instructive and

informs the potential for understanding the resiliency process, even in terms of engagement in the face of traumatic stress. *Engagement* can be defined as a persistent, pervasive, and positive affective–motivational state of fulfillment in individuals who are reacting to challenging circumstances (Schaufeli *et al.*, 2002). Engagement, in turn, is conceptualized as a product of three dimensions – *vigor, dedication*, and *absorption*.

Dedication is seen as the commitment to key life tasks. In the case of terrorism and war, it includes dedication to family, work, organizations, society and the preservation of the self. Absorption is defined as the sense of full involvement and even excitement over life tasks. When we are absorbed in a major challenge, we often lose the sense of time, and problem solving is maximized. In contrast, to the extent that people are worried about what might happen or has happened they become less absorbed in the task before them and are likely to be less capable of performing complex tasks. Vigor, in turn, refers to high levels of energy and mental resilience when meeting life challenge.

Shirom (2004) suggested that vigor is the fundamental element of this process and that, if it occurs, the issues of absorption and commitment are not consequential. When addressing the consequences of terrorism and war, however, the issues of absorption and commitment may be more fundamental, as it is critical that individuals and the society at large continue their involvement and sustaining of key life tasks.

Engagement as both process and outcome

Absorption, commitment, and being vigorous are both processes and outcomes. We can speak of people acting in an absorbed manner and being committed to tasks in their lives. We can likewise view people as acting in a vigorous manner, full of energy and active, and they can also report a sense of vigor. Both the process and the outcomes aid understanding and should be incorporated in future study of resiliency following terrorism and war. In some ways, being both process and outcome is also reflective of depression and anxiety, as these describe and indeed are defined by processes. This perhaps just underscores the key point made by Lazarus and Folkman (1984), that the stress process is transactional and multidirectional with multiple feedback loops and no true outcome point.

Engagement involves central affective components that results from processes that center on peoples' *intrinsic energetic resources*, more specifically emotional robustness, cognitive agility, and physical vigor (Hobfoll & Shirom, 2001; Shirom, 2004). Seen this way, engagement has emotional, cognitive, and behavioral components that are integrally tied to resource investment and its consequences, and which can be quickly drained by loss cycles. It is important to note that resiliency and distress are also not polar opposites. We and others have often depicted them as such (Hobfoll *et al.*, 2009), by calling resiliency and resistance the absence of symptoms, which is one aspect of resilience. Surely, engagement and psychological distress are negatively related. However, when confronting momentous events, distress and engagement, and even high levels of vigor, may be simultaneously experienced. They also may wax and wane, with times of engagement following distress as people reinsert themselves in addressing instrumental, emotional, and cognitive tasks. To the extent that resources remain available and are not critically depleted in loss cycles, they may be reinvested in resiliency processes.

In this regard, Shirom (2004) has posited that the cognitions and behaviors that are closely interrelated with the changes in energetic resources are part of autonomous biobehavioral systems. Hence, one biobehavioral system influences the withdrawal response that accompanies PTSD, depression, and high anxiety levels. At the same time, a second system facilitates and accompanies an approach-oriented behavior facilitation system that produces persistence and resilience-characterizing engagement. Evidence shows that these two biobehavioral systems, too, operate quite independently from one another (Shirom, 2004), which is another reason why distress and engagement should be seen as potentially co-occurring, if negatively associated.

The engagement process underscores that, just as depression and PTSD are typified by a withdrawn or agitated energetic state, engagement is typified by a positive energetic state matched with a positive feeling tone. Energetic states are key to human functioning. Throughout life, people's energetic state needs to be consonant and facilitative of their life tasks to aid in decision making, activity level, information processing, and social action (Gaillard & Wientjes, 1994). Both consciously and unconsciously, there is a constant taxing of the energetic state in order to react to life threat and opportunities. Csikszentmihalyi (1997) has argued that this is mainly not thoughtful or within consciousness, and further that when we are engaged it is inherently a pleasant process. He further has argued

that under optimal conditions such engagement results in the peak experience of flow, where people are fully wrapped up in their activity. This might help to explain why resiliency may be self-perpetuating, as the success of withstanding stress and remaining actively involved in life tasks is self-rewarding in addition to its extrinsic social and material rewards.

Informal and formal support from family, friends, organizations, professional agencies, and government bodies aid engagement by adding key resources at critical junctures following terrorism and war. This positive influx of resources must also be strategic, as resilient individuals are likely to be self-sufficient often yet at other times be quite open to and needy of aid. On a more mesosocial level, public mental health intervention and actions of government to compensate for losses and help to actualize people's use of what resources they have (e.g., making loans available for rebuilding, making sure insurance companies pay their debts to consumers) are critical actions to aid resiliency. We should not fall into the trap of considering resiliency to be a trait or action of the individual, isolated self. Concerning the allocation of sufficient adequate resources, non-governmental and government organizations can aim at compensating lack or loss of individual, family, and business resources (Hobfoll, 2001). A positive interaction between the individual, the family, and organizations will spread resiliency, as gain spirals are shared between these social–structural levels. That is, where families do better, individuals do better, and where individuals at work do better, the organization is more resilient.

Distinguishing resiliency from traumatic growth

Our research has illustrated that attempts at post-traumatic and peritraumatic growth are common, but often backfire. That is, our studies have shown that in most instances, those who report greater post-traumatic growth do worse, and continue to do worse than those who get on with life tasks (Hobfoll *et al.*, 2007). The attempt to grow from trauma is fraught with pitfalls as it leads to expectations that are difficult to achieve, particularly when we are speaking of types of trauma that may be chronic and where there is little that individuals can do other than to get on with their lives.

Resiliency is in many ways a lower bar than traumatic growth. As we have already outlined in this chapter, resiliency involves staying involved in resource gain cycles and minimizing resource loss cycles. It involves keeping psychological distress to a minimum and preserving functioning. Even when we speak of engagement, this involves achieving a state that is normal in most people's lives but that becomes interrupted when people experience high levels of distress.

In this way, the resource gain cycles that people should hope to achieve are the normal ones of their lives and the extraordinary ones demanded by mass casualties and personal trauma. The goal is to return to the engagement that is common in most people's lives when they are doing well. They are committed to their work, families, friends, and even the hobbies and pastimes that they are passionate about. When doing these activities they are absorbed in them fully. That is they commit their energetic, cognitive, and emotional resources to the tasks that involve them. This requires extra effort and will power during and following trauma, but again it is for the most part a return to fairly normal levels of functioning.

Likewise, achieving a sense of vigor is a normal healthy state. It may not be characteristic of all people at all times, but it can and is often achieved even by those with low levels of psychological distress. Sustaining post-traumatic growth, in contrast, may be an extraordinary state as it appears to be achieved with positive effect on other aspects of life by relatively few individuals, at least when facing terrorism and war.

Distinguishing engagement trajectories from distress trajectories

Borrowing largely from seminal work of Bonanno et al. (2007) and Norris et al. (2007), we have examined four key distress-symptom trajectories over time after exposure to ongoing terrorism and war in Israel. This study was during a relative lull in violence, but as is often the case in terrorism and war, ongoing threats imbue the situations with peritraumatic elements and reminders as well. The first trajectory contained individuals who never develop symptoms of disorder, termed the *resistance* trajectory (Layne et al., 2007). A second trajectory was characterized by initial symptoms, followed by recovery: the *resilience* trajectory. The resilience trajectory was seen as characterized by improvement to levels that indicate absence of psychological symptoms from even low levels of earlier symptoms. In using the general term resilience, we followed Bonanno's conceptualization of resilience as the

"ability to maintain relatively stable, healthy levels of psychological… functioning" (Bonanno, 2005, p. 20) in the face of highly disruptive, threatening events. Lacking symptoms means that "ill health" or what Antonovsky (1979) termed "dis-ease" was not occurring. However, in this chapter we are adding to this the concept of engagement as a way to better capture the spirit of Bonanno's thinking.

A third trajectory was one that would reflect sustained lack of resilience: the *chronic distress* trajectory. This trajectory reflects some level of symptoms of disorder even if these symptoms are low in intensity. This is quite different to a chronic disorder, which would mean meeting diagnostic criteria for a disorder or at least having high levels of symptoms, which is the state that has typically been studied. The final trajectory is termed the *delayed distress* trajectory, and it is characterized by initial resistance that is lost, again even if only low symptom levels develop (Bonanno et al., 2007; Layne et al., 2007).

A sizable minority of individuals displayed a resistant trajectory (22.1%), although this is lower than earlier writing on resiliency might have led us to expect (Bonanno et al., 2006). Further, a small group (13.5%) of individuals showed a resilience trajectory, such that they initially were symptomatic but became relatively free of symptoms over time. The chronic distress trajectory was by far the most common pattern, seen in 54.0% of the sample. Finally, a small group of individuals were initially resistant but became symptomatic over time (10.3%). These rates compare more closely to those of another study in Israel (Bleich et al., 2006), which found that 14.4% of an Israeli sample were resistant, as defined by an absence of symptoms assessed at one time point. However, these results reflect much less resiliency and resistance than Bonanno et al. (2006) found among Manhattan residents following the 9/11 attacks: more than 50% of their sample was resistant and even their most exposed groups never fell below 30% showing resistance.

Returning to our sample, the resistance trajectory was predicted demographically by being male, having higher income and education, being secular (versus being traditionally religious), and being a member of the majority ethnic group (Jewish versus Arab). Consistent with COR theory, experiencing less psychosocial resource loss at either time point predicted the resistance trajectory. Moreover, maintaining high levels of social support was related to greater likelihood of displaying resistance.

Predictors of the resilience trajectory were similar to those predicting resistance. Specifically, the resilience trajectory was associated with higher income and being Jewish versus being Arab. Again, consistent with COR theory, psychosocial resource loss at a second time point was associated with lower likelihood of having a resilience trajectory. Illustrating that traumatic growth and engagement are likely not similar processes, lower (not higher) traumatic growth at time point two was associated with the resilience trajectory. Finally, there was a borderline significant association of high social support predicting this resilience pattern. Although the findings for resistance and resilience trajectories were not identical, there was clear support for the association of these resiliency-related processes with lower resource loss, and that possessing greater resources (e.g., having majority status, higher income, and greater social support from friends) was associated with these more favorable outcomes (Hobfoll, 1989, 2002).

We believe our findings on resistance and resilience trajectories add to the existing body of knowledge on resiliency; however, at the same time, our examination of the lack of symptoms is not the same as positive well-being. Not developing symptoms in the face of chronic terrorist attack and threat and war is no small achievement and is integrally related to resiliency. Nevertheless, the study of engagement processes goes significantly further. Indeed, the ability to resist symptom development may be a product of the ability to become engaged. Hence, when individuals are initially affected by terrorism and war, or other trauma, many recover reasonably healthy levels of functioning and low levels of distress in a reasonable amount of time, and they may well do so by being engaged, as well as becoming more capable of engagement as their symptoms subside (Frankl, 1963; Caplan, 1964; Antonovsky, 1979; Norris *et al.*, 2007). This should be distinguished from recovery as it is normally defined, which is to go from diagnostic or high levels of symptoms of a disorder to subclinical levels. In such conceptualizations, considerable symptoms may still exist and there is no evidence about health processes like engagement.

In our current studies in Israel and Palestine, we are adding the examination of resiliency markers. Following Shirom (2004), we feel that vigor is an essential element of engagement. We hope also to examine absorption and commitment, albeit there are difficult issues to resolve in their study. First, it may also be difficult for research to distinguish between absorption and rumination. Second, the time elements relating to

Csikszentmihalyi's (1997) concept of flow have always been difficult to study empirically. The aspect of flow, of losing track of time, whereby individuals find that time flies or does not move will need to be distinguished from the painful processes in PTSD related to dissociation. Indeed, the element of how the flow of time is experienced, positively or negatively, may be the key element. In the case of commitment, we would need to rely on people's assessment of how committed they felt, and, for example, there are many demand characteristics regarding saying that one is committed to family.

How engagement and distress may interact

Following from COR theory, we can speculate on a number of principles that, while speculative, fit the existing research on the interaction of resource loss and gain and are worthy starting points. Hence, what follows discusses three speculative principles of COR theory relating specifically to engagement:

engagement principle 1: engagement processes are a fundamental aspect of human motivation and are, therefore, also primed by role behavior and role obligations

engagement principle 2: resource loss markedly limits engagement and absorption

engagement principle 3: gain cycles and engagement processes are mutually iterative and expansive.

The first engagement principle deals with the processes of engagement. Individuals who face traumatic and highly challenging circumstances will attempt to remain, or re-immerse themselves, in life activities with increasing levels of absorption and commitment. These will include activities relating to family, self, work, and society. This absorption and commitment will result in decreased psychological distress and ill health and increased sense of well-being, including a sense of vigor.

People's involvement in life tasks is consistent with their role behavior, which is deeply ingrained. Further, life tasks have many survival and obligation-based demand characteristics. Hence, unless people become extremely despondent or withdrawn, they will have a drive to continue their involvement in life tasks. This may become robotic at high levels of distress, but even such robotic activity will positively contribute to vigor, albeit in small amounts. It follows from principle 2 of COR theory that these small amounts of increases in vigor can have enormous potential, as resource gains have increased weight and meaning when losses are high.

The second engagement principle considers the effect of resource loss on engagement and absorption. Resource loss cycles will limit individuals' ability to sustain absorption and commitment to life tasks and as such will limit the sense of vigor and diminishment of psychological stress and ill health.

Because resource loss is more powerful than resource gain, and because resource loss has such powerful impact, it will be difficult to sustain or reassert absorption and commitment in life tasks under high levels of resource loss. Rather than a linear, all or nothing process, however, this will appear as a seesaw process, as there is a strong human motivation to be involved, absorbed, and committed to life tasks, and learned helplessness is the exception, even when resource loss is massive in amount or kind.

The third engagement principle considers the interaction of gain cycles and engagement processes. Resource gain cycles will contribute to increased absorption and commitment in life tasks and a sense of vigor. This, in part, will come from the direct association of absorption and commitment, in that when people are absorbed and committed they build and contribute to material, personal, social, condition, and energy resources. It will also occur because, as resource gains are made, more energies and attention will be available for absorption and commitment in life tasks. In this sense, absorption and commitment involve both physical actions and cognitive and emotional task attention.

Conclusions

It would be a step backwards to study engagement without regard to distress. We would expect that engagement will co-occur with stress. At the same time, as individuals are able to become increasingly engaged, their psychological distress should diminish. This process may well be iterative with many loops, as opposed to linear. Even the most resilient individuals will experience dark moments when in the midst or aftermath of disasters with mass casualties. Engagement, however, should be integral to the ability to stay involved in meaningful life processes, to derive joy from them, and to bounce back following difficult times.

Some of the most interesting aspects of engagement following terrorism, warfare and other traumatic stressors may be how even individuals who are deeply distressed remain engaged. A parent who is deeply depressed but continues to nurture and care for his or her children, the soldier who is deeply grieving but continues to fight with his comrades, the employee who goes to work with PTSD because work is important to feed his or her family and because work keeps society going are all showing remarkable resiliency of a kind that we have only begun to appreciate.

References

Agronick, G., Steuve, A., Vargo, S., & O'Donnell, L. (2007). New York City young adults' psychological reactions to 9/11: Findings from the Reach for Health Longitudinal Study. *American Journal of Community Psychology*, **39**, 79–90.

Antonovsky, A. (1979). *Health, stress, and coping*. San Francisco, CA: Jossey-Bass.

Benight, C. C., Ironson, G., Klebe, K., *et al.* (1999). Conservation of resources and coping self-efficacy predicting distress following a natural disaster: A causal model analysis where the environment meets the mind. *Anxiety, Stress, and Coping*, **12**, 107–126.

Bleich, A., Gelkopf, M., & Solomon, Z. (2003). Exposure to terrorism, stress-related mental health symptoms, and coping behaviors among a nationally representative sample in Israel. *Journal of the American Medical Association*, **290**, 612–620.

Bleich, A., Gelkopf, M., Melamed, Y., & Solomon, Z. (2006). Mental health and resiliency following 44 months of terrorism: A survey of an Israeli national representative sample. *BMC Medicine*, **4**, 21.

Bonanno, G. A. (2005). Clarifying and extending the construct of adult resilience. *American Psychologist*, **60**, 265–267.

Bonanno, G. A., Rennicke, C., & Dekel, S. (2005). Self-enhancement among high-exposure survivors of the September 11th terrorist attack: Resilience or social maladjustment? *Journal of Personality and Social Psychology*, **88**, 984–998.

Bonanno, G. A., Galea, S., Bucciarelli, A., & Vlahov, D. (2006). Psychological resilience after disaster- New York City in the aftermath of the September 11th terrorist attack. *Psychological Science*, **17**, 181–186.

Bonanno, G. A., Galea, S., Bucciarelli, A., & Vlahov, D. (2007). What predicts psychological resilience after disaster? The role of demographics, resources, and life stress. *Journal of Consulting and Clinical Psychology*, **75**, 671–682.

Breznitz, S. (1983). Anticipatory stress reactions. In S. Breznitz (ed.), *The denial of stress* (pp. 225–255). New York: International Universities Press.

Caplan, G. (1964). *Principles of preventative psychiatry*. New York: Basic Books.

Carver, C. S. & Scheier, M. F. (1998). *On the self-regulation of behavior*. New York: Cambridge University Press.

Csikszentmihalyi, M. (1997). *Finding flow, the psychology of engagement with everyday life*. New York: Basic Books.

Frankl, V. (1963). *Man's search for meaning*. Boston: Beacon.

Freedy, J. R., Saladin, M. E., Kilpatrick, D. G., Resnick, H. S., & Saunders, B. E. (1994). Understanding acute psychological distress following natural disaster. *Journal of Traumatic Stress*, **7**, 257–273.

Gaillard, A. W. K. & Wientjes, C. J. E. (1994). Mental load and work stress as two types of energy mobilization. *Work and Stress*, **8**, 141–152.

Galea, S., Ahern, J., Resnick, H., *et al.* (2002). Psychological sequelae of the September 11 terrorist attacks in New York City. *New England Journal of Medicine*, **346**, 982–987.

Hall, B. J., Hobfoll, S. E., Palmieri, P., *et al.* (2008). The psychological impact of impending forced settler disengagement in Gaza: Trauma and posttraumatic growth. *Journal of Traumatic Stress*, **21**, 22–29.

Hobfoll, S. E. (1988). *The ecology of stress*. New York: Hemisphere.

Hobfoll, S. E. (1989). Conservation of resources: A new attempt at conceptualizing stress. *American Psychologist*, **44**, 513–524.

Hobfoll, S. E. (1991). Traumatic stress: A theory based on rapid loss of resources. *Anxiety Research*, **4**, 187–197.

Hobfoll, S. E. (1998). *Stress, culture, and community: The psychology and philosophy of stress*. New York: Plenum Press.

Hobfoll, S. E. (2001). The influence of culture, community, and the nested-self in the stress process: Advancing conservation of resources theory. *Applied Psychology*, **50**, 337–370.

Hobfoll, S. E. (2002). Social and psychological resources and adaptation. *Review of General Psychology*, **6**, 307–324.

Hobfoll, S. E. & Lilly, R. S. (1993). Resource conservation as a strategy for community psychology. *Journal of Community Psychology*, **21**, 128–148.

Hobfoll, S. E. & Shirom, A. (2001). Conservation of resources theory. In R. Golembiewski (ed.), *Handbook of organizational behavior* (pp. 57–80). New York: Dekker.

Hobfoll, S. E., Lavin, J., & Wells, J. D. (1999). When it rains it pours: The greater impact of resource loss compared to gain on psychological distress. *Personality and Social Psychology Bulletin*, **25**, 1172–1182.

Hobfoll, S. E., Canetti-Nisim, D., & Johnson, R. J. (2006a). Exposure to terrorism, stress-related mental health symptoms, and defensive coping among Jews and Arabs in Israel. *Journal of Consulting and Clinical Psychology*, **74**, 207–218.

Hobfoll, S. E., Tracy, M., & Galea, S. (2006b). The impact of resource loss and "traumatic growth" on probable PTSD and depression following terrorist attacks. *Journal of Traumatic Stress*, **19**, 867–878.

Hobfoll, S. E., Hall, B. J., Canetti-Nisim, D., *et al.* (2007). Refining our understanding of traumatic growth in the face of terrorism: Moving from meaning cognitions to doing what is meaningful. *Applied Psychology*, **56**, 345–366.

Hobfoll, S. E., Palmieri, P. A., Johnson, R. J., *et al.* (2009). Trajectories of resilience, resistance and distress during ongoing terrorism: The case of Jews and Arabs in Israel. *Journal of Consulting Clinical Psychology*, **77**, 138–148.

Iscoe, I. (1974). Community psychology and the competent community. *American Psychologist*, **29**, 607–613.

Kaniasty, K. & Norris, F. H. (1995). In search of altruistic community: Patterns of social support mobilization following hurricane Hugo. *American Journal of Community Psychology*, **23**, 447–477.

Klingman, A. (2006). Children and war trauma. In A. Renniger & I. E. Sigel (eds.), *Handbook of child psychology*, Vol.4: *Child psychology in practice*, 6th edn (pp. 619–652). Hoboken, NJ: Wiley.

Klingman, A. & Cohen, E. (2004). *School-based multisystemic interventions for mass trauma*. New York: Kluwer Academic/Plenum Press.

Layne, C. M., Warren, J., Shalev, A., & Watson, P. (2007). Risk, vulnerability, resistance, and resilience: Towards an integrative conceptualization of posttraumatic adaptation. In M. J. Friedman, T. M. Kean, & P. A. Resick (eds.), *PTSD: science and practice: A comprehensive handbook* (pp. 497–520). New York: Guilford Press.

Lazarus, R. S. & Folkman, S. (1984). *Stress, appraisal and coping*. New York: Springer.

Norris, F. H. & Kaniasty, K. (1996). Received and perceived social support in times of stress: A test of the social support deterioration deterrence model. *Journal of Personality and Social Psychology*, **71**, 498–511.

Norris, F. H., Stevens, S. P., Pfefferbaum, B., Wyche, K. F., & Pfefferbaum, R. L. (2007). Community resilience as a metaphor, theory, set of capacities, and strategy for intervention. *American Journal of Community Psychology*, **41**, 127–150.

Palmieri, P. A., Canetti-Nisim, D., Galea, S., Johnson, R. J., & Hobfoll, S. E. (2008). The psychological impact of the Israel–Hezbollah war on Jews and Arabs in Israel: The impact of risk and resilience factors. *Social Science and Medicine*, **67**, 1208–1216.

Panamaki, R. L., Komproe, I. H., Qouta, S., Elmasri, M. & de Jong, J. T. V. M. (2005). The role of peritraumatic dissociation and gender in the association between trauma and mental health in a Palestinian community sample. *American Journal of Psychiatry*, **162**, 545–551.

Pynoos, R. S., Steinberg, A. M., Grete, D., *et al.* (2004). Reverberations of danger, trauma and PTSD on group dynamics. In B. Sklarew, S. W. Twemlow & S. M. Wilkinson (eds.), *Analysts in the trenches: Streets, schools, war zones* (pp. 1–22). Hillsdale, NJ: Analytic Press.

Sattler, D. N. (2006). Family resources, family strains, and stress following the Northridge earthquake. *Stress, Crisis, and Trauma*, **9**, 187–202.

Schaufeli, W. B., Salanova, M., Gonzáles-Romá, V., & Bakker, A. B. (2002). The measurement of burnout and engagement: A confirmatory factor analytic approach. *Journal of Happiness Studies*, **3**, 71–92.

Seligman, M. E. P. & Csikszentmihalyi, M. (2000). Positive psychology. *American Psychologist*, **55**, 5–14.

Shalev, A. Y., Tuval, R., Frenkiel-Fishman, S., Hadar, H., & Eth, S. (2006). Psychological responses to continuous terror: A study of two communities in Israel. *American Journal of Psychiatry*, **163**, 667–673.

Shirom, A. (2004). Feeling vigorous at work? The construct of vigor and the study of positive affect in organizations. In P. L. Perrewe & D. Ganster (eds.), *Research in organizational stress and well-being*, Vol. 3 (pp. 135–165). Greenwich, CT: JAI Press.

Smith, B. W. & Freedy, J. R. (2000). Psychosocial resource loss as a mediator of the effects of flood exposure on psychological distress and physical symptoms. *Journal of Traumatic Stress*, **13**, 349–357.

Somer, E., Ruvio, A., Soref, E., & Sever, I. (2005). Terrorism, distress and coping: High versus low impact regions and direct versus indirect civilian exposure. *Anxiety, Stress and Coping*, **18**, 165–182.

Stein, B. D., Elliott, M. N., Jaycox, L. H., *et al.* (2004). A national longitudinal study of the psychological consequences of the September 11, 2001 terrorist attacks: Reactions, impairment, and help-seeking. *Psychiatry: Interpersonal and Biological Processes*, **67**, 105–117.

Resilience in the context of poverty

John C. Buckner and Jessica S. Waters

Introduction

Resilience has been defined as the manifestation of positive outcomes in the face of some form of adversity (Luthar *et al.*, 2000; Masten, 2001), poverty being one such adversity. Poverty, "the state or condition of having little or no money, goods, or means of support," has meaning in both relative and absolute terms. Those who are defined as poor in an affluent country like the USA may not seem impoverished, on a more absolute basis, compared with those living in extreme poverty in regions such as sub-Saharan Africa. Nonetheless, individuals who are poor in a more relative sense may still experience significant distress through the comparative wealth they see around them.

Poverty in developed countries indexes a range of social ills that extend beyond the absolute or relative lack of money and goods. Crowded living conditions, community and family violence, drug trafficking, high crime rates, a weaker civil infrastructure, and higher prevalence rates of mental and substance use disorders are issues that are more commonly found in poor communities. These social conditions are better able to fester in impoverished settings and can feed on themselves, creating a downward spiral or "vicious circle," wherein one problem provokes the emergence or worsening of another. For example, a high crime rate in a neighborhood may lead to businesses deciding to avoid it as a place of investment, leading to higher unemployment and further crime in that area.

Both the manifestations and the ramifications of poverty can be described at different levels of analysis. At a *community* or population level, poverty is associated with increased rates of crime, higher prevalence of mental health and substance use disorders, and higher rates of disease. Also, rates of unemployment, school dropout, and teenage pregnancy are often higher in areas where poverty is widespread. For *individuals*, being poor heightens one's risk of experiencing a negative outcome of some sort, such as the development of a significant physical or mental health disorder. Living in poverty can also increase the likelihood of facing adversities and experiences that are much less common for those with greater financial resources. Such hardships can take the form of *negative life events*, which tend to be discrete in nature (e.g., being the victim of crime or violence), or *chronic life strains*, which are more episodic and enduring (e.g., experiencing hunger, economic insecurity, residential instability, and other adversities related to the lack of material resources). Although it is no surprise that the quantity of life events and chronic strains experienced by persons living in poverty tends to be higher than for more financially advantaged individuals, it is noteworthy that the qualitative nature of these events and strains often stands apart from what individuals with middle and or higher incomes would realistically encounter. For example, while children of all backgrounds may experience physical illness, the divorce of their parents, or some such adversity, children growing up in poor communities are much more likely to become homeless, witness a violent crime, or have a family member incarcerated (Masten *et al.*, 1993; Huston *et al.*, 1994; McLoyd, 1998; Buckner *et al.*, 1999, 2004). Most often children living in poverty have little or no control over such severe negative events.

In addition to the distinction between negative events and chronic strains, stressors have also been differentiated as to whether they are "positive," "tolerable," or "toxic" in nature (National Scientific Council on the Developing Child, 2007). Positive stressors are usually modest in intensity and represent situations that pose challenges, which can lead to successes or growth (e.g., final examinations, music recitals, athletic competitions, applying to college, etc.). Tolerable stressors are

Resilience and Mental Health: Challenges Across the Lifespan, ed. Steven M. Southwick, Brett T. Litz, Dennis Charney, and Matthew J. Friedman. Published by Cambridge University Press. © Cambridge University Press 2011.

more severe but are time limited, thus allowing a person to recover once the stressor has ended (e.g., living through a natural disaster, experiencing the serious, but brief, illness of a loved one). A toxic stressor is extraordinary in nature and/or severe and prolonged, thereby overwhelming a person's ability to cope. Children as well as adults who live in poverty often have many more *toxic* stressors in their lives and fewer *positive* stressors than those who are more affluent.

Poor individuals and families also lack the material resources with which to mitigate some of the effects of stressors. Events or strains that may be tolerable for some individuals – if material resources can be brought to bear to curtail or buffer their effects – may be toxic to persons who have more limited options at their disposal. For example, a fire or natural disaster could displace middle-income families from their homes for a period of time, but they may have savings they can access or insurance to claim that can readily restore them to permanent housing. Facing a similar predicament, low-income families without such safety nets would likely find themselves having to live in a homelessness shelter for an extended period of time or move into crowded housing with extended family or friends (Bassuk *et al.*, 1996). Also, individuals with limited financial resources are often one pay check (or unexpected major expense) away from financial crisis, which can lead to eviction from housing and a resulting cascade of other negative events.

Resilience in children has been defined as "achieving desirable outcomes in spite of significant challenges to adaptation or development" (Masten & Coatsworth, 1998, p. 37). The prerequisite for evidencing "resilience" is to have faced a major adversity of some sort. Without such hardship, a child who manifests "desirable outcomes" would be said to be evidencing "competence." The remainder of this chapter summarizes studies of resilience that have taken place in impoverished settings: studies focusing on children, on adults/ families, and on entire communities. The chapter then attempts to identify common themes about resilience and poverty emerging from these different studies.

Studies of resilience among children living in poverty

Of the many published studies of resilience involving children and adolescents, relatively few have examined children's resilience in the context of poverty. One of the most well-known studies of resilience in children

was conducted by Emmy Werner and colleagues, who followed a cohort of 698 children born in 1955 to families with limited income living on the island of Kauai in Hawaii. The Kauai Longitudinal Study (Werner & Smith, 1982, 1992, 2001) followed these children from before birth into adulthood (data were collected beginning in the prenatal period, at birth and at ages 1, 2, 10, 18, 32, and 40 years). The investigators designated about 200 of their study participants as high-risk children as they were born into low-income families with troubled family environments. About two thirds of these youngsters developed significant behavioral difficulties by childhood, the other third growing up without any significant learning or behavioral problems. The Kauai study focused intently on describing the characteristics of this latter group of children, who the investigators deemed to be resilient.

The extensive longitudinal nature of this study afforded an opportunity to examine resilience at various stages of development and to identify internal characteristics and external factors associated with these adaptive outcomes. In terms of internal characteristics, those evidencing positive adaptation, that is resilience, tended to have easy temperaments as infants and were successful in eliciting positive attention from adults. They were characterized by their caregivers as active, alert, responsive, and sociable babies (Werner, 1993). Similar attributions were used to describe resilient youngsters when they reached their pre-school years. By middle childhood, resilient children began to demonstrate good problem-solving and communication skills as well as a reflective cognitive style, good impulse control, ability to concentrate, and flexibility in their approaches to dealing with stress. Teachers noted them as sociable but also quite independent. When children in the Kauai study reached adolescence, those evidencing resilience had a more internal locus of control and higher self-esteem. Resilient youths of both sexes also tended to be somewhat androgynous in their personality traits and interests. In both adolescence and young adulthood, these resilient individuals seemed to have internalized a positive set of core values and were more responsible, nurturing, and socially perceptive than their less well-adapted peers (Werner, 1993).

In terms of factors external to the child, such as family structure and characteristics, resilient children in the Kauai study tended to have better educated and more competent caregivers. Having a mother who worked at a steady job appeared to be a prominent protective factor for resilient girls. Resilient children typically had the opportunity to establish a close bond with at least one older person in their lives who provided them with stable care and positive attention. This was not always a parent; a close tie with a grandparent or older sibling (usually a sister) appeared to be sufficient to promote resilience in some children (Werner & Smith, 2001). Beyond caregivers and family, ties to adults in school (e.g., a favorite teacher) or in broader community who could serve as positive role models was an important external resource for participants in the Kauai study, both in childhood and adolescence.

Another longitudinal study of resilience involving a sample of low-income youths was the Harvard Medical School Study of Adult Development, reported by Felsman and Vaillant (1987). This investigation, which took place over a 40-year period, focused on a group of 500 males selected from inner city schools in Boston, who were originally enrolled to represent a non-delinquent control group for a prospective study of juvenile delinquency (Glueck & Glueck, 1950). This cohort was re-interviewed at multiple time points in adulthood (ages 25, 31, and 47 years). At age 47, men in the top and bottom quartiles of mental health were compared. Intelligence (as measured in adolescence) and parental socioeconomic status were not useful predictors of outcomes in mid-life. Rather, those who demonstrated competence as adolescents (e.g., held part-time job, participated in school and extracurricular activities, did well in school) were much more likely to evidence positive outcomes at age 47. Also, a rating of "childhood environmental strengths" (e.g., based on relationships with family members and lack of childhood emotional problems) was positively associated with good outcomes in adulthood.

In two related studies, Luthar and colleagues (Luthar, 1991; Luthar et al., 1993) studied resilience and competence among inner city youths, many from a low socioeconomic background, in New Haven, Connecticut. Among ninth grade students identified as resilient (on the basis of experiencing high stress but evidencing good social competence), it was common to find that these youths were experiencing difficulties in other spheres of adjustment, particularly internalizing problems such as symptoms of anxiety and depression. This observation suggests caution in applying the term "resilient" to children upon an assessment of only one domain of functioning.

The Rochester Resilience Project is another study of urban children, many of whom were from low-income families. This project entailed two separate cross-sectional investigations that were conducted approximately a decade apart on different samples (Parker et al., 1990; Wyman et al., 1991, 1999; Cowen et al., 1992; Magnus et al., 1999). The later study of youngsters (aged seven to nine years) had many of the same findings as the original investigation, which focused on those aged 9–12 years. The investigators posited a range of inner resources and parenting variables that would differentiate "stress-resistant" (i.e., resilient) from "stress-affected" youths. Among internal attributes examined in the later study, resilient children scored higher on measures of perceived competence, self-esteem, empathy, and "realistic control" attributions (Magnus et al., 1999). These findings largely replicated their earlier results. Similarly, as reported by Wyman et al. (1999) the two studies had similar findings with regard to temperament and parenting as predictors of resilience status. Like the Kauai study, resilient children were more likely to be rated by their parents as having had an easy going temperament as toddlers. Resilient children were also more likely to have parents who felt competent in their roles, were consistent in disciplinary practices, evidenced an authoritative approach to parenting, and were responsive to their child's emotional needs (Wyman et al., 1999). One strength of the Rochester study is its replication of similar findings at two points in time with different samples. A limitation is the authors' decision to report findings pertaining to inner resources and external (e.g., parenting) factors as they relate to resilience in separate articles rather than considering the relative predictive power of these variables in a single multivariate model.

Buckner et al. (2003) conducted a study comparing 45 resilient with 70 non-resilient youths from families with extremely low incomes in Worcester, Massachusetts. A third of these school-aged children had been homeless within the past two years and all were from households with incomes below the poverty line. Resilience was operationally defined in a multidimensional manner using well-established instruments that measured children's emotional well-being, behavior, competence, and level of functioning. Children deemed resilient showed positive adjustment in each of these realms, whereas those determined to be non-resilient evidenced significant problems in one or more of these areas. Although participants in this study all lived below the poverty line, there was still substantial variation in the quantity of negative events and chronic strains they had experienced in recent years.

Because these adversities were predictive of outcomes in expected directions, it was necessary to statistically control for them in order to understand the independent contributions of inner and external resources for predicting resilience.

While this study was limited to a cross-sectional comparison of children, a decided strength was its extensive assessment battery, which was made up of data collected directly from the child as well as from a parent and an external rater. In combination with multivariate analyses, this allowed the investigators to examine the relative contribution of an array of variables, reflecting both inner and external resources of a child, in predicting their resilience status. Among inner resources, self-esteem and, particularly, self-regulation skills emerged as independent predictors of resilience. Likewise, among external resources that were examined, parental monitoring stood out as a predictor, when controlling for all other explanatory variables. Perhaps surprisingly, children's social support did not predict resilience status. The parental monitoring variable tapped into a parent's proclivity to pay close attention to the whereabouts of a child when away from home and to who the child was with. Of note, the non-verbal intelligence of a child, while associated with resilience status in bivariate analyses, was not a predictor of resilience status in multivariate modeling. Instead, when in the same model, self-regulation (which was positively associated with intelligence) was the much more potent predictor.

Self-regulation and resilience

Over the years, intelligence is a variable that has been found to be predictive of resilience in children across a range of studies. More recently, there has been a growing interest in self-regulation as an important predictor of positive outcomes in children (Masten & Coatsworth, 1998; Buckner *et al.*, 2003; Dishion & Connell, 2006). Both theory and recent empirical findings are supportive of the argument that self-regulation skills may be an important inner resource for children, including those living in poverty (Buckner *et al.*, 2009).

Self-regulation refers to an integrated set of metacognitive skills that draw from both executive function and emotion-regulation capacities, which are invoked in the service of accomplishing both proximal and distal goals. While associated with intelligence, self-regulation is a somewhat separate construct that may have closer links to adaptive functioning. Research on

self-regulation (and executive functions) did not begin in earnest until the mid-to-late 1990s, so researchers who conducted the pioneering studies on resilience in children did not deliberately assess and examine this variable as a predictor. Interestingly, if the findings from the Kauai Longitudinal Study are examined through a self-regulation "lens," it is clear that many of the attributes used to characterize resilient children in this study reflect adept self-regulatory capacities (e.g., strong problem-solving skills, a reflective cognitive style, good impulse control, an ability to concentrate, and flexibility in dealing with stressful circumstances). It is highly likely that, if a precise measure of self-regulation could have been employed in this pioneering longitudinal investigation (unfeasible at the time because the construct had yet to be formed), Werner and colleagues would have found it very effective in distinguishing resilient from non-resilient children.

How is it that self-regulation skills may be important in dealing with stress in an adaptive manner? Aspinwall and Taylor (1997) argued that self-regulatory capacities are behind *proactive* means of coping with stress. An individual who copes in a proactive manner tries to anticipate stressors before they occur, analyzes how to prevent them, and plans a course of action if a stressor is unavoidable. The net result may be a reduction in the number of stressors experienced (or a diminution in their impact), thereby leading to better psychosocial adjustment (Aspinwall & Taylor, 1997). Self-regulation skills may also be important in adaptively dealing with stressors after they have occurred. For example, good emotion regulation, which is a facet of self-regulation, may help to overcome uncontrollable adversities to which one can only react (Eisenberg *et al.*, 1997). Unpreventable losses, such as the death of a loved one through illness, are a type of event that may require good emotion-regulation skills in order to deal with it effectively. Good self-regulation skills are probably useful in handling adversities of different types, although they might be especially helpful for those living in poverty, particularly if they can mitigate controllable stressors (e.g., turn what would otherwise be toxic stressors into more tolerable negative events).

A methodological note to mention for future research on resilience in children, particularly within the context of poverty, is the need to account for substantial variation in stressors that can be experienced by children living within the same impoverished context (or more generally who have experienced a common adverse event). Such variation in the nature and quantity of stress experienced can partly explain differences in outcomes seen in children (or adults). If not measured and accounted for in the study design or statistical analyses, such differences in adverse experiences can act as a confounding variable(s), and distort or misrepresent study findings. For example, as mentioned above, in their study of resilience among children belonging to families with very limited income in Worcester, Massachusetts, Buckner *et al.* (2003) found that children deemed to be resilient had experienced fewer negative life events and chronic strains over the past year than youths who were non-resilient. These researchers statistically controlled for those differences in order to identify more meaningfully internal characteristics and external resources that (also) distinguished the resilient from the non-resilient children.

Studies of resilience among adults and families living in poverty

There are comparatively few published studies of resilience involving adults and families who are economically disadvantaged. In a review of the literature, Bonanno and Mancini (2008) cited several factors linked to resilient outcomes in the face of traumatic events, including male gender, older age, cognitive ability, and greater education. They also cited "adaptive flexibility" as an inner resource that helps some individuals to manage traumatic events. By this they mean, "the capacity to shape and modify one's behavior to meet the demands of given stressor event" (Bonanno & Mancini, 2008, p. 372). (It should be noted that the ability to be flexible in one's problem-solving approach [to select a response that best fits a given situation] is a component of self-regulation.) Social resources are also a predictor of resilient outcomes among persons who have experienced a natural disaster (Bonanno *et al.*, 2007).

In a study of risk and resilience in Denver, involving members of low-income families, Wadsworth and Santiago (2008) found that child family members appeared more negatively impacted than parents by poverty-related stressors that families experienced. Use of primary control coping (problem solving, emotional expression, emotion regulation) and secondary control coping (acceptance, cognitive restructuring, distraction, and positive thinking) by study participants was linked to better outcomes for family members of all ages. High secondary control coping in the face of poverty-related adversities was linked to lower

symptoms of anxiety and depression among both adults and children.

McCubbin and colleagues (McCubbin & McCubbin 1988; McCubbin *et al.*, 1998) have studied factors leading to resilient outcomes in families. Qualities of resilient families they identified include cohesion, commitment, warmth, affection, and emotional support for family members. Several research studies have examined risk and protective factors for family homelessness. In the context of extreme poverty, the ability to remain in permanent housing can be looked at as a resilient outcome for low-income families. Findings from studies in different locales are consistent in identifying resources, specifically Section 8 housing vouchers and certificates in the USA, as a key protective factor in keeping families in permanent housing (Bassuk *et al.*, 1997; Shinn *et al.*, 1998).

Resilient communities

Once again, in contrast to the more substantial literature regarding individual resilience in children, relatively few studies have explored factors associated with resilience at the community level (whether impoverished or not). Nevertheless, drawing from the fields of sociology, community development, and community psychology, several themes emerge regarding constructs that may influence community resilience in the context of poverty.

Focusing on geographic communities as opposed to communities of interest, community has been defined as "a collection of both people and institutions occupying a spatially defined area influenced by ecological, cultural, and sometimes political forces" (Park, 1916, cited in Sampson *et al.*, 2002, p. 445). In practice, many researchers use the local boundaries identified by the US census to define neighborhoods or communities. Residents of a community tend to live within reasonable proximity one to another, and to share physical and social resources. As such, the net worth of individuals in the same community is often similar, which in poorer communities results in a phenomenon known as "concentrated disadvantage" (Sampson, 2004).

Endemic, enduring poverty, and the resulting concentrated disadvantage, presents considerable obstacles to community health and well-being and is often associated with other negative factors such as higher rates of crime, school dropout, and infant mortality (Sampson, 2004). As with individuals, the effects of this type of long-term strain on a community differ from those of a sudden event, and they are often harder to gauge. In addition, a relative lack of economic and institutional resources leads poor communities to experience greater difficulty when confronted with an acute stressor, such as a natural disaster or a terrorist attack (Suarez-Ojeda & Autler, 2003).

Numerous indicators can be used to measure the resilience of communities in the face of poverty or concentrated disadvantage. One process often associated with resilient communities includes economic growth, or the amelioration of poverty itself. However, other desirable outcomes, such as the health of residents or the survival of local customs and values, can be used to characterize resilient communities independent of economic change. Furthermore, community resilience can be demonstrated by either the presence of positive outcomes or by the absence of negative outcomes. As such, many studies have identified resilient communities by their avoidance of the undesirable social conditions often associated with poverty, for example, high crime rates or other forms of social disorder.

In spite of growing interest in this field, few researchers have demonstrated empirical associations between community-level variables and community resilience. As there are a relatively small number of studies addressing community resilience in the face of poverty, anecdotal examples and case studies are mentioned here in addition to empirical research. Some of the studies do not identify poverty as the main adversity faced by a community, but rather as a pre-existing condition when the adversity in question (e.g., natural disaster) arises. However, it is reasonable to assume that the same processes that build resilience against one community stressor may strengthen resistance to the effects of another. Also, the sparse nature of the literature in this area and inconsistency in how terms are defined sometimes makes it difficult to discern important distinctions between the community level variables investigated.

Despite these limitations, a number of studies have linked certain constructs to the resilience of impoverished communities. We have identified several constructs that are repeatedly discussed as pertinent to community resilience. These can be grouped loosely into three categories:

social capital: social and institutional resources

cohesion: collective sense of togetherness and
     connection

collective efficacy: the ability to take empowered
     action).

Social capital

Social capital "refers to features of social organization, such as networks, norms, and trust that facilitate coordination and cooperation for mutual benefit" (Putnam, 1995, p. 67). This sociological construct has been tied to resilience in impoverished areas. For example, the 2004 Pacific Ocean tsunami in Sri Lanka and Hurricane Katrina's 2005 landfall in New Orleans reveal striking differences in local community response (Munasinghe, 2007). In spite of the limited material resources and infrastructure in the poorer nation of Sri Lanka, a rallying of local efforts began within hours of the natural disaster. Well before national or international reinforcements arrived, the residents of the region were searching for survivors, administering medical care, and providing food, water, and shelter to those who were displaced. In New Orleans, by contrast, citizens tended to wait for and rely on the slower and less effective response of the national government. As a result, the American communities in the Gulf Coast area were, overall, not as successful at organizing relief efforts as their Sri Lankan counterparts. Although these case studies focus on responses to natural disaster, it is worth noting that the strength of the social networks and established patterns of providing mutual aid of communities in Sri Lanka led to a more effective response to acute need. In other words, these qualities helped the Sri Lankans to react more effectively to the natural disaster despite the more absolute poverty experienced in their country compared with the Gulf Coast of the USA.

In her pivotal work, *All Our Kin*, Stack (1974) provided a case study of an urban African-American community that exemplifies the adaptive nature of social capital in the face of poverty. According to Stack (p. 32), "black families living in 'The Flats' need a steady source of cooperative support to survive"; they have, thus developed a system for sharing and swapping resources based on a valuing of mutual aid and trust, resulting in a network of individuals, friends, and families bound by both need and kinship. As described by Stack (1974), the expectation that one will share resources, the social pressure to repay favors, and the networks that link donors and recipients provide evidence of how strong social capital helps residents of this community to survive despite entrenched poverty.

Cohesion

While social capital comprises the social resources, norms, and common values that unite members of a community, cohesion denotes a collective sense of togetherness and connection to the community. Buckner (1988) described cohesion as a collective-level variable for which the individual-level "psychological sense of community" (a feeling of belonging and connection to other individuals) is a major indicator. That is to say, the presence of a psychological sense of community among many members of a community suggests a larger phenomenon, namely "cohesion," which transcends the individual. In reviewing the literature, Sampson *et al.* (2002) noted that the construct of cohesion has been found to be related to positive outcomes in impoverished communities in several studies. One investigation, based on the results of the British Crime Survey from 1984 to 1992, demonstrated a negative association between neighborhood cohesion and both burglary rates and social disorder, as measured by resident ratings of problems such as litter in the streets or the presence of loiterers (Markowitz *et al.*, 2001). Steptoe and Feldman (2001) found supporting results in their survey of London residents, which indicated that greater social cohesion was significantly correlated with lower levels of a cluster of neighborhood problems, including vandalism and noise disturbance; this effect remained even when controlled for neighborhood socioeconomic status and individual financial or material deprivation. Similarly, Fagg and colleagues (2008), analyzing data from a national survey in England, found less psychological distress among individuals living in areas with greater social cohesion even after controlling for the effects of poverty. These studies provide examples of the positive impact of social cohesion on impoverished communities.

The ethnographic study of Erikson (1976), which described the collective trauma resulting from the loss of community following the Buffalo Creek flood of 1972, serves as a noteworthy example of the potential outcomes when social cohesion is adversely impacted. Prior to the flood that destroyed their community, the citizens of Buffalo Creek exhibited, despite minimal economic resources, a strong "communality"; in other words, the community evidenced high cohesion and social capital as demonstrated by the routine practice of mutual assistance. However, after the disaster, the inhabitants of this mining community found themselves separated from friends, living in areas assigned by relief workers with no regard for prior social connections, and wielding little control over their situations. Many residents experienced symptoms of depression, anxiety, and trauma from the disaster and the resulting

dislocation. Erikson posited that the "loss of communality" caused by the Buffalo Creek flood was central to the ensuing negative outcomes experienced by residents of the community. The disruption of cohesion through the fragmentation of communities, and the resulting loss of community resilience, demonstrates the importance of this construct in maintaining the health and functioning of impoverished communities.

Collective efficacy

A third factor that appears to contribute to community resilience is the willingness and ability to take collective action; this quality has been described with terms such as collective efficacy (Sampson *et al.*, 1997), empowerment (Norris *et al.*, 2008), and citizen participation (Burkey, 1993). Sampson (2004, p. 108) described collective efficacy as "an emphasis on shared beliefs in a neighborhood's capability for action to achieve an intended effect, coupled with an active sense of engagement on the part of residents." The concept of collective efficacy appears to be distinct from but related to social cohesion and capital. Collective efficacy can depend on context and the specific task at hand, but it generally indicates a community's ability to actively address needs and take action. As Sampson and colleagues define collective efficacy as the combination of social cohesion, trust, and informal social control, their results give further support to the hypothesis that cohesion increases community resilience to poverty.

Using data from the Project on Human Development in Chicago Neighborhoods, which included a cross-sectional study of over 300 Chicago communities, Sampson *et al.* (1997) found that levels of violent crime, as measured by homicide rates and resident reports of victimization, were negatively associated with the construct of "collective efficacy" when controlling for prior violence, individual characteristics, and measurement error. More precisely, collective efficacy was shown to diminish the strength of the relationship between concentrated disadvantage and homicide; although poorer neighborhoods did evidence higher rates of homicide, collective efficacy appeared to be a protective factor, leading to lower than expected levels of violence (Sampson & Raudenbush, 1999; Morenoff *et al.*, 2001).

The construct of collective efficacy also appears applicable to the Sri Lankan response following the tsunami. The swift and concerted action taken by local citizens after the disaster attested to a high level of collective efficacy in response to the disaster, facilitated by pre-existing social networks. In contrast, the residents of Buffalo Creek exhibited a less effective response to the disaster. Erikson suggested that the lack of self-determination in the resettlement of their villages, and the resulting inability to take collective action, contributed to the depression and isolation experienced by so many residents of Buffalo Creek. These observations seem to indicate that the residents' sense of collective efficacy was impaired by the circumstances following the flood. It is important to note that not all nearby citizens were directly affected by the tsunami and so were in a position to offer aid; in contrast, nearly all of the residents of Buffalo Creek suffered significant loss of property and loved ones. This distinction may have contributed to the contrast between the two populations in ability to take action when faced with a need in the face of natural disaster. Many practitioners of psychology and community development attempt to foster the collective efficacy form of active citizen participation by promoting self-government, encouraging democratic processes, or otherwise empowering residents (Burkey, 1993). It is clear that collective efficacy is viewed by these professionals as a positive asset, enhancing the resilience of the communities they work in. However, more research is needed to clarify the relationship between collective efficacy and the resilience of communities to poverty, with the hope of informing future interventions.

Community resilience: summary

The three constructs discussed (social capital, cohesion, and collective efficacy) have been shown, through empirical investigation and case studies, to be linked to community resilience in the context of poverty. Beyond these variables, many people have hypothesized about factors that might protect resilience in impoverished communities. Suggested constructs include shared spirituality or consciousness (Sonn & Fisher, 1998), community hope (Ahmed et al., 2004), collective self-esteem (Suarez-Ojeda & Autler, 2003), and citizen participation (Norris et al., 2008). Further research may provide empirical basis for these ideas, but it is possible that they are tied to the variables above. For example, citizen participation can reasonably be assumed to be related to collective action and social capital, while shared spirituality could be a byproduct of having achieved a high degree of social cohesion. Studies assessing relationships between these constructs

could shed light on the underpinnings of community resilience.

As discussed above, researchers who have studied community resilience have sometimes defined similar terms in diverse manners and used different terms to describe overlapping phenomena. Similarly, distinctions between the characteristics that allow communities to be resilient and the definition of community resilience itself are often blurred. For example, some researchers (Ahmed et al., 2004) conceive of social cohesion as an indicator of community resilience itself rather than as an independent predictor. Further clarification is needed regarding the indicators of community resilience and the factors that distinguish resilient from non-resilient communities. Interdisciplinary collaboration would help both to unify constructs across disciplines and to highlight important differences in the conceptual frameworks of psychology, sociology, and community development. Finally, further investigation could shed light on processes that specifically protect communities from the adverse outcomes associated with poverty. Nonetheless, the studies referenced here offer an intriguing foundation for future research on the characteristics of resilient communities and the processes that facilitate this resilience.

Conclusions

Attributes of individuals that may be associated with resilient outcomes for children and adults often have no clear parallels or do not make sense when examining community-level characteristics that are linked to resilience. It is, therefore, a challenge to draw comparisons across studies that have looked at resilience using different levels of analysis. Nonetheless, it is tempting to point out that qualities that serve the purpose of facilitating adaptive, goal-directed behavior have been found to be linked to resilient outcomes at both the individual and the community level. For individuals, this attribute is self-regulation, while at the community level it is social cohesion/collective efficacy. As mentioned above, individuals invoke their self-regulatory capacities in the service of goal-directed behavior (Karoly, 1993) and good self-regulation skills may be fundamental to effectively coping with stress, either by problem solving or through emotion regulation. Such skills have been linked to resilient outcomes as well as to adaptive coping for impoverished youths (Buckner et al., 2003, 2009), although additional research is needed to buttress these findings. For communities, the capacity of residents to come together to effectively address common problems or crises is a consistent theme in the literature. Such capability seems particularly important when responding to natural disasters, but it likely extends to dealing with the more chronic adversity of poverty.

To survive in conditions of poverty, individuals must play close attention to the acquisition and maintenance of basic resources. The stressors that are part and parcel to poverty can deplete the inner and external resources that promote resilient outcomes. Conservation of resources (COR) theory, as articulated by Hobfoll (1988, 1989; see also Chapter 17), seems particularly well suited to the examination of resilience in the context of poverty. This approach uses a comprehensive theory of stress and adaptation based on the central tenet that individuals strive to obtain, build, and protect things that they value (i.e., resources) and that psychological stress and distress ensue when these resources are lost, threatened with loss, or if individuals fail to replenish resources after having made a significant investment of some form (Hobfoll, 1989). The COR theory highlights the purposeful, goal-directed manner in which individuals, families, and communities struggle to combat the stressors engendered by poverty. For example, strong social ties within a community do not just happen spontaneously; rather, they are constructed over time in a deliberate manner by those individuals involved. Social capital is a resource that low-income individuals and families seek to garner and maintain over time to guard against both personal and possibly collective disaster. While wealthier individuals can draw from savings, a home equity line of credit, or insurance policies to ward off a personal crisis, impoverished individuals must rely on the "good credit" they may have established with relative, friends, and neighbors when faced with comparable difficulties. This highlights the relative importance of community organization and social cohesion as counterbalances to a lack of monetary resources for persons living in poverty. In spite of its relevance, we are unaware of any attempts to apply COR theory to this topic. Future research on resilience in the context of poverty should consider the applicability of COR theory in order to develop hypotheses and explain the mechanisms that engender successful adaptation despite adversities.

Whether examining resilience at the individual, family, or community level, factors associated with resilient outcomes may represent interesting targets of intervention in order to promote resilience. For example, there is a growing interest in developing interventions to teach self-regulation skills in children as a means of promoting positive outcomes (Blair, 2002; Diamond et al., 2007; Buckner et al., 2009). Efforts to promote community organization and social cohesion might be analogous at the family and community levels.

As efforts to promote resilient outcomes in impoverished settings often take the form of individual and family-level interventions, program developers and society at large should be sensitive to what is realistic in a context having few economic resources and opportunities. A pitfall when viewing resilience in the context of poverty is the illusion that if individuals or communities possess the right combination of attributes they can thrive despite economic hardship. A "pull yourself up by your own bootstraps" philosophy that leads to individual-level strengths-based interventions is not sufficient. The vast majority of impoverished people suffer greatly from their lack of material resources and the social consequences of poverty. The longer a community remains in poverty the more difficult it becomes to overcome the vicious cycle that has taken root. Impoverished communities, wherever they may be, often require external forms of assistance to become more viable and break the proverbial "cycle of poverty."

Such external assistance could take the form of helping to build social cohesion and collective efficacy to respond to community needs. It is also likely that external economic aid through federal and state government programs is also needed. In the USA, community development block grants represent aid targeted at the community, whereas assistance programs such as the earned income tax credit, food stamps, Section 8 housing assistance, Medicaid, TANF (cash assistance), and energy assistance are important means by which low-income individuals and families receive vital economic support to address their basic needs.

A key virtue of the concept of resilience is its strengths-based approach. Promoting both individual and community-level factors linked to positive outcomes in the face of poverty is a noble task. The structural problems that engender poverty can sometimes feel overwhelming to address. Yet these factors, whether they be community violence, lack of affordable housing, racial discrimination, insufficient educational and employment opportunity, or lack of basic resources, must be targeted in order to see resilient outcomes at the individual level. Having said this, structural efforts to alleviate poverty and interventions to promote factors leading to resilient outcomes among individuals or families are not mutually exclusive; both types of endeavor have important roles to play in improving the lives of people living in poverty as well as the communities in which they live.

References

Ahmed, R., Seedat, M., van Niekerk, A., & Bulbulia, S. (2004). Discerning community resilience in disadvantaged communities in the context of violence and injury prevention. *South African Journal of Psychology*, **34**, 386–408.

Aspinwall, L. G. & Taylor, S. E. (1997). A stitch in time: Self-regulation and proactive coping. *Psychological Bulletin*, **121**, 417–436.

Bassuk, E. L., Browne, A., & Buckner, J. C. (1996). Single mothers and welfare. *Scientific American*, **275**, 60–67.

Bassuk, E. L., Buckner, J. C., Weinreb, L., *et al.* (1997). Homelessness in female-headed families: Childhood and adult risk and protective factors. *American Journal of Public Health*, **87**, 241–248.

Blair, C. (2002). School readiness: Integrating cognition and emotion in a neurobiological conceptualization of children's functioning at school entry. *American Psychologist*, **57**, 111–127.

Bonanno, G. A. & Mancini, A. D. (2008). The human capacity to thrive in the face of potential trauma. *Pediatrics*, **121**, 369–375.

Bonanno, G. A., Galea, S., Bucciarelli, A., & Vlahov, D. (2007). What predicts psychological resilience after disaster? The role of demographics, resources, and life stress. *Journal of Consulting and Clinical Psychology*, **75**, 671–682.

Buckner, J. C. (1988). The development of an instrument to measure neighborhood cohesion. *American Journal of Community Psychology*, **16**, 771–791.

Buckner, J. C., Bassuk, E. L., Weinreb, L. F., & Brooks, M. G. (1999). Homelessness and its relation to the mental health and behavior of low-income school-age children. *Developmental Psychology*, **35**, 246–257.

Buckner, J. C., Mezzacappa, E., & Beardslee, W. (2003). Characteristics of resilient children living in poverty: The role of self-regulatory processes. *Development and Psychopathology*, **15**, 139–162.

Buckner, J. C., Beardslee, W. R., & Bassuk, E. L. (2004). Exposure to violence and low income children's mental health: Direct, moderated, and mediated relations. *American Journal of Orthopsychiatry*, **74**, 413–423.

Buckner, J. C., Mezzacappa, E., & Beardslee, W. (2009). Self-regulation and its relations to adaptive functioning in low-income youths. *American Journal of Orthopsychiatry*, **79**, 19–30.

Burkey, S. (1993). *People first: A guide to self-reliant, participatory rural development*. London: Zed Books.

Cowen, E. L., Work, W. C., Wyman, P. A., *et al.* (1992). Test comparisons among stress-affected, stress-resilient, and nonclassified 4th-6th grade urban children. *Journal of Community Psychology*, **20**, 200–214.

Diamond, A., Barnett, W. S., Thomas, J., & Munro, S. (2007). Preschool program improves cognitive control. *Science*, **318**, 1387–1388.

Dishion, T. J. & Connell, A. (2006). Adolescents' resilience as a self-regulatory process: Promising themes for linking intervention with developmental science. *Annals of the New York Academy of Sciences*, **1094**, 125–138.

Eisenberg, N., Fabes, R. A., & Guthrie, I. K. (1997). Coping with stress: The role of regulation and development. In S. A. Wolchik & I. N. Sandler (eds.), *Handbook of children's coping: Linking theory and intervention* (pp. 41–70). New York: Plenum Press.

Erikson, K. T. (1976). *Everything in its path: Destruction of community in the Buffalo Creek flood*. New York: Simon & Schuster.

Fagg, J., Curtis, S., Stansfeld, S. A., *et al.* (2008). Area social fragmentation, social support for individuals and psychosocial health in young adults: Evidence from a national survey in England. *Social Science and Medicine*, **66**, 242–254.

Felsman, J. K. & Vaillant, G. E. (1987). Resilient children as adults: A 40-year study. In E. J. Anthony & B. J. Bertram (eds.), *The invulnerable child* (pp. 289–314). New York: Guilford Press.

Glueck, S. & Glueck, E. (1950). *Unraveling juvenile delinquency*. New York: The Commonwealth Fund.

Hobfoll, S. E. (1988). *The ecology of stress*. Washington, DC: Hemisphere.

Hobfoll, S. E. (1989). Conservation of resources: A new attempt at conceptualizing stress. *American Psychologist*, **44**, 513–524.

Huston, A., McLoyd, V. C., & Garcia Coll, C. (1994). Children and poverty: Issues in contemporary research. *Child Development*, **65**, 275–282.

Karoly, P. (1993). Mechanisms of self-regulation: A systems view. *Annual Review of Psychology*, **44**, 23–52.

Luthar, S. S. (1991). Vulnerability and resilience: A study of high-risk adolescents. *Child Development*, **62**, 600–616.

Luthar, S. S., Doernberger, C. H., & Zigler, E. (1993). Resilience is not a unidimensional construct: Insights from a prospective study on inner-city adolescents. *Development and Psychopathology*, **5**, 703–717.

Luthar, S. S., Cicchetti, D., & Becker, B. (2000). The construct of resilience: A critical evaluation and guidelines for future work. *Child Development*, **71**, 543–562.

Magnus, K. B., Cowen, E. L., Wyman, P. A., Fagen, D. B., & Work, W. C. (1999). Correlates of resilient outcomes among highly stressed African-American and white urban children. *Journal of Community Psychology*, **27**, 473–488.

Markowitz, F. E., Bellair, P. E., Liska, A. E., & Liu, J. (2001). Extending social disorganization theory: Modeling the relationships between cohesion, disorder, and fear. *Criminology*, **39**, 293–320.

Masten, A. S. (2001). Ordinary magic: Resilience processes in development. *American Psychologist*, **56**, 227–238.

Masten, A. S. & Coatsworth, D. (1998). The development of competence in favorable and unfavorable environments: Lessons from research on successful children. *American Psychologist*, **53**, 205–220.

Masten, A. S., Miliotis, D., Graham-Bermann, S. A., Ramirez, M., & Neemann, J. (1993). Children in homeless families: Risks to mental health and development. *Journal of Clinical and Consulting Psychology*, **61**, 335–343.

McCubbin, H. I. & McCubbin, M. A. (1988). Typologies of resilient families: Emerging roles of social class and ethnicity. *Family Relations*, **37**, 247–254.

McCubbin, H. I., McCubbin, M. A., Thompson, A. I., & Thompson, E. A. (1998). Resiliency in ethnic families: A conceptual model for predicting family adjustment and adaptation. In H. I. McCubbin, E. A. Thompson, A. I. Thompson, & J. E. Fromer (eds.), *Resiliency in Native American and immigrant families*, Vol. 2 (pp. 3–48). Thousand Oaks, CA: Sage.

McLoyd, V. C. (1998). Socioeconomic disadvantage and child development. *American Psychologist*, **53**, 185–204.

Morenoff, J. D., Sampson, R. J., & Raudenbush, S. W. (2001). Neighborhood inequality, collective efficacy, and the spatial dynamics of homicide. *Criminology*, **39**, 517–560.

Munasinghe, M. (2007). The importance of social capital: Comparing the impacts of the 2004 Asian tsunami on Sri Lanka, and Hurricane Katrina 2005 on New Orleans. *Ecological Economics*, **64**, 9–11.

National Scientific Council on the Developing Child (2007). *The science of early childhood development: Closing the gap between what we know and what we do.* Cambridge, MA: Center for the Developing Child, Harvard University, http://developingchild.harvard.edu/library/reports_and_working_papers/science_of_early_childhood_development/ (accessed February 27, 2011).

Norris, F. H., Stevens, S. P., Pfefferbaum, B., Wyche, K. F., & Pfefferbaum, R. L. (2008). Community resilience as a metaphor, theory, set of capacities, and strategy for disaster readiness. *American Journal of Community Psychology*, **41**, 127–150.

Park, R. (1916). Suggestions for the investigations of human behavior in the urban environment. *American Journal of Sociology*, **20**, 577–612.

Parker, G. R., Cowen, E. L., Work, W. C., & Wyman, P. A. (1990). Test correlates of stress-affected and stress-resilient outcomes among urban children. *Journal of Primary Prevention*, **11**, 19–35.

Putnam, R. D. (1995). Bowling alone: America's declining social capital. *Journal of Democracy*, **6**, 65–78.

Sampson, R. J. (2004). Neighborhood and community: Collective efficacy and community safety. *New Economy*, **11**, 106–113.

Sampson, R. J. & Raudenbush, S. W. (1999). Systematic social observation of public spaces: A new look at disorder in urban neighborhoods. *American Journal of Sociology*, **105**, 603–651.

Sampson, R. J., Raudenbush, S. W., & Earls, F. (1997). Neighborhoods and violent crime: A multilevel study of collective efficacy. *Science*, **277**, 918–924.

Sampson, R. J., Morenoff, J. D., & Gannon-Rowley, T. (2002). Assessing "neighborhood effects": Social processes and new directions in research. *Annual Review of Sociology*, **28**, 443–478.

Shinn, M., Weitzman, B. C., Stojanovic, D., *et al.* (1998). Predictors of homelessness among families in New York City: From shelter request to housing stability. *American Journal of Public Health*, **88**, 1651–1657.

Sonn, C. C. & Fisher, A. T. (1998). Sense of community: Community resilient responses to oppression and change. *Journal of Community Psychology*, **26**, 457–472.

Stack, C. B. (1974). *All our kin: Strategies for survival in a black community.* New York: Harper & Row.

Steptoe, A. & Feldman, P. J. (2001). Neighborhood problems as sources of chronic stress: Development of a measure of neighborhood problems, and associations with socioeconomic status and health. *Annals of Behavioral Medicine*, **23**, 177–185.

Suarez-Ojeda, E. N. & Autler, L. (2003). Community resilience: A social approach. In E. H. Grotberg (ed.), *Resilience for today: Gaining strength from adversity* (pp. 189–210). Westport, CT: Praeger.

Wadsworth, M. E. & Santiago, C. D. (2008). Risk and resiliency processes in ethnically diverse families in poverty. *Journal of Family Psychology*, **22**, 399–410.

Werner, E. E. (1993). Risk, resilience, and recovery: Perspectives from the Kauai Longitudinal Study. *Development and Psychopathology*, **5**, 503–515.

Werner, E. E. & Smith, R. S. (1982). *Vulnerable but not invincible: A study of resilient children.* New York: McGraw-Hill.

Werner, E. E. & Smith, R. S. (1992). *Overcoming the odds: High risk children from birth to adulthood*. Ithaca, NY: Cornell University Press.

Werner, E. E. & Smith, R. S. (2001). *Journeys from childhood to midlife: Risk, resilience, and recovery*. Ithaca, NY: Cornell University Press.

Wyman, P. A., Cowen, E. L., Work, W. C., & Parker, G. R. (1991). Developmental and family milieu correlates of resilience in urban children who have experienced major life-stress. *American Journal of Community Psychology*, **19**, 405–426.

Wyman, P. A., Cowen, E. L., Work, W. C., *et al.* (1999). Caregiving and developmental factors differentiating young at-risk urban children showing resilient versus stress-affected outcomes: A replication and extension. *Child Development*, **70**, 645–659.

19

Resiliency in individuals with serious mental illness

Piper S. Meyer and Kim T. Mueser

Introduction

For many years the original term for schizophrenia, *dementia praecox* (or premature dementia) coined by Kraepelin in 1919 (1971) conveyed the assumption that the course of this disease and other serious mental disorders was invariably a chronic and deteriorating one. People with schizophrenia were informed that there was little they could do with their lives, that they should give up their hopes and dreams (Deegan, 1990), they should focus on following their treatment recommendations, but they had little role to play in actual decision making about their care. Over the past several decades there has been a sea change in the long-term perspective on schizophrenia, and more broadly on the concept of recovery from serious mental illness. These new perspectives have been largely brought about by the rise of the mental health consumer movement (Chamberlin, 1978; Davidson *et al.*, 2009), and the development of new and more personally meaningful definitions of recovery that instill hope, empowerment, and responsibility in individuals with a psychiatric illness, and involve the individual as an active participant in his or her own treatment. As new perspectives on recovery have assumed an increasingly dominant role in the treatment of serious mental illness, the importance of resiliency has been recognized, both in terms of understanding how people meet and cope with the many challenges of their disorder and in terms of helping them to bolster their ability to learn and grow from their experiences in order to experience a full and rewarding life (Roe & Chopra, 2003).

This chapter begins with a brief review of the evolving concept of recovery, and its relevance for elevating considerations of resiliency to the understanding and improvement of outcomes in serious mental illness. Next, the role of resiliency as both an adaptive and a protective factor in serious mental illness is considered, followed by a description of strategies that specifically target resiliency skills for improving long-term outcomes. The chapter concludes with a discussion of how a resiliency-focused approach to treatment could further shift attention to important but neglected areas in serious mental illness, such as the experience of positive emotions, thereby improving quality of life in spite of the potential persistence of symptoms and impairments.

The recovery paradigm

Recovery from schizophrenia and other serious mental disorders was once thought of strictly in medical terms that emphasized the complete remission of all symptoms and associated impairments related to the defining characteristics of the illness (Liberman *et al.*, 2002; Andreasen *et al.*, 2005). More recently, there has been a shift away from such definitions and towards alternative conceptualizations that are more personally meaningful to *consumers* (i.e., individuals with a serious psychiatric disorder) and are not explicitly tied to the defining characteristics of their specific disorders. There are several factors that contributed to consumers' dissatisfaction with traditional medical definitions of recovery from mental illness that led to a re-conceptualization of the word, and the emergence of the recovery paradigm of treatment.

Limitations of medical definitions of recovery

A common experience of consumers was being informed by well-intentioned but misguided mental health professionals that recovery from severe mental illnesses such as schizophrenia was impossible. Mental health consumers were often told that their future prospects of a meaningful life were bleak, that their

Resilience and Mental Health: Challenges Across the Lifespan, ed. Steven M. Southwick, Brett T. Litz, Dennis Charney, and Matthew J. Friedman. Published by Cambridge University Press. © Cambridge University Press 2011.

psychiatric illness was chronic, and that they would be best advised to give up on any personal life goals that required significant effort or competence (Deegan, 1990; Mead & Copeland, 2000). A natural consequence of this message for consumers was initially an overwhelming sense of loss or disbelief, often followed by resentment about being told what they could and could not accomplish with their lives.

Reactions against such information and advice provided by professionals were amplified as evidence emerged that symptomatic and functional recovery over the lifespan of people with serious mental illness was actually much more common than previously believed. For example, long-term outcome studies of schizophrenia have shown that between 40 and 70% of individuals demonstrate partial or complete remission of symptoms and impairment over their lives (Ciompi, 1980; Harding *et al.*, 1987; Harrison *et al.*, 2001). Medical recovery from serious mental illness does, in fact, occur.

Objections to traditional hierarchical decision making

Another factor contributing to a new perspective on recovery was the growing dissatisfaction among consumers to the traditional hierarchical decision-making process that dominated psychiatric treatment of serious mental illness until quite recently. Increasingly, consumers refused to buy the adage that "the doctor knows best" and began to demand more respect and involvement in making decisions about their own treatment (Blaska, 1990; Campbell, 1996), in line with the trend towards shared decision making across the medical spectrum (Wennberg, 1988). Consumers demanded to be recognized by mental health professionals as active participants in their own treatment and to be afforded a lead role in the decision-making process (Carling, 1995). Furthermore, they insisted on a role not only in making treatment decisions but also in defining the goals of intervention, challenging the traditional focus of much treatment on symptoms and relapse, as described below.

Broadening the focus of treatment beyond psychopathology

Historically, much of psychiatric treatment was oriented towards the minimization of symptoms, relapses, and impairments, with less attention paid to other important areas, such as social relationships, role functioning, and satisfaction with life. Rather than focusing on symptoms and deficits, consumers argued that they should be more actively involved in identifying the goals of treatment, and that successful treatment requires a shift in focus away from pathology and towards improved psychological and psychosocial functioning, as defined by the consumer (Madera, 1988; Deegan, 1992). As a part of questioning traditional definitions of recovery based on psychopathology, consumers advocated for a newer, more nuanced, and more personally meaningful definition of recovery.

One widely cited definition of recovery is "Recovery involves the development of a new meaning and purpose in one's life as one grows beyond the catastrophic effects of mental illness" (Anthony, 1993, p. 21). Another influential definition is given by Deegan (1988, p. 13):

> Recovery is a process, a way of life, an attitude and a way of approaching the day's challenges. It is not a perfectly linear process. At times our course is erratic and we falter, slide back, regroup, and start again... The need is to re-establish a new and valued sense of integrity and purpose within and beyond the limits of the disability; the inspiration is to live, work, and love in a community in which one makes a significant contribution.

Although a wide range of different definitions of recovery have been offered (Davidson *et al.*, 2005a; Slade, 2009), most definitions are based on one or two core elements: the subjective experience of the process of recovering and functional aspects of recovery. As illustrated in the two definitions of recovery provided above, recovery is subjectively experienced as an intensely personal process that is not defined by the attainment of the specific end point but rather by the development of meaning and sense of purpose in one's life. Most subjective definitions of recovery place a high priority on the consumer's own perception of whether he or she is in recovery, and what that means to the individual.

In addition to emphasis on the experiential process of recovery, descriptions of recovery often refer to changes in specific functional outcomes. For example, the Deegan (1988) quotation above defines the overriding motive of recovery as "the inspiration is to live, work, and love in a community in which one makes a significant contribution" – a clear reference to functional outcomes such as independent living, quality of social relationships, work, and being a member of a community. Consequently, recovery can be conceptualized as including both subjective aspects, related to the process of coming to grips with and growing past the experience of having developed a mental illness, and objective aspects that tap quality of functioning in areas such as social relationships, work, and community integration.

Themes of recovery

In addition to new and more personally meaningful definitions of recovery, several themes of recovery have emerged from consumers' writings on the topic (Ralph, 2000). Common recovery themes include hope and optimism, self-respect and self-determination, coping, and openness to discovery and new experiences. These are briefly described below.

Hope and optimism

Numerous writings on recovery emphasize that hope and optimism are the wellspring from which motivation to change emerges (Fisher, 1992; Deegan, 1996; Perry *et al.*, 2007). At the most basic level, the belief that change is possible is critical if individuals are to invest the time and effort necessary to improve their lives. Deegan and colleagues (Deegan 1996; Perry *et al.*, 2007) noted that, when people with serious mental illness themselves have no hope, others around them can form a "conspiracy of hope" that is capable of touching and ultimately inspiring hope for those who previously had none.

Self-respect and self-determination

The emphasis in traditional psychiatric treatment on hierarchical decision making, combined with coercive treatment and cultural and institutional stressors related to mental illness (e.g., social extrusion and stigma), has led to personal empowerment and choice as core themes of recovery (Miller, 1990; Beale & Lambric, 1995; Fisher *et al.*, 1996). Consumers have often expressed resentment at not being treated as genuine partners in their own treatment and a feeling of lack of respect from treatment providers, family, and society at large. Lack of respect frequently translates to low levels of self-esteem and self-stigma when individuals adopt negative societal attitudes towards mental illness as their own (Estroff, 1989; MacInnes & Lewis, 2008). *Empowerment* has been defined as "a process by which individuals gain mastery or control over their own lives and democratic participation in the life of their community" (Zimmerman & Rappaport,

1988, p. 726). Empowerment has become an important recovery theme as a process involving respecting oneself, demanding respect from others, expecting and demanding collaboration from treatment providers, and possessing a strong conviction in one's own sense of agency and self-determination.

Coping

Although recovery is not defined by the psychiatric illness per se, a common theme in writings about recovery is the importance of coping strategies for minimizing the effects of symptoms or other aspects of the illness on day to day functioning (Deegan & Affa, 1995; Macdonald *et al.*, 1998; Roe *et al.*, 2006). One consumer wrote the following eloquent description of the importance of coping in her life (Leete, 1989, p. 197):

> More than by any other one thing, my life has been changed by schizophrenia. For the past 20 years I have lived with it and in spite of it – struggling to come to terms with it without giving in to it. Although I have fought a daily battle, it is only now that I have some sense of confidence that I will survive my ordeal. Taking responsibility for my life and developing coping mechanisms has been crucial to my recovery.

Openness to discovery and new experiences

Consumers often describe the experience of recovery as similar to taking a journey or even being on an adventure (Slade, 2009). The development of a serious mental illness can be a life-shattering event that challenges an individual's outlook on the world and on himself or herself. The experience can present a threat to the individual's self-identity, and evoked anxiety about what is perceived to be a less predictable and uncertain future. Accepting the fact of having a mental illness requires the development of a new sense of identity, and an openness to the experience of recovery and the many surprises it may bring (Ralph & Corrigan, 2005). While these experiences involve challenges, they also provide opportunities for personal transformation and growth (Roe, 2001; Roe & Chopra, 2003). Viewed from such a perspective, the recovery process is a learning opportunity that can enrich the individual's life rather then deprive him or her of valuable opportunities.

Summary

The themes described here indicate that recovery is a multidimensional experience that combines elements of both process and outcome. The positive orientation of this new conceptualization of recovery, including the recognition that people can and do recover their lives and establish a sense of purpose after developing a serious mental illness, suggests that resiliency is of central interest to understanding and promoting the recovery process.

Resiliency in serious mental illness

Resiliency is often defined in terms of two key components: the ability to bounce back from adversity or trauma, and the positive adaptations in response to a stressful event, such as developing new insight or strengths that improve functioning or well-being (Luthar & Cicchetti, 2000; Masten, 2001; Atkinson *et al.*, 2009). If recovery is defined as the process of adapting to and growing past disability, and the development of personally meaningful goals, resiliency can be understood as the attributes, strategies, and resources that enable a person to establish a rewarding life. Recovery is a subjective experience shaped by one's personal goals, whereas the strengths and resources that an individual builds upon and further develops are the tools that facilitate engagement in the process of recovery and progress towards recovery goals.

In the context of recovery, resiliency then becomes a bridge between the past qualities, skills, and strategies used to overcome adversity and a person's dreams and aspirations for the future. Resiliency is one process that facilitates recovery and helps clinicians to promote individual competencies, focusing on healthy adjustment and enhancing adaptation (Tedeschi & Kilmer, 2005). Resilient skills and strategies developed in, or employed in, past stressful experiences have the potential to help consumers to broaden the use of their own natural coping strategies. People who are helped to strengthen their resilient qualities may learn to apply these strengths in different situations to promote their confidence, competence, and well-being.

Resiliency factors

The most influential theory associated with the development and course of mental illness is the stress–vulnerability model. This states that the development of symptoms and/or relapses is an interaction between biological and environmental or stress factors (Zubin & Spring, 1977; Nuechterlein & Dawson, 1984). Biologically, alcohol and drug use can worsen biological vulnerability, while medication can reduce it. This model also states that social support and

individual coping skills serve to moderate the noxious effects of stress, providing some protection. While the focus of outcome of the stress–vulnerability model is on psychopathology, resiliency factors (coping, social support) are alluded to for their role in reducing the negative effects of stress.

However, taking a resiliency perspective could broaden both the options for treatment and the goals of treatment. Instead of only focusing on resiliency factors such as coping skills and social support, a wider range of resiliency factors could be developed to minimize the effects of stress on biological vulnerability (Edward & Warelow, 2005). Further, a broader variety of resiliency factors becomes relevant when the focus of treatment shifts from reducing symptoms and relapses to facilitating the recovery process and achieving recovery goals such as improved functioning, sense of purpose, and well-being.

There are numerous resilient qualities described in the literature. Some mentioned often include personal optimism, faith, subjective well-being, creativity, gratitude, forgiveness, perseverance, adaptability, tolerance, self-reliance, and viewing one's life as meaningful; other resources that contribute to resiliency include social and family support (Richardson, 2002; Atkinson *et al.*, 2009). Integrating resiliency into treatment for people with serious mental illness begins by eliciting resilient qualities such as strengths and resources, along with understanding deficits and weaknesses. Through eliciting consumers' own resiliency stories in personal narratives that focus on overcoming past challenges, people can recall and rediscover the strengths they used to deal with setbacks in the past and build on them to spring back from their current predicament. These stories help people to visualize a path to their goals and provide examples of coping strategies based on their strengths. Resiliency stories offer a sense of hope to people with serious mental illness, a common feature of both recovery and resiliency. Hope is critical to people pursuing their own personal pathways to recovery and achieving their goals. Hope is also an agent for change through helping people to conceptualize and sustain motivation for personal goals (Lopez *et al.*, 2004). A person with serious mental illness experiences periods when his or her illness interferes with life and periods when the illness does not. Re-discovering resilient qualities from the past helps individuals to identify strengths that help them "to bounce back." Questions such as "Tell me about a difficult time in your life" and "What helped you get through that time?" can be used to help people to feel more hopeful about future possibilities for recovery (Tedeschi & Kilmer, 2005).

Resiliency in traditional mental health treatment

The concept of resiliency was rarely evoked in the context of early, pathology-oriented treatment approaches for serious mental illness, as described above. When the dominant belief was that people could not get better, the concept of resiliency and of "springing back" from a chronic, disabling illness seemed irrelevant. As a new and more personally meaningful definition of recovery has emerged from the consumer movement, the relevance of resiliency has become apparent. Recovery from serious mental illness is now understood as involving personal growth, expanding abilities, and developing a meaningful life despite illness (Davidson *et al.*, 2005b). The ability to achieve the goals of recovery implies the presence of individual resilience. Similarly, the common themes of recovery, including hope, optimism, and self-determination, are frequently used to characterize resiliency (Brodkin & Coleman, 1996; Andresen *et al.*, 2003; Geanellos, 2005; Atkinson *et al.*, 2009).

As recovery became a legitimate focus of treatment for people with serious mental illness, attention shifted towards developing services that were more in line with the goals of recovery. Recovery-oriented services have been described as being person centered, strengths based, and informed by the needs of the individual (Rodgers *et al.*, 2007). This definition is informative to programs but provides little detail about how to transform services to become more recovery oriented. The relevance of resiliency as a personal attribute to achieving the goals of recovery suggests that resiliency theory may offer some insight into strategies to further promote the transformation of mental health services to make them more recovery focused.

Research on resiliency theory has progressed through three stages to develop recommendations for building resiliency in treatment. The first wave focused on identifying the resilient qualities in people that help them to bounce back from adversity. Some of the most common resilient qualities that had helped people to survive adversity were identified from longitudinal studies of children over 30 years, children of parents with schizophrenia, and studies of character traits in adults. The second wave described the process through which individuals might develop and strengthen resilient qualities, and the insight and growth that occur as a result of adversity. As resiliency theory is now in its third wave, researchers are trying to identify the motivational forces that underlie efforts to be resilient. Research has suggested that the sources of this motivation may stem from ecological triggers such as a belief in God, thoughts or feelings that cause neuropeptide releases in the brain, or increases in cells that fortify the immune system (Richardson, 2002).

The consumer movement has faced some similar challenges and could learn something from the development of resiliency theory. As the definition of recovery has broadened, so has the exploration of individual themes across definitions of recovery (Rodgers *et al.*, 2007; Bonney & Stickley, 2008). This, in turn, has led to the development of models of the recovery process as the consumer movement has moved into a partnership with mainstream mental health services (Andresen *et al.*, 2003). Transforming mental health systems to support recovery requires a better understanding of the motivation for recovery, such as identification and fostering of recovery goals, and of how resilient qualities and resources can help consumers to achieve those goals. Such resources may include, but are not limited to, becoming a contributing member of one's community, connecting with friends and family, and establishing meaning and purpose in life. Researchers have begun to examine one part of recovery through helping consumers to establish personally meaningful goals that can enhance motivation, but understanding the motivation that is integral to the recovery process is still in its early stages (Mueser *et al.*, 2002; Farkas *et al.*, 2005; Clarke *et al.*, 2006). Recovery is defined by a person's goals and their desire and motivation for recovery. Resilient qualities and resources can help a person to access their strengths and build new skills that foster the attainment of recovery goals.

Resilience strategies in existing treatment interventions

Interventions that incorporate a resilience framework into the treatment model have the potential to improve the outcomes for people with serious mental illness. Consumers who enhance existing resilient qualities and learn new resiliency skills have an increased capacity to make greater progress towards their recovery goals (Luthar & Cicchetti, 2000; Tedeschi & Kilmer, 2005). The following paragraphs summarize a number of treatment strategies that contribute to the development of resilient qualities and resources. These strategies represent a selection of what is currently used in the treatment of serious mental illness and some approaches that have not typically been applied in this population but have strong potential for promoting work towards recovery. Descriptions will focus not only on how the strategies reduce distress but also on building competence and positive experiences.

Resilience strategies targeting the effects of stress

Treatment strategies commonly used for people with serious mental illness have tended to focus on managing or reducing psychopathology. Some of these strategies have been influenced by the stress–vulnerability model, and aim at helping people to reduce the effects of stress and the likelihood of stress-induced relapses. Three strategies that are commonly used in treatment are enhancing coping skills, teaching problem-solving skills, and building social support (Mueser et al., 2002). Coping is one of the fundamental components in the resiliency process, such that a person who is resilient has coped successfully in spite of adversity (Tusaie & Dyer, 2004). Research has shown that 50–100% of those with serious mental illness spontaneously use coping strategies to deal with their illness in response to stressors or symptoms, but the strategies that they choose are not always effective (Garcelan & Rodriguez, 2002; Farhall et al., 2007). Coping strategies are often taught to people with serious mental illness because they can be learnt and serve as protective factors that moderate against intense emotion. Individuals who are able to recognize stressful situations can use effective coping strategies before their symptoms become overwhelming (Garcelan & Rodriguez, 2002). Cognitive-behavioral strategies that emphasize cognitive restructuring also have a goal of enhancing coping skills by linking thoughts and feelings about symptoms, normalizing symptoms, and identifying the negative beliefs and assumptions about diagnosis (Fowler et al., 1995; Morrison et al., 2004). The focus of treatment is the individual meaning attached to symptoms along with the person's understanding and coping strategies for symptoms (Turkington et al., 2006; Tai & Turkington, 2009). Fostering the use of effective coping strategies in treatment can increase the individual's resiliency in response to stress or persistent symptoms.

Problem solving is another skill often taught to people with serious mental illness (Falloon et al., 2007). By taking steps to identify and resolve problems, individuals are able to develop a resiliency skill to better enable them to face challenges or adversity, and reduce stress in their lives. As people learn problem-solving skills, they often experience rapid success, feel better about themselves, and become more motivated to change. Within the framework of the stress–vulnerability model, these skills serve as a protective factor that moderates the effects of stress. In the illness management and recovery program, consumers are taught a behavioral problem-solving model at the beginning of treatment that focuses on clearly defining the problem, generating alternative solutions, and trying out the solution best suited to the individual (Mueser et al., 2002). These skills are essential in helping an individual to achieve his or her recovery goal, by presenting a framework that he or she can use when faced with a challenge or obstacle. Problem-solving skills are also a key ingredient in skills training interventions. People with serious mental illness can identify and describe problems in their life and use a problem-solving model to find a manageable solution (Liberman et al., 2001). These strategies have been effective at helping people to function more independently and to manage their symptoms better (Kopelowicz et al., 2006).

Another key factor that moderates stress while also serving as a protective factor is social support. By decreasing interpersonal stress and increasing social support, people can increase their resilient qualities and resources. Social skill deficits are common among people with serious mental illness and strongly associated with the course and outcome of illness (Mueser & Bellack, 1998). Studies have shown that social competence is also highly correlated with increased life satisfaction in people with serious mental illness (Salokangas et al., 2006). Social skills training uses social learning techniques to teach people how to communicate better their needs and emotions to help them to meet their goals, and this has been shown to improve outcomes, including treatment adherence, social role functioning, and self-efficacy (Kurtz & Mueser, 2008). As individuals are better able to interact with others and improve social relationships, so they build social supports that serve as a buffer against stress and future adversities (Bebbington & Kuipers, 1992), leading to increased resiliency. Additionally, social support can lead to an increased support network that provides assurance that the person is not alone and offers some people meaning and purpose in life (Neenan, 2009).

Resilience strategies targeting deficits

The next group of treatment strategies describes methods aimed less at decreasing psychopathology and more on the common deficits associated with serious mental illness. Three areas that have received some attention include improving self-esteem, finding recreational interests and activities, and setting and working towards a meaningful goal. People with serious mental illness are often disempowered by hierarchical treatment decision making that ignores their voice, stigmatizing attitudes that marginalize their potential for contribution, and self-stigma that limits their own efforts to take control of their lives. All lead to feelings of hopelessness, worthlessness, and low self-esteem. Treatments that target improving self-esteem may lead to improvements in coping and competence, which do serve as protective factors against relapse. One program for people with serious mental illness that targeted self-esteem by focusing on improving self-worth, competence, and self-determination found improvements in coping abilities and self-esteem (Lecomte *et al.*, 1999). People who have a healthy self-esteem feel more confident in coping with stressful situations and, as a result, are going to be more resilient. Interventions such as the one described above focus on helping people to feel better about their lives and giving them tools to cope more effectively with adversity in the future.

Having an absorbing interest can be a source of social support, giving life purpose and meaning, and improved well-being, both of which are connected to increased resiliency. A hobby or recreational activity provides a distraction from daily life but can also remind people how to enjoy life. Such an activity offers people the opportunity to become an expert, to increase their happiness, and to pursue goals related to recovery in their lives (Neenan, 2009). People with serious mental illness often have little recreation in their lives, compounded by the lack of motivation that can be associated with their illness. Strategies to enhance leisure and recreational activities can lead to increased motivation towards recovery as people experience more positive emotions. Interventions that have focused on increasing leisure and recreational activities have used both a skills training and a recreational therapy approach for individuals with serious mental illness and have found that they are not only interested in finding leisure activities but are also motivated to change behaviors to maintain these activities after treatment (Roder *et al.*, 1998). Finding activities that are both absorbing

and incorporate a person's strengths builds resiliency by highlighting individual competencies and building resources. These activities also provide direction for treatment and inform the goal-setting process. For example, if people have difficulty setting goals, encouraging them to find an absorbing activity initially can lead to a more meaningful goal later.

Goals are what give life meaning and purpose. Setting and pursuing goals gives someone's life direction, boosts self-esteem and confidence, adds structure and meaning to daily life, helps in accomplishing tasks by breaking them down into smaller steps, and encourages social connections (Lyubomirsky, 2008). People build resilient qualities and resources by setting and working towards goals. Goal setting is an important part of many treatment interventions designed to increase problem-solving abilities, remediate weaknesses, create hope, achieve more effective coping, and facilitate the recovery process (Clarke *et al.*, 2006). Traditionally, most treatment interventions have helped consumers to set goals in order to remediate deficits, but there has been a shift more recently toward ensuring that the goals set are personally meaningful to the consumer. Consumers, in fact, have stated how important goals are to their recovery process (Marshall *et al.*, 2007). Treatment programs such as the illness management and recovery program view goals as critical to the rehabilitation of people with serious mental illness and as one of the core features of recovery to help people to achieve something meaningful in their lives (Mueser *et al.*, 2002).

Novel resiliency treatment strategies

Other resilience-building strategies have rarely been used to treat people with serious mental illness. Savoring and mindfulness, gratitude, practicing acts of kindness, and humor are all strategies that focus on increasing positive emotions and well-being, rather than remediating weaknesses or the ability to manage stress. Positive emotions such as hope and optimism have been found to buffer against depression and have been linked to better life outcomes, mental and physical health, more effective coping, and increased lifespan (Seligman, 2002; Lyubomirsky *et al.*, 2005a). Positive emotions have an important lasting effect on a person's ability to build resilience such that over time these experiences aggregate into life-changing resources. The repeated experience of positive emotions can become habitual, leading to an increase in the personal resources that can be used to cope more effectively in times of stress. In fact, research has shown that short-term effects of positive emotions lead to long-term physical, social, and psychological resources, including resiliency (Cohn *et al.*, 2009). Although interventions have not traditionally used these strategies for people with serious mental illness, engaging in pleasurable activities has been related to improved ability to regulate depressive symptoms, leading to better self-esteem in this population and suggesting that positive emotions can play an important role in recovery (Davidson, 2003).

Savoring can be described as the thoughts that enhance experiences from the past, present, and future. It has been defined as an ability to enjoy positive experiences and the thoughts and behaviors associated with building, engaging in, and lengthening these experiences (Bryant & Veroff, 2007; Lyubomirsky, 2008). In essence, savoring allows a person to bring the positive emotions from past experiences, a current situation, or anticipating future events into the present moment. People who are better able to experience pleasure in the present moment and to hold onto those feelings experience less depression or stress (Lyubomirsky, 2008). Savoring has been shown to improve well-being and self-concept (Bryant *et al.*, 2005). Specific strategies have been developed to enhance savoring, including sharing good news with others, replaying happy moments, and taking pleasure in ordinary experiences (Lyubomirsky, 2008). Mindfulness can be considered an aspect of savoring where a person is open to the present experience or has increased and enhanced attention to the present moment (Bryant & Veroff, 2007). Mindfulness also has been associated with increases in positive emotions, and use of mindfulness over time creates improvements in mood and decreases in stress (Brown & Ryan, 2003). People with serious mental illness often have negative trait affectivity (Blanchard *et al.*, 1998), and strategies that enhance the experience of savoring and mindfulness offer skills to build positive emotions into their daily life. The skills of savoring are relatively easy to learn and can be applied in situations to reduce the effects of stress and symptoms on functioning. People can learn to replay the happy moments from the past, relish positive events in the present, and anticipate positive experiences from their dreams. People with negative symptoms such as anhedonia often have particular deficits in the ability to anticipate and reminisce about pleasurable events (Burbridge & Barch, 2007; Gard *et al.*, 2007), and could benefit from deliberate

practice of these skills. Consumers who use savoring and mindfulness can build resources by experiencing more positive emotions that can enhance resilient qualities and resources.

Gratitude is appreciating the things that are important to a person and stimulates concern for others. When the focus of the gratitude is another person, expressing the associated positive feelings to that person makes them feel appreciated and valued, in much the same way the person expressing the gratitude feels. Enhancing gratitude may serve to build resilient qualities and resources because it is associated with the development of social connections and coping skills that foster well-being in the face of stress (McCullough *et al.*, 2001). Research has shown that gratitude is incompatible with negative emotions and may offer protection against psychiatric disorders (Bono & McCullough, 2006). Teaching skills to increase a sense of gratitude, and inhibit negative emotions, could be particularly important for people with serious mental illness given the amount of depression associated with schizophrenia (Drake & Cotton, 1986; Häfner *et al.*, 2005) and, by definition, with major mood disorders. The lives of those affected are often characterized by multiple setbacks, and at times it may be difficult for them to find the blessings in their daily lives; however, enhancing gratitude may be even more important in addressing these issues given its incompatibility with negative emotions and its role in building of social relationships. Feeling grateful for the good things in one's life and sharing this with others can buoy resilience and serve to buffer the effects of whatever stress the individual is under.

Another strategy that encourages the building of positive emotions is practicing acts of kindness. Social relationships are a key ingredient to well-being and, as discussed above, can serve as a buffer against stress-induced relapses (Buchanan, 1995). Research has suggested that when people help others they rate their moods as more positive (Lyubomirsky *et al.*, 2005a). Indeed, the process of assisting others benefits the helper as much as the person helped (known as the *helper's principle*) (Gartner & Riessman, 1977; Madera, 1988; Campbell, 1989, 1997; Carpinello *et al.*, 1992). People with serious mental illness are often dependent upon other people for many things in their life, such as financial help, housing, and transportation. As a result, they may experience feelings of a loss of control in their lives and may not have as many opportunities to help other people. The benefits of practicing acts of kindness, such as feeling more positive about one's community, increased sense of cooperation, and increased awareness of the good things in one's life, seem even more relevant to people with serious mental illness. Practicing acts of kindness may also result in strengthening feelings of confidence, control, and optimism about the future (Lyubomirsky *et al.*, 2005b).

The benefits of having a sense of humor have been linked to increases in psychological well-being as well as being a means to cope more effectively with stressful situations. Specifically, using affiliative humor, a non-threatening humor style used to enhance relationships, may facilitate the development of social connections and improved well-being (Kuiper & McHale, 2009). Furthermore, the ability to laugh at oneself and one's own human failures can promote health psychological adjustment, even in the face of loss or other stressors (Vaillant, 1977; Taylor *et al.*, 2000). Research has shown that people with serious mental illness display some deficits in detecting humor when the situation is presented but still are able to appreciate humor (Tsoi *et al.*, 2008). Therefore, developing a deeper sense of humor may be adaptive for people with serious mental illness. Adaptive humor strategies focused on effective coping, relating to other people, and looking at a situation from a different perspective can be taught as skills to build resilient qualities and serve as a buffer against stressors. Teaching humor also gives people a chance to experience positive emotions as part of treatment and the recovery process (Davidson *et al.*, 2006).

Conclusions

Resilient qualities and resources are directly associated with helping a person to move past a stressful or traumatic experience while building resources to face future adversities. A person with serious mental illness is faced with many difficult stressors, which can be compounded by illness-related symptoms. The most commonly used elements of treatment have primarily focused on helping to overcome the deficits through strategies such as coping, problem solving, and increasing social support. These treatment methods mainly build resilient qualities and resources by moderating the effects of stress on symptoms and in daily life. As treatment components move away from the psychopathology model, a few interventions have used strategies to target self-esteem, finding absorbing activities, and pursuing meaningful goals. The

development of a broader definition of recovery has led to a wider range of treatment options for people. To help an individual to achieve recovery more fully, treatments need to focus on how to improve well-being outside of the psychopathology model. Interventions that include strategies to build gratitude, savoring and mindfulness, practicing acts of kindness, and humor generate, enhance, and prolong positive emotions, thus building a greater sense of well-being in the process of recovery rather than only minimizing the dysfunction. These strategies represent a picture of treatment that is focused both on enhancing well-being by building positive emotions and on reducing the impact of stress on illness. All of these strategies recognize that the treatment of the illness must also address how a person pursues well-being and happiness, because remittance of symptoms does not always result in positive well-being and outcomes (Fava *et al.*, 2007). Treatments that address a person's meaningful goals and positive life activities and experiences help the person more readily to embrace recovery and build resiliency.

References

Andreasen, N. C., Carpenter, W. T. Jr., Kane, J. M. *et al.* (2005). Remission in schizophrenia: Proposed criteria and rationale for consensus. *American Journal of Psychiatry*, **162**, 441–449.

Andresen, R., Oades, L., & Caputi, P. (2003). The experience of recovery from schizophrenia: Towards an empirically validated stage model. *Australian and New Zealand Journal of Psychiatry*, **37**, 586–594.

Anthony, W. A. (1993). Recovery from mental illness: The guiding vision of the mental health service system in the 1990s. *Psychosocial Rehabilitation Journal*, **16**, 11–23.

Atkinson, P. A., Martin, C. R., & Rankin, J. (2009). Resilience revisited. *Journal of Psychiatric and Mental Health Nursing*, **16**, 137–145.

Beale, V. & Lambric, T. (1995). *The recovery concept: Implementation in the mental health system – A report by the Community Support Program Advisory Committee.* Columbus, OH: Department of Mental Health, Office of Consumer Services.

Bebbington, P. E. & Kuipers, L. (1992). Life events and social factors. In D. J. Kavanagh (ed.), *Schizophrenia: An overview and practical handbook* (pp. 126–144). London: Chapman & Hall.

Blanchard, J. J., Mueser, K. T., & Bellack, A. S. (1998). Anhedonia, positive and negative affect, and social functioning in schizophrenia. *Schizophrenia Bulletin*, **24**, 413–424.

Blaska, B. (1990). The myriad medication mistakes in psychiatry: A consumer's view. *Hospital and Community Psychiatry*, **41**, 993–997.

Bonney, S. & Stickley, T. (2008). Recovery and mental health: A review of the British literature. *Journal of Psychiatric and Mental Health Nursing*, **15**, 140–153.

Bono, G. & McCullough, M. E. (2006). Positive responses to benefit and harm: Bringing forgiveness and gratitude into cognitive psychotherapy. *Journal of Cognitive Psychotherapy*, **20**, 147–158.

Brodkin, A. & Coleman, M. (1996). What makes a child resilient? *Instructor*, **105**, 28–29.

Brown, K. W. & Ryan, R. M. (2003). The benefits of being present: Mindfulness and its role in psychological well-being. *Journal of Personality and Social Psychology*, **84**, 822–848.

Bryant, F. B. & Veroff, J. (2007). *Savoring: A new model of positive experience*. Mahwah, NJ: Erlbaum.

Bryant, F. B., Smart, C. M., & King, S. P. (2005). Using the past to enhance the present: Boosting happiness through positive reminiscence. *Journal of Happiness Studies*, **6**, 227–260.

Buchanan, J. (1995). Social support and schizophrenia: A review of the literature. *Archives of Psychiatric Nursing*, **9**, 68–76.

Burbridge, J. A. & Barch, D. M. (2007). Anhedonia and the experience of emotion in individuals with schizophrenia. *Journal of Abnormal Psychology*, **116**, 30–42.

Campbell, J. (1989). *The Well Being Project: Mental health clients speak for themselves*, Vol. 6. Sacramento, CA: California Network of Mental Health Clients.

Campbell, J. (1996). Toward collaborative mental health outcomes systems. *New Directions for Mental Health Services*, **71**, 69–78.

Campbell, J. (1997). How consumers/survivors are evaluating the quality of psychiatric care. *Evaluation Review*, **21**, 357–363.

Carling, P. J. (1995). *Return to community: Building support systems for people with psychiatric disabilities*. New York: Guilford Press.

Carpinello, S. E., Knight, E., & Jatulis, L. L. (1992). A study of the meaning of self-help, self-help group processes, and outcomes. In *Proceedings of the Third Annual Meeting of the National Association of State Mental Health Program Directors*, Alexandria, VA.

Chamberlin, J. (1978). *On our own: Patient-controlled alternatives to the mental health system*. New York: Hawthorne.

Ciompi, L. (1980). Catamnestic long-term study on the course of life and aging of schizophrenics. *Schizophrenia Bulletin*, **6**, 606–618.

Clarke, S. P., Oades, L. G., Crowe, T. P., & Deane, F. P. (2006). Collaborative goal technology: Theory and practice. *Psychiatric Rehabilitation Journal*, **30**, 129–136.

Cohn, M. A., Fredrickson, B. L., Brown, S. L., Mikels, J. A., & Conway, A. M. (2009). Happiness unpacked: Positive emotions increase life satisfaction by building resilience. *Emotion*, **9**, 361–368.

Davidson, L. (2003). *Living outside mental illness: Qualitative studies of recovery in schizophrenia*. New York: New York University Press.

Davidson, L., Lawless, M. S., & Leary, F. (2005a). Concepts of recovery: competing or complementary? *Current Opinion in Psychiatry*, **18**, 664–667.

Davidson, L., Harding, C., & Spaniol, L. (2005b). *Recovery from severe mental illnesses: Research evidence and implications for practice*, Vol 1. Boston, MA: Center for Psychiatric Rehabilitation of Boston University.

Davidson, L., Shahar, G., Lawless, M. S., Sells, D., & Tondora, J. (2006). Play, pleasure, and other positive life events: "Non-specific" factors in recovery from mental illness? *Psychiatry: Interpersonal and Biological Processes*, **69**, 151–163.

Davidson, L., Tondora, J., Lawless, M. S., O'Connell, M. J., & Rowe, M. (2009). *A practical guide to recovery-oriented practice: tools for transforming mental health care*. New York: Oxford University Press.

Deegan, P. E. (1988). Recovery: The lived experience of rehabilitation. *Psychosocial Rehabilitation Journal*, **11**, 11–19.

Deegan, P. E. (1990). Spirit breaking: When the helping professionals hurt. *Humanistic Psychologist*, **18**, 301–313.

Deegan, P. E. (1992). The Independent Living Movement and people with psychiatric disabilities: Taking back control over our own lives. *Psychosocial Rehabilitation Journal*, **15**, 3–19.

Deegan, P. E. (1996). Recovery and the conspiracy of hope. In *Proceedings of the Sixth Annual Mental Health Conference of Australia and New Zealand*, Brisbane, Australia.

Deegan, P. E. & Affa, C. (1995). *Coping with voices: Self-help strategies for people who hear voices that are distressing*. Lawrence, MA: National Empowerment Center.

Drake, R. E. & Cotton, P. G. (1986). Depression, hopelessness and suicide in chronic schizophrenia. *British Journal of Psychiatry*, **148**, 554–559.

Edward, K.-L. & Warelow, P. (2005). Resilience: When coping is emotionally intelligent. *Journal of the American Psychiatric Nurses Association*, **11**, 101–102.

Estroff, S. E. (1989). Self, identity, and subjective experiences of schizophrenia: In search of the subject. *Schizophrenia Bulletin*, **15**, 189–196.

Falloon, I. R. H., Barbieri, L., Boggian, I., & Lamonaca, D. (2007). Problem solving training for schizophrenia: Rationale and review. *Journal of Mental Health*, **16**, 553–568.

Farhall, J., Greenwood, K. M., & Jackson, H. J. (2007). Coping with hallucinated voices in schizophrenia: A review of self-initiated strategies and therapeutic interventions. *Clinical Psychology Review*, **27**, 476–493.

Farkas, M., Gagne, C., Anthony, W., & Chamberlin, J. (2005). Implementing recovery oriented evidence based programs: Identifying the critical dimensions. *Community Mental Health Journal*, **41**, 141–158.

Fava, G. A., Ruini, C., & Belaise, C. (2007). The concept of recovery in major depression. *Psychological Medicine*, **37**, 307–317.

Fisher, D. B. (1992). Humanizing the recovery process. *Resources*, **4**, 5–6.

Fisher, W. A., Penney, D. J., & Earle, K. (1996). Mental health services recipients: Their role in shaping organizational policy. *Administration and Policy in Mental Health*, **23**, 547–553.

Fowler, D., Garety, P., & Kuipers, E. (1995). *Cognitive behaviour therapy for psychosis: Theory and practice*. Chichester, UK: Wiley.

Garcelan, S. P. & Rodriguez, A. G. (2002). Coping strategies in psychotics: Conceptualization and research results. *Psychology in Spain*, **6**, 26–40.

Gard, D. E., Kring, A. M., Gard, M. G., Horan, W. P., & Green, M. F. (2007). Anhedonia in schizophrenia: Distinctions between anticipatory and consummatory pleasure. *Schizophrenia Research*, **93**, 253–260.

Gartner, A. & Riessman, F. (1977). *Self-help in the human services*. San Francisco, CA: Jossey-Bass.

Geanellos, R. (2005). Adversity as opportunity: Living with schizophrenia and developing a resilient self. *International Journal of Mental Health Nursing*, **14**, 7–15.

Häfner, H., Maurer, K., Trendler, G., *et al.* (2005). Schizophrenia and depression: Challenging the paradigm of two separate diseases – A controlled study of schizophrenia, depression and healthy controls. *Schizophrenia Research*, **77**, 11–24.

Harding, C. M., Brooks, G. W., Ashikaga, T., Strauss, J. S., & Breir, A. (1987). The Vermont longitudinal study of persons with severe mental illness: I. Methodology, study sample and overall status 32 years later. *American Journal of Psychiatry*, **144**, 718–726.

Harrison, G., Hopper, K., Craig, T., *et al.* (2001). Recovery from psychotic illness: A 15- and 25-year international follow-up study. *British Journal of Psychiatry*, **178**, 506–517.

Kopelowicz, A., Liberman, R. P., & Zarate, R. (2006). Recent advances in social skills training for schizophrenia. *Schizophrenia Bulletin*, **32**, S12–S23.

Kraepelin, E. (1971). *Dementia praecox and paraphrenia*. [R. M. Barclay, trans.] New York: Krieger.

Kuiper, N. A. & McHale, N. (2009). Humor styles as mediators between self-evaluative standards and psychological well-being. *Journal of Psychology: Interdisciplinary and Applied*, **143**, 359–376.

Kurtz, M. M. & Mueser, K. T. (2008). A meta-analysis of controlled research on social skills training for schizophrenia. *Journal of Consulting and Clinical Psychology*, **76**, 491–504.

Lecomte, T., Cyr, M., Lesage, A. D., *et al.* (1999). Efficacy of a self-esteem module in the empowerment of individuals with schizophrenia. *Journal of Nervous and Mental Disease*, **187**, 406–413.

Leete, E. (1989). How I perceive and manage my illness. *Schizophrenia Bulletin*, **15**, 197–200.

Liberman, R. P., Eckman, T. A., & Marder, S. R. (2001). Training in social problem solving among persons with schizophrenia. *Psychiatric Services*, **52**, 31–33.

Liberman, R. P., Kopelowicz, A., Ventura, J., & Gutkind, D. (2002). Operational criteria and factors related to recovery from schizophrenia. *International Review of Psychiatry*, **14**, 256–272.

Lopez, S. J., Snyder, C. R., Magyar-Moe, J. L., *et al.* (2004). *Strategies for accentuating hope: Positive psychology in practice* (pp. 388–404). Hoboken, NJ: Wiley.

Luthar, S. S. & Cicchetti, D. (2000). The construct of resilience: Implications for interventions and social policies. *Development and Psychopathology*, **12**, 857–885.

Lyubomirsky, S. (2008). *The how of happiness: A scientific approach to getting the life you want*. New York: The Penguin Press.

Lyubomirsky, S., King, L., & Diener, E. (2005a). The benefits of frequent positive affect: does happiness lead to success? *Psychological Bulletin*, **131**, 803–855.

Lyubomirsky, S., Sheldon, K. M., & Schkade, D. (2005b). Pursuing happiness: The architecture of sustainable change. *Review of General Psychology*, **9**, 111–131.

Macdonald, E. M., Pica, S., McDonald, S., Hayes, R. L., & Baglioni, A. J. J. (1998). Stress and coping in early psychosis: Role of symptoms, self-efficacy, and social support in coping with stress. *British Journal of Psychiatry*, **172**(Suppl. 33), 122–127.

MacInnes, D. L. & Lewis, M. (2008). The evaluation of a short group programme to reduce self-stigma in people with serious and enduring mental health problems. *Journal of Psychiatric and Mental Health Nursing*, **15**, 59–65.

Madera, E. J. (1988). Seven principles in self help: Understanding how self-help groups help. *New Program Initiatives in Mental Health*, May, 3–4 [Newsletter published by the New Jersey State Division of Mental Health & Hospitals.]

Marshall, S. L., Crowe, T. P., Oades, L. G., Deane, F. F., & Kavanagh, D. J. (2007). A review of consumer involvement in evaluations of case management: Consistency with a recovery paradigm. *Psychiatric Services*, 58, 396–401.

Masten, A. S. (2001). Ordinary magic: Resilience processes in development. *American Psychologist*, 56, 227–238.

McCullough, M. E., Kilpatrick, S. D., Emmons, R. A., & Larson, D. B. (2001). Is gratitude a moral affect? *Psychological Bulletin*, 127, 249–266.

Mead, S. & Copeland, M. E. (2000). What recovery means to us: Consumers' perspectives. *Community Mental Health Journal*, 36, 315–328.

Miller, J. S. (1990). Mental illness and spiritual crisis: Implications for psychiatric rehabilitation. *Psychosocial Rehabilitation Journal*, 14, 29–45.

Morrison, A. P., Renton, J. C., Dunn, H., Williams, S., & Bentall, R. P. (2004). *Cognitive therapy for psychosis: A formulation-based approach*. New York: Brunner-Routledge.

Mueser, K. T. & Bellack, A. S. (1998). Social skills and social functioning. In K. T. Mueser & N. Tarrier (eds.), *Handbook of social functioning in schizophrenia* (pp. 79–96). Needham Heights, MA: Allyn & Bacon.

Mueser, K. T., Corrigan, P. W., Hilton, D., *et al.* (2002). Illness management and recovery for severe mental illness: A review of the research. *Psychiatric Services*, 53, 1272–1284.

Neenan, M. (2009). *Developing resilience: A cognitive-behavioural approach*. New York: Routledge/Taylor & Francis.

Nuechterlein, K. H. & Dawson, M. E. (1984). A heuristic vulnerability/stress model of schizophrenic episodes. *Schizophrenia Bulletin*, 10, 300–312.

Perry, B. M., Taylor, D., & Shaw, S. K. (2007). "You've got to have a positive state of mind": An interpretative phenomenological analysis of hope and first episode psychosis. *Journal of Mental Health*, 16, 781–793.

Ralph, R. O. (2000). *Review of recovery literature: A synthesis of a sample of recovery literature 2000*. Portland, ME: Edmund S. Muskie Institute of Public Affairs, University of Southern Maine.

Ralph, R. O. & Corrigan, P. W. (eds.) (2005). *Recovery in mental illness: Broadening our understanding of wellness*. Washington, DC: American Psychological Association.

Richardson, G. E. (2002). The metatheory of resilience and resiliency. *Journal of Clinical Psychology*, 58, 307–321.

Roder, V., Jenull, B., & Brenner, H. D. (1998). Teaching schizophrenic patients recreational, residential and vocational skills. *International Review of Psychiatry*, 10, 35–41.

Rodgers, M. L., Norell, D. M., Roll, J. M., & Dyck, D. G. (2007). An overview of mental health recovery. *Primary Psychiatry*, 14, 76–85.

Roe, D. (2001). Progressing from patienthood to personhood across the multidimensional outcomes in schizophrenia and related disorders. *Journal of Nervous and Mental Disease*, 189, 691–699.

Roe, D. & Chopra, M. (2003). Beyond coping with mental illness: Toward personal growth. *American Journal of Orthopsychiatry*, 73, 334–344.

Roe, D., Yanos, P. T., & Lysaker, P. H. (2006). Coping with psychosis: An integrative developmental framework. *Journal of Nervous and Mental Disease*, 194, 917–924.

Salokangas, R. K. R., Honkonen, T., Stengard, E., & Koivisto, A.-M. (2006). Subjective life satisfaction and living situations of persons in Finland with long-term schizophrenia. *Psychiatric Services*, 57, 373–381.

Seligman, M. E. P. (2002). *Authentic happiness: Using the new positive psychology to realize your potential for lasting fulfillment*. New York: Free Press.

Slade, M. (2009). *Personal recovery and mental illness: A guide for mental health professionals*. Cambridge, UK: Cambridge University Press.

Tai, S. & Turkington, D. (2009). The evolution of cognitive behavior therapy for schizophrenia: Current practice and recent developments. *Schizophrenia Bulletin*, 35, 865–873.

Taylor, S. E., Kemeny, M. E., Reed, G. M., Bower, J. E., & Gruenewald, T. L. (2000). Psychological resources, positive illusions, and health. *American Psychologist*, 55, 99–109.

Tedeschi, R. G. & Kilmer, R. P. (2005). Assessing strengths, resilience, and growth to guide clinical interventions. *Professional Psychology: Research and Practice*, 36, 230–237.

Tsoi, D. T. Y., Lee, K. H., Gee, K. A., *et al.* (2008). Humour experience in schizophrenia: Relationship with executive dysfunction and psychosocial impairment. *Psychological Medicine*, 38, 801–810.

Turkington, D., Dudley, R., Warman, D. M., & Beck, A. T. (2006). Cognitive-behavioral therapy for schizophrenia: A review. *Focus*, 4, 223–233.

Tusaie, K. & Dyer, J. (2004). Resilience: a historical review of the construct. *Holistic Nursing Practice*, 18, 3–10.

Vaillant, G. E. (1977). *Adaptation to life*. Boston: Little, Brown.

Wennberg, J. E. (1988). Improving the medical decision-making process. *Health Affairs*, 7, 99–105.

Zimmerman, M. A. & Rappaport, J. (1988). Citizen participation, perceived control, and psychological empowerment. *American Journal of Community Psychology*, **16**, 725–750.

Zubin, J. & Spring, B. (1977). Vulnerability: A new view of schizophrenia. *Journal of Abnormal Psychology*, **86**, 103–126.

Interventions to enhance resilience and resilience-related constructs in adults

Steven M. Southwick, Robert H. Pietrzak, and Gerald White

Introduction

Most people are exposed to at least one significant trauma during their lifetime. Individuals employed in high-risk occupations, such as soldiers, policemen, and firemen, are typically exposed to many traumas. While numerous training programs have been developed with the goal of increasing resilience and ability to cope with traumatic stress, very few programs and interventions have been subjected to rigorous scientific evaluation. As a result, currently there exists little empirical evidence to support specific approaches to enhancing resilience and preventing the development of psychopathology in the face of stress and trauma. Nevertheless, given recent interest in the development and enhancement of resilience (Meichenbaum & Jaremko, 1983; Meichenbaum, 1985; Maddi, 2002; Davidson *et al.*, 2005; Defense Centers of Excellence, 2009), we believe there is value in reviewing published research on interventions designed to enhance constructs that are related to resilience, such as hardiness, coping self-efficacy, and stress inoculation, as well as factors that are associated with resilience, such as optimism and social support. As noted in earlier chapters, there is no single definition and no agreed upon criteria for resilience. This makes it challenging to evaluate existing treatments and interventions designed to enhance resilience.

The Preface gives a variety of definitions of resilience. Resilience has been defined in terms of protective factors associated with growing up in disadvantaged environments (Garmezy, 1974; Garmezy & Streitman, 1974), successful adaptation to adversity (Luthar *et al.*, 2000), a "class of phenomena characterized by good outcomes in spite of serious threats to adaptation or development" (Masten, 2001, p. 228), enhanced psychobiological regulation of stress hormones (Charney, 2004), and symptom-free functioning following trauma exposure (Bonanno *et al.*, 2006). In general, resilience may be understood as "the process of adapting well in the face of adversity, trauma, tragedy, threats, or even significant sources of stress. Further, it may be understood as the ability to 'bounce back' from difficult experiences" (American Psychological Association, 2010, p. 2).

Resilience to stress has been associated with a host of neurobiological factors (Charney 2004, Southwick 2005, Haglund *et al.*, 2007). The neurobiology of resilience, which is highly complex, involves numerous brain regions and circuits, as well as neurotransmitter and endocrine systems. Some of the more important factors and systems that have been studied to date include the hypothalamic–pituitary–adrenal axis, the sympathetic nervous system, the dopamine-mediated reward system, and the amygdala, hippocampus, and prefrontal cortex. These factors and circuits have been described in detail in an earlier chapter.

Resilience has also been associated with a number of psychosocial factors that appear to have a protective role in highly challenging and stressful situations. Some of the best studied psychosocial factors include realistic optimism and positive emotions, active problem-focused coping, high levels of positive social support, altruism, religious/spiritual practice, attention to physical health and exercise, cognitive flexibility (e.g., cognitive reappraisal, acceptance, positive explanatory style), disciplined focus on skill development, commitment to a valued cause or purpose, and the capacity to extract meaning from adverse situations and from life in general (Southwick, 2005).

Interventions designed to enhance resilience, or constructs associated with resilience, can be directed at the individual, the family, the organization, or the community. Further, interventions can be delivered at various points in time prior to (i.e., preparation/

Resilience and Mental Health: Challenges Across the Lifespan, ed. Steven M. Southwick, Brett T. Litz, Dennis Charney, and Matthew J. Friedman. Published by Cambridge University Press. © Cambridge University Press 2011.

prevention), during or after stress/trauma exposure. Training administered prior to stress/trauma exposure is generally designed to enhance performance during stressful life events or traumas, with the intent to lessen or even prevent the development of stress-related morbidities. Such training typically focuses on increasing familiarity with stressful scenarios that one might encounter, as well as with potential emotional and physiological reactions to these stressors; increasing perceptions of predictability and controllability of both external and internal trauma-related stimuli; developing skills relevant to the specific stressor/trauma (e.g., intensive combat training), as well as more generic stress management skills (e.g., diaphragmatic breathing, muscular-relaxation training); and exposing individuals to intensive, realistic training (e.g., scenario-based training), which may be delivered in graduated doses of intensity (Whealin *et al.*, 2008).

Measurement of resilience

Several measures of resilience and constructs related to resilience (e.g., hardiness, self-efficacy, meaning-making) have been developed and are described below.

The Dispositional Resilience Scale-15 (DRS-15). This is a brief, valid, and reliable 15-item self-report instrument that provides a measure of hardiness (Bartone, 1995, 2007). It assesses three dimensions of resilience related to hardiness: commitment (i.e., tendency to engage fully in life activities), perceived control (i.e., perceived ability to exercise control over life circumstances), and challenge (i.e., tendency to enjoy challenges). This measure, which is derived from longer 30- and 45-item versions of the Dispositional Resilience Scale (DRS; Bartone *et al.*, 1989), has been applied in military and occupational settings. Scores on this measure have been shown to be negatively associated with perceived occupational stress and psychological dysfunction (Bartone *et al.*, 1989; Steinhardt *et al.*, 2003; Bartone, 2006, 2007; McCalister *et al.*, 2006).

The Connor–Davidson Resilience Scale (CD-RISC). This 25-item self-report measure assesses a broad range of resilient characteristics, including hardiness, personal competence, tolerance of negative affect, acceptance of change, personal control, and spirituality (Connor & Davidson, 2003). The CD-RISC is a psychometrically sound measure of resilience that was designed to be used as an outcome measure (Connor & Davidson, 2003). For example, in a randomized trial of patients with post-traumatic stress disorder (PTSD), treatment with venlafaxine was associated with increased scores on dimensions of resilience reflecting hardiness, persistence/tenacity, social support, and faith (Davidson *et al.*, 2008). Abbreviated 10- (Campbell-Sills & Stein, 2007) and 2-item (Vaishnavi *et al.*, 2007) versions of the CD-RISC are also available and may be easily incorporated into treatment studies.

The Response to Stressful Experience Scale (RSES). This 22-item self-report measure was developed by the National Center for PTSD and assesses a broad range of behaviors, thoughts, and actions that individuals characteristically employ when responding to stress, adversity, or trauma (Johnson *et al.*, 2011). The measure consists of a total score and six subscales: active coping, meaning-making, cognitive flexibility, spirituality, self-efficacy, and restoration. To date, the RSES has been used to characterize behaviors, thoughts, and actions that may confer protection against traumatic stress and related psychopathology in military populations. For example, higher scores on the RSES were found to be negatively associated with PTSD symptom severity in military personnel on active duty, as well as in treatment-seeking veterans (Johnson *et al.*, 2011).

The Resilience Scales for Children and Adolescents (RSCA). This 64-item self-report measure assesses resilience-related attributes of children and adolescents, including sense of mastery, sense of relatedness, and emotional reactivity (Prince-Embury, 2008). The RSCA consists of three global scales: (1) sense of mastery (optimism, self-efficacy, adaptability); (2) sense of relatedness (trust, support, comfort, tolerance); and (3) emotional reactivity (sensitivity, recovery, impairment). Each global scale comprises 20–24 questions, and there are 10 subscales. The RSCA has been used to screen for psychological vulnerability in children and adolescents. Higher scores on the emotional reactivity scale have been found to be associated with greater symptoms of depression, anxiety, anger, and disruptive behavior, while higher scores on the sense of mastery and sense of relatedness scales were negatively associated with these variables (Prince-Embury, 2008).

Measures of resilience may have different applications in studies of resilience-enhancing interventions. For example, the CD-RISC may be most useful as an outcome measure in interventions purporting to enhance resilience (e.g., Vaishnavi *et al.*, 2007; Davidson *et al.*, 2008; Steinhardt & Dolbier, 2008), while the DRS-15, RSES, and RSCA may be most useful in assessing characteristics of resilience (e.g., hardiness, self-efficacy, sense of mastery) that may buffer or protect against traumatic stress and related psychopathology (Steinhardt *et al.*, 2003; McCalister *et al.*, 2006; Prince-Embury, 2008; Johnson *et al.*, 2011). Given that research on the measurement of resilience is in its early stages, additional studies are needed to validate these instruments in a broader range of stress- and trauma-exposed populations; to evaluate their similarities and differences in assessing aspects of resilience; to determine their relative sensitivity in predicting response to resilience-enhancing interventions; and to evaluate their role in mediating treatment-related change, as well as in assessing the effects of these interventions.

Interventions designed to enhance resilience

This section describes three interventions designed specifically to enhance resilience: hardiness training, stress inoculation training (SIT), and psychoeducational resilience enhancement training.

Hardiness training

Psychological hardiness is a construct that was developed to describe an inner resource (Florian *et al.*, 1995) or constellation of personality characteristics (Westphal *et al.*, 2008) associated with good health and optimal performance under conditions of high stress (Eid & Morgan, 2006). As defined by Kobasa *et al.* (1982), hardiness is composed of three primary, interrelated components: (1) control, or the belief that one can influence events in life; (2) commitment, or the ability to feel deeply involved in one's existence, relationships, activities, and self; (3) challenge, or the tendency to view adverse events and change as challenges rather than threats (Maddi & Khoshaba, 2005). Hardiness is believed to develop early in life and remain relatively stable over time, although changes in hardiness are possible (Kobasa *et al.*, 1982). As noted above, Kobasa and Maddi constructed the Hardiness Scale to measure this attribute (Kobasa, 1979; Kobasa *et al.*,

1982) and the scale has undergone a number of revisions designed to shorten the original measure (e.g., the DRS) (Bartone *et al.*, 1989; Bartone, 2006).

Summarizing several decades of research, Maddi (2007, p. 61) described hardiness as "a pattern of attitudes and skills that provides the courage and strategies to turn stressful circumstances from potential disasters into growth opportunities instead." He also wrote that hardiness requires the "courage and motivation to face stressors accurately rather than to deny or catastrophize" (Maddi, 2005, p. 261). Such courage and motivation may well lead to active coping, problem solving, and the giving and receiving of social support. In a study of a nationally representative sample of 1632 Vietnam veterans, King and colleagues found that higher level of hardiness in veterans was negatively related to PTSD symptoms and that hardiness was associated with increased resistance to PTSD through its association with functional social support (King *et al.*, 1998). Studies in a variety of populations have shown that hardiness is positively associated with good mental and physical health (Westphal *et al.*, 2008), that hardiness is a significant modifier or buffer of combat stress (Bartone, 1993; Westphal *et al.*, 2008) and occupational stress (Kobasa & Puccetti, 1983; Kobasa *et al.*, 1985; Contrada, 1989), and that hardy individuals tend to appraise or evaluate potentially negative events as less threatening (Kobasa *et al.*, 1981, 1982) and remain more optimistic about their ability to cope with the situation (Allred & Smith, 1989) compared with less hardy individuals.

Khoshaba and Maddi (2001) have developed a training program to increase hardiness. The program takes place in small groups led by a trainer, involves weekly sessions, and addresses the core elements of the hardiness construct. Trainees are taught techniques to handle stress and practice exercises designed to enhance attitudes of commitment, control, and challenge (Maddi & Khoshaba, 2005; Maddi, 2008). In addition, they learn problem-solving skills. In what is termed *transformational coping*, trainees learn to broaden their perspective and deepen their understanding of the stressful experience they face, and then develop and carry out a decisive course of action. Finally, trainees learn how to build two-way social support relationships where they give and receive encouragement and assistance from others (Maddi & Khoshaba, 2005).

The effects of hardiness training have been examined in working adults and college students. In 1981, the US Federal Court ordered the deregulation of the

American Telephone and Telegraph (AT&T) monopoly. Maddi and colleagues (2006) studied the effects of this deregulation, as well as the effects of hardiness training at Illinois Bell Telephone (IBT) (a subsidy of AT&T) from 1975 to 1987. Massive layoffs and a dismantling of long-standing norms and policies resulted in high levels of stress among most employees. This longitudinal study of over 450 male and female IBT employees examined the differences between the one third who thrived (i.e., one third of the employees took the changes as opportunities to grow and they rose to the top of the company, with some even starting companies of their own) compared with the remaining two thirds who demonstrated overt signs of stress during the transition (e.g., physical and mental health problems, marital problems). The thriving group demonstrated the "three Cs" of commitment, control, and challenge to a significantly greater degree than the other workers.

Based on findings from this initial study of IBT employees (Maddi & Kobasa, 1984; Maddi & Khoshaba, 2005), Maddi and colleagues (2006) developed and applied a hardiness training method (*HardiTraining*) to enhance hardiness in this population of IBT employees. Compared with employees who did not receive hardiness training, those who completed training experienced greater reductions in stress, depression, anxiety, and blood pressure, and had better job satisfaction and job performance (Maddi & Khoshaba, 2005). Of the workers who completed the training, 93% reported an improvement in their ability to cope with stressful situations, with these group differences persisting at a six-month follow-up.

Hardiness training has also been applied in college students where it has been associated with increases in grade point averages and retention in school (Maddi *et al.*, 2002; Maddi & Khoshaba, 2005). Hardiness training has been recommended as a potential method to enhance performance, leadership, and health in military personnel, and to help with recovery from stress-related difficulties (Maddi, 2007). To date, however, we are unaware of any studies that have examined the efficacy of hardiness training in this population.

Stress inoculation training

Stress inoculation training is based on a transactional model of stress and coping that was first described by Lazarus and Folkman (1984). In this model, stress is viewed as a bidirectional and dynamic transaction between the individual and the environment. For any given life event, each person will interpret or appraise that event in his or her own unique manner depending on a complex array of biological, developmental, psychological, social, and spiritual factors. The individual experiences the event as stressful when he or she believes that the skills and resources needed to deal with the event exceed his or her ability. Thus, in the transactional model, appraisal of environmental demands and of one's capacity to handle and cope with those demands determines how an individual responds to stress.

The SIT approach was originally developed as a treatment for anxiety by Meichenbaum and colleagues (Meichenbaum, 1975, 1985; Meichenbaum & Jaremko, 1983). It was later adapted by Kilpatrick and colleagues (1982) to treat trauma survivors. The program typically consists of 8 to 22 weekly sessions and is composed of what Meichenbaum describes as three overlapping phases (Meichenbaum & Deffenbacher, 1988). Beginning with the conceptual and educational phase, a collaborative therapeutic relationship is established and the neurobiological and psychological impact of trauma and stress-related symptoms is discussed and normalized. Individuals are taught to self-monitor by learning to recognize emotional, behavioral, physical, and cognitive responses to trauma-related cues or triggers. Then, signs of strength and resilience are identified to help to facilitate changes in how stressors are perceived (i.e., challenging rather than overwhelming).

During the second phase (the skills acquisition and rehearsal phase), individuals are taught new coping skills and are helped to consolidate skills they already possess. Examples of coping skills include relaxation training, thought stopping, guided self-dialogue, identification and replacement of irrational and maladaptive thinking, and problem solving.

In the third phase of SIT, the individual is encouraged to practice the skills acquired in the first two phases through role playing, modeling, imagery rehearsal, and behavioral rehearsal in situations that are stressful and anxiety provoking. These stressful situations are graduated (i.e., graded in vivo exposure) so that they become increasingly challenging (i.e., creating an inoculating effect). Once one situation is mastered, the individual moves on to the next most challenging one. Throughout this phase, emphasis is placed on accurately discriminating dangerous from safe situations, managing fear, problem solving, and staying actively engaged in the situation through the use of relaxation, cognitive restructuring, guided self-dialogue, and other coping strategies. There is also a focus on extending into the future what was learned during the training program through booster sessions and follow-up.

The SIT approach has been studied primarily in female victims of sexual assault (Foa *et al.*, 1991, 1999). Results of these studies suggest that SIT is associated with reductions in PTSD and depressive symptoms that are largely maintained at follow-up one year later. Magnitudes of these reductions are comparable to those associated with prolonged exposure and with the combination of prolonged exposure and SIT (Foa *et al.*, 1999).

Psychoeducational resilience enhancement

College is often seen as a period of rapid growth but also of psychological vulnerability. Students are faced with many new challenges at a time when they have not fully developed their coping abilities. To help to address this period of vulnerability, Steinhardt and Dolbier (2008) designed a four-week psychoeducational intervention to enhance resilience to stress as well as decrease psychological and psychosomatic symptoms by reducing maladaptive coping mechanisms, fostering adaptive coping skills, and enhancing factors that protect against the deleterious effects of stress (e.g., positive affect, self-esteem). This study was conducted during a period of increased academic stress (i.e., the final weeks of classes). Students were randomized into the experimental group (30) or the waitlist control group (27). The intervention consisted of four sessions of two hours each that were psychoeducational in nature: (1) transforming stress into resilience, (2) taking responsibility, (3) focusing on empowering interpretations, and (4) creating meaningful connections. After the intervention, the experimental group had significantly higher resilience scores (CD-RISC), lower negative psychological symptom scores, higher scores on effective coping strategies, and higher scores on measures of positive affect, self-esteem, and self-leadership compared with the waitlist control group. Results of this study suggest that this intervention may be useful in managing stress and enhancing resilience. Additional research is needed to examine the durability of these changes over time, as well as whether the changes associated with this intervention generalize to other life stressors.

Interventions designed to enhance constructs related to resilience

This section describes three interventions designed specifically to enhance constructs related to resilience: social support interventions, learned optimism training, and well-being therapy. A number of other constructs, such as altruism and positive religious coping, have also been associated with resilience, but will not be reviewed in this chapter.

Social support interventions

A large body of literature has examined the relationship between social support, resilience, and physical and mental health. Higher perceived social support, which has been conceptualized as an individual's perception or experience of helpful social interactions, is associated with better physical functioning (Moak & Agrawal, 2010), as well as decreased symptoms of PTSD (King *et al.*, 1998; Brewin *et al.*, 2000; Ozer *et al.*, 2008) and depression (Charuvastra & Cloitre, 2008). For example, in a nationally representative sample of 34 653 US adults, Moak and Agrawal (2010) found that high perceived social support was negatively associated with depression, generalized anxiety disorder, and social phobia, as well as with physical health problems. Higher perceived social support also buffered the relationship between traumatic life events and psychopathology.

The importance of social support has also been examined in military samples. For example, as described above, King and colleagues (1998), in a nationally representative sample of 1632 Vietnam veterans, found that hardiness and post-war social support were negatively associated with PTSD symptoms, and that functional social support (i.e., emotional sustenance and instrumental assistance) accounted for a substantial amount of the indirect effect of hardiness on PTSD. More recently, a study of 272 Iraq/Afghanistan veterans found that greater perceptions of unit support were associated with greater psychological resilience (CD-RISC scores), and that both psychological resilience and post-deployment social support were inversely associated with PTSD symptoms, even after adjusting for combat exposure (Pietrzak *et al.*, 2010).

To address the finding that low perceived social support in patients with heart disease may be related to cardiac morbidity and mortality, investigators in the Enhancing Recovery in Coronary Artery Heart

Disease (ENRICHD) research group developed a treatment designed to enhance social support in 2481 patients who had recently experienced an acute myocardial infarction (Writing Committee for the ENRICHD Investigators, 2003). A psychosocial intervention based on cognitive-behavioral therapy was used to address cognitions, emotions, and behaviors associated with low perceived social support. The intervention included counseling to address behavioral and social skill deficits, as well as social outreach and social network development. The primary focus was to strengthen and improve existing social networks as well as to create new relationships. At a six-month follow-up assessment, the intervention group reported significantly greater improvement in depression and social isolation, but no differences in cardiac event-free survival were observed. Results of this study suggest that a psychological intervention based on cognitive-behavioral methods may be useful in reducing depressive symptoms and enhancing perceptions of social support in individuals who recently suffered an acute myocardial infarction, but that this intervention may not affect rates of recurrent infarction or death. Additional research has also been done on the role of social support in myocardial infarction (Lett et al., 2007, 2009).

In addition to the robust positive relationship between health and the receiving of social support, there is emerging evidence for a positive association between health and the giving of social support. In a five-year, prospective study of 846 older married adults who had experienced a recent myocardial infarction, Brown et al. (2003) compared the effects on longevity of receiving versus providing support. Results indicated reduced risk of mortality among individuals who reported providing support to others. This was true whether individuals provided emotional support to a spouse or instrumental support (e.g., housework, child care, etc.) to neighbors, friends, and relatives. When providing support was taken into consideration, there was no effect of receiving support on mortality. Taken together, these results suggest that *providing* social support may have a positive effect on longevity and that this effect may be independent of received social support.

Interventions designed to increase social support have been shown to enhance physical and mental health and may be useful in promoting resilience to stress (King et al., 1998; Kaniasty & Norris, 2008). While we are aware of no published studies that have specifically examined the effect of social support interventions on enhancing resilience to stress, numerous studies have examined the impact of social support interventions on a variety of physical and mental health outcomes.

In a comprehensive review of the literature, Hogan and colleagues (2002) reviewed 100 studies that were designed to test the effect of interventions to enhance social support on a broad range of physical and mental health outcomes. Social support interventions had been delivered in group, individual, and combined formats, with outcomes comparable across these modalities. Individuals who participated in these intervention studies were drawn from several populations, including individuals with cancer, substance abusers, as well as those preparing for surgery. The authors of this review found that 83% of studies reported at least some benefits of social support relative to no treatment or another active treatment, benefits including reductions in psychological distress, depression, and substance abuse.

A number of research and treatment programs for individuals with alcohol dependence include strategies designed to change the patient's social network from one that reinforces drinking to one that supports sobriety. Examples include Alcoholics Anonymous (AA), the community reinforcement approach, and the UK Alcohol Treatment Trial Social Behavior and Network Therapy Study (Litt et al., 2007). Studies by Bond and colleagues (Kaskutas et al., 2002, 2009; Bond et al., 2003) have found that benefits from AA appear to be mediated, at least in part, by changes in social network. Similarly, Litt and colleagues (2007) developed a manualized treatment for the Network Support Project that consists of once weekly outpatient sessions over 12 weeks. The program focused on attending AA meetings as a way to avoid drinking and to make new acquaintances, assertiveness training, engaging in enjoyable activities other than drinking, re-establishing contact with relatives and friends who do not drink, and exploring ways to change one's social network. Peer-support and self-help interventions, particularly for reducing specific symptoms, have been found to be effective in enhancing well-being, improving coping skills, and expanding social networks.

Litt and colleagues (2007) tested the network support intervention in 210 alcohol-dependent individuals, who were randomized to one of three outpatient treatments: network support, network support plus contingency management, and case management. Over two years of follow-up, individuals who received network support treatment reported no change in number of drinking friends but an increase in the number of abstinent people in their social network; they also experienced a better drinking outcome compared with a control group. Changes in social network were associated with increases in self-efficacy and coping, which, in turn, predicted better long-term drinking outcomes.

Many studies evaluating the association between social support and physical and mental well-being have measured perceived social support, or an individual's appraisal of being reliably connected to others, as opposed to actual enacted social support (Barrera, 1986). The mechanism by which increased perceived social support might increase physical and psychological well-being as well as resilience is not well understood. Brand and colleagues (1995) began to address these questions using a 13-week preventive psycho-educational intervention they developed to enhance perceived social support in 51 community residents with low perceived social support. The intervention, which involved training in social skills and cognitive reframing, focused on recognizing one's positive qualities, correcting cognitive distortions about oneself, reconceptualizing relationships with family members, addressing negative cognitive biases when interpreting supportive behaviors, and improving social competence. Compared with a waitlist control group, the active treatment group reported increased perceived social support from family, but not friends. Results further indicated that increases in perceived social support may be mediated by changes in self-esteem and frequency of self-reinforcement.

The giving and receiving of social support constitutes an important aspect of Maddi's hardiness training, described above (Maddi & Khoshaba, 2005). Building two-way social support involves the exchange of assistance and encouragement, as well as minimizing destructive competition and overprotection. In the hardiness model, critical elements of social support include empathy, sympathy, and showing appreciation for the other person. Communicating faith in the other person's ability to handle problems and helping with responsibilities when the other person is overwhelmed, yet providing some breathing room for him/her to deal with problems, is an important aspect of this model. Resources such as expertise and contacts are also offered when needed. Concrete steps to increase social support include creating a social interaction map, which involves recording the names, frequency of contact, degree of interaction and intimacy for all of the important people in one's life. This is followed

by recording whether and to what degree each of these relationships involves conflict. Conflicts are subsequently solved through assistance and encouragement while carrying out an action plan that includes responding to feedback.

It is important to note that not all studies have reported that social support interventions yield beneficial mental and physical health outcomes. In some cases, relying on others for support may increase dependence, feelings of guilt and anxiety, and the feeling that one is a burden to others (Hogan et al., 2002, Litt et al., 2007). It is also not clear which elements of social support are most important for enhancing health and functioning. While most studies have focused on receiving support, very few have evaluated the effects of providing social support on health outcomes. Given the great variability in subject populations, methodology, interventions, assessments, and outcome measures employed in studies of social support interventions, it is difficult to draw specific conclusions from an analysis of these studies (Hogan et al., 2002). Nevertheless, accumulating evidence from both epidemiological and treatment research suggests that interventions designed to enhance social support may be helpful in enhancing resilience to stress as well as factors associated with resilience, such as coping self-efficacy.

Learned optimism training

The teaching of optimistic thinking has been operationalized in a 12-week program called Learned Optimism (Seligman, 1991). This program is based largely on Beck and colleagues' cognitive models of treatment for depression (Beck et al., 1979). In Learned Optimism, an individual learns to recognize the connections between adversity, beliefs, and consequences in everyday life. He or she begins by keeping a diary to record examples of daily adversities, even minor ones such as disagreeing with a co-worker. The writing exercise begins by describing what happened as objectively as possible without evaluating the event. Next, thoughts and beliefs about the adverse event are recorded. Finally, the individual describes consequences of the event (i.e., feelings and/or actions) and his or her subsequent beliefs about it.

In an intervention study designed to prevent anxiety and depression, Seligman and colleagues recruited 231 college students who were assessed to be at risk based on their scores in the bottom quartile (i.e., the most pessimistic explanatory style) of the Attributional

Style Questionnaire (Seligman *et al.*, 1999). Half of the students were randomized into a control group, which completed an initial assessment but did not participate in the prevention workshop, while the other half completed the same assessment and then participated in the eight-week prevention workshop. Workshop trainers all had experience working at the Beck Center for Cognitive Therapy. The workshop covered a number of cognitive-behavioral topics, including the cognitive theory of change, identification of automatic negative thoughts and beliefs, empirical hypothesis testing to question and dispute automatic negative thoughts and irrational beliefs, and generation of more constructive interpretations. The workshop also covered behavioral activation techniques such as creative problem solving and assertiveness training, training in interpersonal skills, relaxation training, and the application of these coping skills to a variety of situations. Participants were followed for three years. During the study period, participants who completed the workshop reported fewer symptoms of anxiety and depression than participants in the control group, although there was no difference in frequency of major depressive episodes. The workshop group also experienced significant improvements in measures of hopelessness, dysfunctional attitudes, and cognitive explanatory style. At 6–30 months after entry into the study, participants in the workshop group reported fewer illness-related visits to student health centers, fewer doctor visits, and fewer symptoms of physical illness (Seligman *et al.*, 1999).

The Penn Resiliency Program has tested a similar intervention to prevent depression in a large group of US middle school children (Cutuli *et al.*, 2006). The intervention was based on a failure model where repetitive failures in important domains of life are seen as contributing to later symptoms of depression. Over the course of 12 sessions, children learned cognitive-behavioral techniques to challenge inaccurate negative self-perceptions and learned techniques to regulate emotions and enhance social skills. While the intervention was described as generally beneficial to all participants, it was most effective for young adolescents with elevated levels of conduct problems.

Well-being therapy

Well-being therapy is a short-term structured psychotherapeutic intervention designed to enhance well-being. While it shares many therapeutic features found in cognitive-behavioral therapies for the treatment of mood and anxiety disorders, its primary goal is to engender positive outcomes (i.e., well-being, resilience) rather than to alleviate psychological distress. Well-being therapy is based on Ryff's multidimensional model where well-being is viewed as more than the absence of psychological distress (Ryff, 1989). In this model, well-being incorporates six dimensions: autonomy, personal growth, environmental mastery, purpose in life, positive relations, and self-acceptance (Ryff, 1989; Fava, 1999; Fava & Ruini, 2003).

Well-being therapy has been described as structured, directive, and problem oriented (Fava, 1999; Fava & Ruini, 2003). It is generally conducted over eight sessions of 30–50 minutes that are spaced one to two weeks apart. The initial sessions focus on learning to recognize personal episodes of well-being, identifying the context in which these episodes occur, and rating the intensity of each episode, even if the episode is very brief in duration. Patients record their observations in a structured diary.

In the intermediate phase of treatment, the individual learns to recognize beliefs and thoughts that trigger premature interruption of the episode of well-being. For example, an individual may observe that he is feeling positive about a comment from a friend, but also notices that the positive feeling is short lived because he imagines that the friend feels sorry for him and that the compliment was not genuine but instead an attempt to make him feel better. As in traditional cognitive-behavioral therapies, the individual learns to challenge irrational beliefs and automatic thoughts, but in this case the irrational beliefs are related to episodes of well-being rather than to episodes of distress. The therapist also assigns the individual to engage in pleasurable activities and tasks and to self-monitor these experiences.

In the final phase, the therapist teaches the individual about the six dimensions in Ryff's multidimensional model and provides guidelines for enhancing these dimensions (Ryff, 1989; Fava, 1999; Fava & Ruini, 2003). Individuals learn to take greater control of their environment (environmental control); recognize and acknowledge self-improvement (personal growth); search for a sense of meaning and develop life goals (purpose in life); become more assertive and resistant to social pressures (autonomy); recognize unrealistically high self-standards and develop a more accepting and positive attitude toward self (self-acceptance); and to value and strive for closer, warmer, and more trusting relationships (positive relations with others). Throughout this phase of treatment, correction of irrational and automatic thoughts as well as errors in thinking and alternative interpretations are emphasized.

The formal study of well-being therapy is in the preliminary stage. So far, well-being therapy has been used in a number of small studies for treating the residual phase of affective disorders (Fava *et al.*, 1998a), the prevention of recurrent depression (Fava *et al.*, 1998b) and residual symptoms in remitted patients with panic disorder with agoraphobia (Fava *et al.*, 2001). For example, in a small controlled study of patients who had been treated successfully for affective disorders but who continued to experience residual symptoms, patients were randomized either to cognitive-behavioral treatment or well-being therapy (Fava *et al.*, 1998a). While both treatments resulted in a significant reduction in depression and a significant improvement in well-being, the improvements in the well-being therapy group were significantly greater, particularly in the area of personal growth. Well-being therapy has also been found to increase psychological well-being, decrease distress, and improve long-term outcomes in individuals with generalized anxiety disorder (Fava *et al.*, 2005) and PTSD (Belaise *et al.*, 2005).

Well-being therapy has also been tested in children and adolescents. In a sample of 111 junior high school students, Ruini and colleagues (2006) implemented a four-session version of well-being therapy that included psychoeducation, cognitive-behavioral techniques, and Ryff's model of psychological well-being. Participation in the program was associated with increased well-being and decreased anxiety among the students. In a subsequent intervention adapted for adolescents, 227 high school students were randomized to a well-being intervention or an attention-placebo protocol (Ruini *et al.*, 2009). Both interventions involved six weekly sessions of two hours each conducted in a group format. The well-being therapy included cognitive-behavioral techniques and focused on the six dimensions of Ryff's model. In the well-being therapy group, significant improvement (although a modest effect size) was reported in personal growth and physical well-being, while significant reductions were noted in somatization, anxiety, and physiological anxiety. When taken together, these studies provide encouraging preliminary evidence that it may be possible to enhance psychological well-being and possibly resilience through school-based interventions.

Preparatory interventions

Many organizations whose personnel routinely face potential traumatic stressors have developed preparatory training programs to provide information and teach skills to facilitate optimal performance under conditions of high stress. Examples of these programs include military basic and advanced training, police and firefighter training academies, and first-responder training. While these programs are widely employed and believed to be useful, there is little scientific evidence supporting their effectiveness (Whealin *et al.*, 2008).

Preparatory interventions are designed to provide information and to familiarize and expose personnel to stressful situations that they are likely to encounter in their occupations. These programs are thought to increase familiarity; increase controllability and predictability of internal emotions and physical sensations, and promote the development of greater perceptions of control and self-efficacy (Salas & Cannon-Bowers, 2001; Salas *et al.*, 2006; Whealin *et al.*, 2008).

One of the most common preparatory interventions is scenario-based training. Scenari-based training involves learning through doing, where trainees apply what they have learned in the classroom to realistic and challenging situations (Salas & Cannon-Bowers, 2001; Salas *et al.*, 2006; Whealin *et al.*, 2008). It is theory based and requires careful scripting of scenarios so that trainees must have mastered the information and skills they have been taught if they are to succeed.

Scenario-based training has been shown to be an effective form of learning that can be adapted to a wide variety of settings and learning tasks. These include practice of learned skills, assessment of accurate skill acquisition, and real-time constructive feedback. Salas and colleagues (Salas & Cannon-Bowers, 2001; Salas *et al.*, 2006), who have written extensively on scenario-based training, believe that it is ideal for training in military tasks and for skill acquisition and performance that involves complex team work. Scenario-based training is commonly used with professionals such as police officers and firemen who are involved in highly stressful work. Research has shown that scenario-based training can be used to enhance test flight performance (Gopher *et al.*, 1994), train pediatric critical care clinicians (Nishisaki *et al.*, 2009), and improve skills and operating-room performance among surgeons (Goff, 2010).

Seven interrelated stages have been described in scenario-based training (Cannon-Bowers & Salas, 1998).

Step 1: collect past performance data and conduct a skills inventory to determine what skills trainees have already acquired

Step 2: determine the competencies and tasks that the scenario-based training will be designed to enhance

Step 3: develop training objectives based on competencies and job/task needs; objectives can be based on either the need to accomplish a specific task or the need to develop skills that are transferrable to a variety of settings

Step 4: embed scenarios, which should be carefully crafted with the goal of promoting training objectives and targeting specific desired competencies

Step 5: develop performance measures that assess performance and training effectiveness

Step 6: provide constructive and timely feedback so that the trainee can learn rapidly and correctly, as well as improve performance

Step 7: modify future training programs to eliminate ineffective components while retaining and possibly improving effective components.

Scenario-based training is most effective when partnerships are formed between subject matter experts and experts in the science of learning, and when trainees practice with close supervision, guidance, and immediate feedback.

Case example: landmine survivors

This final section of the chapter presents a more in-depth description of a specific program to foster resilience. The program was developed by Survivor Corps and was primarily targeting survivors of war trauma.

In 1995, Jerry White and Ken Rutherford, who both lost limbs to landmine explosions, founded Landmine Survivors Network, the first international organization created by and for survivors to prevent future mine injuries and offer peer support to victims of the weapon. White and Rutherford are recognized leaders of the International Campaign to Ban Landmines and co-laureates of the 1997 Nobel Prize for Peace. They helped to draft three major international treaties to address the rights of people with disabilities, including victims of particular weapons: the 1997 Landmine Ban Treaty, the 2008 Convention on the Rights of Persons with Disabilities, and the 2009 Cluster Munitions Convention. White and Rutherford have worked in over 20 war-affected countries to train survivor leaders as co-advocates and peer role models. When the Landmine Survivors Network later grew into the Survivors Corp, White and Rutherford stated, "We focus on the unique contributions and leadership of conflict survivors because we believe no one is better positioned to break cycles of violence and victimization than those who have survived war." For over a decade, this survivor network helped victims of war rebuild their lives and communities. The signature peer-support programs connected survivors with survivor role models to offer the encouragement and motivation critical to helping new survivors to find hope, get jobs, and get on with their lives.

The challenge is to transform victims into survivor leaders. Through the support of those around them (peers and family), these traumatized people mentor, teach, coach, and support others on their path to survivorship. White defines "survivorship" simply as, "choosing to live positively and dynamically in the face of death, disaster and disability. Survivorship is a healthy and pragmatic approach to quality living even after traumatic adversity or loss." His philosophy is shared by many types of survivors, from genocide and torture to breast cancer and bereavement, from war and disability to addiction and human betrayal.

White himself survived a landmine explosion and lost his right leg at the age of 20 while studying abroad as an undergraduate in Israel. Ten years after recovery, White began his professional outreach to other war victims. He has since observed, in countries as diverse as Bosnia–Herzegovina, El Salvador, Ethiopia, Jordan, and Vietnam, that it is not uncommon for trauma survivors to get stuck for years in a victim mentality where they tend to pity themselves, resent their circumstances, live in the past, and/or blame others. Even worse, they might become the next victimizers: "This was done to me, now I will do it to the next person." White believes that a victim-minded person is generally inflexible, stuck in his or her grievances, and seemingly unable to let go, find hope, or move forward. Over time, a victim's intense focus on their own personal suffering can interfere with his or her ability to take positive action, relate to others in a healthy manner, or participate more fully in daily life.

After establishing more than a dozen peer-support programs working with thousands of victims of landmines and violence, White believes each survivor has something to teach about resilience. Drawing from personal experience and lessons learned in the field, he recommends five "steps" to help trauma survivors to tap their innate resilience and grow stronger.

1. Face facts: accept what has happened, the suffering and loss
2. Choose life: live for the future, not in the past
3. Reach out: connect to others who have "been there"
4. Get moving: set goals and take action for a healthy recovery
5. Give back: be thankful for what you do have, contribute to your community.

These five steps to overcoming crisis do not necessarily take place in a specific order; not everyone experiences each step; some steps may evolve over the course of years; and sometimes the trauma survivor may tackle more than one step simultaneously. The following material, excerpted interviews and recommendations were adapted from the book by Jerry White, *Getting up when life knocks you down: five steps to overcoming a life crisis* (2008).

The five steps to overcoming a life crisis

Face facts

When something threatens our very being and way of life, we often try to deny or avoid it. We may actively avoid memories of the trauma or forget important aspects of what happened; we may shut down emotionally and numb ourselves; we may detach emotionally from our family, friends, and environment. Rape survivors may shower repeatedly hoping to wash away the violation. War-injured veterans may drink or take drugs to numb painful memories. Individuals permanently paralyzed and in wheelchairs may pray fervently for years to walk again. This is natural. However, the Survivor Corps approach encourages survivors to "face facts" by acknowledging what has happened and then finding a way to live with it.

Talking through a personal trauma is one way to help to integrate the experience. That is why Survivor Corps trained peer outreach workers to listen actively to other trauma survivors who describe, in their own words, their traumas and subsequent attempts to cope. In order to facilitate acceptance and assimilation of the painful facts, it is often necessary to repeat this process of telling the traumatic story in the presence of an active listener, perceived to be empathetic.

This was the case for Zainab Salbi, who grew up in Iraq as the daughter of Saddam Hussein's pilot (Salbi & Buckland, 2005). Her family lived close to the inner circle of power in the shadows of dictatorship. Being close to Saddam was often harrowing and horrifying, and Zainab spent years suppressing the facts of her life. Since childhood, Zainab's mother had always told her to "erase from your memory" anything too scary, like the kidnapping and killing of friends who were also in Saddam's employ. Zainab was a grown woman in her thirties before she started to face these facts, a little at a time. And it was only after Saddam Hussein was captured in 2003, that the "dam finally broke." Zainab experienced a nervous breakdown, telling a female paramedic, "Nothing is wrong. Everything is going right in my life. I just don't know how to stop crying." (Salbi & Buckland, 2005, p. 231). Zainab reflected (p. 5):

> I wanted to make myself whole again. I wanted to come clean. I wanted to do my job without feeling like a hypocrite. But I had been afraid for so long I didn't know how to get rid of the layers of fear inside me. Because I had survived by hiding my past, even from myself, I had never really pieced together the story of my own life. Which of the things that had happened to me were causes, and which were the effects?

Writing about her experiences proved cathartic, "It felt like the heavy, dark stone in my chest finally passed through me; it's gone now," she said, "Taking the time to piece together my personal story and my family's history has given me new energy" to face the future with more optimism and resilience (White, 2008, p. 49).

Choose life

Trauma survivors have the ability to choose life, even though this choice may be enormously difficult, particularly in the immediate aftermath of the trauma. In 1989, Jesús Martinez was 17 and living through civil war in El Salvador. He had a job in the city and had to take a bus to work. Because of roadblocks set up by guerillas, Jesús had to get off his bus, walk around the roadblock, and get on another bus to continue his journey to work. White (2008, p. 61) quotes him as saying:

> I was a teenager, and not aware of the danger of mines. Everyone just got off the buses and walked on the side of the road. I don't know why I was walking where no one else was, but I remember someone saying there might be mines. I didn't think about it much.

Walking along the side of the road, he stepped on a mine that blew off both his legs on the spot. The explosion was so powerful that others walking near him were wounded. He never lost consciousness, but he did lose hope. He went on to say

> I fell in a hole. Both of my legs were blown off. I had blood in my mouth. My arm was wounded, and really, I thought it was all a bad dream. I tried to kill myself with an explosive that was lying on the ground near me. It didn't explode when I picked it up. When the soldiers arrived, I took a gun from one of them and begged him to kill me with it. I remember being so desperate to die, and saying over and over, "Please kill me."

Jesús did not die that day. Instead he chose life (White, 2008, p. 62):

> The healing process was very difficult for me. There was the healing of my body, and also the trauma in my mind. I am thankful that I had the support of my family. It was very important for me to meet other disabled people, and seeing how they lived their lives. Sports had always been a part of my life, and I was very happy when I saw people practicing wheelchair sports in the hospital. It has been a long journey from wanting to die to getting where I am now. I am very happy and excited about many aspects of my life. I have a wife, my children, a family, my parents and siblings, and a very wide circle of friends.

Initially, Jesús could not imagine living his life as a severely physically disabled young man. But somehow he was able to reach deep inside, find the courage and power to reframe his tragic experience, and ultimately chose to embrace his life. For many survivors, this choice is supported by faith, spirituality, religion, hope, and/or an optimistic outlook. The survivor who chooses life understands that he or she is far more than their scars and circumstances.

Reach out

Reaching out to peers, friends, and family is a key to building resilience. Many survivor groups, from cancer to disability to veterans, attest to the power of peer support to build resilience. Mental Health America (2008) concurs that peer support is

> … a unique and essential element of recovery-oriented mental health and substance abuse systems. MHA [Mental Health America] calls on states and communities to incorporate peer-support services into community-based mental health and substance abuse services, both as stand-alone entities and in conjunction with other services. The provision of mental health and substance abuse support services by persons who have experienced

mental and substance abuse conditions make use of empathy and empowerment to help support and inspire recovery.

Cancer peer-support groups have been shown to enhance emotional functioning, quality of life, strategies for coping with illness, and attitudes toward treatment (Glajchen & Magen, 1995). Peer support has been used effectively for large numbers of people struggling with a host of health issues and disabling conditions, including physical and sexual abuse, substance abuse, breast cancer, chronic medical illnesses, and landmine injuries.

Given the fundamental importance of social support, particularly in communities fragmented by war, Survivor Corps spent most of its programmatic energy and resources building networks of peer supporters as a way for survivors to reconnect. By 2002, Survivor Corps had pioneered peer-to-peer-support networks in Bosnia–Herzegovina, Jordan, El Salvador, Ethiopia, Mozambique, and Vietnam. More recently, it has trained partner survivor groups in Colombia, Rwanda, Burundi, and the USA.

Get moving

Climbing out of horrific crises often requires Herculean effort, physically and emotionally. To assist the survivor in their efforts to move forward, the Survivor Corps approach required that each survivor developed his or her own *individual action plan*. The survivor must identify his or her life priorities (objectives) in the areas of health, livelihood, and community, and then, with the help of a peer-support worker, develop a realistic plan with concrete steps to reach each objective.

Creating an individual action plan, believing that the objectives can be achieved, and successfully completing concrete steps tends to engender hope and build self-confidence. By measuring these objectives and the completion of specific steps, peer-support workers can more effectively evaluate progress and, when needed, re-evaluate and change objectives. Developing and working on the individual action plan calls for specificity of objectives, identification of activities, and measurable outputs relevant to the survivor's life goals – all achievable within a reasonable period of time. The individual action plan is a contract of sorts that is used as a guide to track each survivor's progress. Understandably, livelihood or work objectives tend to become the strongest focus for survivors with disabilities living in poverty. Survivors know well how work affects their self-esteem, standing in the community, structure for the day, social companionship, and sense of purpose.

Give back

Gratitude (thanking people who have helped) and generosity (giving more than taking) both promote resilience. The acts of thanking and giving indicate the survivor has begun to emerge from the depths of their trauma. Survivor Corps hired survivors who have struggled with their disabilities but found positive ways to cope, and then trained these survivors to visit and listen to newer victims. By serving as an inspiration and motivating force for other survivors, veteran survivors help to accompany newer survivors out from the darkness of their isolation. Veteran survivors benefit as well when they see how far they have come and rediscover their own strength. Survivor Corps observed that the survivor who learns to focus energy on more than their own survival is more likely to thrive. That is why community service has been incorporated as a principle mode of recovery.

Community service refers to service that an individual survivor or group of survivors provides for the benefit of his or her community. The objective is to provide meaningful and productive opportunities for survivors to contribute to other members of the community. By moving from *beneficiary* to *benefactor*, the survivor no longer feels like a social burden but, instead, a contributing member of the community. Making a difference in the lives of other survivors and community members tends to evoke a sense of satisfaction, pride, and personal growth. By performing community service, a survivor can change the community's perception of survivors and motivate other survivors and community members to become active in worthwhile community projects. It is expected that the survivor will decide on a service project within the first 18 months of working on their individual action plan and complete their service project before graduating from their peer-supported program. While some survivors are ready to participate in a community service project early in their recovery process, many need more time to heal and recover first and, therefore, do not participate until later in the process.

Giving is a particularly healing practice for individuals who have survived war and witnessed the fragmentation and destruction of their communities. The act of giving is a sign of resilience.

In 1994, Ramiz stepped on a landmine in Bosnia–Herzegovina. White (2008, p. 124) tells his story. He lost his right leg. He wondered how he would feed his wife and six-month-old son. His young family had no home. So Ramiz moved in with his parents, but he avoided his family, drank heavily, and fell into a deep depression. Then Ramiz met Adnan, another amputee and peer outreach worker. Adnan listened for hours to Ramiz and gently encouraged him to get back to his life, his responsibilities. Ramiz told Adnan he felt overwhelmed with the responsibility of taking care of his family. But Adnan persisted, showing up weekly in support of his fellow amputee survivor.

It took over a year, but finally peer-to-peer support began to pay off. Ramiz joined a survivor economic support group and attended meetings for six months. Armed with a business plan and new confidence, Ramiz built a greenhouse and a thriving tomato business. He became known in the community as honest and hardworking, and people lined up to buy his produce. White (2008, p. 124) quotes him as saying:

> I feel like I have eliminated that horrible feeling of uncertainty and insecurity. If it weren't for this opportunity, I would still be wasting my days drinking and my future would be uncertain. Thanks to the support from my community, my family has a strong husband and father again, and with my new business, our future is no longer uncertain.

But Ramiz took his growth even a step further. He planned to build a second greenhouse and hire other survivors. He also gave out produce to his neighbors in need: "The day I first donated 200 kilograms of fresh tomatoes to the local orphanage was an incredible moment for me. After so many years, I could now help others in need. I was no longer the beneficiary, but the benefactor" (White, 2008, p. 125).

The challenge of monitoring and evaluation

Increasingly, civil society organizations use a version of peer support in efforts to promote resilience. However, very few organizations define or operationalize "peer support" and very few measure its efficacy, which has limited the impact of these peer-support interventions within the clinical and scientific community.

In partnership with the Centers for Disease Control and Prevention, Survivor Corps set out to measure the efficacy of its program using the Medical Outcomes Study 36-Item Short Form Health Survey (SF-36; http://www.sf-36.org/tools/sf36.shtml), a commonly used and well-validated instrument that measures self-perceived health-related quality of life. The SF-36 has been has been translated into numerous languages and used to assess self-perceived health in many countries across a wide cross-spectrum of socioeconomic contexts. Survivors entering Survivor Corps programs were administered the SF-36 at the beginning of the program and again when they "graduated" or discontinued from the program, up to two years after entry. Preliminary data analysis with 280 survivors suggests that the Survivor Corps approach has significant positive effects on subjective assessments of physical and mental well-being.

Conclusions

This chapter has described a broad range of interventions that have been designed to enhance resilience or constructs associated with resilience, such as social support. These interventions are delivered in various formats (e.g., in a classroom setting, over the Internet, or as part of a therapy modality), are commonly psychoeducational and cognitive-behavioral in nature, and have been applied in a diverse range of populations. Although some of these interventions have received preliminary empirical support (e.g., psychoeducational resilience enhancement training, well-being therapy), the majority have received little or no such support.

While the interventions described have been designed to foster resilience in individuals, interventions to enhance resilience can be targeted toward families, organizations, and communities. For example, the Walsh family resilience framework (Chapter 10) focuses on fostering family strengths in response to stressful life events, adversity, and life transitions. It does so in three domains of family life: organizational processes, family belief systems, and communication processes. Walsh and colleagues stress the variety and complexity of families and the ways in which they function, and believe that no single strategy for enhancing resilience applies to all families.

Just as resilience differs from one individual to another and from one family to another, communities differ in their capacity to respond and adapt to adversity. Norris and colleagues (Chapter 11) have proposed that community resilience can be bolstered by developing economic resources and using these resources to assist areas of greatest social vulnerability by coordinating relevant organizational networks (e.g., fire, police, mental health, rescue and recovery) prior to adverse events, by supporting naturally occurring social supports, by involving local citizens in community preparedness and responses to adversity, and by preparing for the unexpected.

Interventions designed to enhance resilience can be targeted at preventing risk factors; bolstering resources; developing skills; supporting cultural, religious, and spiritual rituals; promoting organizations that focus on developing competence (i.e., schools, fire and police departments, disaster response organizations, and the military); limiting stressful/traumatic exposure; and providing rapid evidence-based treatment for traumatized individuals. Interventions to enhance resilience can be directed to the individual, the family, and/or the community and may involve the bolstering of internal and external resources. As noted by Masten and others (Chapter 7), interventions can be initiated at one or more levels within a multi-level model. Finally, interventions to enhance resilience should take into account other critical variables such as age, physical and mental health, and cultural dynamics and norms, as well as personal beliefs and values. For example, specific cultural and spiritual practices may enhance resilience in one group of individuals but not in another.

The second part of this chapter presented a more in-depth description of a program developed by an international organization, Survivor Corps, to foster resilience in war-traumatized individuals. Survivor Corps built a global network of survivors and partners, helping thousands of victims of war to heal and rebuild their communities. Peer support formed the core delivery vehicle in the program to foster and strengthen coping mechanisms that are known to be associated with resilience. Survivors themselves recommend building resilience through five steps, which include facing the facts, choosing life, reaching out to connect with others, getting moving (e.g., setting goals and taking action), and giving back.

In conclusion, research on resilience-enhancing interventions is in its infancy, but growing rapidly. More research is needed to refine measurement of resilience and related constructs, to examine factors that mediate the development of resilience in intervention studies, and to carefully consider outcome variables (e.g., reductions in psychopathology, functioning, coping, self-efficacy) that are sensitive to change. Most importantly, controlled trials are needed to examine the efficacy of resilience-enhancing interventions in a broad range of populations.

References

Allred, K. D. & Smith, T. W. (1989). The hardy personality: cognitive and physiological responses to evaluative threat. *Journal of Personality and Social Psychology*, **56**, 257–266.

American Psychological Association (2010). *The road to resilience*. Washington, DC: American Psychological Association, http://www.apa.org/helpcenter/road-resilience.aspx (accessed June 25, 2010).

Barrera, M. Jr. (1986). Distinctions between social support concepts, measures, and models. *American Journal of Community Psychology*, **14**, 413–445.

Bartone, P. T. (1993). Psychosocial predictors of soldier adjustment to combat stress. In *Proceedings of the Third European Conference on Traumatic Stress,* Bergen, Norway, June.

Bartone, P. T. (1995). A short hardiness scale. In *Proceedings of the 103rd Annual Convention of the American Psychological Association,* New York, July.

Bartone, P. T. (2006). Resilience under military operational stress: Can leaders influence hardiness? *Military Psychology*, **18**(Suppl.), S131–S148.

Bartone, P. T. (2007). Test-retest reliability of the dispositional resilience scale-15, a brief hardiness scale. *Psychological Reports*, **101**, 943–944.

Bartone, P. T., Ursano, R. J., Wright, K. M., & Ingraham, L. H. (1989). The impact of a military air disaster on the health of assistance workers. A prospective study. *Journal of Nervous and Mental Disease*, **177**, 317–328.

Beck, A. T., Rush, A. J., Shaw, B. F., & Emery, G. (1979). *Cognitive therapy of depression*. New York: Guilford Press.

Belaise, C., Fava, G. A., & Marks, I. M. (2005). Alternatives to debriefing and modifications to cognitive behavior therapy for posttraumatic stress disorder. *Psychotherapy and Psychosomatics*, **74**, 212–217.

Bonanno, G. A., Galea, S., Bucciarelli, A., & Vlahov, D. (2006). Psychological resilience after disaster: New York City in the aftermath of the September 11th terrorist attack. *Psychological Science*, **17**, 181–186.

Bond, J., Kaskutas, L. A., & Weisner, C. (2003). The persistent influence of social networks and alcoholics anonymous on abstinence. *Journal of Studies on Alcohol*, **64**, 579–588.

Brand, E. F., Lakey, B., & Berman, S. (1995). A preventive, psychoeducational approach to increase perceived social support. *American Journal of Community Psychology*, **23**, 117–135.

Brewin, C. R., Andrews, B., & Valentine, J. D. (2000). Meta-analysis of risk factors for posttraumatic stress disorder in trauma-exposed adults. *Journal of Consulting and Clinical Psychology*, **68**, 748–766.

Brown, S. L., Nesse, R. M., Vinokur, A. D., & Smith, D. M. (2003). Providing social support may be more beneficial than receiving it: results from a prospective study of mortality. *Psychological Science*, **14**, 320–327.

Campbell-Sills, L. & Stein, M. B. (2007). Psychometric analysis and refinement of the Connor–Davidson Resilience Scale (CD-RISC): Validation of a 10-item measure of resilience. *Journal of Trauma and Stress*, **20**, 1019–1028.

Cannon-Bowers, J. A. & Salas, E. (eds.) (1998). *Making decisions under stress: Implications for individual and team training*. Washington, DC: American Psychological Association.

Charney, D. S. (2004). Psychobiological mechanisms of resilience and vulnerability: implications for successful adaptation to extreme stress. *American Journal of Psychiatry*, **161**, 195–216.

Charuvastra, A. & Cloitre, M. (2008). Social bonds and posttraumatic stress disorder. *Annual Review of Psychology*, **59**, 301–328.

Connor, K. M. & Davidson, J. R. (2003). Development of a new resilience scale: the Connor–Davidson Resilience Scale (CD-RISC). *Depression and Anxiety*, **18**, 76–82.

Contrada, R. J. (1989). Type A behavior, personality hardiness, and cardiovascular responses to stress. *Journal of Personality and Social Psychology*, **57**, 895–903.

Cutuli, J. J., Chaplin, T. M., Gillham, J. E., Reivich, K. J., & Seligman, M. E. (2006). Preventing co-occurring depression symptoms in adolescents with conduct problems: the Penn Resiliency Program. *Annals of the New York Academy of Sciences*, **1094**, 282–286.

Davidson, L., Payne, V. M., Connor, K. M., *et al.* (2005). Trauma, resilience and saliostasis: effects of treatment in post-traumatic stress disorder. *International Clinical Psychopharmacology*, **20**, 43–48.

Davidson, L., Baldwin, D. S., Stein, D. J., *et al.* (2008). Effects of venlafaxine extended release on resilience in posttraumatic stress disorder: an item analysis of the Connor–Davidson Resilience Scale. *International Clinical Psychopharmacology*, **23**, 299–303.

Defense Centers of Excellence (2009). *Defense Centers of Excellence for Psychological Health and Traumatic Brain Injury: Annual Report 2009*. Silver Springs MD: Defense Centers of Excellence.

Eid, J. & Morgan, C. A. 3rd (2006). Dissociation, hardiness, and performance in military cadets participating in survival training. *Military Medicine*, **171**, 436–442.

Fava, G. A. (1999). Well-being therapy: conceptual and technical issues. *Psychotherapy and Psychosomatics*, **68**, 171–179.

Fava, G. A. & Ruini, C. (2003). Development and characteristics of a well-being enhancing psychotherapeutic strategy: well-being therapy. *Journal of Behavioral Therapy and Expimental Psychiatry*, **34**, 45–63.

Fava, G. A., Rafanelli, C., Cazzaro, M., Conti, S., & Grandi, S. (1998a). Well-being therapy. A novel psychotherapeutic approach for residual symptoms of affective disorders. *Psychological Medicine*, **28**, 475–480.

Fava, G. A., Rafanelli, C., Grandi, S., Conti, S., & Belluardo, P. (1998b). Prevention of recurrent depression with cognitive behavioral therapy: preliminary findings. *Archives of General Psychiatry*, **55**, 816–820.

Fava, G. A., Rafanelli, C., Ottolini, F., *et al.* (2001). Psychological well-being and residual symptoms in remitted patients with panic disorder and agoraphobia. *Journal of Affective Disorders*, **65**, 185–190.

Fava, G. A., Ruini, C., Rafanelli, C., *et al.* (2005). Well-being therapy of generalized anxiety disorder. *Psychotherapy and Psychosomatics*, **74**, 26–30.

Florian, V., Mikulincer, M., & Taubman, O. (1995). Does hardiness contribute to mental health during a stressful real-life situation? The roles of appraisal and coping. *Journal of Personality and Social Psychology*, **68**, 687–695.

Foa, E. B., Rothbaum, B. O., Riggs, D. S., & Murdock, T. B. (1991). Treatment of posttraumatic stress disorder in rape victims: A comparison between cognitive-behavioral procedures and counseling. *Journal of Consulting and Clinical Psychology*, **59**, 715–723.

Foa, E. B., Dancu, C. V., Hembree, E. A., *et al.* (1999). A comparison of exposure therapy, stress inoculation training, and their combination for reducing posttraumatic stress disorder in female assault victims. *Journal of Consulting and Clinical Psychology*, **67**, 194–200.

Garmezy, N. (1974). Children at risk: the search for the antecedents of schizophrenia. Part II: Ongoing research programs, issues, and intervention. *Schizophrenia Bulletin*, **1**, 55–125.

Garmezy, N. & Streitman, S. (1974). Children at risk: the search for the antecedents of schizophrenia. Part I. Conceptual models and research methods. *Schizophrenia Bulletin*, **1**, 14–90.

Glajchen, M. & Magen, R. (1995). Evaluating process, outcome, and satisfaction in community-based cancer support groups. In M. J. Galinsky & J. H. Schopler (eds.), *Support groups: Current perspectives on theory and practice* (pp. 27–40). New York: Haworth Press.

Goff, B. A. (2010). Training and assessment in gynaecologic surgery: the role of simulation. *Best Practice in Research and Clinical Obstetrics and Gynaecology*, **24**, 759–756.

Gopher, D., Weil, M., & Bareket, T. (1994). Transfer of skill from a computer game trainer to flight. *Human Factors*, **36**, 387–405.

Haglund, M. E., Nestadt, P. S., Cooper, N. S., Southwick, S. M., & Charney, D. S. (2007). Psychobiological mechanisms of resilience: Relevance to prevention and treatment of stress-related psychopathology. *Development and Psychopathology*, **19**, 889–920.

Hogan, B. E., Linden, W., & Najarian, B. (2002). Social support interventions: Do they work? *Clinical Psychological Reviews*, **22**, 383–442.

Johnson, D. C., Polusny, M. A., Erbes, C. R., *et al.* (2011). Development and initial validation of the Response to Stressful Experiences Scale (RSES). *Military Medicine*, **176**, 161–169.

Kaniasty, K. & Norris, F. H. (2008). Longitudinal linkages between perceived social support and posttraumatic stress symptoms: sequential roles of social causation and social selection. *Journal of Traumatic Stress*, **21**, 274–281.

Kaskutas, L. A., Bond, J., & Humphreys, K. (2002). Social networks as mediators of the effect of Alcoholics Anonymous. *Addiction*, **97**, 891–900.

Kaskutas, L. A., Bond, J., & Avalos, L. A. (2009). 7-year trajectories of Alcoholics Anonymous attendance and associations with treatment. *Addictive Behavior*, **34**, 1029–1035.

Khoshaba, D. M. & Maddi, S. R. (2001). *HardiTraining.* Newport Beach, CA: Hardines Institute.

Kilpatrick, D. G., Veronen, L. J., & Resick, P. A. (1982). Psychological sequelae to rape: Assessment and treatment strategies. In D. M. Dolays & R. L. Meredith (eds.), *Behavioral medicine: Assessment and treatment strategies* (pp. 473–497). New York: Plenum Press.

King, L. A., King, D. W., Fairbank, J. A., Keane, T. M., & Adams, G. A. (1998). Resilience-recovery factors in post-traumatic stress disorder among female and male Vietnam veterans: hardiness, postwar social support, and additional stressful life events. *Journal of Personality and Social Psychology*, **74**, 420–434.

Kobasa, S. C. (1979). Stressful life events, personality, and health an inquiry into hardiness. *Journal of Personality and Social Psychology*, **37**, 1–11.

Kobasa, S. C. & Puccetti, M. C. (1983). Personality and social resources in stress resistance. *Journal of Personality and Social Psychology*, **45**, 839–850.

Kobasa, S. C., Maddi, S. R., & Courington, S. (1981). Personality and constitution as mediators in the stress-illness relationship. *Journal of Health and Social Behavior*, **22**, 368–378.

Kobasa, S. C., Maddi, S. R., & Kahn, S. (1982). Hardiness and health: a prospective study. *Journal of Personality and Social Psychology*, **42**, 168–177.

Kobasa, S. C., Maddi, S. R., Puccetti, M. C., & Zola, M. A. (1985). Effectiveness of hardiness, exercise and social support as resources against illness. *Journal of Psychosomatic Research*, **29**, 525–533.

Lazarus, R. & Folkman, S. (1984). *Stress, appraisal, and coping*. New York: Springer.

Lett, H. S., Blumenthal, J. A., Babyak, M. A., *et al.* (2007). Social support and prognosis in patients at increased psychosocial risk recovering from myocardial infarction. *Health Psychology*, **26**, 418–427.

Lett, H. S., Blumenthal, J. A., Babyak, M. A., *et al.* (2009). Dimensions of social support and depression in patients at increased psychosocial risk recovering from myocardial infarction. *International Journal of Behavioral Medicine*, **16**, 248–258.

Litt, M. D., Kadden, R. M., Kabela-Cormier, E., & Petry, N. (2007). Changing network support for drinking: initial findings from the network support project. *Journal of Consulting and Clinical Psychology*, **75**, 542–555.

Luthar, S. S., Cicchetti, D., & Becker, B. (2000). The construct of resilience: a critical evaluation and guidelines for future work. *Child Development*, **71**, 543–562.

Maddi, S. R. (2002). The story of hardiness: Twenty years of theorizing, research, and practice. *Consulting Psychology Journal: Practice and Research*, **54**, 173–185.

Maddi, S. R. (2005). On hardiness and other pathways to resilience. *American Psychology*, **60**, 261–262; discussion 265–267.

Maddi, S. R. (2007). Relevance of hardiness assessment and training to the military context. *Military Psychology*, **19**, 61–70.

Maddi, S. R. (2008). The courage and strategies of hardiness as helpful in growing despite major, disruptive stresses. *American Psychologist*, **63**, 563–564.

Maddi, S. R. & Khoshaba, D. M. (2005). *Resilience at work* New York: AMACOM.

Maddi, S. R. & Kobasa, S. C. (1984). *The hardy executive: Health under stress*. Homewood, IL: Dow Jones-Irwin.

Maddi, S. R., Khoshaba, D. M., Jensen, K., *et al.* (2002). Hardiness training for high-risk undergraduates. *NACADA Journal*, **22**, 45–55.

Maddi, S. R., Harvey, R. H., Khoshaba, D. M., *et al.* (2006). The personality construct of hardiness, III: Relationships with repression, innovativeness, authoritarianism, and performance. *Journal of Personality*, **74**, 575–597.

Masten, A. S. (2001). Ordinary magic. Resilience processes in development. *American Psychologist*, **56**, 227–238.

McCalister, K. T., Dolbier, C. L., Webster, J. A., Mallon, M. W., & Steinhardt, M. A. (2006). Hardiness and support at work as predictors of work stress and job satisfaction. *American Journal of Health Promotion*, **20**, 183–191.

Meichenbaum, D. (1975). A self-instructional approach to stress management: A proposal for stress inoculation training. In C. Spielberger & I. Sarason (eds.), *Stress and anxiety*, Vol. 2 (pp. 237–264). New York: Wiley.

Meichenbaum, D. (1985). *Psychology practitioner guidebooks: Stress inoculation training*. New York: Pergamon Press.

Meichenbaum, D. & Jaremko, M. E. (eds.) (1983). *Stress reduction and prevention*. New York: Plenum Press.

Meichenbaum, D. H. & Deffenbacher, J. L. (1988). Stress inoculation training. *Counseling Psychologist*, **16**, 69–90.

Mental Health America (2008). *Position Statement 37: The role of peer support services in the creation of recovery-oriented mental health systems*. Alexandria, VA: Mental Health America (accessed February 28, 2011). http://www.nmha.org/go/position-statements/37 (accessed February 28, 2011).

Moak, Z. B. & Agrawal, A. (2010). The association between perceived interpersonal social support and physical and mental health: results from the national epidemiological survey on alcohol and related conditions. *Journal of Public Health*, **32**, 191–201.

Nishisaki, A., Hales, R., Biagas, K., *et al.* (2009). A multi-institutional high-fidelity simulation "boot camp" orientation and training program for first year pediatric critical care fellows. *Pediatric Critical Care Medicine*, **10**, 157–162.

Ozer, E. J., Best, S. R., Lipsey, T. L., & Weiss, D. S. (2008). Predictors of posttraumatic stress disorder and symptoms in adults: A meta-analysis. *Psychological Trauma: Theory, Research, Practice, and Policy*, **1**(Suppl. 1), 3–36.

Pietrzak, R. H., Johnson, D. C., Goldstein, M. B., *et al.* (2010). Psychosocial buffers of traumatic stress, depressive symptoms, and psychosocial difficulties in veterans of Operations Enduring Freedom and Iraqi Freedom: the role of resilience, unit support, and postdeployment social support. *Journal of Affective Disorders*, **120**, 188–192.

Prince-Embury, S. (2008). The Resiliency Scales for Children and Adolescents: Psychological symptoms, and clinical status in adolescents. *Canadian Journal of School Psychology*, **23**, 41–56.

Ruini, C., Belaise, C., Brombin, C., Caffo, E., & Fava, G. A. (2006). Well-being therapy in school settings: a pilot study. *Psychotherapy and Psychosomatics*, **75**, 331–336.

Ruini, C., Ottolini, F., Tomba, E., *et al.* (2009). School intervention for promoting psychological well-being in adolescence. *Journal of Behavioral Therapy and Experimental Psychiatry*, **40**, 522–532.

Ryff, C. D. (1989). Happiness is everything, or is it? Explorations on the meaning of psychological well-being. *Journal of Personality and Social Psychology*, **57**, 1069–1081.

Salas, E. & Cannon-Bowers, J. A. (2001). The science of training: a decade of progress. *Annual Reviews in Psychology*, **52**, 471–499.

Salas, E., Priest, H. A., Wilson, K. A., & Burke, C. S. (2006). Scenario-based training: Improving military mission performance and adaptability. In A. B. Adler, C. A. Castro, & T. W. Britt (eds.), *Military life: The psychology of serving in peace and combat,* Vol. 2: *Operational stress.* Westport: Praeger Security International.

Salbi, Z. & Buckland, L. (2005). *Between two worlds – Escape from tyranny: Growing up in the shadow of Saddam.* New York: Penguin.

Seligman, M. E. P. (1991). *Learned optimism.* New York: Pocket Books.

Seligman, M. E. P., Schulman, P., DeRubeis, R. J., & Hollon, S. D. (1999). The prevention of depression and anxiety. *Prevention and Treatment*, **2**, 8.

Southwick, S. M., Vythilingam, M., & Charney, D. S. (2005). The psychobiology of depression and resilience to stress: Implications for prevention and treatment. *Annual Reviews of Clinical Psychology*, **1**, 255–291.

Steinhardt, M. A. & Dolbier, C. (2008). Evaluation of a resilience intervention to enhance coping strategies and protective factors and decrease symptomatology. *Journal of the American College of Health*, **56**, 445–453.

Steinhardt, M. A., Dolbier, C. L., Gottlieb, N. H., & McCalister, K. T. (2003). The relationship between hardiness, supervisor support, group cohesion, and job stress as predictors of job satisfaction. *American Journal of Health Promotion*, **17**, 382–389.

Vaishnavi, S., Connor, K., & Davidson, J. R. (2007). An abbreviated version of the Connor–Davidson Resilience Scale (CD-RISC), the CD-RISC2: psychometric properties and applications in psychopharmacological trials. *Psychiatry Research*, **152**, 293–297.

Westphal, M., Bonanno, G. A., & Bartone, P. T. (2008). Resilience and personality. In B. J. Lukey & V. Tepe (eds.), *Biobehavioral resilience to stress* (pp. 219–244). Boca Raton, FL: CRC Press.

Whealin, J. M., Ruzek, J. I., & Southwick, S. (2008). Cognitive-behavioral theory and preparation for professionals at risk for trauma exposure. *Trauma, Violence, and Abuse*, **9**, 100–113.

White, J. (2008). *Getting up when life knocks you down: Five steps to overcoming a life crisis.* New York: St. Martin's Press.

Writing Committee for the ENRICHD Investigators (2003). Effects of treating depression and low perceived social support on clinical events after myocardial infarction: the Enhancing Recovery in Coronary Heart Disease Patients (ENRICHD) Randomized Trial. *Journal of the American Medical Association*, **289**, 3106–3116.

Chapter

21

Childhood resilience: adaptation, mastery, and attachment

Angie Torres, Steven M. Southwick, and Linda C. Mayes

Introduction

Exposure to adversity, challenge, and day to day stress is an inevitable aspect of nearly every child's development. For some children, these challenges are acute, uncontrollable, and immediately overwhelming. Others are exposed on a daily basis to chronic stressors such as poverty, parental psychopathology, and environmental chaos. Still others experience the stress of moving to a new school or a new home and grow adaptively from the experience. The ability to cope with, even grow in response to, novel or threatening situations is essential to healthy development and to survival.

The capacity to respond to and manage novelty and potential threat is based in brain circuits whose development is influenced by multiple experiences beginning in the first years of life. Experiences or environmental conditions that activate these circuits are considered stressors and, under optimal or usual conditions, the body's response to such stressors promotes learning so that the child has developed a set of adaptive responses for subsequent exposures.

At the same time, findings from a growing body of research suggest that exceptionally stressful experiences early in life may have long-term consequences for a child's cognitive, social, and emotional health, and long-term consequences for both physical and mental health (Gunnar & Vazquez, 2006). So-called "toxic stress" (Loman & Gunnar, 2010) may lead to a detrimental impact on developing brain architecture and on the physiological regulatory systems that help children to respond to and learn from challenge and adversity. What makes a situation detrimental or toxic relates to whether the stressful experience is controllable, how often and how long the stress-response system has been activated (e.g., chronic stress), and whether or not the child has a dependable, stable set of relationships that is

able to provide support and protection, and buffer the impact of the experience.

How challenging circumstances promote adaptation or are sufficiently toxic to lead to enduring changes in the neural circuitry of stress-response systems is a critical question for studies of childhood resilience. This chapter focuses on how the relationships in a child's life serve to moderate and buffer the potentially detrimental impact of stress and adversity, as well as how these relationships may promote the development of skills needed to master subsequent stress and adversity. There is an explicit decision not to frame the discussion in terms of children who are more or less resilient but rather in terms of those environmental conditions and experiences that potentially enhance every child's ability to respond adaptively to and learn from stress (Luthar & Cicchetti, 2000). The environment is defined as primarily the child's parenting and home caregiving environment but also, particularly as children mature, their caregiving environments outside of the home, including schools and communities, which may also be positively supportive. Accumulating data suggest that environmental/caregiving conditions are critical for establishing "set-points" for stress-system activation and also for the ability of the system – and the body – to return to baseline after a stressful condition has resolved or the child is no longer in the situation.

The later part of the chapter reviews those prevention and intervention programs that, while not expressly focused on "promoting resilience," have positive effects on children's stress-regulatory abilities through their impact on children's caregiving environment, their ability to develop social supports and networks, their ability to adaptively seek out and use social relationships, and their ability to master challenges and develop a strong sense of self-efficacy. The discussion is

Resilience and Mental Health: Challenges Across the Lifespan, ed. Steven M. Southwick, Brett T. Litz, Dennis Charney, and Matthew J. Friedman. Published by Cambridge University Press. © Cambridge University Press 2011.

framed particularly on the concept of allostasis and of allostatic load (McEwen, 2000).

Allostasis refers to the ability to maintain stability throughout change or to maintain homeostasis. Adaptation in response to stressful situations involves activation of neural, endocrine, and immune mechanisms that permit the body to respond to the challenge and then to return to a homeostatic baseline. Allostatic load refers to the physiological impact of chronic activation of neural, endocrine, and immune systems in response to chronic stress. The higher the allostatic load, or the longer the activation of the body's stress response, the greater the damage to the body in the long run. The main hormonal mediators of the stress response, cortisol and epinephrine, have both protective and damaging effects. In the acute situation, both are essential for adaptive response and maintaining homeostasis in the face of challenge. However, if activated frequently and for long periods of time (i.e., an increase in allostatic load), the same system that under a lower allostatic load is protective becomes damaging and can accelerate a number of disease processes, including cardiovascular disease, diabetes, depression, and anxiety.

Systems for maintaining homeostasis develop in early childhood and are particularly sensitive to the allostatic load placed on the child at any given time in early development. That is, a greater allostatic load earlier in childhood may permanently alter the responsiveness of stress-regulatory systems throughout life. Hence, those experiences (e.g., caregiving relationships) and conditions that moderate a child's allostatic load are critical to the long-term development of adaptive homeostasis. Converging research findings from many sources suggest that early care and attachment relationships are the major developmental contributors to moderating the allostatic load in a child's life (Loman & Gunnar, 2010). In turn, when allostatic load is appropriately moderated, children develop a strong sense of self-efficacy and mastery, which helps to moderate future adversity.

Attachments as stress regulating

Healthy development depends on the quality and stability of a child's relationships with the caring adults in his or her life, including parents, other family caregivers, and adults outside the family. Such relationships lay the foundation for a range of developmental outcomes and skills that significantly impact children's lives and adaptation to the world around them. These include a motivation to learn; the ability to regulate emotions, including aggressive impulses; the capacity to soothe the self; the ability to solve problems under stress; knowing the difference between right and wrong; having the capacity to form and sustain friendships and intimate relationships; and, ultimately, to care for a child as a parent. Each of these capacities, in turn, promotes positive, healthy adaptation to challenge and adversity.

In the earliest interactions with parents, there is an essential reciprocity of exchanges – what some have called "serve and return" (Shonkoff & Phillips, 2000) – in which infants and young children naturally make bids for interactions through their babbling, facial expressions, and gestures. Adults respond often with the same kind of vocalizations, gestures, or expressions – sometimes even more marked for emphasis. The consistency, reliability, and affective tone of these types of early exchange are fundamental to creating relationships in which the infant's social communication abilities are nurtured and their exploration and learning about the world around them is supported. Accumulating evidence also underscores the importance of these early interactions for the development of the brain, particularly in enhancing neural networks and in supporting learning (summarized by Shonkoff & Phillips, 2000). Perhaps most salient in the effects of early relationships appears to be the long-term impact on stress reactivity and allostatic capacities in the face of challenge. Chronic adversity in young children's lives is related to greater permeability and reactivity to stress in later childhood and adolescence (Nachmias et al., 1996; Loman & Gunnar, 2010), whereas secure, consistent caregiving is related to more flexible allostatic or stress-response capacities, which, in turn, may facilitate children in growing from stress and challenge.

Attachment perspectives offer models for conceptualizing how relationships or "internalized working models" can be stress buffering and can enhance positive adaptation (Southwick et al., 2008). Attachment perspectives are essentially models of stress and emotion regulation (Cassidy & Shaver, 1999) and of how children (and adults) use important persons in their lives to downregulate negative affective states and upregulate positive or rewarding states. In this way, attachment perspectives are readily integrated into neurobiological models of the balance between stress regulation and reward systems that are relevant to processes with negative outcomes, such as drug use and addiction (Brady & Sinha, 2005), and positive outcomes, such as enhanced mastery and self-efficacy. There are a number of key features of an attachment perspective relevant to allostasis and stress reactivity: how early caregiving does or does not enhance secure and trusting attachments in infants, how these early experiences of being cared for shape templates of what one might expect generally from relationships with others, and how relationships with others do and do not provide expected safety and security. In the language of attachment theory, these early templates are thought of as "internalized working models"; in social cognitive theory, they are considered as social schemas or models for social interactions.

Secure models of attachment emerge from early relationships that are appropriately contingent to a child's needs and buffer the child from overwhelming stress but at the same time give the child sufficient challenge and opportunities to solve problems and regulate his or her own feelings; this allows the child to begin to develop a sense of autonomy and individuality as well as agency and mastery. Importantly, too-perfect contingency or too much protection is just as distorting of relationship schemas as too little or neglectful care with frequent exposure to overwhelming stress and chaos. From these early experiences and developing templates, children begin to develop a perspective on the world of relationships and other persons as trustworthy, responsive, caring, and helpful, or as frightening, unsafe, uncaring, and not reliable under challenge or extreme stress.

Indeed, these templates of social relationships come into play for the child or the adult particularly in times of stress. That is, at times of distress and fright, children and adults call on their individual schemas of how important caregivers have responded in the past. If a child's internalized map is secure, he or she is able to use real people in the external world for comfort and for companionship during stress – and is also able to learn from others around in these challenging circumstances. If that template is insecure or disorganized, the individual child or adult is left more isolated, more anxious in the face of challenge, and hence with increased allostatic load and dysfunctional allostasis mechanisms; these, in turn, perpetuated and activated again at the next stressful time. These circumstances also interfere with a child's ability to develop a sense of mastery of the specific challenge and an individual sense of efficacy for their capacity to respond adaptively in the future. In this point of view, positive adaptation to challenge is based largely on the security of one's internalized working models or social schema of relationships.

This notion also ties into the idea of "good enough parenting," where caregivers provide sufficient protection, emotional buffering, and responsiveness, which change with the developmental needs of the child, but at the same time provide the child with sufficient exposure to the challenges and stressors that promote growth and mastery. As children mature, their capacity to tolerate negative affective experiences and meet both challenge and acutely stressful situations changes. The source of that change is not only maturation but also how parents buffer the environment just enough that the child is not overwhelmed but at the same time has the experience of mastery which, in turn, contributes to a sense of individuality, efficacy, coping, and optimism.

Related capacities shaped by early care and relationships that are relevant to response and adaptation to challenge include flexibility; imagination, or the ability to cognitively reframe or think through alternative possibilities for an experience or considered choice; and curiosity, as a manifestation of flexibility. Each of these abilities is, in turn, central to positive adaptation or resilience. Further, research has shown that secure children are more curious, more flexible, and generally have greater access to imagination and an adaptive playfulness than insecure children (Sroufe, 2005; Sroufe et al., 2005), and that these differences are based in developmental changes in specific neural systems.

Neurobiological models of caregiving and stress reactivity

There are now considerable supporting data from pre-clinical models for the relationship between early experiences and individual differences in caregiving behavior as these affect individual differences in children's ability to modulate their response to stress and adversity (Kaufman et al., 2000; Southwick et al., 2008). Developing animals that are forced to confront overwhelming and uncontrollable stressors tend to display an exaggerated or sensitized sympathetic nervous system and/or hypothalamic–pituitary–adrenal (HPA) axis response to stress as adults (reviewed by Kaufman et al. [2000] and Southwick et al. [1999]). For example, separating rat pups or infant monkeys from their mother for substantial periods of time results in long-term increases in corticotropin-releasing hormone

(CRH), reduced central benzodiazepine binding, altered neuron development (reduced fiber densities) in some areas of the brain, increases in anxiety-like behaviors, impaired cognitive performance, and decreases in social interaction (reviewed by Kaufman et al., 2000).

Primate studies show similar effects of early uncontrolled or chronic stress, including studies in rhesus and squirrel monkeys exposed to varying degrees of maternal deprivation (Suomi, 1997; Levine, 2005). Rhesus infants reared only with peers showed larger cortisol responses to psychological stressors as adults and were more reactive (Higley et al., 1992); they also consumed more alcohol when given access (Fahlke et al., 2000). In a non-human primate brain imaging study, Rilling and colleagues (2001) showed that separation of juvenile rhesus monkeys from their mothers was associated with activation of cortical brain circuits that are susceptible to stress hormones.

Indeed, the behavioral profiles of mistreated monkeys (normative reactivity with normal care versus high-stress reactivity with disrupted maternal care) are remarkably similar to Bowlby's original description of anxious versus secure attachment in human infants (Suomi, 1995). In addition, studies of human infants reared in orphanages, malnourished, and/or exposed to prenatal stress suggested similar long-term effects on stress-regulatory HPA systems, which endured into adulthood (reviewed by Gunnar, 2000). Consequently, it appears that under early exposure to chronic, uncontrollable stress individuals develop stress-sensitized systems that hyperrespond to future stressors with exaggerated physiological and biochemical responsiveness (Kaufman et al., 2000). Further, it is also clear that the effects of early maternal deprivation in primates may be difficult to reverse, such that many maternally deprived monkeys are able to function normally as adults under normal conditions but are unable to cope with psychosocial stressors (Suomi et al., 1976).

As discussed earlier in this chapter, parenting is key to buffering children from uncontrollable or overwhelming stress. Recent advances in our understanding of the genetic, epigenetic, and neurobiological substrates of maternal behavior in model mammalian species are relevant to processes contributing to resilient and non-resilient adaptations. Pre-clinical studies suggest that the nature of the maternal behavior in the days following birth serves to establish the the level of HPA responsiveness to stress in pups, as well as "programming" the subsequent maternal behavior

of the adult offspring (Denenberg et al., 1969; Levine, 1975; Francis et al., 1999). Although many of the recent data are from rodent studies, investigations in social primates also highlight the importance of early mothering in determining how the daughters will mother (Harlow, 1963; Suomi et al., 1983). This complex programming through maternal care also appears to influence aspects of learning and memory.

Models relating maternal care to developing neural stress-response systems and to subsequent parenting use both experimental manipulations and naturally occurring variations. Repeated handling of pups in conjunction with *prolonged* maternal separations induces deranged maternal behavior, including a reduction in licking and grooming by the rat dams and reduced maternal aggression. Similarly, the adult offspring show increased neuroendocrine responses to acute restraint stress and airpuff startle, including elevated levels of mRNA for CRH in the paraventricular nucleus and elevated plasma levels of adrenocorticotropic hormone (ACTH), corticosterone and mRNA for steroid. These animals also show an increased acoustic startle response and enhanced anxiety or fearfulness to novel environments (Ladd et al., 2000, 2004).

In contrast, developing animals exposed to mild to moderate stressors that are under their control and that they can master tend to become stress inoculated, with a reduced overall response to future stressors (reviewed by Kaufman et al., 2000) and more efficient mastery of novelty and/or future challenges. Repeated handling of rodent pups in conjunction with *brief* maternal separations induces more licking and grooming by the rat dams (Liu et al., 1997). As adults, the offspring of mothers that exhibited more licking and grooming of pups during the first 10 days of life showed reduced plasma ACTH and corticosterone responses to acute restraint stress, as well as increased hippocampal glucocorticoid receptor mRNA expression, and decreased levels of hypothalamic CRH mRNA (Plotsky & Meaney, 1993; Liu et al., 1997). Subsequent studies have shown that the offspring of these mothers with high licking and grooming activity also show reduced acoustic startle responses and enhanced spatial learning and memory (Ladd et al., 2000; Liu et al., 2000). It appears in these models that, in the face of controllable stressors, enhanced maternal care serves to facilitate more robust stress-response capacities as adults.

Naturally occurring variations in licking, grooming, and arched back nursing have also been associated with the development of individual differences in behavioral responses to novelty in adult offspring. Adult offspring of the nursing mothers with low levels of licking, grooming, and arched back show increased startle responses, decreased open-field exploration, and longer latencies to eat food provided in a novel environment (Francis *et al.*, 1999). Importantly, these differences pertain in cross-fostering designs when offspring of mothers with high licking and grooming habit are cross-fostered to mothers with a low habit and vice versa. In the cross-fostering experiments, offspring of mothers with a high licking and grooming habit cared for by mothers with a low habit show similar increased startle and decreased open-field exploration to those of the offspring of the mothers with a low licking and grooming habit (Francis *et al.*, 1999).

Furthermore, Francis and co-workers (1999) demonstrated that the influence of maternal care on the development of stress reactivity was mediated by changes in gene expression in regions of the brain that regulate stress responses. For example, adult offspring of dams with high licking, grooming, and arched back nursing habit showed increased mRNA expression for the hippocampal glucocorticoid receptor and brain-derived neurotrophic factor, and increased production of the N-acetyl-D-aspartate (NMDA) receptor subunit and cholinergic innervation of the hippocampus. In the paraventricular nucleus, there is decreased CRH mRNA. These adult pups also show a number of changes in receptor density in the locus ceruleus, including increased α_2-adrenoceptors, reduced $GABA_A$ receptors, and decreased CRH receptors (Caldji *et al.*, 2000).

In sum, despite genetic constraints, data from animal studies indicate that the interval surrounding the birth of the rat pup or the rhesus infant is a critical period in the life of the animal that likely has enduring neurobiological and behavioral consequences. In particular, the nature of early caregiving experiences can have enduring consequences on individual differences in subsequent anxiety regulation and patterns of stress response, occurring through specific neuropharmacological mechanisms (reviewed by Weaver *et al.*, 2004).

Turning to humans, increasing clinical and epidemiological data support the view that exposure to early adverse environments underlies vulnerability to altered physiological responses to stress and the later expression of mood and anxiety disorders (Brown *et al.*, 1987; Ambelas, 1990; Kendler *et al.*, 2002, 2006). Among the most important early environmental influences is the interaction between the primary caregiver

and the infant. Building on the early work of Bowlby and colleagues (Bowlby, 1969), efforts to characterize this reciprocal interaction between caregiver and infant and to assess its impact have provided a powerful theoretical and empirical framework for social and emotional development (Cassidy & Shaver, 1999). Since the 1970s, clear evidence has emerged that significant disturbances in the early parent–child relationship (reflected in such things as child abuse and neglect or insecure attachments) contribute to an increased risk for developing both internalizing and externalizing disorders over the entire life (Sroufe *et al.*, 1999; Sroufe, 2005). While early adversity and insecure attachment may not be a proximal cause of later psychopathology, it appears to confer risk.

Conversely, longitudinal studies of high-risk infants suggest that the formation of a special relationship with a caring adult in the perinatal period confers a degree of resiliency and protection against the development of psychopathology later in life (Werner, 1997). Similar to the findings in rodents by Liu, Francis, and colleagues (Liu *et al.*, 1997; Francis *et al.*, 1999), there is accumulating evidence indicating that human caregivers' levels of response to their children can be traced in part to the caregivers' own childrearing histories and attachment-related experiences (Miller *et al.*, 1997). Caregivers' attachment-related experiences are encoded in "internal working models," described above, and establish styles of emotional communication that either buffer the individual in times of stress or contribute to maladaptive patterns of affect regulation and behavior (Bretherton & Munholland, 1999).

Self-efficacy, mastery, and stress

Self-efficacy, defined as a positive belief in one's ability to perform optimally in a situation, has wide-reaching effects in children's (and adult's) functioning. Perceived self-efficacy impacts how children feel, their motivation to learn and meet challenges, and their perception of their world and day to day experiences. For example, individuals with a strong sense of self-efficacy approach novel tasks or difficult situations as challenges that can be mastered, rather than as threats or dangers to be avoided. Indeed, individuals with a strong sense of efficacy may seek out challenges, set goals, and maintain a high commitment to these goals. In the face of failure or set-back, individuals with high perceived self-efficacy redouble their efforts to master the situation at hand. They also approach stressful or uncertain situations with a perception that they will be able to meet whatever the situation requires. In turn, such an efficacious outlook diminishes the experience of stress and lowers the likelihood of the detrimental experience of chronic stress. Consequently, perceived self-efficacy reflects both a response to challenges that have been met and mastered and a capacity that facilitates stress management.

As discussed above, early adversity and stress that is well buffered by parents not only contributes to the development of a well-regulated stress-response system but also to a developing sense of mastery and self-efficacy in the child; these, in turn, promote positive adaptation to subsequent adversity and stress. In other words, not all stress and adversity is associated with a negative impact on development. Instead, early exposure to controlled stress may enhance mastery and coping skills later in development (Southwick et al., 2008; Dienstbier & Zillig, 2009). As noted above, controlled exposure to stress as a means to enhance future adaptation and allostasis capacities is often referred to as stress inoculation. For example, in studies of squirrel monkeys, Parker et al. (2004) found that brief intermittent maternal separation in postnatal weeks 17–27 led to diminished anxiety responses on subsequent exposure to novel environments. "Stress-inoculated" monkeys were also found to have lower basal plasma ACTH and cortisol, as well as lower stress-induced cortisol. In follow-up at 18 months of age, these same monkeys performed better on a response-inhibition task than their age-matched, non-stress-inoculated peers (Parker et al., 2005).

Similarly, as also addressed above, rodents reared in a nurturing environment have been found to demonstrate enhanced tolerance to stress in adulthood (reviewed by Lyons & Parker, 2007). Rat pups that received 15 minutes of handling per day during the first three weeks of life were less reactive to stress and less fearful in novel environments as adults than the adults that had not been handled as pups (Ladd et al., 2005). They also had reduced ACTH and corticosterone responses to stress and demonstrated a more rapid return of corticosterone levels to baseline after exposure to stress. Further, cross-fostering studies, also cited above, suggest that even after stress-induced neurobiological and behavioral alterations have occurred it may be possible to modify these alterations by subsequent supportive, maternal caregiving and/or pharmacological interventions (Caldji et al., 1998; Kuhn & Schanberg, 1998).

Far less is known about the so-called stress-inoculation effect in humans. In one study, pediatric inpatients with previous positive separation experiences such as staying with grandparents for short periods of time experienced less stress during their hospital stay (Stacey, 1970). Childhood exposure to mild stress has also been associated with reduced heart rate and blood pressure responses during stressful laboratory tests in adolescents (Boyce & Chesterman, 1990). Norris and colleagues have also reported better psychiatric outcomes among adult survivors of natural disaster who had experienced similarly traumatic events earlier in their lives (Basoglu et al., 1997; Knight et al., 2000). The idea that manageable and controlled doses of stress can have "steeling" or inoculating effects has been incorporated into a number of clinical therapeutic approaches both for the treatment of and the prevention of trauma effects. Wells et al. (1986) demonstrated that preoperative stress inoculation was associated with less postoperative pain and anxiety, as has been the finding now in a number of perioperative educational programs for children and families (Kain et al., 1996, 1998, 2007).

While the literature specifically linking manageable stressful experiences to increased mastery in children is still emerging, there are more findings regarding the factors associated with a well-developed sense of efficacy and mastery in children and adults (Bandura et al., 2001; Thompson et al., 2004; Jones & Prinz, 2005; Davis-Kean et al., 2008). Notably these include, among others, supportive caregiving environments that provide encouragement to meet age-appropriate challenges, support during times of failure and stress, and opportunities to practice and subsequently succeed. As children grow up, a similarly supportive community (e.g., teachers, coaches, counselors) and peer networks provide key contexts for developing and enhancing self-efficacy. Hence, as with the promotion of a range of capacities central to positive adaptation to stress, parental care and social networks are key.

Intervention approaches that enhance capacities for healthy allostasis

We suggest that, while there are few to no explicit "resilience promoting" interventions for children, interventions that seek to enhance parents' ability to care appropriately for their children are in and of themselves resilience-enhancing interventions through their effects on children's stress modulation or capacities for healthy allostasis. Interventions that promote children's mastery of challenges or enhance emotional regulatory skills also have effects on capacities for responding to adversity and are, thus, likely to promote positive adaptation to challenge. This section of the chapter discusses intervention areas, with specific examples of approaches that may be considered to have a direct impact on children's ability to respond adaptively to stress and challenge – and hence increase their likelihood of reduced allostatic load and more resilient adaptation. These interventions are divided into those that work directly with parents in an effort to diminish parental stress, and thus child stress, and those that focus on the child's broader environment, schools, and community – specifically interventions that focus on mastery, self-efficacy, and effective use of social relationships. The division of the interventions into those for parents and those taking place in communities and schools moves from the more proximal approaches that impact the child's day to day caregiving to efforts that offer children more role models and a broader community of caring adults, and that promote life skills (e.g., mastery and self-efficacy skills) to strengthen, both directly and indirectly, children's ability to respond to stress and challenge.

Interventions with parents

A comprehensive review of the range of parenting interventions reported in the clinical and research literature is beyond the scope of this chapter. The discussion here focuses on two intervention models that have demonstrated effective outcomes and target infancy and early childhood. Since the mid 1980s, several intervention trials have suggested that well-designed intervention programs may have significant effects on both children's health and their psychological adaptation, particularly in the areas of emotional regulation and stress reactivity (Olds et al., 2007). For example, perhaps the most well-studied set of early interventions included home visits by nurses that began prenatally and continued for 30 months after birth. This has shown a number of positive outcomes as late as 15 years of age (Olds et al., 1997, 1998, 1999). Outcomes include a reduction in the number of subsequent pregnancies, use of welfare, child abuse and neglect, and criminal behavior on the part of low-income, unmarried mothers 15 years after the birth of the first child. Although the mechanism by which these effects are achieved remains in doubt, Olds and colleagues

have argued that one key element is the length of time between the first and second pregnancies by the mothers participating in the home visitation program (Olds et al., 1999; Eckenrode et al., 2000). On average, the time to the second pregnancy was more than 60 months in the experimental group that participated in the home visitation program and less than 40 months in the comparison group. With a delay of subsequent pregnancy, there is more time for the mother to attend to her developing infant and less family disruption and stress, which can often accompany the rapid birth of a second child. Over the three separate randomized control trials with different populations and contexts, there was less abuse and improved infant emotional and language development in the intervention group (Olds, 2006).

Another model program that also began prenatally and continued through to the child's second birthday is Minding the Baby (Slade et al., 2005), a model that integrates advanced practice nursing and mental healthcare in home visits for first time at-risk parents and builds on the principles from the Olds model as well as the attachment-based approaches of Heinicke and colleagues (2006). The Minding the Baby program aims to enhance the capacity of a young parent to understand her infant's mental and emotional needs as well as her own needs as a parent. Based in attachment theory and the notion of parental reflective functioning (Fonagy & Target, 1997), the program is directed specifically toward young parents living in communities affected by the many stressors associated with poverty. The intervention approach helps mothers to keep both the physical and emotional needs of their infants in mind as they provide daily care. The approach acknowledges the parent's own emotional and cognitive needs as a parent and explicit attention is given to the parent's own mental health needs. Early findings suggest that this very intensive relationship-focused approach may be particularly beneficial for families where chronic stress and early adversity precludes response to less-intensive interventions, and that this model may have a significant impact on both parental and child emotional regulatory abilities (Olds et al., 2007).

In sum, findings from selective early intervention programs suggest that these programs are likely to reduce a variety of maladaptive outcomes later in development, as well as improving proximal infant outcomes such as language/emotion development and enhanced attachment security. Less clear is the impact of these early interventions on the later rates of depression and anxiety disorders as the children reach adolescence. What seems clear from the range of early intervention programs for parents and infants is that starting early, even prenatally, is most effective. Further, the effectiveness of the intervention may be facilitated by targeting not just parental education or child care practices but the developing relationship between parent and child, and even more specifically those stressors and challenges that come from parenting children and that may impede effective parenting, including responding effectively to a child's distress.

Interventions in schools and community

Interventions based in schools and communities can have a critical impact on children, particularly those living in poverty and/or with parental discord. Also, as children's peer networks broaden, there are greater opportunities for learning from others and for learning mastery and emotional regulation skills. The focus here is on selected examples of school- and community-based interventions that are organized around facilitating mastery and improved coping and emotional regulatory skills.

Several decades of research show strong evidence for the role of schools and school-related programs (e.g., sports, community programs for students) in promoting mastery and self-efficacy in children and youth (Masten *et al.*, 1990; Wang & Gordon, 1994; Rutter & Maughan, 2002; Condly, 2006; Luthar, 2006). Research on how schools effectively promote childhood mastery and efficacy parallels studies in families, where positive effects are linked to stable and nurturing relationships, a supportive climate in the face of challenge, high expectations, and an expectable structure with consistent rules (Masten, 2006). Schools present many potentially positive opportunities for children to experience challenge and master failure as well as to succeed, learn from role models, and benefit from mentors and supportive adult relationships. Further, for at-risk students, schools offer a relatively asset-rich opportunity compared with their homes or the communities in general. These include after-school programs, libraries, sports, recreational activities in the community, and opportunities to explore talents in, for example, music, athletics, and writing. Specific examples of school- and community-based programs that particularly facilitate developing positive self-efficacy and mastery in children follow.

Emotional literacy

Learning to regulate emotions is an essential skill that dramatically impacts one's ability to manage stress and trauma. Emotions are often associated with high levels of physiological and psychological arousal. When faced with a challenge or stressor, the child who underreacts emotionally may allocate too few internal and external resources to solve the problem. On the other hand, the child who overreacts emotionally may be physiologically and psychologically flooded or overwhelmed, disrupting his or her ability to process information and make good decisions.

The ability to regulate emotions derives from a complex interaction of genetics, development, and environment. A number of school-based programs have been developed to help children to improve what some have termed "emotional literacy." For example, Maurer and colleagues (2004) have designed an emotional literacy program for middle school children that teaches students to recognize and evaluate their own and others' thoughts, feelings, and actions. This classroom-based program, which is recommended for fifth through eighth grade, conforms to the guidelines of the Collaborative for Academic, Social and Emotional Learning (2002) and focuses on social and emotional learning as well as academics. One of its goals is to teach children to cope more adaptively with modern-day stresses, and, in the process, to decrease behaviors that can be destructive.

The program has six steps: introducing feeling words, designs and personified explanations, real world association, personal/family association, classroom discussions, and creative writing assignments. These steps are intended to help students to learn to control their emotions by understanding the relationship between thoughts, feelings, and behaviors, thus increasing self- and social awareness and learning to choose emotional and behavioral responses that are adaptive rather than destructive. An important goal of the program is to teach students to express their feelings more freely, through writing and through conversation, in an environment that is challenging yet caring and supportive. Another goal is to promote school, family, and community partnerships.

A second example of a program for strengthening social and emotional competence in young children is the Incredible Years Teacher program for teachers and the accompanying Child Training Programs (Webster-Stratton *et al.*, 2008). The program was originally developed to treat children aged three to seven years with early-onset conduct problems and oppositional defiant disorder, but it has been expanded to be used as a preventive intervention by school teachers for young students. Its goal is to strengthen the capacity of young children to manage their emotions and behaviors and to develop the social skills needed to make meaningful relationships. These skills are seen as critical for success in cognitive and academic preparedness, success in school, and for dealing with stress, particularly for children who are exposed to multiple life stressors.

The intervention involves four days of training workshops where teachers learn skills related to classroom management strategies (e.g., methods to develop positive relationships with students and parents, effective use of encouragement and praise, incentive programs targeted to specific prosocial skills, and discipline plans when needed), promoting self-regulation of emotions in students, teaching class members how to solve problems, and promoting social competence among students. In addition to teacher training the intervention follows the Dina Dinosaur Social Skills and Problem Solving Curriculum for children, which includes the following seven units: learning school rules, how to be successful in school, emotional literacy including perspective taking and empathy, interpersonal problem solving, anger management, social skills, and communication skills. Lessons are typically delivered in a large group circle of students, two to three times each week in 15–20 minute time periods, followed by practice activities of approximately 20 minutes in a smaller group setting. Teachers also promote skill development throughout the course of the day during meals, recess, and so on. Parents are regularly informed about the concepts and skills that are being taught to the children and are asked to help their child to complete Dina Dinosaur home activity books. Randomized controlled studies (Webster-Stratton & Hammond, 1997, Webster-Stratton & Reid 2004; Webster-Stratton et al., 2004, 2008) of the Incredible Years Child Training Program have been conducted in both clinic-based and school-based populations. For example, in one clinic-based study (Webster-Stratton et al., 2001), chidren aged four to eight years and with early-onset conduct problems were randomly assigned to receive training using the Incredible Years Dinosaur Social Skills and Problem Solving Curriculum or to be in a waitlist control group. After treatment, children in the intervention group demonstrated statistically and clinically significant improvement in non-compliant and aggressive behaviors as well as in social problem-solving strategies compared with children in the control group. At one year follow-up, most of the improvements were maintained. In a 30-lesson school-based study involving 120 classrooms, Webster-Stratton and colleagues (2008) randomly assigned schools to intervention or control conditions. Results indicated that the intervention had a robust effect on changing teachers' approaches to classroom management and resulted in significantly fewer critical statements by teachers to students. Compared with children in the control school group, those in the intervention group showed significant improvements in conduct problems, social competence, and emotion regulation. The intervention had a particularly large effect in schools with high conduct problems and very low levels of school readiness. Both teachers and parents in the intervention schools reported being very satisfied with the program.

Team sports

In addition to its well-known positive effects on physical health and development, regular physical activity, and in some cases participation in team sports, has also been associated with psychological health. Studies have found a positive relationship between regular physical activity and self-esteem, perceptions of competence, life satisfaction, and well-being (Steptoe & Butler, 1996; Fox, 2000; Valois et al., 2004, Pedersen & Seidman 2004; Bailey, 2006). For example, in a study of 247 urban adolescent girls, Pedersen and Seidman (2004) found that achievement in team sport during early adolescence was positively associated with self-esteem in middle adolescence. In addition, reduced depression, anger, anxiety, and stress have been associated with regular physical activity (Hassman et al., 2000; Valois et al., 2004). Sports programs, with their focus on strengths and resilience, have even been employed as psychosocial interventions in countries that have suffered from disasters and wars (Colliard, 2005; Heninger & Meuwly, 2005).

In addition to increasing physical toughness, team sports can build heart and enhance mental toughness (Bell & Suggs, 1998). To be a successful team member, the young athlete must master a set of physical and emotional skills, endure challenging and unpleasant training sessions, learn to control negative emotions and cooperate during times of high stress, learn to "go the extra mile," sacrifice personal goals for team goals, and learn to face and then tolerate the stress of competition. This requires dedication, hard work, and discipline (Bell & Suggs, 1998; Tofler & Butterbaugh, 2005).

Team sports provide a powerful venue for learning lessons in ethical and moral behavior under conditions of high arousal and stress. To be fully successful in team sports, children must learn to maintain ethical standards in the context of hard work, determination, frustration, anger, and the drive to win (Tofler & Butterbaugh, 2005). They must grapple with numerous moral issues such as fair play, sportsmanship, self-aggrandizing behavior, integrity, and character (Stuart, 2003; Tofler & Butterbaugh, 2005). They must also resist the temptation to bend or exploit the rules or to win at all costs. These lessons are often difficult to learn, particularly if parents and coaches have not themselves fully embraced a mature and ethical approach to team sports.

Physical activity and team sports each have been associated with academic performance (Sallis *et al.*, 1999; Fox, 2000). For example, in a survey of over 4000 middle and high school students, Fox and colleagues (Fox, 2000) found that team sport participation was associated with higher grade point average among both boys and girls, and that physical activity was associated with higher grade point average among girls but not boys. There is also some evidence that increased physical activity at school, even if it means reduced time for academic activities, may result in improved academic performance (Shephard, 1997).

As noted earlier in this chapter, higher levels of positive social support are strongly associated with resilience. Social development, social competence, and the fostering of prosocial skills and behaviors are among the most positive effects of team sport participation (Tofler & Butterbaugh, 2005; Bailey, 2006). Children and adolescents learn the importance of communicating with peers and coaches, playing by the rules, cooperating and sharing, and placing the goals of the team above their own personal goals. Team members often develop strong and supportive relationships with fellow team members and coaches. Team sports also tend to foster peer respect and relationships across a broad range of ethnic, racial, and cultural groups (Tofler & Butterbaugh, 2005). Inclusion on a team provides an opportunity to create social networks and may create a sense of belonging (Bailey, 2004).

It is important to note that sport is not always positive and resilience enhancing for children and adolescents. Sport can be detrimental when it excludes some youth or groups of youth, when it focuses on excessive negative feedback and criticism, and when expectations are inappropriate or excessive, as may be the case with unrealistic outcome-driven parenting and coaching (Tofler & Butterbaugh, 2005, Bailey, 2006). In some cases, sport can also exploit youth (Tofler & Butterbaugh, 2005).

Outdoor education programs

Outdoor education/adventure programs may also have a role in enhancing resilience. These programs typically are physically and emotionally challenging and emphasize the importance of character, teamwork, problem solving, skill building, endurance, discipline, and courage. In some programs, altruism is also encouraged. To date, there have been hundreds of studies measuring the efficacy of outdoor education programs and at least five published meta-analyses. The most comprehensive meta-analysis, which was conducted by Hattie and colleagues (1997), included 96 studies from 1968 to 1994 with 12 057 unique participants; 72% of programs lasted between 20 and 26 days. Programs were located in wilderness or backcountry settings where small groups (generally less than 16 participants) were taught a variety of skills and then challenged by physically and mentally demanding objectives that required intense problem solving and decision making among group members.

The meta-analysis carried out by Hattie *et al.* (1997) evaluated the following six main outcome variables: leadership, self-concept, academic achievement, personality, interpersonal skills, and adventuresomeness. Adventure programs had the greatest immediate impact on a number of dimensions that have been associated with resilience, including assertiveness, emotional stability, flexibility, confidence, self-efficacy, problem solving, achievement motivation, internal locus of control, and maturity. The overall effect size was small to moderate (0.34). However, for those programs that included a long-term follow-up evaluation, the overall effect size increased by an additional 0.17. This raised the overall long-term effect size to 0.51, which is generally considered to be moderate. The greatest increase was seen for self-concept, which increased from 0.28 immediately after the program to 0.51 at long-term follow-up. In a review of outdoor education meta-analytic studies, Neill (2002) suggested that the relatively large increase in self-concept over time might indicate a "sleeper effect," meaning that changes in self-concept may begin during a program and then continue to develop after the program.

While it is difficult to draw firm conclusions about specific mediators of success in outdoor/adventure programs, the available evidence suggests that outcomes are related to the specific organizations running the programs (e.g., Outward Bound Australia appears to be particularly effective), the duration of the programs (i.e., programs greater than 20 days appear to be more successful than programs less than 20 days), and perhaps age (i.e., self-concept may change more among younger compared with older adolescents). There is additional evidence to suggest that educational/adventure programs have positive effects on academic performance and may be particularly effective for specific populations with emotional, behavioral, and psychological problems (Cason & Gillis 1994; Neill, 2002), including juvenile delinquents.

While the construct of resilience has not specifically been assessed before and after outdoor education/adventure programs, the available published data suggest that a number of these programs have a positive impact on domains associated with the capacity to deal with adversity. Further, unlike many education programs, the positive effects experienced during these programs may trigger further positive change after adolescent participants have left the program.

Training in moral courage

Just as moral courage, altruism, and giving to others have been associated with resilience in adults, they also appear to be associated with resilience in children. In her classic study of at-risk children on the Hawaiian island of Kauai, Emmy Werner (1992) found that children who were most likely to lead successful lives as adults were those who helped others in meaningful ways (e.g., assisting a family member, a neighbor, or some other community member). Similarly, Zimrin (1986) reported that Israeli children who had been physically abused fared better if they assumed responsibility for someone else, such as a sibling or a pet.

Many parents and teachers instruct children about the value of ethical and moral principles and altruism. One example of a structured approach to teaching moral courage is the Giraffe Project, whose motto is "moving people to stick their necks out for the common good." In a classroom setting, students are introduced to the stories of "heros" who have been morally courageous. These stories are discussed in detail so that children can learn what it means to be morally

courageous. Next children are asked to find examples of such heroes in their own families and communities. Finally, students identify a need in their community and work to address it though a service-learning project. In this way, they themselves become morally courageous heroes. As of 2007, the Giraffe Project had reached more than 30 000 US students in K-12 schools (www.giraffe.org).

Penn Resiliency Program

The Penn Resiliency Program is described in Chapter 20 and so is only touched upon briefly here. As noted above, optimism, particularly realistic optimism, has been associated with resilience in a host of studies involving numerous populations of adults and children (Southwick et al., 2005). The Penn Resiliency Program is largely based on the cognitive models of treatment for depression developed by Beck and colleagues (1979) and on Seligman's learned optimism training, where the participant learns to monitor beliefs about everyday adversity and to connect those beliefs to consequences in his or her daily life. For example, in one study of middle school children, Cutuli and colleagues (2006) used a 12-session cognitive-behavioral intervention to teach children how to challenge inaccurate self-perceptions and perceived failures. The intervention was particularly helpful for young adolescents with conduct problems.

Conclusions

This chapter has primarily focused on caregiving relationships and environments (e.g., home and school) as key to children's response to adversity and challenge. Positive, nurturing, supportive relationships moderate and buffer the potentially detrimental impact of stress and adversity and consequently may promote enhanced mastery skills for subsequent stress challenge. When relationships promote self-efficacy and mastery, they afford children skills for responding to stress and challenge that permit a more positive or "resilient" adaptation. Promoting enhanced self-efficacy and an ability to weather adversity, even to find positive opportunity in negative circumstances, requires also that children be protected from chronic, toxic stress. Environmental/caregiving conditions are critical for establishing "set-points" for stress-system activation and also for the allostatic ability of the system – and the body – to return to baseline after a stressful condition has resolved or the child is no longer in the situation. The concept of stress inoculation requires far more careful study in humans as to how stress and challenge can enhance children's self-efficacy and also prepare the stress-response system for future adversity. That said, a number of interventions ranging from specific efforts to enhance parental abilities to working with children in schools and communities are examples of efforts that implicitly, and sometimes explicitly, promote mastery and stress-weathering abilities in children. In the future, it will be important to consider more explicitly how interventions and educational programs for children can be designed to target key capacities for positive adaptation to and mastery of challenge and adversity.

References

Ambelas, A. (1990). Life events and the onset of mania. *British Journal of Psychiatry*, **157**, 450–451.

Bailey, R. (2004). Evaluating the relationship between physical education, sport and social inclusion. *Education Reviews*, **56**, 71–90.

Bailey, R. (2006). Physical education and sport in schools: a review of benefits and outcomes. *Journal of School Health*, **76**, 397–401.

Bandura, A., Barbaranelli, C., Vittorio Caprara, G., & Pastorelli, C. (2001). Self-efficacy beliefs as shapers of children's aspirations and career trajectories. *Child Development*, **72**, 187–206.

Basoglu, M., Mineka, S., Paker, M., *et al.* (1997). Psychological preparedness for trauma as a protective factor in survivors of torture. *Psychological Medicine*, **27**,1421–1433.

Beck, A. T., Rush, A. J., Shaw, B. F., & Emery, G. (1979). *Cognitive therapy of depression*. New York: Guilford Press.

Bell, C. C. & Suggs, H. (1998). Using sports to strengthen resiliency in children: Training "Heart". *Child and Adolescent Psychology Clinics*, **7**, 859–865.

Bowlby, J. (1969). *Attachment and loss,* Vol. 1: *Attachment*. London: Hogarth Press.

Boyce, W. T. & Chesterman, E. (1990). Life events, social support, and cardiovascular reactivity in adolescence. *Journal of Developmental Behavioral Pediatrics*, **11**, 105–111.

Brady, K. T. & Sinha, R. (2005). Co-occurring mental and substance use disorders: the neurobiological effects of chronic stress. *American Journal of Psychiatry*, **162**,1483–1493.

Bretherton, I. & Munholland, K. A. (1999). Internal working models in attachment relations: A construct revisited. In J. Cassidy & P. R. Shaver (eds.), *Handbook of attachment:*

Theory, research, and clinical implications (pp. 89–111). New York: Guilford Press.

Brown, G. W., Bifulco, A., & Harris, T. O. (1987). Life events, vulnerability and onset of depression: some refinements. *British Journal of Psychiatry*, **150**, 30–42.

Caldji, C., Tannenbaum, B., Sharma, S., *et al.* (1998). Maternal care during infancy regulates the development of neural systerns mediating the expression of fearfulness in the rat. *Proceedings of the National Academy of Sciences of the USA*, **95**, 5335–5340.

Caldji, C., Francis, D., Sharma, S., Plotsky, P. M., & Meaney, M. J. (2000). The effects of early rearing environment on the development of GABAA and central benzodiazepine receptor levels and novelty-induced fearfulness in the rat. *Neuropsychopharmacology*, **22**, 219–229.

Cason, D. & Gillis, H. L. (1994). A meta-analysis of outdoor adventure programming with adolescents. *Journal of Experiential Education*, **17**, 40–47.

Cassidy, J. & Shaver, P. R. (1999). *Handbook of attachment*. New York: Guilford Press.

Collaborative for Academic, Social and Emotional Learning (2002). *Guidelines for social and emotional learning: Quality programs for school and life success* (pp. 1–4). Chicago, IL: Collaborative for Academic, Social and Emotional Learning, http://www.casel.org/downloads/Safe%20and%20Sound/2A_Guidelines.pdf (accessed February 28, 2011.)

Colliard, C. (2005). *Mission Report. Evaulation of the Tdh psychosocial programme of recreational centres in Bam, Iran*. Geneva: Center for Humanitarian Psychology.

Condly, S. J. (2006). Resilience in children: A review of literature with implications for educators. *Urban Education*, **41**, 211–236.

Cutuli, J. J., Chaplin, T. M., Gillham, J. E., Reivich, K. J., & Seligman, M. E. (2006). Preventing co-occurring depression symptoms in adolescents with conduct problems: the Penn Resiliency Program. *Annals of the New York Academy of Sciences*, **1094**, 282–286.

Davis-Kean, P. E., Huesmann, L., Jager, J., *et al.* (2008). Changes in the relation of self-efficacy beliefs and behaviors across development. *Child Development*, **79**, 1257–1269.

Denenberg, V. H., Rosenberg, K. M., Paschke, R., & Zarrow, M. X. (1969). Mice reared with rat aunts: effects on plasma corticosterone and open field activity. *Nature*, **221**, 73–74.

Dienstbier, R. A. & Zillig, L. M. P. (2009). Toughness. In S. J. Lopez & C. R. Snyder (eds.), *Oxford handbook of positive psychology*, 2nd edn (pp. 537–548). New York: Oxford University Press.

Eckenrode, J., Ganzel, B., Henderson, C. R. Jr., *et al.* (2000). Preventing child abuse and neglect with a program of nurse home visitation: the limiting effects of domestic violence. *Journal of the American Medical Association*, **284**, 1385–1391.

Fahlke, C., Lorenz, J. G., Long, J., *et al.* (2000). Rearing experiences and stress-induced plasma cortisol as early risk factors for excessive alcohol consumption in nonhuman primates. *Alcoholism: Clinical and Experimental Research*, **24**, 644–650.

Fonagy, P. & Target, M. (1997). Attachment and reflective function: their role in self-organization. *Development& Psychopathology*, **9**, 679–700.

Fox, K. (2000). The effects of exercise on self-perceptions and self-esteem. In S. Biddle, K. Fox, & S. Boutcher (eds.), *Physical activity and psychological well-being* (pp. 88–117). London: Routledge.

Francis, D. D., Diorio, J., Liu, D., & Meaney, M. J. (1999). Nongenomic transmission across generations of maternal behavior and stress responses in the rat. *Science*, **286**, 1155–1158.

Gunnar, M. R. (2000). Early adversity and the development of stress reactivity and regulation. In C. A. Nelson (ed.), *The Minnesota symposia on child psychology*, Vol. 31: *The effects of early adversity on neurobehavioral development* (pp. 163–200). Mahwah, NJ: Erlbaum.

Gunnar, M. & Vazquez, D. M. (2006). Stress neurobiology and developmental psychopathology. In D. Cicchetti & D. Cohen (eds.), *Developmental psychopathology*, Vol. 2: *Developmental neuroscience,* 2nd edn (pp. 533–577). New York: Wiley.

Harlow, H. F. (1963). The maternal affectional system of rhesus monkeys. In H. L. Rheingold (ed.), *Maternal behavior in mammals* (pp. 254–281). New York: Wiley.

Hassman, P., Koivula, N., & Uutela, A. (2000). Physical exercise and psychological well-being: a population study in Finland. *Preventive Medicine*, **30**, 17–25.

Hattie, J., Marsh, H. W., Neill, J. T., & Richards, G. E. (1997). Adventure education and outward bound: Out-of-class experiences that make a lasting difference. *Reviews of Educational Research*, **67**, 43–87.

Heinicke, C. M., Goorsky, M., Levine, M., *et al.* (2006). Pre- and postnatal antecedents of a home-visiting intervention and family developmental outcome. *Infant Mental Health Journal*, **27**, 91–119.

Heninger, J.-P. & Meuwly, M. (2005). *Movement, games and sports: Developing coaching methods and practices for vulnerable children in the Southern hemisphere.* Lausanne: Foundation Terre des Hommes.

Higley, J. D., Suomi, S. J., & Linnoila, M. (1992). A longitudinal assessment of CSF monoamine metabolite and plasma cortisol concentrations in young rhesus monkeys. *Biological Psychiatry*, **32**, 127–145.

Jones, T. L. & Prinz, R. J. (2005). Potential roles of parental self-efficacy in parent and child adjustment: A review. *Clinical Psychology Review*, **25**, 341–363.

Kain, Z. N., Mayes, L. C., and Caramico, L. A. (1996). Preoperative preparation in children: A cross-sectional study. *Journal of Clinical Anesthesia*, **8**, 508–514.

Kain, Z. N., Mayes, L. C., Caramico, L. A., *et al.* (1998). Preoperative preparation programs in children: a comparative examination. *Anesthesia and Analgesia*, **87**, 1249–1255.

Kain, Z. N., Caldwell-Andrews, A. A., Mayes, L. C., *et al.* (2007). Family-centered preparation for surgery improves perioperative outcomes in children: a randomized controlled trial. *Anesthesiology*, **106**, 65–74.

Kaufman, J., Plotsky, P. M., Nemeroff, C. B., & Charney, D. S. (2000). Effects of early adverse experiences on brain structure and function: Clinical implications. *Biological Psychiatry*, **48**, 778–790.

Kendler, K. S., Gardner, C. O., & Prescott, C. A. (2002). Toward a comprehensive developmental model for major depression in women. *American Journal of Psychiatry*, **159**, 1133–1145.

Kendler, K. S., Gardner, C. O., & Prescott, C. A. (2006). Toward a comprehensive developmental model for major depression in men. *American Journal of Psychiatry*, **163**, 115–124.

Knight, B. G., Gatz, M., Heller, K., & Bengtson, V. L. (2000). Age and emotional response to the Northridge earthquake: A longitudinal analysis. *Psychology and Aging*, **15**, 627–634.

Kuhn, C. M. & Schanberg, S. M. (1998). Responses to maternal separation: Mechanisms and mediators. *International Journal of Developmental Neuroscience*, **16**, 261–270.

Ladd, C. O., Huot, R. L., Thrivikraman, K. V., *et al.* (2000). Long-term behavioral and neuroendocrine adaptations to adverse early experience. *Progress in Brain Research*, **122**, 81–103.

Ladd, C. O., Huot, R. L., Thrivikraman, K. V., Nemeroff, C. B., & Plotsky, P. M. (2004). Long-term adaptations in glucocorticoid receptor and mineralocorticoid receptor mRNA and negative feedback on the hypothalamo-pituitary-adrenal axis following neonatal maternal separation. *Biological Psychiatry*, **55**, 367–375.

Ladd, C. O., Huot, R. L., Thrivikraman, K. V., & Plotsky, P. M. (2005). Differential neuroendocrine responses to chronic variable stress in adult Long Evans rats exposed to handling–maternal separation as neonates. *Psychoneuroendocrinrology*, **30**, 520–533.

Levine, S. (ed.) (1975). *Psychosocial factors in growth and development.* London: Oxford University Press.

Levine, S. (2005). Developmental determinants of sensitivity and resistance to stress. *Psychoneuroendocrinology*, **30**, 939–946.

Liu, D., Diorio, J., Tannenbaum, B., *et al.* (1997). Maternal care, hippocampal glucocorticoid receptors, and hypothalamic–pituitary–adrenal responses to stress. *Science*, **277**, 1659–1662.

Liu, D., Diorio, J., Day, J. C., Francis, D. D., & Meaney, M. J. (2000). Maternal care, hippocampal synaptogenesis and cognitive development in rats. *Nature Neuroscience*, **3**, 799–806.

Loman, M. & Gunnar, M. R. (2010). Early experience and the development of stress reactivity and regulation in children. *Neuroscience and Biobehavioral Reviews*, **34**, 867–876.

Luthar, S. S. (2006). Resilience in development: A synthesis of research across five decades. In D. Cicchetti & D. J. Cohen (eds.), *Developmental psychopathology*, Vol. 3: *Risk, disorder, and adaptation*, 2nd edn (pp. 739–795). New York: Wiley.

Luthar, S. S. & Cicchetti, D. (2000). The construct of resilience: Implications for interventions and social policies. *Developmental Psychopathology*, **12**, 857–885.

Lyons, D. M. & Parker, K. J. (2007). Stress inoculation-induced indications of resilience in monkeys. *Journal of Traumatic Stress* **20**, 423–433.

Masten, A. S. (2006). Promoting resilience in development: A general framework for systems of care. In R. J. Flynn, P. Dudding, & J. G. Barber (eds.), *Promoting resilience in child welfare* (pp. 3–17). Ottawa: University of Ottawa Press.

Masten, A. S., Best, K. M., & Garmezy, N. (1990). Resilience and development: Contributions from the study of children who overcome adversity. *Development and Psychopathology*, **2**, 425–444.

Maurer, M., Brackett, M. A., & Plain, F. (2004). *Emotional literacy in the middle school: A 6-step program to promote social, emotional and academic learning*. Port Chester, NY: Dude.

McEwen, B. S. (2000). Allostasis and allostatic load: implications for neuropsychopharmacology. *Neuropsychopharmacology*, **22**, 108–124.

Miller, L., Kramer, R., Warner, V., Wickramaratne, P., & Weissman, M. (1997). Intergenerational transmission of parental bonding among women. *Journal of the American Academy of Child and Adolescent Psychiatry*, **36**, 1134–1139.

Nachmias, M., Gunnar, M. R., Mangelsdorf, S., Parritz, R., & Buss, K. A. (1996). Behavioral inhibition and stress reactivity: Moderating role of attachment security. *Child Development*, **67**, 508–522.

Neill, J. T. (2002). Meta-analytic research on the outcomes of outdoor education. In *Proceedings of the 6th Biennial Coalition for Education in the Outdoors Research Symposium*, Bradford Woods.

Olds, D. L. (2006). The nurse-family partnership: an evidence based preventative intervention. *Infant Mental Health Journal*, **27**, 5–25.

Olds, D. L., Eckenrode, J., Henderson, C. R. Jr., *et al.* (1997). Long-term effects of home visitation on maternal life course and child abuse and neglect. Fifteen-year follow-up of a randomized trial. *Journal of the American Medical Association*, **278**, 637–643.

Olds, D., Henderson, C. R. Jr., Cole, R., *et al.* (1998). Long-term effects of nurse home visitation on children's criminal and antisocial behavior: 15-year follow-up of a randomized controlled trial. *Journal of the American Medical Association*, **280**, 1238–1244.

Olds, D. L., Henderson, C. R. Jr., Kitzman, H. J., *et al.* (1999). Prenatal and infancy home visitation by nurses: recent findings. *Future Child*, **9**, 44–65, 190–191.

Olds, D. L., Sadler, L., & Kitzman, H. (2007). Programs for parents of infants and toddlers: Recent evidence from randomized trials. *Journal of Child Psychology and Psychiatry*, **48**, 355–391.

Parker, K. J., Buckmaster, C. L., Schatzberg, A. F., & Lyons, D. M. (2004). Prospective investigation of stress inoculation in young monkeys. *Archives of General Psychiatry*, **61**, 933–941.

Parker, K. J., Buckmaster, C. L., Justus, K. R., Schatzberg, A. F., & Lyons, D. M. (2005). Mild early life stress enhances prefrontal-dependent response inhibition in monkeys. *Biological Psychiatry*, **57**, 848–855.

Pedersen, S. & Seidman, E. (2004). Team sports achievement and self-esteem development among urban adolescent girls. *Psychology of Women Quarterly*, **28**, 412–422.

Plotsky, P. M. & Meaney, M. J. (1993). Early, postnatal experience alters hypothalamic corticotropin-releasing factor (CRF) mRNA, median eminence CRF content and stress-induced release in adult rats. *Brain Research, Molecular Brain Research*, **18**, 195–200.

Rilling, J. K., Winslow, J. T., O'Brien, D., *et al.* (2001). Neural correlates of maternal separation in rhesus monkeys. *Biological Psychiatry*, **49**, 146–157.

Rutter, M. & Maughan, B. (2002). School effectiveness findings, 1979–2002. *Journal of School Psychology*, **40**, 451–475.

Sallis, J. F., McKenzie, T. L., Kolody, B., *et al.* (1999). Effects of health-related physical education on academic achievement: project SPARK. *Research Quarterly in Exercise and Sport*, **70**, 127–134.

Shephard, R. J. (1997). Curricular physical activity and academic performance. *Pediatric Exercise Science*, **9**, 113–126.

Shonkoff, J. P. & Phillips, D. (eds.) (2000). *From neurons to neighborhoods: The science of early childhood development*. Washington, DC: National Academy Press for the Committee on Integrating the Science of Early Childhood Development.

Slade, A., Sadler, L. S., & Mayes, L. C. (2005). Minding the baby: Enhancing parental reflective functioning in a nursing/mental health home visiting program. In L. J. Berlin, Y. Ziv, L. Amaya-Jackson, & M. T. Greenberg (eds.), *Enhancing early attachments: Theory, research, intervention, and policy* (pp. 152–177). New York: Guilford Press.

Southwick, S. M., Bremner, J. D., Rasmusson, A., *et al.* (1999). Role of norepinephrine in the pathophysiology and treatment of posttraumatic stress disorder. *Biological Psychiatry*, **46**, 1192–1204.

Southwick, S. M., Vythilingam, M., & Charney, D. S. (2005). The psychobiology of depression and resilience to stress: Implications for prevention and treatment. *Annual Reviews of Clinical Psychology*, **1**, 255–291.

Southwick, S. M., Ozbay, F., & Mayes, L. C. (2008). Psychological and biological factors associated with resilience to stress and trauma. In H. Parens, H. P. Blum, & S. Akhtar (eds.), *The unbroken soul: Tragedy, trauma, and resilience* (pp. 130–151). Lanham, MD: Jason Aronson.

Sroufe, L. A. (2005). Attachment and development: a prospective, longitudinal study from birth to adulthood. *Attachment and Human Development*, 7, 349–367.

Sroufe, L. A., Carlson, E. A., Levy, A. K., & Egeland, B. (1999). Implications of attachment theory for developmental psychopathology. *Developmental Psychopathology*, **11**, 1–13.

Sroufe, L. A., Egeland, B., Carlson, E., & Collins, W. A. (2005). Placing early attachment experiences in developmental context: The Minnesota Longitudinal Study. In K. E. Grossmann, K. Grossmann, & E. Waters (eds.), *Attachment from infancy to adulthood: The major longitudinal studies* (pp. 48–70). New York: Guilford Press.

Stacey, M. (1970). *Hospitals, children, and their families: report of a pilot study*. London: Routledge & Paul.

Steptoe, A. & Butler, N. (1996). Sports participation and emotional wellbeing in adolescents. *Lancet*, **347**, 1789–1792.

Stuart, M. E. (2003). Moral issues in sport: the child's perspective. *Research Quarterly in Exercise and Sport*, **74**, 445–454.

Suomi, S. J. (1995). Influence of Bowlby's attachment theory on research on non-human primate biobehavioral development. In S. Goldberg, R. Muir, & J. Kerr (eds.), *Attachment theory: social, developmental, and clinical perspectives* (pp. 185–201). Hillside, NJ: Analytic.

Suomi, S. J. (1997). Early determinants of behaviour: evidence from primate studies. *British Medical Bulletin*, **53**, 170–184.

Suomi, S. J., Delizio, R., & Harlow, H. F. (1976). Social rehabilitation of separation-induced depressive disorders in monkeys. *American Journal of Psychiatry*, **133**, 1279–1285.

Suomi, S. J., Mineka, S., & DeLizio, R. D. (1983). Short- and long-term effects of repetitive mother-infant separations on social development in rhesus monkeys. *Developmental Psychology*, **19**, 770–786.

Tofler, I. R. & Butterbaugh, G. J. (2005). Developmental overview of child and youth sports for the twenty-first century. *Clinical Sports Medicine*, **24**, 783–804.

Thompson, A. H., Barnsley, R. H., & Battle, J. (2004). The relative age effect and the development of self-esteem. *Educational Research*, **46**, 313–320.

Valois, R. F., Zullig, K. J., Huebner, E. S., & Drane, J. W. (2004). Physical activity behaviors and perceived life satisfaction among public high school adolescents. *Journal of School Health*, **74**, 59–65.

Wang, M. C. & Gordon, E. W. (1994). *Educational resilience in inner-city America: Challenges and prospects*. Hillsdale, NJ: Erlbaum.

Weaver, I. C., Diorio, J., Seckl, J. R., Szyf, M., & Meaney, M. J. (2004). Early environmental regulation of hippocampal glucocorticoid receptor gene expression: characterization of intracellular mediators and potential genomic target sites. *Annals of the New York Academy of Sciences*, **1024**, 182–212.

Webster-Stratton, C. & Hammond, M. (1997). Treating children with early onset conduct problems: A comparison of child and parent training interventions. *Journal of Consulting and Clinical Psychology*, **65**, 93–109.

Webster-Stratton, C. & Reid, J. M. (2004). Strengthening social and emotional competence in young children, The Foundation for Early School Readiness and Success: Incredible years classroom social skills problem-solving curriculum: *Infants and Young Children*, **17**, 96–113.

Webster-Stratton, C., Reid, M. J., & Hammond, M. (2001). Social skills and problem solving training for children with early-onset conduct problems: Who benefits? *Journal of Child Psychology and Psychiatry*, **42**, 943–952.

Webster-Stratton, C., Reid, M. J., & Hammond, M. (2004). Treating children with early-onset conduct problems: Intervention outcomes for parent, child, and teacher training. *Journal of Clinical Child and Adolescent Psychology*, **33**, 105–124.

Webster-Stratton, C., Reid, M. J., & Stoolmiller, M. (2008). Preventing conduct problems and improving school readiness: Evaluation of the incredible years teacher and child training programs in high-risk schools. *Journal of Child Psychology and Psychiatry*, **49**, 471–488.

Wells, J. K., Howard, G. S., Nowlin, W. F., & Vargas, M. J. (1986). Presurgical anxiety and postsurgical pain and adjustment: Effects of a stress inoculation procedure.

Journal of Consulting and Clinical Psychology, **54**, 831–835.

Werner, E. E. (1992). The children of Kauai: Resiliency and recovery in adolescence and adulthood. *Journal of Adolescent Health*, **13**, 262–268.

Werner, E. E. (1997). Vulnerable but invincible: high-risk children from birth to adulthood. *Acta Paediatrica Supplement*, **422**, 103–105.

Zimrin, H. (1986). A profile of survival. *Child Abuse and Neglect*, **10**, 339–349.

Military mental health training: building resilience

Carl Andrew Castro and Amy B. Adler

> For learning to take place with any kind of efficiency students must be motivated. To be motivated, they must become interested. And they become interested when they are actively working on projects which they can relate to their values and goals in life.
>
> *Gus Tuberville, President, Penn College*

Introduction

There is no debate that combat places tremendous psychological and physical demands on those involved. And as we learn more about how combat affects the psychological well-being of those involved, a set of central questions emerge. What can we do to prepare service members for the psychological demands of combat? What can we do to sustain the mental health and well-being of those deployed in a combat environment? What can we do to facilitate the return of these service members from the combat environment to home? In short, what do service members need to know about how combat can affect them?

In response to these questions, the US Army developed the Battlemind Training System, a mental health resilience building program (US Army Medical Command, 2007). This system established several fundamental principles of mental health training, identified key implementation principles, and defined several important terms. Throughout this chapter, the Battlemind Training System will be used as an exemplar to highlight how a military mental health training program can be created that employs theses principles of mental health training and implementation.

Before beginning a discussion of these key principles and terminology, it will be useful to provide an historical perspective on the status of mental health training in the US military prior to Battlemind

Training. To be sure, the task confronting us was by no means an easy one. Imagine, a brigade combat team comprising over 3500 soldiers getting ready to deploy to combat for over a year. You have one hour. What are you going to tell them about the psychological demands of combat in order to prepare and sustain them for that year? That was our task.

Prior to Battlemind Training, none of the services in the US military had developed an empirically based mental health training program for preparing service members for the psychological demands of combat. Of course, some service members did receive mental health training prior to deploying, but this mental health training was generic and non-specific to the actual demands of the combat environment, and it was not conducted in a systematic manner (McKibben *et al.*, 2009). Typically, the mental health training consisted of "home-grown" PowerPoint presentations containing theoretical information on stress that had little or questionable value to service members getting ready to go into combat. For example, these home-grown mental training efforts typically included a discussion of the Yerkes–Dodson model of stress, along with a discussion of the distinction between eustress, astress, and distress, material of interest perhaps to first-year graduate students but not necessarily interesting to soldiers about to deploy to Iraq or Afghanistan.

Even more remarkable, soldiers and marines would receive exactly the same PowerPoint presentations about "combat stress" that they had received prior to deploying upon returning home from a year-long deployment. That is, mental health training was not tailored to where the service members were in the deployment cycle. It is reasonable to assume that the psychological needs of service members would be different upon returning home from combat than when going into combat. While this assumption seems

Resilience and Mental Health: Challenges Across the Lifespan, ed. Steven M. Southwick, Brett T. Litz, Dennis Charney, and Matthew J. Friedman. Published by Cambridge University Press. © Cambridge University Press 2011.

obvious now, it was not until the development of the Battlemind Training System that the content was keyed to the deployment cycle and the concept was acted upon. Indeed, subsequent mental health training programs developed by both the US Marines and US Air Force are now also linked to the phase of the deployment cycle (e.g., the Marine Corps' Warrior Resilience Program).

One of the fundamental questions that existed at the time the Battlemind Training System was being developed was whether mental health training was effective in either preventing or reducing mental health problems, particularly for soldiers deploying to and from combat. Indeed many mental health professionals were understandably skeptical of such an approach. There was little evidence in the scientific literature to suggest that large-scale one-hour programs of any sort could have any significant impact on the resilience of service members (Sharpley *et al.*, 2008). Consequently, the mental health training that was developed should have measurable, long-term effects. That is, the mental health training needed to be based on scientific evidence, but should also be validated scientifically to demonstrate its efficacy. Insisting on scientific validation is critical on several levels. First, it demonstrates that the intervention provides some benefit and is therefore worth time and personnel resources. Second, it demonstrates the limits to the effects of such training so that important outcomes can be targeted in other ways. Third, it provides a standard that can be used to guide decision making for senior leaders faced with a myriad of well-intentioned programs and requests for funding and access to troops. In effect, additional validated training can ensure that opportunists are less likely to be successful in selling unsubstantiated training to the military.

A brief history of Battlemind Training

The Battlemind concept was originally articulated by General Crosbie Saint in a senior leader training guide (*Battlemind guidelines for battalion commanders*) while he was serving as the Commanding General of the US Army, Europe (Saint, 1992). In this guide, Saint emphasized the role of the senior leader in preparing the soldier for the human dimensional aspects of combat. Saint's message described Battlemind as "a warrior's fortitude in the face of danger." Consequently, Battlemind was originally a concept created by the warfighter for the warfighter.

Once Saint left his post upon retirement, the Battlemind concept languished and, therefore, initially did not continue to have an impact on how the US Army prepared for combat. In 2005, the Battlemind Training guide was "re-discovered" and re-shaped as a mental health training program for soldiers and junior leaders (e.g., Castro, 2006; Castro *et al.*, 2006a). Numerous training modules were developed that encompassed the entire deployment cycle, providing soldiers and leaders with mental health training and education tailored for where they were in the deployment cycle. Scientific rigor was also applied where possible to evaluate whether the various Battlemind Training modules accomplished the intended goals (Adler *et al.*, 2007, 2009a; Mental Health Advisory Team, 2008; Thomas *et al.*, 2007). Equally important, however, at the direction of the Secretary of the Army, the Battlemind Training System was integrated into the institutional army via the Deployment Cycle Support Program and the army's formal officer and non-commissioned officer career training courses (Department of the Army, 2007). For this reason, Battlemind Training has been chosen to illustrate the concepts of developing and implementing mental health training within an occupational health context.

Recently, the Battlemind Training System was selected as one of the three programs to be integrated into Comprehensive Soldier Fitness (CSF), a broad US Army initiative (Cornum *et al.*, 2011). This initiative ensures in-depth resilience training that integrates fundamental resilience skills based on work from the Pennsylvania Resiliency Program, performance psychology techniques from the Center for Enhanced Performance, and resilience skills focused on the military occupational context (the former Battlemind Training System). The training and implementation principles discussed in this chapter are also exemplified by the efforts taken with CSF, including the need for evidence-based training and program evaluation (Lester *et al.*, 2011).

Definitions

Before beginning a discussion of the principles of mental health training and implementation considerations, it is useful to provide a few key definitions in order to clarify what is being discussed and prevent confusion.

Mental health training

The central concept to be defined is mental health training. The Technical Cooperation Program Technical Panel 13 (TP-13) defined it as: "Mental health training is an intervention primarily designed to mitigate mental health problems and/or promote good mental health through skills and knowledge. It is armor for the mind. Mental health training/education involves prevention, or early intervention, not clinical treatment" (Castro, 2008).[1] Two things are important to note in this definition. First, the focus is on training, which implies that the training must contain a skills component. That is not to say mental health training does not include education; it most certainly will have educational components, but education is not the exclusive focus. Second, mental health training is not clinical treatment. So, mental health training should not include a discussion of mental health diagnoses nor should it involve treatment intervention suggestions.

Battlemind

Battlemind is the warrior's inner strength to face the realities of the environment with courage, confidence, and resilience.[2] This means meeting the mental challenges of training, operations, combat, and transitioning home. Warriors with Battlemind take care of themselves, their buddies, and those they lead. Two key components of Battlemind are self-confidence and mental toughness; strengths that all soldiers must have to successfully perform in combat and to navigate between training, operations, combat, and home. Both of these concepts comprise a behavior and an attitude. Self-confidence involves taking calculated risks (the behavior) and having the belief in one's self to handle future challenges (the attitude). Mental toughness demands overcoming obstacles and setbacks (the behavior) and maintaining positive thoughts during times of adversity and challenge (the attitude). The goal of Battlemind Training is to build and foster self-confidence and mental toughness (Castro, 2004, 2005).

Resilience

Resilience has many definitions, spanning many dimensions, including psychological, spiritual, physical, and emotional, among others. For the purposes of this chapter, the definition developed by TP-13 (Castro, 2008) is adopted, defining resilience from a psychological perspective: "Resilience comprises the sum total of the psychological processes that permit individuals to maintain or return to previous levels of well-being and functioning in response to adversity."

Similarly, the panel rejected definitions that focused on resilience as a collection of attributes or risk/protective factors that confer susceptibility/resistance to the harmful effects of adversity, such as the presence or absence of childhood adversity. While such attributes are interesting and important as covariates, the panel was mainly interested in the *psychological or behavioral mechanisms by which these attributes confer risk or protection*. The driving consideration here is the pragmatic aspect of being better able to enhance resilience using psychological or behavioral interventions, and to examine potential interactions between individual characteristics and interventions to enhance resilience (Zamorski, 2008).

As the paragraph above suggests, the panel included behavioral aspects of psychological process in its definition of resilience. This definition reflects the fact that the panel viewed resilience as a latent construct that is *inferred* through the preservation of well-being and functioning in response to adversity. The panel felt that other definitions imply more than is really known about resilience by focusing on one or more specific processes, which may indeed contribute to resilience *but are not necessarily the only such processes*. There may come a time when the processes that confer such protection will be understood sufficiently well that resilience can be defined as such processes rather than as the consequence of their application, but the field is not yet ready for such distinctions.

The latency of the resilience construct means that its presence can only be convincingly demonstrated after exposure to adversity. Nevertheless, it seems likely that resilience must exist in some form prior to the experience of adversity, even if it cannot yet be demonstrated convincingly. The panel conceptualized resilience as being processes specific to the person, rather than the sum total of factors (including environmental and social factors) that contribute to the capacity to experience adversity without long-lasting harm (Zamorski, 2008). Environmental and social factors (such as social support) are certainly important factors that merit study, but the panel's interest in such factors was in the role that such factors play as covariates, mediators, or moderators.

Resilience is important for both traumatic and non-traumatic stressors, although the former has attracted much more attention, particularly in the military context. Similarly, the distress or dysfunction that occurs in response to adversity can take many forms beyond the well-known symptom complex of post-traumatic stress disorder (PTSD). For example, depression, risk-taking behavior, acting out, alcohol abuse, and other behaviors can emerge following stressful experiences, and the impact of these behaviors on quality of life and functioning may be greater than PTSD. Despite the importance of broadening the way in which outcomes are considered, the TP-13 panel viewed the measurement of resilience as the assessment of those psychological processes that contribute to recovery after adversity and did not exclusively focus on outcomes. While measurement of the outcomes of distress and dysfunction are critical for the *validation* of resilience measures, such outcome assessment should not be confused with the processes inherent in resilience itself. For example, if an individual is resilient, then they may not experience depression in the presence of some stressor. This lack of depression is not resilience but rather a marker that a resilient process has occurred.

The concept of resilience has become increasingly attractive to mental health specialists. It is consistent with the positive psychology movement (e.g., Seligman & Csikszentmihalyi, 2000) and provides researchers with an alternative approach to understanding why some individuals falter under stress, by focusing on why some individuals do not. For the purposes of this discussion, we do not distinguish between resilience training and mental health training; good mental health training should be the same thing as good resilience training. To make a distinction at this point would be to imply a level of specificity, which neither concept can yet claim. The specific terms may be adopted for meeting the needs of specific organizational goals.

Mental fitness

A new term that is emerging and that also requires a working definition is mental fitness. Mental fitness can be viewed as the psychological equivalent of physical fitness and can be defined as "an individual's capacity to sustain mental health and performance in a demanding environment" (Adler, 2009, p. 5). In contrast to resilience, mental fitness is not a process but a characteristic or state of an individual that can be measured before, during, or after mental health training.

Integrating the definitions

The four key definitions in this chapter – mental health training, Battlemind, resilience, and mental fitness – are clearly interrelated. From the perspective of an organization such as the military, the goal is to develop mental health training, like Battlemind Training, that can increase resilience and mental fitness. Both resilience and mental fitness can be measured as a way to determine the efficacy of mental health training. Resilience, however, can only be inferred in the presence of significant stressors, whereas mental fitness can be measured directly by the presence of skills and capacity. Both resilience and mental fitness, however, demonstrate the potential for mental health training to have an impact on well-being. Effective mental health training is not only based on the content of the training but also on overarching principles that can be used to guide the development of mental health training content.

Fundamental principles of mental health training

The foundations of effective mental health training rest on several fundamental principles (Box 22.1). In developing the mental health training modules for the Battlemind Training System, care was taken to adhere to each of these principles. One could easily argue that these principles are not unique to mental health training, but to all good training, regardless of the topic or domain. However, explicitly stating these principles can guide the development of new modules, thus contributing to the coherency of an integrated training system. Furthermore, without being cognizant of these specific principles, one or more of them may be more likely to be overlooked or violated by those who attempt to develop mental health training. It should be kept in mind that, while the principles of mental health training and the principles of implementation are discussed separately, these principles certainly influence each other. In the following sections, each is discussed in the context of the US Army. Other organizations, however, should be able to easily adapt these concepts for application with their population.

Strength-based approach

Effective mental health training should build on skills and strengths that soldiers and military families already possess. A strength-based approach explicitly rejects a deficit or medical model. Practically, being strength-based means providing a positive approach that sets the expectation of success for the individual and does not reinforce stereotypes that individuals are weak or will become sick as a result of some stressful experience like deployment.

Principles of mental health training

- Strength based
- Relevant purpose and content
- Based on experience
- Explanatory
- Team-based approach
- Action-based strategies
- Developmental approach
- Comprehensive and integrated training
- User acceptability
- Evidence-based and validated methodology

Principles of implementation

- Integration into the organizational culture
- Appropriate in timing
- Quality control
- Train-the-trainer program
- Exportable and scalable
- Training guidelines
- Refresher training
- Mobile training teams
- Sustainability
- Program improvement
- Policy
- Leader supported
- Verifiable claims
- Packaging and multimedia
- Ownership

The strength-based approach also explicitly builds on existing skills and abilities. In the case of the Battlemind Training System, individuals are reminded of the skills that they already possess, and new skills tap into these existing skills. For example, the training emphasizes the importance of building relationships back home. The individuals are reminded that they already have the skills to build relationships, as evidenced by the strong bonds they have formed with their battle buddies. Existing strengths and skills provide a scaffold by which new skills and information can contribute to the resilience of an individual. In addition, since a medical model is rejected, mental health training does not need to include a list of mental health symptoms or include a discussion of mental health diagnosis, as is found in many military mental health training programs.

There is a fine line, however, between avoiding a medical model in which symptoms are prescribed, or at least elucidated, and providing individuals with enough information about typical reactions so that they know what is normal and what might be a sign that professional help is warranted. This balance must be maintained throughout the training and continually re-examined. One way to maintain this balance is to obtain feedback from participants about their perception of the training message and to ensure that the training addresses how existing strengths and new skills can be applied, and that it provides sufficient time to practice those skills before they are needed.

Relevant purpose and content

All training should have a clear purpose or objective, and all the training content should support that purpose. Consistent with this principle, the content for mental health training should be based on documented needs. In the case of the Battlemind Training System, the topics covered in the training modules were based on extensive surveys and interviews with deployed and re-deploying soldiers, as well as with family members. Rather than making assumptions about what soldiers experienced, or what they needed to know, the training was informed by an ongoing systematic assessment. Feedback from this research then influenced the development of the content of each of the Battlemind Training modules. By using this kind of rigorous approach, the training can avoid being the product of a trainer's idiosyncratic experience, which can lead to a training program of limited value.

One example from Battlemind Training's pre-deployment module illustrates this point. The purpose of the module provided right before deployment is to prepare soldiers mentally for what to expect in a combat environment, and to remind them about specific actions that they can take to mitigate the impact of these experiences on their psychological health. The need for this pre-deployment module emerged from focus groups with soldiers who described not being prepared mentally for what they encountered on deployment. Moreover, the content of this preparation was based on surveys and focus group interviews with soldiers when they were asked about their deployment experiences. Thus, in pre-deployment Battlemind Training, the focus is on what soldiers can expect to encounter in the deployed environment that may affect them, and not on how the deployment is going to change them, or on what to expect when they return from deployment. Certainly these other issues are important, but they are reserved for when soldiers return home as part of the post-deployment modules. Relevance refers not only to content but to the timing of the training so that the training matches the needs of the group at that time.

Based on experience

Good mental health training should also include scenarios and situational training that reinforces the information and skills being trained (Thompson & McCreary, 2006). For every skill or educational point addressed in the training, there should be a real-world example that can be used to reinforce that point. In the case of the Battlemind Training, examples should be used that the soldiers and/or families can relate to and that use the language of the military. These examples should be based on experiences of soldiers, not on the experiences of the trainer. When trainers are mental health professionals, their personal examples may undermine their credibility. The trainers may appear misguided if they appear to think that their experience of deployment or stress mirrors the experience of a junior soldier on patrol, a non-commissioned officer in logistics, or an officer in command of a combat arms unit. The Battlemind Training System sought to overcome this problem by developing detailed speaker notes that contain numerous real-world examples from experienced soldiers that the mental health trainer could use in conducting the training.

Explanatory

Good mental health training is explanatory; it highlights conflicted or misunderstood reactions that service members might experience. The Battlemind Training System includes numerous examples of how soldiers might experience mixed or contradictory reactions and emphasizes that these reactions are normal. For example, while soldiers are happy to be home from a long combat deployment, they also often report being angry and on edge. The training normalizes this dual experience and explains that while many soldiers report being happy to see their family and friends, they are often angry about being deployed for a year or angry about how they were treated during the deployment. Providing soldiers with the words to understand

this mixed reaction can help them to understand and normalize it. The development of explanations for such complex and conflicted reactions requires professional expertise in behavioral health.

A team-based approach

The military organization is fundamentally based on teams, on leadership, and on unit cohesion. Any mental health training with the military needs to integrate these fundamental components of the organization. Military mental health training should take advantage of the natural camaraderie and hierarchy that exists within all military cultures. For example, in Battlemind Training, unit cohesion is one of the core elements of all of the training modules. Each module teaches how to look after other unit members and uses this buddy focus as a way to also increase self-awareness. The Battlemind Training modules also highlight the role of leaders and the leaders' responsibilities for ensuring that their subordinates get the mental healthcare they need. The training is typically also provided in a unit context in order to reinforce the material across the group. Battlemind trainers also report anecdotally that unit members will comment to one another during the group training and point out particular reactions that relate to a unit member, interacting in a way that enhances the relevance of the material.

Action-based strategies

Mental health training should address specific actions individuals can take, not just be a theoretical description of stress responses. These actions should be able to guide the behavior of soldiers and spouses. The Battlemind Training System is designed to focus on such behaviors, and future iterations of Battlemind Training modules are being fielded to test the efficacy of teaching specific skills. In keeping with the team-based approach mentioned above, these actions include behaviors that soldiers can take to help themselves, their buddies, and those they lead.

One of the key components to teaching action-based strategies is the need for flexible and adaptive coping in response to a myriad of potential stressors. The training needs to specifically advance the idea that there are different types of stressor and which coping mechanism is best depends on how much direct control the individual has over the stressor. For many military personnel, significant stressors are outside of their direct control and so they need to practice action-based strategies that are not "action" in the sense of getting rid of the stressor. The action may involve a change in cognitive coping, a reduction in physiological arousal, seeking social support, or acceptance. Redefining action as incorporating each of these kinds of skill, and emphasizing the need to match the appropriate coping response to the situation, is a key part of an integrated mental health training system.

Developmental approach

Effective training builds on prior training or upon existing strengths and skills and progressively adds new concepts and skills. Ideally, we believe that a mental health training system should strive to develop skills of increasing complexity, beginning with simple concepts. For example, the training can introduce a simple approach to cognitive restructuring in managing the stressors of basic combat training while waiting until later in the career of a soldier to teach how cognitive restructuring can be used to manage a high-stress environment such as combat deployment. Another example of the developmental approach is to introduce the concepts of PTSD without detailing the complexities of the diagnostic criteria. The initial training could include an overall appreciation for how PTSD-related reactions can interfere with getting along with friends, family, and at work without discussing the disorder itself. This approach avoids the temptation of presenting PTSD criteria in an oversimplified manner that might inadvertently lead soldiers to think that they have PTSD if they have only a few PTSD symptoms. In subsequent courses for certain personnel, such as leaders or medics, more information could be presented about symptoms, symptom clusters, and time course. Such information underscores the need for content to be informed by experts in mental health, as will be discussed under implementation principles.

Comprehensive and integrated training

Implicit throughout this chapter is the assumption that mental health training needs to be more than a single session. Mental health training should not be one-off training that occurs only once a year, only when the service member gets ready to deploy, or only when the service member returns from deployment. It needs to provide the target population with an integrated and comprehensive system that builds skills, reinforces concepts, and targets areas of relevance to the group at the right time. In addition, of course, the fundamental

framework, mental health vocabulary, and actions should be consistent across the training system.

Although the first module of the Battlemind Training System developed was an immediate post-deployment intervention, it was clear that a broader approach was needed. For example, the development team recognized that the training needed to include a follow-up post-deployment module and a spouse module, prior to deployment. Later, based on feedback from training and from army leaders, the Battlemind Training System was expanded to target leadership, medics, mental health providers, and soldiers in various career courses, beginning with basic combat training. By conceptualizing mental health training as an integrated system, the lesson plans can build on one another and can reinforce the points of each training module as exemplified by the CSF initiative.

At this point in the development of the Battlemind Training System, the modules provide a comprehensive and integrated mental health training approach. For example, the deployment-related modules build upon and reinforce each other. The pre-deployment modules prepare soldiers and leaders to deploy to a combat environment (McGurk *et al.*, 2007); the in-theater psychological debriefings sustain soldiers throughout the deployment and reinforce Battlemind Training principles (Adler *et al.*, 2009b); the post-deployment module prepares soldiers and leaders for the reintegration process immediately upon returning home from combat (Adler *et al.*, 2009a; Thomas *et al.*, 2007); and the follow-up module allows soldiers and leaders to reassess their mental health status to determine if they are in need of additional mental healthcare (Adler *et al.*, 2007). Spouse training was also developed for before and after deployment (see also Chapter 16). Finally, modules have been developed that target medical providers; leadership in junior, mid-level, and senior leaders (non-commissioned officers and officers); and soldiers first entering military service. The Battlemind Training System was the first training program in the military to take a comprehensive approach to mental health training across the entire deployment and life cycle.

The Battlemind Training System is well recognized and has been a vehicle for communicating deployment-related mental health literacy among a wide range of military personnel (e.g., Slone & Friedman, 2008). The demand for these deployment and life cycle modules by the military has at time presented the development team at the Walter Reed Army Institute of Research with a dilemma: wait for group randomized trials to be completed or derive the essential elements from modules that have been studied, implement the training, and then follow this implementation with program evaluation and randomized trials to improve training. In order to meet the immediate need, the development team, along with members of the Battlemind Training Office at the Army Medical Department Center and School, produced a series of Battlemind Training modules.

User acceptability

Mental health training must be perceived to be useful by those being trained in order for the training to become accepted into the organizational culture. Even if the training is efficacious, if it is not face valid, the audience does not accept it, and the trainers do not support it, then the training quality is likely to deteriorate or drift and resentment may preclude it from being helpful. In the case of the Battlemind Training System, surveys and interviews with soldiers and spouses after training found that the modules were relevant and useful. However, while user acceptability is necessary, it is not sufficient for establishing good mental health training (Iverson *et al.*, 2008; Sharpley *et al.*, 2008; McKibben *et al.*, 2009). In order to demonstrate that mental health training improves mental fitness, randomized controlled studies must be conducted.

Evidence-based and validated methodology

What does it mean to say "evidence based?" The material in the training needs to be based on research evidence and the training itself needs to be validated. This validation extends beyond satisfaction ratings or demonstration of changes from pre- to post-training. The standard needed for demonstrating mental health training efficacy is a randomized controlled trial. For training that is conducted in intact groups, randomization needs to occur at the level of the group, not the individual. Therefore, group randomized trials are needed (Donner & Klar, 2004; Varnell *et al.*, 2004). This approach can be difficult, time consuming, and complex statistically but the end result is evidence assessing the training's effectiveness. Exactly what these studies assess as markers of effectiveness depends on the goal of the training.

There are many possible markers of a successful mental health training program. Typically, in order to assess a program's effectiveness, the outcomes should match the intent of the program. Historically, much of the research on early interventions has focused on PTSD symptoms, and other researchers have criticized this limited view (Deahl *et al.*, 2001). For our purposes, military mental health training outcomes should include measures of (1) attitude, (2) skill attainment, (3) mental health fitness, (4) training satisfaction, and (5) unit climate and leadership.

First, in terms of attitudes, mental health training should target self-confidence in handling challenges and monitoring positive thoughts during times of adversity. Second, in terms of skill sets, outcomes should address the specific skills and knowledge addressed in the training. For example, training may address knowledge about anxiety management and providing buddy aid. Third, in terms of mental health fitness, outcome indicators should include measures of distress that go beyond traditional PTSD symptoms as well as measures of positive well-being. Outcomes of relevance to the organization should be included, such as aggression, sleep, relationship qualities, and risk-taking behaviors. Fourth, as mentioned above, measures of training satisfaction and user acceptability should be included. Fifth, measures of unit climate should be included because the training can have an impact on the way the unit climate is perceived and because the training can have an impact on the leadership itself. Therefore, these measures should address the degree to which mental health training may have had an impact on cohesion and leadership quality. Indeed research has found that the Battlemind Training System increased soldier perception of organizational support (Thomas *et al.*, 2007). Similarly, the training should also assess the degree to which leaders support the mental health skills and training provided by the organization. Without support from the leadership, the training will likely be less effective.

One outcome measure that may be considered but that is difficult to interpret is whether or not individuals seek help for clinical services as a function of training. On the one hand, if seeking help for mental health problems increases, then this outcome may be an indicator of greater openness to help-seeking, greater awareness of mental health problems, and less stigma associated with seeking care. On the other hand, seeking help for mental health problems could be an indicator of greater distress. Consequently, without a clear rationale, this outcome can lead to results that are difficult to disentangle.

To date, there have been three group randomized controlled trials conducted with post-deployment Battlemind Training. In these studies, platoons recently returned from a year in Iraq were randomly assigned to either a Battlemind Training condition or a comparison condition. For the immediate post-deployment training studies (Adler *et al.*, 2009a; Thomas *et al.*, 2007), the comparison condition was traditional stress education. Follow-up surveys were administered about four months later. For the study in which Battlemind Training was provided four months after returning home, follow-up surveys were administered six months later (Adler *et al.*, 2009). In terms of training satisfaction, all Battlemind Training interventions have received high ratings in terms of user acceptability.

In terms of attitudes, these studies have found that soldiers reported fewer stigma-related attitudes toward seeking help for mental health problems after participating in Battlemind Training. In terms of mental health fitness, for the most part, these studies have found that Battlemind Training is associated with fewer PTSD symptoms (Adler *et al.*, 2007, 2009a; Thomas *et al.*, 2007), depression symptoms (Adler *et al.*, 2007, 2009a), anger problems (Adler *et al.*, 2007), and sleep problems (Adler *et al.*, 2009a). In the Adler *et al.* (2009a) study, effects on PTSD symptoms and sleep problems were found only for those soldiers reporting high levels of combat experiences, although main effects for intervention condition were found for depression symptoms. Main effects were found for the other two group randomized controlled trials. In terms of unit climate, Thomas *et al.* (2007) reported that Battlemind Training resulted in improved perceived organizational support relative to traditional stress education.

While effect sizes were small (e.g., Cohen's *d* values of 0.20–0.30), these studies demonstrate the potential for single-session mental health interventions to improve the adjustment of soldiers returning from combat. Small effect sizes are typically found in field research (Bliese *et al.*, 2011) because the overall model error is larger than in experimental studies (McClelland & Judd, 1993), and a small effect size may have important practical significance. For example, while an effect size of 0.21 is usually considered small, Rosenthal and Rubin (1982) argued that the effect size represents a success rate of 45% versus 55% between two groups. When this effect is assessed in the context of training large numbers of soldiers, the effect size can be considered practically meaningful from a public health perspective. Future studies will examine the impact of Battlemind Training on specific initiatives such as managing intrusive thoughts (Shipherd & Salters-Pedneault, 2008), expressive writing (Adler *et al.*, 2008), and specific coping skill attainment (e.g., Adler, 2009).

Fundamental principles of implementation

When mental health training content is being developed and validated, how the training will be implemented should be considered. While distinct, the training content and processes (the implementation strategy) dramatically influence each other. The key implementation principles regarding mental health training in organizations are given in Box 22.1 and discussed below. While this is not an exhaustive list of all the implementation issues that need to be considered when developing mental health training, it does represent the common issues that arise.

Integration into the organizational culture

Military mental health training must be integrated into the organization's culture (Thomas & Castro, 2003). In the case of the US Army, this means that Battlemind needs to be called "training" and not "education," as the military leadership understands and promotes "training" but not necessarily "education." In fact, many military leaders view education as an unnecessary use of valuable soldier time. This distinction does not mean that mental health training cannot contain educational material, but it does mean that the mental health training needs to involve skill strengthening or skill development. In the context of a military academy, however, the terminology may need to emphasize "education" rather than "training." In other nations, for example Germany and the Netherlands, the two concepts are regarded as sequential. The first phase of the program has to be termed "education" and the second phase in which the skills are practiced is termed "training." The larger issue is that the language used to describe and promote the program needs to make sense within the organizational context.

Mental health training should also be conducted within existing units, preferably at the platoon or company level in order to optimize the impact of small group dynamics and leadership. Conducting mental health training in small, pre-existing groups ensures group members will have the opportunity to share their experiences with each other, and feel comfortable enough to do so. Training conducted in large groups in an auditorium or gymnasium runs the risk of being too impersonal, and too large for focused skill development to occur. In general, mental health training conducted in large groups is likely to become educational or didactic in nature, with little interaction or sharing of the group members' personal experiences. In the case of Battlemind Training, the training was deliberately designed to be conducted in small groups, with group members sharing their experiences. The role of the trainer is to facilitate these group interactions. The degree to which group size actually influences the efficacy of the training remains unclear. Indeed, Thomas *et al*. (2007) compared small and large group Battlemind Training and did not find reliable differences between the two types.

Appropriate in timing

Mental health training should be relevant to the deployment cycle or the stage of professional development. This point has been made above but it deserves repeating. For example, mental health training designed to be given prior to deploying should not be given during the deployment, nor should mental health training designed to be given at post-deployment be given during the deployment or prior to deploying. Since the content of mental health training should vary depending on the phase of the deployment, it stands to reason that the training cannot be used interchangeably.

When training programs are promoted as useful regardless of when they are implemented in the deployment cycle phase, the training itself becomes suspect in terms of its relevance to the organizational context. Training that is independent of the deployment cycle appears to underestimate the importance of the different stressors associated with the deployment cycle phases and how these stressors influence the well-being of service members. Creating a one-size-fits-all approach to the training cycle is not likely to meet the needs of service members and families, as their needs change depending on the phase of the deployment. Proponents and/or developers of such global approaches to mental health training fail to recognize the organizational context and may not have ensured that the needs of the service members are adequately addressed.

In the Battlemind Training System, mental health training modules are distinct for each phase of the development cycle and are focused on the specific needs of the soldier and spouse. This tailored approach was an outcome based on the scientific evidence obtained by the development team at the Walter Reed Army Institute of Research regarding soldier and family deployment-related health and the team's real-world experience working with soldiers before, during, and after combat deployments. The team's multidisciplinary expertise (psychiatry, psychology, sociology, and social work) and experience enabled the development of the US Army's first integrated and comprehensive mental health training program.

Quality control

Any standardized training program requires a robust quality control program to ensure that the training is being conducted as intended. Constant vigilance is required to ensure that the content of the mental health training is maintained; the content should not be altered nor should additional material be inserted into the training modules. Further, the mental health training needs to be conducted using the procedures that have been validated. For the Battlemind Training System, this would mean that that the training needs to be conducted in small, intact groups, with a trained facilitator to guide the group interactions. A mental health training quality control program should systematically ensure that trainers are prepared to conduct the training, that the training materials and lesson plans are clear and detailed, and that the training conducted remains consistent. Maintaining quality training can be difficult in a large organization such as the military. Mechanisms such as refresher courses, team teaching, training evaluation, and spot checking by a mobile team responsible for training quality can facilitate quality sustainment over time.

Train-the-trainer program

The first step in preventing drift in the content and implementation is to develop a train-the-trainer program in which each mental health trainer receives formal training and certification which confirms that they are capable of delivering the training program to standard. At a minimum, a train-the-trainer program should include the training material, a detailed course syllabus, and detailed speaker notes. A train-the-trainer course should also include practice for the individuals who are being certified as trainers and an evaluation of their training performance. Only after the individual being trained has shown competence in giving the mental health training, and in answering anticipated questions regarding the training, should they be certified. A train-the-trainer program, however, does not preclude the need for a quality control program, as drift in training can still occur.

Obviously during the development of a mental health training program, it must be decided who will be conducting the training. For example, will the mental health training be conducted by behavioral healthcare providers, chaplains, experienced combat arms service members, or some other group? This decision needs to be addressed early in the training development process because the decision regarding who conducts the training is likely to shape the content of the training material. Regardless of what decision is made regarding who conducts the mental health training, it should be noted that, while individuals may have a personal preference for one type of trainer, in terms of Battlemind Training at least, trainer effects were not associated with differential rates of training efficacy. In one study, for example, trainers included behavioral health officers, enlisted soldiers with behavioral health training, and civilians (Adler *et al.*, 2009a). Some had combat deployment experience; others did not. In the immediate aftermath, when individuals rated the training atmosphere and their satisfaction with the training, there were differences in the way trainers were rated. Therefore, at this point, there were indeed statistical differences across trainers in the post-session ratings. However, when outcomes were assessed four months later, there were no significant differences across trainers. The training material itself drove the effects, not the trainer. This distinction is important because when training is implemented in an organization on a large scale it will be difficult to ensure that only the best trainers are used; the training material itself needs to be the key ingredient rather than a trainer's personal style. Personal style cannot be dictated in a set of lesson plan instructions.

In examining the question of who should provide the training, we have also noted that soldiers have different opinions on what constitutes an ideal mental health trainer. Some soldiers say they would prefer an experienced combat veteran; others prefer knowing that the information is being provided by an expert in mental health. Consequently, the train-the-trainer program should address how individual trainers can

best manage these conflicting preferences. Regardless of who these trainers are, they will need to acknowledge what they are not. If they are not experts in mental health, they can talk about how the material has been developed by mental health professionals experienced in working with the military. If they have not been deployed, they can talk about how the material has been developed based on what soldiers have said is important to know. Even if the trainer has deployment experience, this experience can be misleading – establishing a link to the service members that is not really there. For example, most trainers with deployment experience are not likely to have been a junior enlisted combat arms soldier out on patrol every day. The train-the-trainer course needs to underscore the reality that the trainers cannot be everything to all people. The trainers can acknowledge what they do bring to training in terms of their expertise, but most importantly they can bring their level of commitment, their enthusiasm, and their professionalism.

Exportable and scalable

Regardless of who conducts the mental health training, a mental health training program must be designed with the average trainer in mind, not the ideal trainer. Whatever the mental health training program, it must be exportable and scalable. For example, a mental health training program will be of little utility to large organizations such as the military if only a handful of people in the world are capable of conducting the training or if it takes years to train others to conduct the training. Surprisingly, this obvious criterion for a useful military mental health program is often not considered or is dismissed by various advocates of mental health training programs, who insist that trainers of various mental health training programs require many years of experience. In one example, outside experts offering a training program to the US Army patiently explained that the only people able to provide the specific training would have to embrace the training on a personal level and spend years of their life attaining "deep experience" with the material before they could train others, and this experience might be obtained in remote sites in other countries. Even if the training content could be validated, such approaches to mental health training are of questionable value to the military because they cannot be implemented across a million or more soldiers in any kind of realistic time frame.

Training guidelines

Another means to ensure that mental health training is conducted consistently across military installations and over time is to develop clear guidelines as to how the training is to be conducted. In military language, this approach to training is known as establishing "task, condition, and standard." Task, conditions, and standards are applied to every form of training conducted in the military, regardless of the type. The task component of this approach specifies exactly what needs to be accomplished. The conditions specify the context or the variables in a situation that may affect performance. Finally, the standards delineate the markers of success. Consequently, a "task, condition, standard" approach to mental health training details the exact training that is to be conducted, who is to be trained, who is to conduct the training, the environment in which the training is conducted, and the means for assessing the effectiveness of the training. This standardized approach to mental health training will also facilitate a rigorous quality control program that can evaluate if the training is being conducted as intended.

Here again, some proponents of mental health training programs proposed for use in the military state that their training should not or cannot be subjected to such rigid procedures. On inspection, proposed mental health training programs that cannot be standardized are programs that have not been scientifically validated. Indeed, there is a common ground between the rigor required in a military's "task, condition, standard" approach and the rigor required of a randomized trial, in which the methods have to be stated clearly so as to facilitate replication and critical review. It appears that the non-standardized programs tend to drift in their approach from one set of procedures to another, or from one trainer to another. Needless to say, such non-standardized programs cannot be expanded on a large scale, nor are they easily amendable to scientific investigation.

Refresher training

Like most effective training, mental health training should contain refresher training modules. Service members should not be repeatedly subjected to the exact same mental health training material because the training will inevitably become stale, which will likely blunt its effectiveness. Various modules provided over time and over the course of the deployment cycle serve to reinforce the key principles, but refresher modules should certainly also be developed. We are unaware of refresher courses being integrated into other organization-based mental health training programs, although a mental health course in Australian recruit training is being developed to integrate a "booster" session midway through basic training.

Mobile training teams

Implementing mental health training on a large scale can be facilitated through the use of mobile training teams. These teams can train service members directly but, more importantly, they can also conduct train-the-trainer courses to certify other trainers. In the case of the Battlemind Training System, for example, the Battlemind Training Office at the Army Medical Department Center and School successfully used mobile training teams to accomplish both of these objectives. The new CSF also uses mobile training teams.

Sustainability

Whatever mental health training program is adopted, it must be sustainable and supportable. The importance of the trainer and standardization has already been discussed in some detail. Equally important is how long the training needs to be in order for it to be effective in increasing mental fitness. In the military context, training time is a valuable commodity that must compete with a myriad of other demands. The modules contained in the Battlemind Training System were deliberately developed to be given in one-hour sessions in order to integrate the modules into busy unit schedules. In developing the modules, the development team recognized that a mental health training program could easily be developed that could consume upwards of 40 hours of training time. However, it was felt that commanders would resist a program that was so time consuming, particularly if this time occurs during the pre-deployment train-up phase.

The fact that a one-hour session has been found in three studies to reduce mental health symptoms related to combat exposure supports the feasibility of this economical approach. The key question now becomes how the one-hour modules can be enhanced to increase effectiveness. Although one-hour modules are effective, judicious use of additional training should be tested in order to improve the efficacy of the entire system. Whatever system results, it must remain cognizant of the issue of time as well as other resources, such as personnel, equipment, and coordination. If too many resources are required, then the training program may not be sustainable in the long run.

Program improvement

Along with ensuring that the training program can be sustained in terms of implementation, there also needs to be a vigorous system for continually assessing whether the mental health training program is achieving its stated goals and to identify how the program can be improved. Unfortunately, military leaders may be reluctant to commit resources for program assessment and improvement. Without such a program in place, however, there will be no systematic, ongoing analyses to ensure that the mental health needs of service members and families are still being met. Such improvement efforts are not only important for ensuring the program remains effective but also provide another way to ensure that service members do not become bored by the same material.

Policy

Even the most effective mental health training cannot be successful without a parallel effort on the part of the organization to institutionalize its implementation (Thomas & Castro, 2003). In the case of the military, policy must be developed that supports and directs that mental health training be conducted. There must also be guidance issued that describes how the training will be implemented (see the discussion of the "task, condition, standard" approach above). In short, orders must be given that mandate that military mental health training occur. Otherwise, such training will be left up to the discretion of each commander, usually with the result that the training is not conducted to the standard that has been shown to be effective, or it will not be conducted at all. Regarding the Battlemind Training System, the Secretary of the Army mandated that it should be conducted for all deploying and re-deploying soldiers and that training opportunities be provided to spouses. The CSF initiative was implemented with similar policy directives.

Leader supported

Whether the training is mandated or not, leaders are critical for the successful implementation of mental health training. Leaders at all levels play an important role in the mental health of service members, both directly and indirectly (Britt *et al.*, 2004; Castro *et al.*,

2006b). Consequently, their explicit and implicit support for a program can mean the difference between a supportive training environment and one in which the training is conducted as a way to "check the block" – simply meeting a specific organizational requirement. Leaders can demonstrate their support for mental health training by attending the training themselves, by emphasizing the importance of the mental health training to their subordinates, and by ensuring that the training is a priority on the unit calendar. Research evidence demonstrating the efficacy of mental health training can directly impact the leader's endorsement of the program. If scientific findings can be provided to leaders showing them that mental health training is effective in increasing the mental fitness of their unit, then they are more likely to support the training. Obtaining high-profile endorsements from senior enlisted service members and officers can also enhance the acceptability of mental health training. The Battlemind Training System received endorsements from senior Army leaders and has served to change the Army culture regarding mental health training. Similarly, CSF has received Army support from high levels.

Verifiable claims

Credibility requires that any claims made regarding mental health training be consistent with verifiable facts that are based on scientific evidence (for a review of military mental health prevention efforts, see Castro *et al.* [2004] and Mulligan *et al.* [2010]). Unfortunately, developers or proponents of various mental health training programs sometimes make unsubstantiated claims regarding what their training program can achieve. These unsubstantiated claims range from preventing PTSD to improving decision making in combat. Perhaps the proponents for these programs become caught up in an enthusiastic attempt to implement their work and neglect the lack of scientific evidence. Perhaps they are more focused on being sure to present their product in a way that is relevant to the organization and they underestimate the degree to which scientific evidence matters. Regardless of their motivation, the end effect is that proponents of these unsubstantiated claims are able to prey upon the hope, fear, and ignorance of unit leaders to gain access to service members, usually with the unit paying for the training. Such unethical behavior should not be tolerated by the organization or by the professionals promoting their training programs. Leaders need to be provided with realistic expectations about what mental health training will achieve and what it will not; the organization needs to make decisions based on science in order to differentiate between effective training and another good idea.

Packaging and multimedia

Effective mental health training needs good packaging. While this implementation principle may sound superficial, it is critical because it ultimately means that the information will be presented in such a way that the organization and the individual service member are more likely to accept it. Furthermore, good packaging through catchy slogans or the use of easy-to-remember phrases and acronyms enhances the degree to which individuals are likely to remember the training content. The use of humor can also make mental health training more engaging. Still, care must be exercised to avoid the training becoming so slick that the trainees are put off by the training or the style distracts from the training objective or message.

Wherever possible, multimedia (e.g., interactive computer simulations, video scenarios, music, gaming technology) should be considered in developing a mental health training program. While there is no clear evidence that mental health training is more effective if it employs multimedia, the training is likely to be more engaging, which increases the likelihood that individuals will attend to the training content. Appropriately incorporated and researched multimedia training can also enhance standardization of training. Multimedia approaches also help to underscore a central tenet of training: training should be conducted to engage the three fundamental types of learner: visual learners, who prefer to be able to see the point written out or visually depicted in a diagram; auditory learners, who prefer to listen and discuss the information; and experiential learners, who prefer to practice a concept and grapple with some task related to the concept.

Ownership

The final implementation principle reviewed here is ownership: who actually controls the content of the training program and retains the right to revise it. Mental health and mental fitness issues facing service members and their families are complex and varied. How to build resilience and increase mental fitness in order to help these people meet the demands of combat

and deployment are equally complex and nuanced. Consequently, the content of the mental health training program needs to belong to military behavioral healthcare experts. The content of mental health training must be determined by behavioral health experts. They are the subject matter experts, not the commander, not the chaplains, not the policy makers, and not others who are interested in helping service members. Obviously, these individuals are expert in their own areas and their input is invaluable for ensuring that the training material addresses issues in a way that is relevant to the audience. In fact, the training development process should actively solicit input from a variety of domains, such as operational leadership, the chaplaincy, military families, and soldiers themselves. However, caring about service member mental health or having been deployed to a combat environment does not make one an expert in mental health training; the behavioral care experts should own the content of the training.

Conclusions and future directions

Lessons learned

Despite using the Battlemind Training System throughout this chapter as a way to illustrate mental health training and implementation principles, it is important to note that the training system encountered significant implementation difficulties. These problems included launching many modules before scientific validation could be conducted, not having a system in place to certify instructors and track who received the training, and not focusing enough on building specific resilience skills. Other mental health training programs have also been fielded prior to proper validation studies being conducted and without a full implementation plan. Such difficulties are part of fielding programs in a real-world setting in which senior leaders demand that something be done immediately.

At some level, these stumbling blocks may be a sign that the mental health training is so meaningful to the leadership that they are willing to direct its implementation without all the training pieces being finalized and validated. It may also partly reflect a lack of communication to leadership about the importance of such plans and studies.

We also recognize that even with dedicated resources to develop and validate mental health training, it is difficult to create training that is interesting, meaningful, and useful. Group randomized trials take years to execute, and the team effort and expertise required should not be underestimated. No doubt, it is for these reasons that there are few examples of validated mental health training modules.

To counteract this common problem, the fielding of mental health training should routinely include a plan to conduct validation research and to address the broader implementation issues identified in this chapter. The awareness of the importance of addressing these concerns appears to be increasing. To date, for example, programs such as CSF and the Australian Defence Force's BattleSMART program are being developed with such plans.

The way ahead

There are numerous occupational hazards associated with serving in the military. One of the greatest physical hazards associated with combat are bullets, fragments, or other explosive munitions; therefore, service members are required to wear body armor for protection. However, there is a limit to the extent that such body armor can protect. Soldiers and marines are still wounded and die from bullets and fragments even when they wear their body armor. Similarly, mental health problems are also an occupational hazard for service members in combat. While mental health training can reduce the symptoms associated with PTSD, it certainly cannot protect every service member from developing a diagnosis of PTSD. Like body armor, there are limits as to what mental health training can achieve – and no matter how much we would like to think otherwise, there are limits to what organizations can do to prevent the negative mental health effects of combat. One useful approach to enhance what can be done to prevent PTSD symptoms and other mental health problems associated with deployment is to view these mental health disorders within an occupational health framework.

Much like the soldier adaptation model developed by Bliese and Castro (2003), an occupational health framework for the military proposes a model for examining the way in which occupational demands have an impact on individual adaptation. While many pre-existing, individual and personality factors may influence the relationship between occupational demands and outcomes, the focus of an occupational health model is on the nature of the occupational stressors (their duration, variability, intensity, predictability, etc.), the training that can be provided to moderate the impact of the demands, the influence of the occupational context on the way in which demands are appraised, and the way in which demands affect outcomes. These organizational factors include multiple levels of moderators from the individual, small group, leader, and organization (Castro & Adler, 2005). By incorporating an occupational perspective into the model, we can take into account factors that can be taught in a mental health training program, such as successful coping strategies and behaviors, the role of professional identity, and finding meaning in one's job. In this way, adopting an occupational health framework can facilitate the development of mental health training targeted specifically on mental health issues inherent within a military context.

This kind of occupational health model does not mean that military mental health training should exclusively focus on deployment-related mental health problems. The focus on mental health problems should be broad enough to address other topics that can adversely impact on service member readiness, such as family readiness and resilience. Both service-related and non-service-related mental health training can be part of a comprehensive, integrated program.

At present, mental fitness does not enjoy the same focus that physical fitness does. Still, the concept of mental fitness is included in the Soldier's Creed: "I am disciplined, physically and mentally tough, trained and proficient in my warrior tasks and drills." By including "mentally tough," the US Army explicitly assumes that mental fitness is a necessary and important element to being a soldier. Within the army, soldiers are required to conduct physical fitness training three times per week and are given time out of the duty day to do so. They are also encouraged to do physical training on their own for the other two days of the week. Physical fitness is taken so seriously in the army that soldiers must pass a physical fitness examination twice a year, and their scores on this examination are used to determine promotion potential. If soldiers receive the maximum score possible on the physical fitness examination then they are often given a four-day pass. Can we ever envision a time when mental fitness is viewed on par with physical fitness? When training time is regularly allotted to maintain mental fitness? When soldiers are tested to ensure they are mentally fit and when they are formally recognized for this resilience? Through defining what we mean by terms such as resilience, mental fitness, and mental health training, and by establishing fundamental principles of mental health training and implementation, we can build toward delivering a system of mental health training for service members that is integrated, relevant, and effective.

Acknowledgement

The views expressed in this chapter are those of the author and do not reflect the official position of the Walter Reed Institute of Research, the US Army, or the US Department of Defense.

References

Adler, A. B. (2009). *Protocol 1543: Basic training and mental fitness study: enhancing performance and mental health.* Silver Spring, MD: Walter Reed Army Institute of Research.

Adler, A. B., Castro, C. A., Bliese, P. D., McGurk, D. & Milliken, C. (2007). The efficacy of Battlemind Training at 3–6 months post-deployment. In *Symposium of the Annual Meeting of the American Psychological Association on the Battlemind Training System: Supporting soldiers throughout the deployment cycle,* San Francisco, August.

Adler, A. B., Bliese, P. D., McGurk, D., *et al.* (2008). Writing about the transition from combat to home: Initial analysis. In *Proceedings of the Force Health Protection Conference,* Albuquerque, August.

Adler, A. B., Bliese, P. D., McGurk, D., Hoge, C. W., & Castro, C. A. (2009a). Battlemind debriefing and battlemind training as early interventions with soldiers returning from Iraq: Randomization by platoon. *Journal of Consulting and Clinical Psychology,* 7, 928–940.

Adler, A. B., Castro, C. A., & McGurk, D. (2009b). Time-driven Battlemind psychological debriefing: A group-level early intervention in combat. *Military Medicine,* 174, 22–28.

Bliese, P. D. & Castro, C. A. (2003). The soldier adaptation model (SAM): applications to peacekeeping research. In T. W Britt & A. B. Adler (eds.), *The psychology of the peacekeeper: Lessons from the field* (pp. 185–204). Westport, CT: Greenwood Publishing.

Bliese, P. D., Adler, A. B., & Castro, C. A. (2011). The deployment context: Psychology and implementing mental health interventions. In A. B. Adler, P. D. Bliese, & C. A. Castro (eds.), *Deployment psychology: evidence-based strategies to promote mental health in the military* (pp. 103–124). Washington, D.C.: American Psychological Association.

Britt, T. W., Davison, J., Bliese, P. D., & Castro, C. A. (2004). How leaders can influence the impact that stressors have on soldiers. *Military Medicine,* 169, 541–545.

Castro, C. A. (2004). How to build Battlemind. *NCO Journal,* April, 23–24.

Castro, C. A. (2005). Building Battlemind. *Countermeasures,* 26, 6–8.

Castro, C. A. (2006). Military courage. In T. W. Britt, A. B. Adler, & C. A. Castro (eds.), *Military life: the psychology of serving in peace and combat,* Vol. 4: *Military culture* (pp. 60–78). Westport, CT: Praeger.

Castro, C. A. (2008). *Symposium of the Annual Meeting of the International Military Testing Association on Military Resiliency: Perspectives from an international technical panel.* Amsterdam, September.

Castro, C. A. & Adler, A. B. (2005). Preface to the special issue. *Military Psychology,* 17, 131–136.

Castro, C. A., Engel, C. C., & Adler, A. B. (2004). The challenge of providing mental health prevention and early intervention in the US military. In B. T. Litz (ed.), *Early intervention for trauma and traumatic loss* (pp. 301–318). New York: Guilford Press.

Castro, C. A., Hoge, C. W., & Cox, A. L. (2006a). Battlemind training: building soldier resiliency. In *Proceedings of RTO-MP-HFM-134, Human dimensions in military operations: Military leaders strategies for addressing stress and psychological support* (Paper 42, pp. 42–1–42–6). Neuilly-sur-Seine, France: NATO Research and Technology Association.

Castro, C. A., Thomas, J. L., & Adler, A. B. (2006b). Towards a liberal theory of military leadership. In A. B. Adler, C. A. Castro, & T. W. Britt (eds.), *Military life: the psychology of serving in peace and combat,* Vol. 2: *Operational stress* (pp. 192–212). Westport, CT: Praeger.

Cornum, R., Matthews, M. D., & Seligman, M. E. P. (2011). Comprehensive soldier fitness: Building resilience in a challenging institutional context. *American Psychologist,* 66, 4–9.

Deahl, M. P., Srinivasan, M., Jones, N., Neblett, C., & Jolly, A. (2001). Commentary. Evaluating psychological debriefing: Are we measuring the right outcomes? *Journal of Traumatic Stress,* 14, 527–529.

Department of the Army (2007). *Deployment cycle support (DCS) directive.* Washington, DC: Department of the Army, http://www.apd.army.mil/pdffiles/ad2007_02.pdf (accessed February 16, 2011).

Donner, A. & Klar, N. (2004). Pitfalls and controversies in cluster randomized trials. *American Journal of Public Health,* 94, 416–422.

Iversen, A. C., Fear, N. T., Hacker Huges, J., *et al.* (2008). Risk factors for post-traumatic stress disorder among UK armed forces personnel. *Psychological Medicine,* 29, 1–12.

Lester, P. B., McBride, S. A., Bliese, P. D. & Adler, A. B. (2011). Bringing science to bear: An empirical assessment of the Comprehensive Soldier Fitness program. *American Psychologist*, **66**, 77–81.

McClelland, G. H. & Judd, C. M. (1993). Statistical difficulties of detecting interactions and moderator effects. *Psychological Bulletin*, **114**, 376–390.

McGurk, D., Castro, C. A., Thomas, J. L., & Hoge, C. W. (2007). Pre-deployment Battlemind Training. In *Symposium of the Annual Meeting of the American Psychological Association on the Battlemind Training System: Supporting soldiers throughout the deployment cycle*, San Francisco, August.

McKibben, E. S., Britt, T. W., Hoge, C. W., & Castro, C. A. (2009). Receipt and rated adequacy of stress management training is related to PTSD and other outcomes among Operational Iraqi Freedom veterans. *Military Psychology*, **21**(Suppl. 2), S68–S81.

Mental Health Advisory Team (2008). *Operation Iraqi Freedom 06–08: Iraq, Operation Enduring Freedom 8.* [Afghanistan Report February 14, 2008.] Washington, DC: US Army Medical Department, http://www.armymedicine.army.mil/reports/mhat/mhat.html (accessed August 30, 2009).

Mulligan, K., Fear, N. T., Jones, N. Wesseley, S. & Greenberg, N. (2011). Psycho-educational interventions designed to prevent deployment-related psychological ill-health in armed forces personnel: A review. *Psychological Medicine*, **41**, 673–686.

Rosenthal, R. & Rubin, D. B. (1982). A simple, general purpose display of magnitude of experimental effect. *Journal of Educational Psychology*, **74**, 166–169.

Saint, C. E. (1992). Battlemind guidelines for battalion commanders. *United States Army, European OPE, and Seventh Army Training Manual*, Heidelberg, Germany: US Army European OPE.

Seligman, M. E. P. & Csikszentmihalyi, M. (2000). Positive psychology: An introduction. *American Psychologist*, **55**, 5–14.

Sharpley, J. G., Fear, N. T., Greenberg, N., Jones, M., & Wessely, S. (2008). Pre-deployment stress briefing: does it have an effect? *Occupational Medicine*, **58**, 30–34.

Shipherd, J. C. & Salters-Pedneault, K. (2008). Attention, memory, intrusive thoughts, and acceptance in PTSD: An update on the empirical literature for clinicians. *Cognitive and Behavioral Practice*, **15**, 349–363.

Slone, L. B. & Friedman, M. J. (2008). *After the war zone: A practical guide for returning troops and their families.* Cambridge, MA: Da Capo Press.

Thomas, J. L. & Castro, C. A. (2003). Organizational behavior and the US peacekeeper. In T. W Britt & A. B. Adler (eds.), *The psychology of the peacekeeper: lessons from the field* (pp. 127–146). Westport, CT: Greenwood.

Thomas, J. L., Castro, C. A., Adler, A. B., *et al.* (2007). The efficacy of Battlemind at immediate post deployment reintegration. In *Symposium of the Annual Meeting of the American Psychological Association on the Battlemind Training System: Supporting soldiers throughout the deployment cycle*, San Francisco, August.

Thompson, M. M. & McCreary, D. R. (2006). Enhancing mental readiness in military personnel. In A. B. Adler, C. A. Castro, & T. W. Britt (eds.), *Military life: The psychology of serving in peace and combat,* Vol. 2: *Operational stress* (pp. 54–79). Westport, CT: Praeger Security International.

US Army Medical Command (2007). *Operations Order 07–48: Implementation of the Battlemind Training System.* Washington, DC: US Army Medical Command.

Varnell, S. P., Murray, D. M., Janega, J. B., & Blitstein, J. L. (2004). Design and analysis of group-randomized trials: A review of recent practices. *American Journal of Public Health*, **94**, 393–399.

Zamorski, M. (2008). Defining resilience: An international perspective. In *International Military Testing Association Meeting Symposium on Military Resiliency: Perspectives from an International Technical Panel,* Amsterdam, September.

Endnotes

1. The concept of mental health training was a topic of the symposium Technical Panel (TP) 13 (Castro, 2008), which examined the psychological health and operational effectiveness domains. The symposium was part of the activities of the Technical Cooperation Program, which is an international collaboration between the USA, Canada, Australia, New Zealand, and the UK. The TP-13 members who prepared the definitions of training and resilience and who participated in dicussions regarding fundamental principles of mental health training are Mark Zamorski, Carl Castro, Neil Greenberg, Amy Adler, Paul Cawkill, Delwyn Neill, Kerry Sudom, and Alan Twomey.

2. Note that this definition differs from the initial definition presented in post-deployment Battlemind Training. The initial definition was "Battlemind is the Soldier's inner strength to face fear and adversity in combat with courage." The definition presented in this chapter more accurately reflects the scope of the Battlemind Training System. It was co-developed by Carl Castro, Amy Adler, Dennis McGurk, and Michael Rinehart in 2009.

Public health practice and disaster resilience: a framework integrating resilience as a worker protection strategy

Dori B. Reissman, Kathleen M. Kowalski-Trakofler, and Craig L. Katz

Introduction

The disciplines of emergency management and public health share objectives in hazard identification and the application of control or prevention strategies in the advent of disasters. This chapter defines resilience as it pertains to workers converging at a disaster site to perform response, recovery, or clean-up operations. A conceptual framework will be applied to disaster situations to highlight intervention avenues to preserve or enhance the resilience of the workers. Possible interventions include worker training and education, medical and emotional support services, disaster safety management, and alignment of organizational culture, policy, and procedures.

The disciplines of public health and emergency management

Public health is "the science and art of preventing disease, prolonging life and promoting health and efficiency through organized community effort" (Winslow, 1920). Epidemiology is the basic science of public health research, policy, and practice; which provides methods to study factors affecting the health and illness of populations (Institute of Medicine, 2002). Modern public health practice requires alliance among many disciplines and emotionally charged points of view, particularly when health and safety become challenged by disasters. Public health and emergency management share the objectives of identifying hazards and managing risk, particularly before a disaster strikes (Haddow & Bullock, 2006). When looking across these disciplines, risk would be defined as susceptibility to death, injury, and illness to people; damage or destruction of the human-built or natural environment; and disruption or stoppage of services that support people from a population perspective. The

purview of both disciplines has varied over time and in response to events, legislative initiatives, and leadership styles. For the purposes of this chapter, a disaster is defined as a serious disruption in the functioning of a local jurisdiction that poses a significant level of threat to life, health, property, or the environment and requires outside assistance to manage or cope with the event (International Federation of Red Cross and Red Crescent Societies, 2000). In common parlance, disasters are local events and directly impact communities.

Community resilience

The term community resilience is used in multiple, and often vaguely defined, ways. Emergency management uses the term "disaster-resilient community" to describe buildings, bridges, and roadways designed to withstand expected weather and geological hazards. Public policy circles use the term resilience to encourage a degree of self-sufficiency for defined jurisdictions to provide immediate emergency services and adequate food, water, medical help, and law enforcement to preserve social order in the face of disaster. National preparedness planning has applied the concept of resiliency to macro-level systems redundancy, equipment back-up, and alternative sources for raw materials, final goods and services, including information management (US Department of Homeland Security, 2009). However, these approaches focus on hardening the human-built environment and enhancing the systems that sustain people, but they do not address human behavior directly. The disaster literature is full of accounts where poor planning and lack of preparedness for the emotional, social, and behavioral consequences were likely to have delayed or compromised recovery efforts (Flynn, 2003). Disaster events have been associated with health-risk behaviors, exacerbation of chronic medical conditions, incitement of new psychiatric disturbances, and unexplained physical symptoms associated with decrements in function or quality of life (Katz *et al.*, 2002; Fullerton *et al.*, 2003; Institute of Medicine, 2003; Engel, 2004). However, inadequate planning, personnel, and resources for this arena continue to plague emergency managers (Flynn, 2006).

In 2006, the term community resilience was directly introduced in the Pandemic Influenza and All Hazards Preparedness Act (Public Law number 109–417) and the Homeland Security Presidential Directive 21 (US Department of Homeland Security, 2007). Community resilience was contextualized (paragraph 20) as:

> Where local civic leaders, citizens, and families are educated regarding threats and are empowered to mitigate their own risk, where they are practiced in responding to events, where they have social networks to fall back upon, and where they have familiarity with local public health and medical systems, there will be community resilience that will significantly attenuate the requirement for additional assistance.

This led the US Department of Health and Human Services (DHHS) to convene a federal advisory committee (the National Biodefense Science Board) for assistance with strategy and implementation. A special expert subcommittee was initiated to provide guidance to the Secretary of the DHHS about operationalizing community resilience as a health protection strategy (US Department of Homeland Security, 2007).[1] A report capturing the deliberations of this expert advisory body was passed to DHHS in November 2008 (Disaster Mental Health Subcommittee of the National Biodefense Science Board, 2008); it began with the following paragraph:

> Disaster mental and behavioral health…, includes the interconnected psychological, emotional, cognitive, developmental, and social influences on behavior and mental health and the impact of those factors on preparedness, response, and recovery from disasters or traumatic events. These factors directly and indirectly influence individual and community risks for health and safety outcomes such as substance use and abuse, aggression and non-adherence to public health recommendations (e.g., medication regimens, infection control, and evacuation or restricted movement), and the success of emergency response strategies and public directives…

Community resilience is sometimes used in multiple, and often vaguely defined ways to imply that the health and/or safety of community members can be influenced through interventions aimed at defined social networks, local governance, and critical infrastructure pathways supplying products and services needed to sustain a community in the face of disaster (Schoch-Spana, 2008). A recent review of the literature across several disciplines led Norris and colleagues (2008, p. 130) to define community resilience as "a process linking a set of adaptive capacities to a positive trajectory of functioning and adaptation after a disturbance" (such as a disaster). Their framework defined adaptation in terms of an ability to function and they went on to comment (p. 132) that post-disaster function is "not necessarily superior in level or character or effectiveness to pre-event functioning; it is simply different." This is a departure from other conceptualizations of collective resilience, which incorporates the element of learning and growth from the disaster, a transformative process catalyzed by the disaster experience (Brown & Kulig, 1996/97; Tedeschi *et al.*, 1998; Paton & Johnston, 2006; Masten & Obradović, 2008). Norris and colleagues (2008) provided a theoretical model that defines economic development (continuity of business, availability of jobs), social capital (collective value of social networks), information and communication, and community competence (ability to address the challenges) as the dynamic domains of adaptive capacity at the collective community level. Their model utilizes an ecological framework of the interdependencies between people, institutions, and organizations to mobilize resources to adapt to the new reality created by the disaster. It incorporates the process of collective problem solving and a common understanding about respective roles and responsibilities of various private, public, and volunteer entities in advance of a disaster. In a book on disaster resilience, Paton and Johnston (2006, p. 8) define the challenge of adapting to the new reality as "a measure of how well people and societies can adapt to a changed reality and capitalize on the new possibilities offered."

A framework to guide interventions promoting resilience in disaster workers

The remainder of this chapter will focus on the resilience of workers (affiliated and volunteer) converging at disaster sites to perform response, recovery, and/or clean-up operations. In essence, the concept of community will be targeted to the workers, their organizations,

Table 23.1 The Haddon matrix template.

	Host	Agent or vehicle	Physical environment	Sociocultural environment
Pre-event				
Event				
Post-event				

and the dynamic disaster work environment. The willingness and ability for workers to comply with safe work practices is greatly influenced by each worker's awareness of the hazards, the existence of a safety plan and availability of personal protective equipment, the culture of the responding and affected organizations, and the peculiarities of the incident itself (Jackson *et al.*, 2004; Qureshri *et al.*, 2005; Zohar, 2010). As such, it will be important to integrate resilience within the organizational culture and the activities designed to protect the health and safety of workers (Flynn, 2006; Reissman *et al.*, 2006a; Ursano *et al.*, 2006; Reissman & Howard, 2008). The approach to interventions that preserve or enhance disaster resilience for workers must be tailored to the work organization, the anticipated disaster scenario, and the training and experience of the workers themselves. This requires systematic analysis and evaluation as part of intervention planning. The analysis benefits from combining expertise in a public health practice framework: specifically applying classic models of causation from epidemiology within the fields of occupational health and safety and behavioral and psychological health.

The Haddon matrix: a tool for developing interventions to enhance resilience in the disaster worker community

Designing interventions for public health practice requires the development of a logic model to ascertain reasonable opportunities for intervention and to evaluate the impact of the resources applied. William Haddon, Jr. developed such a model to enable a systematic multidisciplinary analysis of the contributing factors to injury from traffic crashes, which enabled a comprehensive program of highway safety to be developed. This is known as the Haddon matrix (Haddon, 1968, 1970, 1972) and is illustrated in Table 23.1. The columns capture the contributing factors using basic epidemiology as the underpinning: namely identifying who is harmed (host), what is causing the harm (agent),

and how it is transmitted (vehicle), and defining the circumstances or settings that bring the host and agent together resulting in the adverse health or safety outcome (environment). The rows represent time phases (i.e., before, during, and after) in relation to a defined event (e.g., car crash, infectious disease, or disaster).

This systematic approach has broad application for public health practice (Institute of Medicine, 2003; Runyan, 2003; Barnett *et al.*, 2005). The following text outlines how to use the Haddon matrix to define a health or safety outcome under evaluation. The chapter will then give two case studies where the Haddon matrix is applied to two disasters to explore possible interventions to preserve or enhance resilience for workers involved in disaster response, recovery, and clean-up operations.

The disaster literature describes the following potential outcomes: health-risk coping behaviors (smoking, drinking, recklessness), exacerbation of underlying medical conditions (e.g., hypertension, peptic ulcer disease, asthma, chronic anxiety, thought or mood disorders), and the incidence of new anxiety and mood disorders (Katz *et al.*, 2002; Fullerton *et al.*, 2003; Institute of Medicine, 2003; Engel, 2004). For the purpose of this chapter, the rows can be assigned according to the disaster cycle in emergency management: preparedness and mitigation (pre-event), response (during the event), and recovery (post-event). The adverse health and safety outcomes of concern are stipulated as influenced by perceived threats to resilience: the "agent", such as traumatic loss (e.g., sudden death of a co-worker or loved one), harm (e.g., serious injury), or change (e.g., loss of job/income, home/place) resulting from the disaster. As mentioned above, the "environment" is defined collectively as the work site(s) associated with the disaster event. So, in looking more closely at the host, one could define intrapersonal and interpersonal factors for the worker as having a bearing on vulnerability and resilience. The environment is broken into a physical (human-built or natural landscape) and the social and cultural components. The sociocultural aspects may include the interaction within (co-worker or management support, communication, resources, safety and administrative policies) and between (coordination and control) the work organizations involved in the disaster, the community and workforce behavioral norms and beliefs, and the influence of regulatory aspects (laws and enforcement).

There are several typologies used to classify disasters for the purpose of studying mental and behavioral response. Disasters may be caused by forces of nature or by human action. Examples of natural forces include extreme weather events (hurricanes, tornados, cyclones), geological disturbances (earthquakes, volanic eruptions), or severe infectious epidemics (severe acute respiratory syndrome, pandemic influenza). Technological or industrial disasters may occur from human neglect, error, or by deliberate and harmful actions. People who perceive a loss of control (no warning, unable to avoid, lack of coping skills) or have inadequate social support in relation to the disaster are more likely to have more severe or longer lasting psychopathology (Fullerton *et al.*, 2003; Kaniasty & Norris, 2004). Box 23.1 provides some key observations gleaned from prior disasters, which serve as a context for the case studies to be discussed in the next section.

CASE 1: the World Trade Center terrorist attack on September 11, 2001

At least 40 000 individuals are estimated to have responded to the World Trade Center (WTC) site following the September 11 2001 (9/11) terrorist attacks, encompassing a broad array of traditional first responders, workers as diverse as laborers and morgue staff, and affiliated and unaffiliated volunteers (Herbert *et al.*, 2006). These responders encountered well-characterized physical hazards (including chemical toxins) and emotional traumatogens. It is for this reason and others that their experience provides an ideal lens through which to look at the public health dimensions of resilience amid catastrophe.

Public health observations about the responder population may in fact be particularly generalizable to other catastrophic events because of the vast size of this population and its associated heterogeneity. As responders are members of the broader "disaster community" that grows up around a disaster (Wright *et al.*, 1990), lessons regarding their resilience should be

---

Box 23.1 Lessons from prior disaster responses

- It is difficult to prepare responders for everything they might encounter
- Even seasoned responders can face situations and issues that cause uneasiness and distress
- It is not unusual for responders to be asked to work outside their areas of expertise
- Concerns about family and friends rank high on responders' lists of priorities
- Timely, accurate, and candid information should be shared to facilitate decision making
- Managers, at every level, need to consider the health, safety, and resiliency of workers on the job as part of situation awareness and for staged planning (implies needs for occupational health and wellness monitoring)
- Resiliency is an integral component of occupational safety and health, which requires pre-planning to maximize worker recovery
- Self-care plans and peer-support activities are essential to mission completion
- Everything possible should be done to safeguard responders' physical and emotional health
- Responders do not need to face response challenges alone; they may share their experiences with buddies, teammates, family members, and colleagues
- It is particularly difficult for responders to maintain emotional distance when they witness the deaths of children
- Organizational differences among groups of responders and cultural differences between victims and responders can impede the timely and efficient provision of emergency services
- Individuals may be thrust into leadership roles for which they have had little to no formal training

---

relevant to non-responders as well. The 9/11 responders also have had access to a unique long-term medical follow-up program, the information from which has led to much published discussion about issues relevant to the well-being of the responder community in the event of future large-scale catastrophic events.

Although not intended to be exhaustive, Table 23.2 and the following discussion exemplifies the application of the Haddon matrix to the subject of resilience in responders. When the 9/11 rescue and recovery response is overlaid with the Haddon matrix, the

Table 23.2 Haddon matrix of public health measures promoting the resilience of responders to the World Trade Center attacks.

	Host (WTC responders)	Agent	Physical environment	Social environment
Pre-event	Integrate routine mental health services into employee health programming	Emergency response training, including clear role definition	Biohazard training	Promote workplace environment of openness and support around mental health and resilience
Event	Train and deploy providers of psychological first aid; identify high-risk responders	Institute policies for monitoring and limiting exposure to Ground Zero	Promote/require use of personal protective equipment	Promote a disaster response environment that emphasizes responder, workplace, and family well-being
Post-event	Establish a system for long-term mental health follow-up and care	System of financial support and vocational rehabilitation for affected responders	Establish a system for long-term physical health follow-up and care	Involve families in long-term mental health follow-up and care

boxes highlight true accomplishments, missed opportunities, and lessons learned regarding public health measures relevant to resiliency.

Pre-event

Host

Planning in the pre-disaster peroid affords the opportunity to deploy a robust cohort of responders in the event of disaster. A responder base that begins from a healthy position is best positioned to manage itself and the response in a healthy and effective manner (Bills *et al.*, 2008). In a sample of the first 1138 participants in a medical/mental health screening and treatment program for 9/11 responders, ultimately known as the WTC Medical Monitoring Program, only 3% reported ever having previously seen a mental health professional (Smith *et al.*, 2004).

Ensuring better access to mental health services to responders pre-disaster should enhance resiliency when disaster strikes. To achieve this requires a system of capable and available mental health providers who can be reimbursed for their services. This may be easier for disaster response agencies that rely on employees rather than volunteers, but voluntary agencies could also mandate receiving proof of a "mental health check up" for all potential volunteers.

Agent

Adequate training in disaster response is essential for ensuring not only an effective response but also the well-being of responders themselves. An analysis of 28 962 registrants in the WTC Health Registry who identified themselves as having been rescue or recovery workers at the WTC site found that rates of post-traumatic stress disorder (PTSD) were lowest in police and highest in unaffiliated volunteers (Perrin *et al.*, 2007). This seems to underscore the importance of training and experience in bolstering mental health and coping during disaster. Indeed, the study also found that risk of PTSD was heightened if responders reported having performed tasks at "Ground Zero" atypical for their occupation.

Public health-oriented management of future disaster responses would, therefore, include better gatekeeping around unaffiliated volunteers ill prepared to handle what awaits them. In addition, emergency management agencies can work to ensure that partner agencies provide fully trained and credentialed responders and that these responders adhere to their roles as best as circumstances permit.

Physical environment

The attacks on the WTC generated exposure to physical contaminants, which has been the subject of much subsequent discussion (Herbert *et al.*, 2006). The toxins derived from the thousands of liters of exploded jet fuel and the tons of coarse and fine particular matter generated by the collapse of the towers themselves, airborne exposure to which was perpetuated by days to weeks of smoldering fires. Emergency response training must include consideration of the potential biohazards to which responders may be exposed. Although it may be impossible to anticipate, or at least meaningfully educate about, all possible physical exposures, anyone who trains to participate in disaster response should at least be trained to ask two general questions: what are the potential physical exposures and who is monitoring occupational safety? This will be particularly important in the event of a nuclear, chemical, or biological terrorist attack, although it may be those very cases where the issue is most salient. Emergency response agencies can mandate basic "all-hazards" training to be an element of the training programs of their partner agencies.

Social environment

Even if employers provide for capable, available, and affordable pre-event mental health services for disaster responders, another hurdle remains – stigma. The challenge therein lies to create a workplace environment that promotes mental well-being and characterizes the action of seeking out mental health professionals as not only acceptable but also desirable. This challenge likely extends beyond the purview or capacity of any one employer to that of a community as a whole, including its departments of health or mental health. A discussion of de-stigmatization is beyond the scope of this paper, but, for example, models for addressing workplace depression have been developed (Bilsker *et al.*, 2007).

Event

Host

The evidence base for mental health interventions in the acute aftermath of disaster is limited, leading to reliance on general principles for intervention, including promoting a sense of safety, calm, hope, self-efficacy, and connectedness (Hobfoll *et al.*, 2007). Consensus exists around a set of basic interventions known as "psychological first aid" for addressing the psychological equivalent of the bumps and scrapes of trauma (Brymer *et al.*, 2006). However, little is known about the nature and extent of mental health services provided to responders in the course of their rescue and recovery work at the WTC, despite anecdotal reports of the availability of these services. One organization, Disaster Psychiatry Outreach, did "staff" Ground Zero after the 9/11 attacks with volunteer psychiatrists, although minimal documentation is available regarding the interventions (McQuistion & Katz, 2001).

The experience of 9/11 responders has suggested the need for a comprehensive mental health program that spans the immediate and long-term aftermath of disaster and that includes real-time surveillance, treatment, and study of service utilization and impact (Bills *et al.*, 2008). This program should smoothly link immediate and long-term mental health services (Garakani *et al.*, 2004). Psychological first aid was widely promulgated in the aftermath of 9/11, providing a standard for basic mental health intervention that public health authorities may implement in future disasters. In keeping with a key aspect of psychological first aid, and in the setting of scarce resources, future peri-event mental health interventions can be targeted at higher-risk groups within the responder and general population. A host of well-documented risk factors for developing post-disaster psychopathology have been established in the general psychiatric literature (Garakani *et al.*, 2004) and in the 9/11 responder literature (Katz *et al.*, 2009). These span prior psychiatric history, extent of exposure to a disaster such as 9/11, and availability of post-disaster social supports; this suggests a picture of who among a disaster-affected population may be less resilient and need more assistance.

Agent

The disaster literature is replete with evidence that "dose of exposure" to a disaster or other trauma correlates with likelihood of suffering psychiatrically in its aftermath (Katz *et al.*, 2002). This association has also been shown in 9/11 responders, where exposure was reflected in such dimensions as having directly witnessed the attacks, been exposed to the dust cloud, lost someone, or spent more time at Ground Zero (Bills *et al.*, 2008). Regarding the last, among the WTC Health Registry's 28 962 responders, arriving at the WTC site soon after 9/11 and total duration of time spent working at the site (from 1 to 200 days) were each an exposure variable that correlated with likelihood of having PTSD in all responders except police (Perrin *et al.*, 2007).

Emotional exposure represents a multifaceted construct that includes at least one major modifiable factor – duration of exposure. Communities need their responders to rush in quickly. However, the scientific literature suggests that limiting responders' subsequent duration of exposure at places like the WTC site should promote the resilience of the responders and, therefore, be in the interest of the community that has a stake in their well-being. Responders' time of exposure to a disaster could be monitored according to at least two parameters: total time spent on-site and how much time off occurs within that time period. While further study will be required to calibrate the former threshold, common sense should be of more use in guiding public health decision making on the latter.

Physical environment

One of the major exposures suffered by WTC responders, toxins, has already been alluded to. In a study of the first 9442 WTC responders who participated in a medical and mental health screening program, the WTC Worker and Volunteer Screening Program, 69% reported new or worsened respiratory symptoms at the time of working at the WTC site and 59% reported persistent complaints at the time of their examination up to two and a half years later (Herbert et al., 2006). As with emotional exposure, earlier time of arrival correlated with respiratory symptoms and findings. Likewise, in the WTC Health Registry's cohort, time of arrival as well as duration of exposure at the WTC site correlated with the likelihood of newly diagnosed asthma (Wheeler et al., 2007).

Importantly, the WTC Health Registry study found that delays in use of respiratory masks, and to a lesser degree total days without using masks, correlated with the likelihood of developing asthma (Wheeler et al., 2007). The authors of the study concluded that timely and appropriate use of respiratory masks, along with programs that enforce this usage, should reduce future respiratory exposures in the event of disasters that involve airborne contaminants. This reflects a hard-learned lesson from 9/11 that can inform future public health planning around disasters.

Social environment

In the necessary rush to respond and help after a disaster such as 9/11, there is great potential for neglect of life beyond the disaster site. Self, family, and workplace may all be neglected in the course of becoming immersed in rescue and recovery efforts. When the length of a disaster response spans months, as it did at the WTC site, this neglect may have significant ill consequences in any or all of these domains. For example,

family tensions may become exacerbated (Katz et al. 2006a). In addition, it must be considered whether the immersion in disaster response represents, at least in part, an unhealthy flight from personal problems (Katz & Nathaniel, 2002).

It should be possible for response agencies to "preach" balance to their responders in the course of training and emergency response planning, thereby making it easier to "practice" balance during the inherently unbalanced state of eventual disaster. Attempts can be made to foster disaster response environments that accentuate the need for decisive action without siphoning excessively from the responder's self, home, or workplace. Specific approaches to this include inviting responders to examine their motivations, devising "buddy systems" for responders to look after one another in the course of a disaster, and prioritizing literal lines of communication between responders and their home environments.

Post-event

Host and physical environment

The WTC Worker and Volunteer Medical Screening Program and the associated WTC Worker and Volunteer Mental Health Screening Program were established in July 2002 through a combination of federal and philanthropic funding in order to screen WTC responders for physical and mental health conditions associated with the disaster (Herbert et al., 2006; Katz et al., 2006a). Originally funded as a one-year program, what is now called the WTC Medical Monitoring and Treatment Program (MMTP) has evolved into an ongoing multiyear program that includes physical and mental health screenings, follow-up examinations, on-site treatment services, and case management services (Katz et al., 2006b). A similar but separate program exists for firefighters from the Fire Department of New York. As of May 2008, over 24 000 WTC responders had undergone initial screenings across the consortium of non-fire department clinical sites in the metropolitan New York City area, funded by the National Institutes of Occupational Safety and Health. Details of the clinical programming are described elsewhere (Smith et al., 2004; Herbert et al., 2006; Katz et al., 2006a).

To the best of our knowledge, the MMTP and its forerunner, the WTC Worker and Volunteer Medical Screening Program, represent programs of unprecedented scope and magnitude in addressing the medical and mental health needs of disaster responders.

Congress appropriated $323 million to support both responder and non-responder WTC medical surveillance and treatment programs between 2003 and 2008 (Gerberding, 2008), reflecting the magnitude and the cost of these programs. The MMTP represents a post-event public health safety net to capture 9/11-associated health and mental health problems arising despite whatever pre-event and event-related health measures were undertaken, and because of those measures that perhaps were overlooked. Although future research will be needed to determine the full impact of these WTC programs, the MMTP serves as the best available working model for addressing post-event resiliency through public medical and mental healthcare.

Agent

We are not aware of any peer-reviewed publications on the issue of disability related to working or volunteering as a 9/11 responder. However, clinical observations from the MMTP by one of the authors (CLK) suggest that it is a major issue for many patients, with workers' compensation claims constituting a frequent dimension of both physical and mental healthcare. The inability to work as a result of their exposure at the WTC site deprives 9/11 responders of both income and fulfillment.

As of 2006, Congress had awarded $105 million to New York State in support of 9/11-related worker compensation claims (Gerberding, 2008). A portion of this funding has also gone toward planning for future disasters. The public health impact of providing workers' compensation on the resilience of 9/11 responders remains to be investigated but can be predicted to be a significant ingredient in post-event recovery. Clinical observations suggest that, whatever the magnitude of this impact it could be increased by better pairing of compensation with vocational rehabilitation programming.

Social environment

The need for better connections between responders and their families during a catastrophic event has already been discussed. In a similar fashion, families should be involved in post-event mental health treatment programming for responders. The rationale is twofold: the mental health problems of responders after 9/11 may affect their partners and children, while mental health issues in the family may exacerbate the 9/11-related mental health issues of the responders. Experts have generally agreed that a multifaceted approach to

problems such as PTSD is necessary, particularly given the modest effect and evidence base for most pharmacological and psychotherapeutic treatment modalities (Shalev *et al.*, 1996).

One clinical center within the MMTP has created a family intervention program based on a recent New York State Office of Mental Health initiative for involving families in the treatment of patients with chronic mental illness (Salerno *et al.*, 2008; McKay, personal communication, 2009). Having such a specialized unit within a broader medical/mental health program may serve as a model for broad-based public health planning around future disasters.

CASE 2: the Sago Mine disaster on January 2, 2006

Background

It is useful for the reader to have some understanding of the mine environment in order to appreciate the inherent danger of the workplace and relate to the case study. A mine is broadly defined as an opening or excavation in the earth created for the purpose of extracting minerals (Thrush *et al.*, 1968). Coal is mined either on the surface of the earth or underground. To extract coal from an underground mine, the coalbed (or seam) must be accessed from the surface. The term "portal" is generally given to any entrance that provides access to a coal mine. In hilly terrain, such as is found in the Appalachian coalfields in the eastern USA, the coal may form an outcrop on a hillside, which allows direct entry to the coal seam via a horizontal tunnel or "drift" opening. At other locations, it may be possible to open a "slope" tunnel that angles down from the surface and intersects with the coal seam. If the coal seam is too deep for a slope to be feasible, a "shaft" must be constructed. The shaft, which may be 20 feet (12.5 m) or more in diameter, extends vertically from the surface to the seam and is accessed via a large elevator. Once inside the underground mine, miners are transported to various worksites underground, sometimes miles away. The transportation system is installed for moving workers, supplies, equipment, and the extracted coal.

In an underground coal mine, workers must contend with poorly illuminated work areas that can be dusty, uneven, and wet and muddy depending upon the amount of water present. Work areas can be extremely confined, particularly in mines with a low seam coal height (i.e., less than 5 feet [1.5 m] high). In low seams, coal miners work on their knees or backs during their entire shift. To extract the coal, miners must operate large, noisy, technically sophisticated equipment in these confined work areas. The only lighting available comes from the miner's battery-operated cap lamp and from localized sources on various mining machines. In addition, the coal mining process releases dangerous gases, including methane, which is highly explosive and needs to be monitored. Miners may also have to deal with carbon monoxide should there be a fire or explosion underground and be aware of oxygen deficiency in locations that may not be adequately ventilated. As per federal regulation, miners are required to carry emergency respirators – self-contained self-rescuers (SCSRs) – whenever they are inside the mine. The SCSRs are closed system breathing devices designed to provide the miner with a protected oxygen supply that lasts one hour. Miners are mandated to receive appropriate training on when and how to properly use the SCSRs. The SCSR is for emergency escape from the mine when the air is thought to be contaminated with toxic gas (i.e., carbon monoxide).

In summary, the mining environment is dangerous and the hazards are dynamic in nature – constantly changing as the mining process creates new space (Kowalski-Trakofler & Barrett, 2003). Our example, the Sago Mine disaster in West Virginia, is a drift mine opening into the Middle Kittanning coal seam through five drift openings. Battery-powered track-mounted personnel carriers (mantrips) and locomotives were used to move the men and materials throughout the mine. Coal was transported to the surface by a series of conveyor belts.

Historical trends

The safety of miners is dependent upon many inter-related factors including knowledge of the dynamic, ever-changing environment, the ability to recognize and respond to hazards, training, experience, and communication. In the USA, mine operators, federal and state mine safety agencies, and researchers have looked at numerous aspects of miner injuries and fatalities with regard to mitigating future incidents and increasing resilience amongst the population. The most intense efforts in this area have occurred following major mine emergencies. Mining has a history of disasters. From 1900 to 2007, some 11 612 underground coal mine workers died in 514 different mining disasters, with most disasters resulting from explosions or fires (DeMarchi, 1997; Mine Safety

and Health Administration 1998a, 1998b; Kowalski-Trakofler et al., 2009).

During a five-month period in 2006, three underground coal mining incidents in the USA resulted in the deaths of 19 miners. All three incidents received nationwide attention, particularly the Sago Mine disaster in West Virginia. These incidents represented a departure from the recent trends in underground coal mining safety (Figure 23.1). Before 2006, the number of mining disasters had decreased from a high of 20 in 1909 to an average of one every four years during 1985–2005.

The events of the Sago Mine disaster

On Monday, January 2, 2006, at approximately 6:30 a.m., an explosion occurred at Wolf Run Mining Company's Sago Mine in West Virginia, leading to the death of 12 miners. Thirteen miners were working in the vicinity of the explosion. One miner was working alone about 1500 feet (450 m) from the others and was killed instantly by the forces from the explosion. The other 12 were members of a coal production crew: of this group, 11 perished from carbon monoxide poisoning. The sole survivor from the production crew was able to give testimony in the ensuing investigations conducted by the Mine Safety and Health Administration (Gates et al., 2007) and the West Virginia Office of Miners' Health, Safety, and Training (2006). These official reports conflicted in some aspects in the description of events.

What is understood is that following the explosion the crew attempted to escape by their transport vehicle (mantrip) but soon encountered debris that made their route impassable. The crew then entered their primary escapeway on foot, a tunnel that would lead them to a portal and out of the mine. They walked approximately 1000 feet (305 m) through a potentially deadly atmosphere before donning their SCSRs. They returned to their original location at the coal face and erected a barricade of plastic sheeting – which is part of standard training when escape is not possible. Reportedly, the miners took off their SCSRs while they were building the barricade.

After the barricade was finished, all 12 men went behind it to wait for rescue teams to arrive. The only survivor reported that there were not enough SCSRs to go around since after a time four miners were not able to make their's work, so individuals shared with each other, trading off SCSRs between them. Besides removing and replacing mouthpieces while sharing the apparatus, members of the crew also removed their

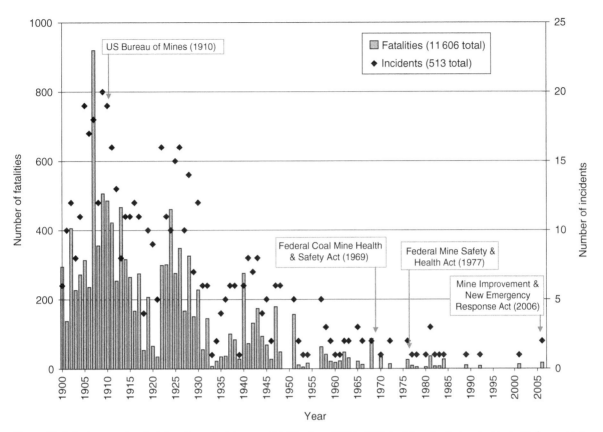

Figure 23.1 Underground coal mining disaster incidents and fatalities from 1900 to 2006. A mining disaster is an incident with five or more fatalities. (Data from http://www.cdc.gov/niosh/mining/statistics/disasters.htm MSHA, accessed February 22, 2011.)

mouthpieces to talk. The West Virginia Office of Miners' Health, Safety, and Training Report of Investigation concluded that the 11 miners succumbed to carbon monoxide poisoning.

Given the way that the SCSRs were utilized during the building of the barricade, it seems apparent that they were not used correctly, at least not in that instance. Evaluation of SCSRs removed from the mine revealed all were working. Lack of expectations and training in how the devices work may have had something to do with their misuse, which, in turn, led to the miners' inability to utilize the equipment fully. In addition, carbon monoxide poisoning may have affected the miners' reasoning and decision-making abilities and may have contributed to how they utilized the SCSRs during the building of the barricade.

The first mine rescue teams arrived about four and a half hours after the explosion, but they did not reach the barricaded miners until 40 hours after the explosion. This proved to be a critical issue. In mining, the miners themselves are actually the "first responders" as

the logistics of escape and rescue in an underground coal mine are complex, involving time and distance to the portal. All miners are trained in emergency response. It takes time to assemble a mine rescue team, who sometimes must travel a distance, assemble, be briefed, and don their equipment. There is a basic mine rescue protocol that has developed over the years based on rescue efforts made during previous mine disasters, with a focus on the safety of the rescuers, monitoring of the environment such as toxic gases, and constructing roof support as needed; consequently forward progress can be slow. However, each mine disaster is unique and presents its own challenges.

To complicate matters, and create a second tragedy, families and the media were told that "all are okay behind barricade – 12 men" (West Virginia Office of Miners' Health, Safety, and Training, 2006). The devastating news came to the families and media over an hour later, that there was only one survivor and that he was in serious condition. Communications were problematic because of the need to pass information

349

Table 23.3 Application of the Haddon matrix to the Sago Mine disaster, 2006.

	Host (underground coal miners; mine emergency response personnel including mine rescue, mine incident command)	Agent/vehicle (death, injury, loss of income, penalty fines, psychological consequences)	Physical environment (underground coal mine)	Social environment (safety culture at mine/in the industry; mine policies; legal environment; community norms)
Pre-event	Promote mental health and resilience behaviors; travel escape routes; teach proper behavior and use of personal protective equipment in mine emergency response	Develop site emergency plans (mandated); emergency response training, know the law; clearly marked escapeways; assigned roles; teach decision-making points to escapees; security and media plan	Prevention through engineering; monitor gases; design emergency communication and protocols; provide equipment at mandated intervals (i.e., SCSRs, refuge shelters, etc.)	Promote workplace support around mental health and resilience; provide community with ways to support each other; provide specific disaster mental health resources. Develop cooperation with local emergency rescue teams, state and federal personnel
Event	On-site response immediate; trapped miners follow escape procedures; mine rescue protocol and incident monitoring take leadership; psychological first aid	Mandates and policies provide structure for response	Monitor mine conditions; build barricade; utilize refuge chamber	Provide information (shift/fatigue) and support to incident command; provide protection and support for families and community
Post-event	Long-term mental health follow-up and care; SCSR training;	Official report; cause; lessons learned; rescue policy evaluation; develop interventions	Evaluate cause; make appropriate engineering interventions to make the mine safe; close mine;	Involve miners, families, mine rescue, and community in long-term mental health follow-up; facilitate evaluation of policies; cooperation; positive support; MINER Act passed

SCSR, self-contained self-rescue.

through multiple individuals. On the surface, there were two pager phones in the mine office, one in the dispatcher's building and one just inside the mine portal, in addition to one near the mine rescue truck. There were over 100 people on the surface, many with cell phones. Although the site was being secured by police, the national media had set up observation positions for their camera crews; what was not known at the time was that some of these media crews had directional listening devices pointed at the mine portal and could hear the pager phone, further complicating official communication from the command center to the affected families.

Analysis of the disaster using the Haddon matrix

To determine mine emergency prevention and intervention strategies, the Haddon matrix is helpful in organizing and examining the various aspects of pre-event, event, and post-event activities (Table 23.3). There are more pre-event activities than in most other emergency situations, mainly because of legal mandates and constraints, both state and federal, concerning types of hazard, enforcement of safety regulations, allowable technology, and particularly mandated training in the mining industry. While the discussion of the WTC disaster was covered by considering events before, during, and after the attack, the mine disaster here is better illlustrated by considerations based on the matrix column heads – host, agent, physical environment, and social environment – at various stages within the disaster pathway.

Host

The population or host for the Sago disaster is defined as the actors involved. All played a part in the event response from the moment the event was identified. The actors are highly dependent upon each other. Underground coal miners are actually their own first responders, as they may be miles from the surface. It may takes hours to assemble a mine rescue team, command center, and support personnel. Therefore, the host or responder is defined broadly to include the escaping miners, the mine office initial response personnel (dispatcher), the eventual incident command (mine management, federal, state, union personnel) and the mine rescue teams, plus of course the miners' families and the community. Pre-event for the host is focused on training for emergencies, including understanding escapeways, practicing with equipment, and reviewing emergency plans and procedures. The Sago miners completed mandated training, yet *during the event* they struggled with the use and operation of their SCSRs. Mine rescuers, who are highly trained, took 40 hours to reach the miners because of the environment and the established protocols for advancement in toxic air.

Agent

The loss or harm (or agent) that results from an incident such as Sago is substantial. At Sago, there were 12 deaths; one injured miner; closure of the mine, resulting in loss of livelihood for many in the community; legal and financial penalties for the mine company; and long- and short-term mental health consequences. Pre-event development of site-specific emergency plans is mandated. All miners must complete emergency response training annually. Mine operators are expected to know the law. Teaching miners decision-making points in escape should be an important component in the training. During the event, escapeways should be clearly identified and emergency roles assigned. Sago Mine provided the lesson that extensive security and media plans need to be in place. Mines have plans in the event of an emergency to cordon-off the mine property. Mine personnel provide this function until local

or state police arrive on scene. In addition, mines designate an area for families to gather and provide space for media at a separate location. The essential goals are to protect incident command in order to focus on the emergency, provide for the families, and maintain official communications. Sago showed the industry that with the advent of sophisticated technology, revisiting security of both property and information communication is important.

Post-event, the matrix can put into perspective the need for SCSR training and the development of a switch-over procedure from one SCSR unit to another, as the units are designed to last one hour. There is also need for expectations training for miners so that they understand what they can anticipate when wearing a working unit. There were two ex-Sago miners who committed suicide eight months after the disaster. The company had provided "grief counseling" after the disaster and renewed the offer after the two suicides. There is no formal ongoing disaster mental health counseling after a mine disaster. The Sago disaster emphasized the need for such a service and the Mine Safety and Health Administration has recognized this need.

The physical environment

Much is known about the *pre-event* physical environment in most mine disasters. Specific mine hazards such as fires and explosions or inundations of gas or water are well known and continuously studied. Underground coal mines are inspected by both federal and state inspectors regularly. Maintaining a safe mining environment is a key component to a safe and resilient workforce. At Sago, the explosion was most likely caused by a lightning strike on the surface. It is believed that energy from the lightning propagated through the earth to a sealed, abandoned working area, igniting methane gas that had accumulated in the old workings, blasting out the walls between the abandoned and active mine areas. *During the event*, the mine rescue team monitors the air in addition to drilling surface bore holes to lower sensors. The major focus of *post-event* interventions in the mining industry are engineering controls. The first line of defense is to engineer out the hazard in the environment.

The social environment

Less is known about the *pre-event* social environment: the safety climate at the mine. Most miners work within a crew and buddy system and are taught to stay together in the event an escape is necessary. The Sago crew exemplified their training. As the Haddon matrix defines social environment, policies and the legal environment are included, which are well defined in the mining industry. Therefore, the social environment pre-event at Sago Mine can be defined and understood more than in many other types of disaster. Mines are in rural locations and most members of the mining community live in rural or small communities. This provides a support system during and after an event – one which is already in place through community interaction.

Lessons from the Sago Mine disaster

Examination of the Sago Mine disaster utilizing the Haddon matrix helps to define the response strengths and to focus on key issues to target for intervention with the goal of developing a more resilient host, including miners, mine operators, mine emergency response and command personnel, and the overall mining community itself. Clearly as the model illuminates, further training on SCSR use is warranted. In addition, since SCSRs last approximately one hour, switching SCSRs in a toxic environment became an issue after Sago. Why some miners thought their SCSRs did not function when testing after the incident showed that the units were not empty remains a concern.

Within six months of the Sago disaster, the US Congress enacted the 2006 Mine Improvement and New Emergency Response Act (MINER Act, 2006). This legislation contained provisions to improve safety, health, preparedness, and emergency response in US mines. The MINER Act requires mine operators to develop and maintain an emergency response plan. Prior to the Sago incident, mines were only required to provide miners with a single self-contained breathing apparatus affording the wearer one hour of protection. Regulators felt miners needed to be provided with sufficient quantities of breathing apparatus to give them at least two hours of protection in the event of a prolonged escape. The legislation requires mines to store extra emergency breathing apparatus along escapeways in sufficient quantities that miners will have oxygen breathing apparatus available to them the entire length of their escapeways. The Mine Safety and Health Administration developed SCSR switchover training along with expectations training, based on a study by researchers at the National Institutes of Occupational Safety and Health (Kowalski-Trakofler et al., 2008)

The inability of trapped miners to communicate with rescuers during the Sago Mine disaster led to another feature in the MINER Act, which called for installation and maintenance of flame-resistant directional lifelines in escapeways. Mine operators must install wireless two-way communication and tracking systems between underground and surface workers. Congress subsequently passed an emergency supplemental appropriation to accelerate implementation of (1) emergency oxygen supplies, (2) underground refuge chambers, and (3) communications and tracking systems.

Communication quality surfaced as a major issue in the Sago disaster, in the mine, mine to surface, and personal communication with families and media. Since Sago, resources have been applied to the development of wireless communications, and procedures have been put in place to communicate with families and secure the media. Evaluations of mine rescue policies are ongoing. Of major interest in terms of developing a resilient workforce is the need for training on psychological aspects of human response and behaviors in disaster, in addition to a program such as psychological first aid during the event and afterwards (Brymer et al., 2006).

Conclusions

The tools for impacting resilience at the workforce (population) level share strategies with those used for occupational health and safety and public health practice, such as leadership training, public education, worker training, legislation, engineering design codes and standards, land use management, and research regarding human behavior and intervention effectiveness. During the pre-event period, workers must acquire and maintain appropriate education, training, and certification (credentials) specific to their potential deployment roles. Medical, emotional, and cognitive readiness are important dimensions of workforce health protection planning. This may be enhanced by improving coping skills through training and by building social support networks before the disaster strikes. Leadership training is a critical element of force protection as team cohesion, buddy relations, and operations are all leadership dependent.

In addition, the employers can implement organizational changes to preserve and maintain worker resilience by encouraging and supporting safe work practices and adopting policies that better enable workers to balance competing work and life demands. Boxes 23.2 and 23.3 are organizational tools for use pre-event to improve leadership and resiliance in workers,

Box 23.2 Organizational Leadership Self-Assessment Tool: adapting existing worker support services to provide enhanced workforce support during public health emergencies

The Organizational Leadership Self-Assessment Tool is designed to help state and local health departments, healthcare facilities, and first-responder organizations to develop plans for ensuring the availability of workforce support services during an influenza pandemic. These plans may be developed by existing employee assistance programs, occupational health services, or human resource departments and can be used as the basis for other disaster scenarios. The tool consists of a series of questions.

- What are the most essential or mission critical functions performed by your organization? How might they be impacted by pandemic influenza? What is your organization's plan for protecting workers and maintaining essential functions? What is your organization's role in the response to pandemic influenza?

- What psychosocial issues might arise within your organization and workforce because of pandemic influenza (i.e., consider increases in workload [absenteeism], alternative work strategies such as telework, just-in-time training, currency of information, exchange of ideas, grief leadership to help with death of co-workers or others in personal life, management flexibility, increased challenge of disseminating current, accurate, timely information, etc.)?

- What significant aspects of your organization's structure, business practices, workforce demographics, and culture should be considered in planning for pandemic influenza?

- What hurdles might your organization encounter in attempting to provide services to your workforce during different phases of pandemic influenza? What strategies might be employed to overcome those hurdles (e.g., alternative service delivery methods)?

- How might your organization assist your covered workforce in preparing for and dealing with these psychosocial issues?

- How might your organization assist its executive leaders in preparing for and dealing with these psychosocial issues?

- What might your organization be doing now to promote the resiliency of your workforce and coping ability in the event of a pandemic emergency (prepare and mitigate)?

Source: Reissman *et al.*, 2006b.

Box 23.3 Organizational actions supporting resiliency for essential service workers

Actions supporting worker resiliency at the organizational level require dedicated resources and an alignment of management practices and administrative policies. The following list provides guidance about how to achieve this level of support for both workforce and organizational resiliency:

- monitoring workforce needs for stress management and healthcare

- planning for continuity of medical care (specialists, medicines) for workers with chronic illnesses (physical and psychological)

- monitoring for emerging needs (e.g., stress-related, depression, grief, idiopathic medical conditions)

- providing education about stress-related conditions and anticipated health and safety concerns

- providing family assistance programs (most coping will come from family/friends/faith and programs within workplaces and schools)

- providing/receiving leadership, management, and supervisory training

- anticipating needs and work pace over time (think of the metaphor of a marathon not a sprint)

- providing/receiving grief leadership, ceremony, support (fatality management)

- improving perceptions of collective efficacy (i.e., ability to handle problems as a team) through education, training, and drills

- promoting integrated health, safety, and security culture/climate (hardiness, resiliency)

- using role modeling by leadership

- enabling workers to balance work and home demands through flexible work schedules and other administrative policies

- reinforcing organizational commitment to worker safety and health through appropriate supervision, training, and access to services

- implementing continuity of information and communication systems (FEMA Emergency Management Guide for Business and Industry, http:www.fema.gov/business/guide/index.shtm; Continuity of Operations, http:www.fema.gov/government/coop/index.shtm#0)

- ensuring continuity of essential operations (organizational resiliency)

- ensuring redundancy and cross-training of critical tasks/roles providing alternative worksites and innovative use of technology to maintain operations.

Sources: Reissman *et al.*, 2006a; Ursano *et al.*, 2006.

Box 23.4 The Worker Resiliency Program

The Worker Resiliency Program was created by the US Centers for Disease Control and Prevention (CDC) as an internal workforce strategy in 2004, during the humanitarian response to the Indian Ocean earthquake and tsunami, to safeguard the health, safety, and resiliency of staff members deployed to dangerous locations. It was further expanded during the 2005 responses to Hurricane Katrina along the Gulf Coast in the USA and to a large outbreak of Marburg hemorrhagic fever in Angola. The program, which continues to evolve, currently performs the following activities:

- identifies and anticipates stressors that responders are likely to encounter
- develops field resources and conducts predeployment briefings on how to use self-care strategies to minimize anticipated stressors
- ensures access to healthcare and counseling services during and after deployment
- recommends organizational strategies to assist responders deployed to harsh settings, such as administrative leave, just-in-time training, tactical logistical assistance, clarifying mission assignments
- provides support materials for families of those deployed using Internet technology and a peer-support (family buddy) system
- assists in interim and after-action reporting
- supports development of routine training courses for team leaders and deployment personnel
- facilitates external expert consultation with senior leadership and employee assistance professionals on strategic and operational policies, training, and behavioral healthcare practices
- institutes an integrated health, safety, and resiliency function as part of command staffing within the CDC incident management system
- supports a pilot field-support program, ranging from field support by peers (buddy) and tactical deployment, safety and resiliency team members, with linkage to CDC emergency operations for technical support and situation awareness
- provides field training involving the basics of safety, peer support, and psychological first aid.

respectively. Box 23.4 outlines the Worker Resiliency Program developed by the US Centers for Disease Control and Prevention to support its workers during a disaster and in its aftermath. This program is being presented to demonstrate how the principles presented in this chapter have been applied to a particular workplace setting and organizational culture. Organizational changes may include flexible schedules, portable communication devices (and air time), leadership and team building, regulating the operational tempo or staff rhythm, monitoring worker health, fatigue and safety practices, and providing services to meet work-related physical and emotional healthcare needs. Supervisors should be aware that fatigue and sleep deprivation can have serious negative consequences in the workplace and lead to recklessness or unsafe work practices during an emergency, particularly if shift length and duration of mandated service are long and rest periods are inadequate (Caruso *et al.*, 2006). Fatigue management becomes increasingly important when workers face multiple or hazardous work demands, threats to personal safety, and/or traumatic and psychologically challenging experiences, such as witnessing mass fatalities or handling affected persons who are angry or emotionally distraught.

It is helpful to anticipate needs for psychological interventions within the workplace and do the homework required to ensure that potential techniques are based on empirically defensible and evidence-based practices – and are conducted by qualified individuals. It is also important to tailor any intervention strategy to the ecology of the workplace and workforce (e.g., when and how the intervention unfolds) (Hobfoll *et al.*, 2007). These are all essential elements for organizational continuity. The cost of not doing this can be quite high, including loss of specialized workers, with a need to recruit and train new staff; interim loss of productivity; worker compensation costs for job-related injury, illness, or disability; and other potentially cascading organizational effects (e.g., loss of morale). Effective disaster safety management requires appropriate infrastructure and interagency planning and coordination before the emergency arises. Pre-deployment and preparedness activities shape and influence the overall success of the emergency response efforts, and, in turn, the disaster recovery process. As seen in the WTC disaster, workers who assume roles to which they are not accustomed, or for which they are psychologically unprepared, may experience significant interpersonal and organizational stresses (Perrin *et al.*, 2007). The same may be true for workers who shoulder extra responsibilities to ensure the continuity of businesses, governmental offices, or critical community services (e.g., energy, food, and water supply; waste management; telecommunications; and transportation).

Finally, expert consultation (advisor) to the incident or crisis leadership regarding the resilience, health, and safety of the affected workers would greatly benefit the efficiency of the combined operations. Behavioral expertise in a command staff advisory role may also serve to minimize decision-making errors stemming from the impact of the traumatic events on the leaders themselves.[2] Psychologically and behaviorally informed advice is likely to improve information analyzed about when and why leadership should implement major decisions: such as when to transition from *response* (rescue and life safety activities) to *recovery* (managing the losses) operations. There are cascading and enduring consequences that can occur when such a transition is delayed (Jackson *et al.*, 2004).

References

Barnett, D. J., Balicer, R. D., Lucey, D. R., *et al.* (2005). A systematic analytic approach to pandemic influenza preparedness planning. *PLoS Medicine*, **2**, 1235–1241.

Bills, C., Levy, N., Sharma, V., *et al.* (2008). The mental health of workers and volunteers responding to the events of 9/11: a review of the literature. *Mount Sinai Journal of Medicine*, **75**, 115–127.

Bilsker, D., Gilbert, M., & Samra, J. (2007). *Anti-depressant skills at work: Dealing with mood problems in the workplace.* Vancouver: British Columbia Mental Health and Addiction Services, Provincial Health Services Authority, British Columbia, http://www.comh.ca/antidepressant-skills/work/ (accessed July 31, 2009).

Brown, D. & Kulig, J. (1996/97). The concept of resiliency: Theoretical lessons from community research. *Health and Canadian Society*, **4**, 29–52.

Brymer, M., Jacobs, A., Layne, C., *et al.* (2006). *Psychological first aid: Field operations guide*, 2nd edn. Los Angeles, CA: National Child Traumatic Stress Network and National Center for Posttraumatic Stress Disorder.

Caruso, C. C., Bushnell, T., Eggerth, D., *et al.* (2006). Long working hours, safety, and health: Toward a national research agenda. *American Journal of Industrial Medicine*, **49**, 9300–9342.

DeMarchi, J. (1997). *Historical mining disasters* (pp. 34–44). Beckley, WV: National Mine Health and Safety Academy, Mine Safety and Health Administration.

Disaster Mental Health Subcommittee of the National Biodefense Science Board (2008). *Disaster mental health recommendations.* Washington, DC: National Biodefense Science Board, http://www.phe.gov/Preparedness/legal/boards/nbsb/meetings/Documents/dmhreport-final.pdf (accessed February 15, 2011).

Engel, C. C. (2004). Somatization and multiple idiopathic physical symptoms: Relationship to traumatic events and posttraumatic stress disorder. In P. P. Schnurr & B. L. Green (eds.), *Trauma and health: Physical health consequences of exposure to extreme stress* (pp. 191–216). Washington, DC: American Psychological Association.

Flynn, B. W. (2003). Leadership, mental health, and bioterrorism. In *Bioterrorism and public health: Communities and leaders preparing for psychological and behavioral responses to a biological attack*. Bethesda, MD: Center for the Study of Traumatic Stress.

Flynn, B. W. (2006). Facing the future: Who will own readiness for our emerging threats. In *Proceedings of the 22nd Annual Rosalynn Carter Symposium on Mental Health Policy*, Atlanta, http://www.cartercenter.org/documents/nondatabase/sym06_flynn.ppt (accessed August 30, 2009).

Fullerton, C. S., Ursano, R. J., Norwood, A. E., & Holloway, H. H. (2003). Trauma, terrorism, and disaster. In R. J. Ursano, C. S. Fullerton, & A. E. Norwood (eds.), *Terrorism and disaster: Individual and community mental health interventions* (pp. 1–22). New York: Cambridge University Press.

Garakani, A., Hirschowitz, J., & Katz, C. L. (2004). General disaster psychiatry. *Psychiatric Clinics of North America*, **27**, 391–406.

Gates, R. A., Phillips, R. L., Urosek, J. E., *et al.* (2007). *Report of investigation: Fatal underground coal mine explosion, January 2, 2006, Sago Mine, Wolf Run Mining Company, Tallmansville, Upshur County, West Virginia.* [ID No. 46–087910.] Arlington, VA: Mine Safety and Health Administration, US Department of Labor.

Gerberding, J. L. (2008). *World Trade Center health effects.* [Testimony to the Committee on Energy and Commerce, Subcommittee on Health of the US House of Representatives.] Atlanta, GA: Centers for Disease Control and Prevention, http://www.hhs.gov/asl/testify/2008/07/t20080731d.html (accessed on September 5, 2009).

Haddon, W. Jr. (1968). The changing approach to the epidemiology, prevention, and amelioration of trauma: The transition to approaches etiologically rather than descriptively based. *American Journal of Public Health*, **58**, 1431–1438.

Haddon, W. Jr. (1970). On the escape of tigers: an ecologic note. *American Journal of Public Health, Nations Health*, **60**, 2229–2234.

Haddon, W. Jr. (1972). A logical framework for categorizing highway safety phenomena and activity. *Journal of Trauma*, **12**, 193–207.

Haddow, G. D. & Bullock, J. A. (2006). The historical context of emergency management. In *Introduction to emergency management*, 2nd edn (pp. 1–18). Burlington MA: Elsevier Butterworth-Heinemann,

Herbert, R., Moline, J., Skloot, G., *et al.* (2006). The World Trade Center disaster and the health of workers: Five year assessment of a unique medical screening program. *Environmental Health Perspectives*, **114**, 1853–1858.

Hobfoll, S. E., Watson, P. J., Bell, C., *et al.* (2007). Five essential elements of immediate and mid-term mass trauma intervention: Empirical evidence. *Psychiatry*, **70**, 283–315.

Institute of Medicine (2002). *The future of the public's health in the 21st century*. Washington, DC: National Academies Press.

Institute of Medicine (2003). Institute of Medicine, National Academy of Sciences. A. Stith Butler, A. M. Panzer, & L. R. Goldfrank (eds.), *Preparing for the psychological consequences of terrorism: A public health strategy*. Washington, DC: National Academies Press.

International Federation of Red Cross and Red Crescent Societies (2000). *Introduction to disaster management*. Geneva: International Federation of Red Cross and Red Crescent Societies, http://www.ifrc.org/Docs/pubs/disasters/resources/corner/dp-manual/all.pdf (accessed July 11, 2009).

Jackson, B. A., Baker, J. C., Ridgely, M. S., Bartis, J. T., & Linn, H. I. (2004). *Protecting emergency responders*, Vol. 3: *Safety management in disaster and terrorism response*. [DHHS publication 2004–144.] Santa Monica, CA: RAND Corporation for the National Institute for Occupational Safety and Health, http://www.cdc.gov/niosh/docs/2004–144/ (accessed July 11, 2009).

Kaniasty, K. & Norris, F. H. (2004). Social support in the aftermath of disasters, catastrophes, and acts of terrorism: altruistic, overwhelmed, uncertain, antagonistic, and patriotic communities. In R. Ursano, A. Norwood, & C. Fullerton (eds.), *Bioterrorism: psychological and public health interventions* (pp. 200–229). Cambridge, UK: Cambridge University Press.

Katz, C. L. & Nathaniel, R. (2002). Disasters, psychiatry, and psychodynamics. *Journal of the American Academy of Psychoanalysis*, **30**, 519–530.

Katz, C. L., Pellegrino, L., Pandya, A., Ng, A., & DeLisi, L. (2002). Research on psychiatric outcomes subsequent to disasters: a review of the literature. *Psychiatry Research*, **110**, 201–217.

Katz, C. L., Smith, R., Herbert, R., Levin, S., & Gross, R. (2006a). The World Trade Center worker/volunteer mental health screening program. In Y. Neria, R. Gross, R. Marshall, & E. Susser (eds.), *9/11: Public mental health in the wake of a terrorist attack* (pp. 355–377). New York: Cambridge University Press.

Katz, C. L., Smith, R. P., Silverton, M., *et al.* (2006b). A mental health program for Ground Zero rescue and recovery workers: cases and observations. *Psychiatric Services*, **57**, 1335–1358.

Katz, C. L., Levin, S., Munro, S., Pandya, A., & Smith, R. (2009). Prevalence and predictors of psychiatric symptoms in Ground Zero iron workers: the aftermath of the World Trade Center attacks of September 11, 2001. *Psychiatric Bulletin*, **33**, 49–52.

Kowalski-Trakofler, K. M. & Barrett, E. A. (2003). The concept of degraded images applied to hazard recognition training in mining for reduction of lost-time injuries. *Journal of Safety Research*, **34**, 515–523.

Kowalski-Trakofler, K. M., Vaught, C., & Brnich, M. J. (2008). Expectations training for miners using self-contained self-rescuers. *Journal of Occupational and Environmental Hygiene*, **5**, 671–677.

Kowalski-Trakofler, K. M., Alexander, D. A., Brnich, M. J., McWilliams, L., & Reissman, D. B. (2009). Underground coal mining disasters and fatalities: United States, 1900–1906. *Morbidity and Mortality Weekly Report*, **57**, 1379–1383.

Masten, A. S. & Obradović, J. (2008). Disaster preparation and recovery: Lessons from research on resilience in human development. *Ecology and Society*, **13**, 1–9.

McQuistion, H. & Katz, C. L. (2001). The September 11, 2001 disaster: some lessons learned in mental health preparedness. *Emergency Psychiatry*, **7**, 61–64.

MINER Act (2006). Mine Improvement and New Emergency Response Act of 2006, Pub. L. No. 108–236 (S 2803), http://www.msha.gov/MinerAct/MinerActSingleSource.asp (accessed February 28, 2011).

Mine Safety and Health Administration (1998a). *Historical summary of mine disasters in the United States*, Vol. II: *Coal Mines 1959–1998*. Arlington, VA: Mine Safety and Health Administration, US Department of Labor.

Mine Safety and Health Administration (1998b). *Historical summary of mine disasters in the United States*, Vol. I: *Coal Mines 1810–1958*. Arlington, VA: Mine Safety and Health Administration, US Department of Labor.

Norris, F. H., Stevens, S. P., Pfefferbaum, B., Wyche, K. F., & Pfefferbaum, R. L. (2008). Community resilience as a metaphor, theory, set of capacities and strategy for disaster readiness. *American Journal of Community Psychology*, **41**, 127–150.

Paton, D. & Johnston, D. (eds.) (2006). *Disaster resilience: An integrated approach*. Springfield, IL: Charles C. Thomas.

Perrin, M. A., DiGrande, L., Wheeler, K., *et al.* (2007). Differences in PTSD prevalence and associated risk factors among World Trade Center rescue and recovery workers. *American Journal of Psychiatry*, **9**, 1385–1394.

Qureshri, K., Gerson, R. R. M., & Sherman, M. F., *et al.* (2005). Health care workers ability and willingness to report to duty during catastrophic disasters. *Journal of Urban Health,* **82***,* 378–388.

Reissman, D. B. & Howard, J. (2008). Responder safety and health: Preparing for future disasters. *Mount Sinai Journal of Medicine,* **75***,* 135–141.

Reissman, D. B., Schreiber, M., Klomp, R. W., *et al.* (2006a). The virtual network supporting the front lines: Addressing emerging behavioral health problems following the tsunami of 2004. *Military Medicine,* **171***,* 40–43.

Reissman, D. B., Watson, P. J., Klomp, R. W., Tanielian, T. L., & Prior, S. D. (2006b). Pandemic influenza preparedness: adaptive responses to an evolving challenge. *Journal of Homeland Security and Emergency Management,* **3***,* 13.

Runyan, C. W. (2003). Introduction: back to the future: Revisiting Haddon's conceptualization of injury epidemiology and prevention. *Epidemiological Review,* **25***,* 60–64.

Salerno, A., Margolies, P., & Cleek, A. (2008). *Wellness and self-management personal workbook,* 2nd edn. New York: New York State Office of Mental Health and the Urban Institute for Behavioral Health.

Schoch-Spana, M. (2008). Editorial: Community resilience for catastrophic health events. *Biosecurity and Bioterrorism: Biodefense Strategy, Practice, and Science* **6***,* 2.

Shalev, A. Y., Bonne, O., & Eth, S. (1996). Treatment of post-traumatic stress disorder: A review. *Psychosomatic Medicine,* **58***,* 165–182.

Smith, R. P., Katz, C. L., Holmes, A., *et al.* (2004). Mental health status of World Trade Center rescue and recovery workers and volunteers: New York City, July 2002–August 2004. *Morbidity and Mortality Weekly Report,* **53***,* 812–815.

Tedeschi, R. G., Park, C. L., & Calhoun, L. G. (1998). Posttraumatic growth: Conceptual issues. In R. Tedeschi & L. Calhoun (eds.), *Posttraumatic growth: Positive changes in the aftermath of crisis* (pp. 1–22). Mahwah, NJ: Earlbaum.

Thrush, P. W. & staff of the U. S. Bureau of Mines (1968). *A dictionary of mining, mineral and related terms.* Washington, DC: Bureau of Mines.

Ursano, R. J., Vineburgh, N. T., Gifford, R. K., Benedek, D. M., & Fullerton, C. S. (2006) *A leadership document to inform planning, response and policy for workplace preparedness and behavioral risk management of disaster and terrorism.* Bethesda, MD: Center for the Study of Traumatic Stress, http://www.centerforthestudyoftraumaticstress.org/downloads/CSTS%20Leadership%20Planning%20for%20Workplace%20Preparedness.pdf (accessed July 11, 2009).

US Department of Homeland Security (2007). *Homeland Security Presidential Directive 21. Public health and medical preparedness.* Washington, DC: US Department of Homeland Security, http://www.dhs.gov/xabout/laws/gc_1219263961449.shtm (accessed September 5, 2009).

US Department of Homeland Security (2009). *Homeland Security Presidential Directive 7. National infrastructure protection plan: Partnering to enhance protection and resiliency.* Washington, DC: US Department of Homeland Security, http://www.dhs.gov/xlibrary/assets/NIPP_Plan.pdf (accessed September 5, 2009).

West Virginia Office of Miners' Health, Safety, and Training (2006). *Report of investigation into the Sago Mine explosion.* Charleston, WV: West Virginia Office of Miners' Health, Safety, and Training.

Wheeler, K., McKelvey, W., Thorpe, L., *et al.* (2007). Asthma diagnosed after 11 September 2001 among rescue and recovery workers: Findings from the World Trade Center Health Registry. *Environmental Health Perspectives,* **115***,* 1584–1590.

Winslow, C. E. A. (1920). The untilled field of public health. *Modern Medicine,* **2***,* 183–191.

Wright, K. M., Ursano, R. J., Bartone, P. T., & Ingraham, L. H. (1990). The shared experience of catastrophe: an expanded classification of the disaster community. *American Journal of Orthopsychiatry,* **60***,* 35–42.

Zohar, D. (2010). Safety climate: Conceptual and measurement issues. In J . Campbell Quick & L. E. Tetrick (eds.), *Handbook of occupational health psychology,* 2nd edn (Ch. 8). Washington, DC: American Psychological Association.

Endnotes

1. The National Biodefense Science Board was established by the Secretary of the US Department of Health and Human Services (DHHS) pursuant to section 319M of the Public Health Services Act (42 USC. 247d-7f) as added by section 402 of the Pandemic and All Hazards Preparedness Act (PAHPA) (Pub. L. 107–417), effective December 19, 2006. The Board provides expert advice and guidance to the Secretary on scientific, technical, and other matters of special interest to HHS regarding current and future chemical, biological, nuclear, and radiological agents, whether naturally occurring, accidental, or deliberate. The Board may also provide advice and guidance to the Secretary on other matters related to public health emergency preparedness and response. It is an established Federal Advisory Committee with both legal and discretionary authorities.

2. Under the Homeland Security Presidential Directive 21, paragraph 31 (US Department of Homeland Security, 2007), the Secretary of Health and Human Services, in coordination with the Secretaries of Defense, Veterans Affairs, and Homeland Security, was directed to establish a Federal Advisory Committee for Disaster Mental Health. The directive stated that the committee shall consist of appropriate subject matter experts and, within 180 days after its

establishment, shall submit to the Secretary of Health and Human Services recommendations for protecting, preserving, and restoring individual and community mental health in catastrophic health event settings, including pre-, intra-, and post-event education, messaging, and interventions. To execute this directive, the Disaster Mental Health Subcommittee was established under the National Biodefense Science Board, an established Federal Advisory Committee with both legal and discretionary authorities providing advice and guidance to the Secretary of Health and Human Services.

Index

5-HT, *see* serotonin
5-*HTTLPR, see* serotonin transporter
    gene
absorption, 257
abyss experience, 182–183
acceptance and commitment therapy,
    97
acculturation, 177
achievement, 66
active coping, 17
acts of kindness, 283–284
acute stress response
    modulating agents, 10–18
        brain-derived neurotrophic factor,
            12–13
        epigenetic mechanisms, 13–14
        neural circuitry of fear, 14–15
        psychological processes, 15–18
        sex hormones, 10–12
    systems, 2–10
        corticotropin-releasing hormone,
            4–5
        dopamine, 7–9
        hypothalamic–pituitary–adrenal
            axis, 2–4
        neuropeptides, 9–10
        norepinephrine, 5–6
        serotonin, 6–7
adaptive capacities, 163
adaptive systems, 111–114
    attachment relationships, 112
    cultural systems, 113
    improving or mobilizing, 115
    intelligence and problem-solving
        systems, 112
    motivation to adapt, 112–113
    self-regulation systems, 113
adolescents
    well-being therapy, 297,
        see also children
adrenocorticotropin hormone, 2
    estrogens and, 12
    α_2-adrenoceptor, 5
African-Americans' resiliency systems,
    179–180
aging, *see also* older adults
    mental health and, 136
    resilience theories, 136–138

burden perspective, 137
    inoculation perspective, 137
    maturation hypothesis, 137–138
    mortality hypothesis, 138
    vulnerability theory, 137
aging population, 135
    increased diversity, 135,
    see also older adults
Alaska Natives' resiliency systems, 180
alcohol dependence, 294–295
allostasis, 1–2, 80, 308
    enhancement in children, 312–313
        emotional literacy, 314–315
        interventions in schools and
            communities, 314
        interventions with parents,
            313–314
        moral courage training, 317
        outdoor education programs,
            316–317
        Penn Resiliency Program, 317
        team sports, 315–316
allostatic load, 2, 81, 308
American-Indian/Alaska Native
    resiliency systems, 180
amygdala
    role in fear, 14
    stress response and, 16
a-priori beliefs, appraisal theory, 31–32,
    46
    primary appraisal, 46
    secondary appraisal, 46
    self-appraisal, 47
Arab American resiliency systems, 180
arginine vasopressin, 4–5
Asian cultural resiliency systems,
    180–181
Asian Indian cultural resiliency
    systems,
attachment relationships, 112
attention control, 32–33, 40
    adaptive, 35
    cognitive reappraisal, 37–40
    distraction, 36
    resilience and, 33–37
    rumination, 36
    selective attention, 35–36
attentional bias, 34

training, 35–36
avoidance, 195–196, 230

baseline function, 208–209
Battlemind, 325
Battlemind Training System, 323–324
    comprehensiveness, 329
    future directions, 336–338
    history, 324
    implementation, 331–336
        exportability and scalability, 333
        integration into organizational
            culture, 331–332
        leader support, 335
        mobile training teams, 334
        ownership issues, 336
        packaging and multimedia, 336
        policy, 335
        quality control, 332
        refresher training, 334
        sustainability, 334
        timing, 332
        training guidelines, 333–334
        train-the-trainer program,
            332–333
        verifiable claims, 335–336
    mental health training
        action-focused, 328
        developmental nature, 328–329
        evidence-based, 330–331
        experience-based, 327–328
        explanatory nature, 328
        relevant purpose and content, 327
        strength-based, 327
        team-based approach, 328
        user-acceptability, 329–330
    program improvement, 334–335
bereavement, 121, 189
    delayed reactions, 123
    grief counseling, 129
    individual differences, 189
        ethnic and cultural differences,
            197
        implications of, 196–197
        variation in grief reactions, 123
    older adults, 125–126, 139–140
    positive emotions and, 127–128
    trajectories

bereavement (*cont.*)
    chronic grief, 194–196
    recovery, 219
    resilience, 192–194, *see also* grief
beta-blockers, 6
Bosnian refugees, 157
brain-derived neurotrophic factor,
    12–13
breast cancer, benefits of social ties,
    82, 83
    resilience promotion, 84
Brief Multidimensional Measure of
    Religion/Spirituality (BMMRS),
    93–94, 99
Buddhism, 181
Buffalo Creek flood, 270, 271
burden hypothesis, 137

CAFES program, 157
cancer, benefits of social ties, 82, 83
    resilience promotion, 84
cardiovascular stress response, 79–80
    social ties and, 79–80
caregiving, 139
    stress reactivity in children and,
    309–311
Caribbean black resiliency system,
    181
catechol-*O*-methyl-transferase, 5–6
causal attributions, 46
CDC Worker Resiliency Program, 354
challenge, 63
change, models of, 114–115
Chicago Center for Family Health
    programs, 156
    Bosnian and Kosovar refugees, 157
    job loss stresses, 156–157
    Kosovar Family Professional
        Educational Collaborative,
        157–158
children, 307–308
    adaptive systems, 111–114
        attachment relationships, 112
        cultural systems, 113
        intelligence and problem-solving
            systems, 112
        motivation to adapt, 112–113
        self-regulation systems, 113
    allostasis enhancement, 312–313
        emotional literacy, 314–315
        interventions in schools and
            communities, 314
        interventions with parents,
            313–314
        moral courage training, 317
        outdoor education programs,
            316–317
        Penn Resiliency Program, 317
        team sports, 315–316
developmental research, 108–111

competence and cascades,
    166–167
    intervention models, 110
    person-focused approaches, 108
    variable-focused approaches,
    108–110
developmental tasks, 105
grief in, 123
    intervention issues, 128–129
    grief counseling, 129
    PTSD, 124–125
    resilience, 103–104, 111–114, 123,
    265
        attachments and, 308–309
        poverty effects, 265–268
    resilience development
        good adaptation, 105
        promotive and protective factors,
        106
        threats, 105–106
    resilience framework, 114–115
    resilience promoting factors, 128
    self-efficacy
        promotion of, 314
        stress relationships, 311–312
    stress reactivity related to caregiving,
    309–311
    trauma responses, 123
    well-being therapy, 297
Chinese culture, 180
chronic disease, 122–123
    older adults, 139
    physiological adjustment, 76
    psychological adjustment, 76
    social ties and
        behavioral effects, 79
        evidence for effects, 81–83
        physiological benefits, 79–81,
        82–83
        psychological benefits, 78, 81–82
        resilience promotion, 83–85
chronic grief, 194–195
    qualitative aspects, 195–196
chronic life strains, 264
citalopram, 7
citizen participation, 165
coal mining, *see* mining
cognitive approaches, 45, 46–47
    challenges, 52
    see also social cognitive theory
cognitive-behavioral stress
    management, 38, 40
cognitive-behavioral therapy, 40
    following rape, 233
    serious mental illness, 281
cognitive disorganization, 190
cognitive emotion regulation, 32–33,
    40–41
    attention control, 32–37, 40
    cognitive reappraisal, 32–33, 40–41

cognitive reappraisal, 32–33, 40–41
    resilience and, 37–40
collective efficacy, 47–49, 270–271
collectivism, 177
combat, *see* warfare
combat and operational stress
    continuum model, 243–246
    core leader functions, 246–249
Combat and Operational Stress Control
    program. *see* US Marine Corps
combat and operational stress first aid,
    248
commitment, 63
communication, community resilience
    and, 165–166
communities
    definition, 207–208, 268
    disaster impact on, 206
Community Assessment of Resilience
    (CART), 167–168
community competence, 166–167
community preparedness, 170
community resilience, 162, 203, 209–
    210, 340–341
    assessment of capacities, 167–170
        participatory approaches,
        167–168
        social indicator research, 168–170
    enhancement, 170–172
    multiple meanings of, 340–341
    poverty effects, 268–271
        cohesion, 269–270
        collective efficacy, 270–271
        social capital, 269
    predictors of, 203–204
    resources, 163
        community competence,
        166–167
        economic development,
        163–164
        information and communication,
        165–166
        social capital, 164–165
competence, 166–167
complicated grief, 189
Comprehensive Soldier Fitness (CSF),
    324, 335
conditionability, 66–67
Confucianism, 181
Connor–Davidson Resilience Scale
    (CD-RISC), 290
conservation of resources theory,
    254–257, 272
    defensive responding with resource
        lack, 257
    engagement/distress interactions,
        260–261
    primacy of resource loss, 254
    resource investment, 254–255
    resource loss and gain spirals, 256

constraint/impulsivity, 57
   see also personality factors
control, 63
coping self-efficacy, 47, 48–49
   demands and, 50–51
      traumatic demands, 49–50
coping strategies
   active coping, 17
   avoidance coping, 67
   emotion-focused coping, 67
   following rape, 229–230
   personality and, 67
   pragmatic coping, 126–127
   problem-focused/approach coping, 67
   recovery and, 278
   religious coping, 94–95, 98
      negative religious coping, 95
   with serious mental illness, 281
coronary heart disease, 79
   benefits of social ties, 81–83
      resilience promotion, 84
corticotropin-releasing hormone, 4–5
   allostatic contribution, 4
   allostatic load, 4
   factors promoting resilience, 4–5
   neuropeptide Y interaction, 9
   receptors, 4
cortisol, 2
   allostatic contribution, 2
   DHEA ratio, 3–4
   dysregulation, 2–3
   social ties and, 81
critical incident stress debriefing, 128
cultural diversity, 151
cultural systems, 113
   African-American, 179–180
   American-Indian/Alaska Native, 180
   Arab-American, 180
   Asian cultural, 180–181
   Asian Indian, 181
   Caribbean black resiliency system, 181
   Hawaiian Native, 182
   Latin-American, 182
culture, 176–178
   monocultural ethnocentrism, 178
   resiliency and, 177–178
   in trauma recovery, 182–183
   see also cultural systems; ethnic considerations
cumulative risk, 105

dedication, 257
dehydroepiandrosterone (DHEA), 2
   allostatic contribution, 2
   cortisol ratio, 3–4
   treatment, 3–4
demands, 50–51
   traumatic demands, 49–50

depression,
   attentional bias and, 34
   distraction and, 33
   in chronic disease, benefits of social ties, 81–82
   rumination and, 33–34
   see also manic depressive disorder
developmental cascades, 111
developmental psychopathology, 103–104
developmental tasks, 105
dexamethasone suppression test, 3
dialectical behavior therapy, 97
disaster management, 170–172
   resilience promotion in disaster workers, 341–343, 352–355
      Haddon matrix, 342–343
      Sago Mine disaster, 347–352
      World Trade Center case study, 343–347
   see also emergency management
disaster research, 200–202
   resilience concept in, 203–204
disasters, 200, 203–204, 340
   challenges in applying resilience, 207–213
      baseline function, 208–209
      defining communities, 207–208
      defining value-neutral resilience and failure, 211–212
      resilience for whom, 209–211
   multilevel consequences of, 204–207
      community impact, 206
      displacement, 205–206
      economic and political impact, 206–207
      environmental health, 205
      family impact, 206
      physical health, 204
      psychological health, 204–205
      rescue and clean-up operations, 205
   typologies, 343
   see also disaster management
displacement, 205–206
Dispositional Resilience Scale-15 (DRS-15), 290
distraction, 33, 36
distress
   engagement/distress interactions, 260–261
   trajectories, 259–260
dopamine, 7–9
   allostatic contribution, 8
   allostatic load, 8–9
   factors contributing to resilience, 9
dopamine D_2 receptor gene (*DRD2*), 9
dysphoric emotions, 190–191

economic development, 163–164
   index of, 169
   measurement, 169–170
economic disparity, 151
economic impact of disasters, 206–207
elderly, *see* older adults
emergency management, 170–172, 340
   see also disaster management
emotion regulation, 16, 30
   active coping, 17
   humor, 17
   meaning-making, 17
   moderator model, 31
   optimism, 17
   promotion in children, 314–315
   reframing/reappraisal, 16
   social competence, 17–18
   see also cognitive emotion regulation
emotional literacy, 314–315
emotional support, 77
emotions, 15–18
   dysphoric, following bereavement, 190–191
   elements of, 15
   see also emotion regulation; negative emotions; positive emotions
empathy, 17–18
empowerment, 278
engagement, 257
   as both process and outcome, 257–258
   engagement versus distress trajectories, 259–260
   engagement/distress interactions, 260–261
engagement theory, 254, 257
Enhancing Recovery in Coronary Artery Heart Disease (ENRICHD), 293–294
environmental context
   demands, 50–51
      traumatic demands, 49–50
   genetic–environmental interactions, 178–179
      religiosity as an environmental influence, 179
epigenetic changes, 13–14
epinephrine (E)
   social ties and, 81
estrogens, 11–12, 13
   stress response and, 11–12
ethnic considerations
   African-American resiliency systems, 179–180
   American-Indian/Alaska Native resiliency systems, 180
   Arab-American resiliency systems, 180

ethnic considerations (*cont.*)
Asian cultural resiliency systems, 180–181
Caribbean black resiliency system, 181
Hawaiian Native resiliency system, 182
Latin-American cultural resiliency systems, 182
see cultural systems
executive function, 113

faith, loss of
see also religion/spirituality
families
disaster impact on, 206
structure, 150–151
family resilience, 149–150
assessment of family function, 152–155
genograms, 153
Walsh Family Resilience Framework, 153–155
developmental perspective, 151–152
family life cycle stressors, 152
intergenerational legacies, 152
pile-up of stressors, 152
varied pathways in resilience, 151–152
family resilience-oriented practice, 155–158
approaches to traumatic loss and major disaster, 158
Chicago Center for Family Health programs, 156
key processes, 154
poverty effects, 268
research challenges and opportunities, 158
sociocultural context, 150–151
family impact of broader social trauma, 151
family transformations in changing societies, 150–151
fear
conditioning, 14–15
neural circuitry of, 14–15
fight or flight response, 80
FKBP5 gene, 4
flexible adaptation, 127
fluoxetine side-effects, 7
forgiveness, lack of, 95
intervention studies, 97

galanin, 10
allostatic contribution, 10
allostatic load, 10
factors promoting resilience, 10

GAL-3 receptor, 10
gender roles, 150–151
genetic approaches, 116
genetic–environmental interactions, 178–179
religiosity as an environmental influence, 179
genograms, 153
Giraffe Project, 317
glucocorticoids, 2
glucocorticoid receptor sensitivity,
goal-setting, with serious mental illness, 282
good adaptation, 105
gratitude enhancement, 283
grief
children, 123
complicated grief, 189
delayed reactions, 123
individual difference implications, 196–197
phenomenology, 189–192
cognitive disorganization, 190
dysphoric emotions, 190–191
health deficits, 191–192
social and occupational dysfunction, 192
trajectories, 192–195
chronic grief, 194–196
recovery, 219
resilience, 192–194
variation in grief reactions, 123
contextual factors, 197
see also bereavement
grief counseling, 129
gross domestic product (GDP), 169
guilt, 95

Haddon matrix, 342–343
application to Sago Mine disaster, 347–352
application to World Trade Center disaster, 343–347
hardiness, 63–64, 142, 178, 291
personality trait relationships, 64
training for resilience enhancement, 291–292
HardiTraining, 292
Hawaiian resiliency system, 182
health
bereavement impact on, 191–192
disaster impact on, 204
environmental health, 205
psychological health, 204–205
social support and, 293–294
hippocampus role in fear, 14
HIV, benefits of social ties, 82, 83
resilience promotion, 84–85
Holocaust survivors, 140

homeostasis, 1, 2
hope, 278
HPA, *see* hypothalamic–pituitary–adrenal axis
Human Development Index, 169
humor, 17, 284
Hurricane Andrew, 124–125, 128
Hurricane Katrina, 141, 200–201, 208, 210
hypothalamic–pituitary–adrenal axis, 2–4, 80–81
allostatic contribution, 2
allostatic load, 2–3
factors promoting resilience, 3–4
axis feedback, 4
cortisol to DHEA ratio, 3–4
single nucleotide polymorphisms, 3

immune function, 80
Incredible Years Teacher and Child Training Programs, 314–315
Indian Ocean tsunami, 200
Sri Lankan response, 269, 270–271
individualism, 177
information, community resilience and, 165–166
informational support, 77
inoculation perspective, 137
stress inoculation training, 292–293
instrumental support, 77
intelligence, 112
IQ, 109
intergenerational legacies, 152
intervention models, 110
IQ, 109

Job Demands–Control model (JD-C), 50
job loss, 156–157

Kauai Longitudinal Study, Hawaii, 265–266
Kosovar Family Professional Educational Collaborative, 157–158
Kosovar refugees, 157

Landmine Survivors Network, 298–302
latent growth mixture modeling, 122
Latin-American cultural resiliency systems, 182
learned helplessness, 5
learned optimism training, 295–296
life course, 151
locus coeruleus, 5
allostatic contribution, 5
allostatic load, 5
loneliness, 191

loss of faith, 95
Lower Manhattan Community
        Recovery Project, 158

manic depressive disorder (MDD)
    cortisol dysregulation, 2–3
    5-HTTLPR polymorphism and, 7
    reward responses, 8
maturation hypothesis, 137–138
meaning-making, 17
mediating effects, 110
mental fitness, 326
mental health training, 324, 326–331
    action-focused, 328
    developmental nature, 328–329
    evidence-based, 330–331
    experience-based, 327–328
    explanatory nature, 328
    implementation, 331–336
        exportability and scalability, 333
        integration into organizational
            culture, 331–332
        leader support, 335
        mobile training teams, 334
        ownership issues, 336
        packaging and multimedia, 336
        policy, 335
        quality control, 332
        refresher training, 334
        timing, 332
        training guidelines, 333–334
        train-the-trainer program,
            332–333
    relevant purpose and content, 327
    strength-based approach, 327
    team-based, 328
    user-acceptability, 329–330
mental illness, *see* serious mental illness
mental toughness, 66
Mexico City earthquake, 207, 212
military personnel, 238, 323
    resilience challenges, 238–242
        operational resilience, 239–240
        post-deployment resilience,
            240–241
        psychological resilience, 241–242
    social support importance, 293
    US Navy and Marine Corps
        approach, 242–249
        core leader functions, 246–249
        program goals, 242
        rationale, 242–243
        stress continuum model, 243–246,
            see also Battlemind Training
            System
mindfulness, 97–98, 283
mindfulness-based cognitive therapy,
        97–98
mindfulness-based stress reduction, 98

Minding the Baby program, 313
mining, 347–348
    disaster incidents, 349
    safety history, 348
    see also Sago Mine disaster
mirror neurons, 18
monocultural ethnocentrism, 178
moral courage training, 317
mortality hypothesis, 138
mortality, following bereavement,
        191–192
motivation to adapt, 112–113

National Vietnam Veterans
        Readjustment Study, 63
negative attentional bias, 34
negative emotions, 15
    negative emotionality/neuroticism,
        56–57
        post-traumatic adjustment and,
            64–65
        see also emotions; personality
            factors
negative life events, 264
networks, 164
neural circuitry of fear, 14–15
neural plasticity, 115
neuroendocrine activity, 80–81
    social ties and, 81
neuropeptide Y, 9–10
    allostatic contribution, 9
    allostatic load, 9
    factors promoting resilience, 9–10
neuroticism, 56–57, 141–142
    post-traumatic adjustment and,
        64–65
norepinephrine, 5–6
    allostatic contribution, 5
    allostatic load, 5
    factors promoting resilience, 5–6
    social ties and, 81

occupational stress, 50
older adults, 125, 126, 135
    mental health problems, 136
    resilience in, 138–143
        bereavement and, 139–140
        caregiving and, 139
        chronic illness and, 139
        former combatants and prisoners
            of war, 140
        future directions, 143
        Holocaust survivors, 140
        in daily life, 138–139
        personality factors, 141–142
        social support and, 142–143
        trauma-specific variables, 142
    resilience theories, 136–138
        burden perspective, 137

inoculation perspective, 137
    maturation hypothesis, 137–138
    mortality hypothesis, 138
    vulnerability theory, 137
trauma recovery, 136–138
operational resilience, 239–240
Operational Stress Control (OSC)
        program, *see* US Navy
optimism, 17, 35, 278
    learned optimism training,
        295–296
Organizational Leadership Self-
        Assessment Tool, 353
outdoor education programs, 316–317
oxytocin, 17–18

Penn Resiliency Program, 296, 317
personality factors, 51–52, 56–57
    future research, 68–69
    hardiness and, 63–64
    mediators of the link with resilience,
        66–68
        conditionability, 66–67
        coping style, 67
        social support, 67–68
    older adults, 141–142
    post-trauma prospective studies,
        60–63
    post-traumatic adjustment
        relationships, 64–66
    pre-trauma prospective studies,
        58–60
    research challenges, 57–58
    resilience promotion, 126–127
person-focused approaches, 108
place attachment, 165
political impact of disasters, 206–207
positive emotions, 15–16
    mechanisms of effects, 128
    positive emotionality/extroversion,
        56
        resilience relationship, 66
    resilience promotion, 127–128
    serious mental illness treatment,
        282–283
        acts of kindness, 283–284
        gratitude enhancement, 283
        savoring, 283
        sense of humor, 284,
            see also emotions; personality
            factors
positive goals, 114
post-deployment resilience, 240–241
post-traumatic growth, 143
    versus resiliency, 258–259
post-traumatic stress disorder (PTSD),
        121
    children, 123, 124–125
    coping dysfunction, 67

post-traumatic stress disorder (PTSD)
    (*cont.*)
    cortisol dysregulation, 2–3
    delayed reactions, 123
    dopamine and, 9
    following rape, 218–219, 222–223
        future research, 231–232
        methodological issues, 219–220,
            221
        peritraumatic factors, 225–228
        post-assault factors, 230–231
        pre-trauma factors, 223–225
        resilience promotion, 232–233
    Holocaust survivors, 140
    intervention issues, 129
    older adults, 125
    personality factors, 65–66
        hardiness, 63,
    prevention, 6
    reward responses, 8
    risk factors, 221–222
    social support relationship, 68
    trauma intensity significance,
        68–69
    variation in trauma response, 122
potentially traumatic events, 120, 122
    heterogeneous trajectories following
        exposure, 121–123
        chronic dysfunction, 122–123
        delayed reactions, 123
        resilience and recovery, 123
    intervention implications across the
        lifespan, 128–129
    resilience promoting factors
        demographic and contextual
            factors, 126
        in children, 128
        personality, 126–127
        positive emotions, 127–128
        worldview, 127
    see also trauma
poverty, 264–265
    resilience and, 271–273
        adults and families, 268
        children, 265–268
        communities, 268–271
pragmatic coping, 126–127
preparatory interventions, 297–298
primary appraisal, 46
prisoners of war, 140, *see also* warfare
problem-solving systems, 112
problem-solving therapy, 281
Project on Human Development in
    Chicago Neighbourhoods, 270
promotive factors, 106, 126–128
    demographic and contextual factors,
        126
    in children, 128
    personality, 126–127

positive emotions, 127–128
    worldview, 127
propranolol, 6
prosocial behavior, 17–18
protective factors, 106, 176
psychoeducational resilience
    enhancement, 293
public health, 340
    see also disaster management;
        emergency management

racial variation, 177–178
    see also ethnic considerations
rape
    consequences of, 218–219
    definitions, 219
    future research directions, 231–233
    methodological issues, 219–221
        ideal study, 219–220
        unacknowledged rape, 220–221
    peritraumatic factors associated with
        post-rape function, 225–228
        acknowledgement of rape,
            227–228
        assault characteristics, 225–226
        peritraumatic reactions, 226–227
        post-assault concerns, 228
    post-assault factors associated with
        post rape function, 228–231
        additional stresses and trauma,
            230–231
        coping strategies, 229–230
        social support, 229
    pre-trauma factors associated with
        post-rape function, 223–225
        demographics, 223–224
        mental health history, 225
        prior assault history, 224–225
    prevalence, 218–219
    PTSD risk and protective factors,
        222–223
    resilience promotion, 232–233
rapidity, 163
RCOPE, 99
reappraisal, 16, *see also* cognitive
    reappraisal
recovery, 107, 123, 124
    culture significance, 182–183
    definitions, 277–278
    following bereavement, 219
    from serious mental illness, 276
        limitations of medical definitions,
            276–277
        themes, 278–279
            coping, 278
            hope and optimism, 278
            openness to new experiences, 278
            self-respect and self-
                determination, 278

recreational interests, with serious
    mental illness, 282
redundancy, 163
reframing, 113
    see also cognitive reappraisal
        religion; religion/spirituality
    Buddhism, 181
    Confucianism, 181
    definition, 90, 91
    religiosity as an environmental
        influence, 179
    Taoism, 180
religion/spirituality (RS), 90, 91, 178
    dynamic nature of, 91
        trauma response and, 91–92
    future directions, 98–99
    interventions, 97–98
        spirituality group therapy module,
            96–97
    measurement of, 98–99
    multidimensional representation,
        93–94
    religious coping, 94–95, 98
        negative religious coping, 95
    resilience relationships, 94–95
        relilience development, 93
    spiritual "red flags", 95, 98
        guilt, 95
        lack of forgiveness, 95
        loss of faith, 95
        negative religious coping, 95
    spiritual development, 92
    model, 91
rescue and clean-up operations, 205
resilience, 30, 45, 136, 289, 325–326
    across the lifespan, 124–126
    as a process, 162–163
    bereavement and, 192–194
    capacities for, 163
    children, 103–104, 111–114, 123,
        265
        attachments and, 308–309
        poverty effects, 265–268
    community, *see* community
        resilience
    construct development, 123–124
    definition, 2, 91, 103, 202–203
        controversies, 106–108
        criteria, 106–107
        developmental approaches, 104
        following rape, 219
        good adaptation, 105
        narrow versus broad definition,
            107
        threats, 105–106
        time frame, 107
    definitions, 325
    development, 93
        late-emerging resilience, 107

promotive and protective factors, 106
trauma impact, 120
dynamic perspective, 92–93, 104
enhancement interventions, 289–290, 291–293, 302
case example, 298–302
children, 312–317
disaster workers, 341–343, 352–355
hardiness training, 291–292
psychoeducational resilience enhancement, 293
stress inoculation training1052
enhancement of related constructs, 293–298
learned optimism training, 295–296
social support interventions, 293–295
well-being therapy, 296–297
family, *see* family resilience
framework, 31–33, 114–115
measures, 115
methods, 115
mission, 114
models of change, 114–115
multilevel approaches, 115
future directions, 115–116
in disaster research, 203–204
individual resilience, 149
measurement, 290–291
multilevel concept, 200, 202–203
older adults, 138–143
bereavement and, 139–140
caregiving and, 139
chronic illness and, 139
former combatants and prisoners of war, 140
future directions, 143
Holocaust survivors, 140
in daily life, 138–139
resilience theories, 136–138
social support and, 142–143
trauma recovery and, 136–138
trauma-specific variables, 142
predictors of, 104
preparatory interventions, 297–298
promotion, *see* promotive factors
religion/spirituality relationships, 93, 94–95
reorienting, 212–213
research, 1
competence and cascades, 166–167
developmental research, 108–111
intervention models, 110
person-focused approaches, 108

variable-focused approaches, 108–110
see also resiliency
Resilience Scales for Children and Adolescents (RSCA), 290
resiliency, 108
African-American resiliency systems, 179–180
American-Indian/Alaska Native resiliency systems, 180
Arab-American resiliency systems, 180
Asian cultural resiliency systems, 180–181
Caribbean black' resiliency system, 181
characteristics of, 176
cultivation, 179–182
culture and, 177–178
in serious mental illness, 279
resiliency factors, 279–280
Hawaiian Native resiliency system, 182
Latin-American cultural resiliency systems, 7–9
versus post-traumatic growth, 258–259, *see also* resilience
resistance, 107
resource dependency, 164
resources, boosting, 115
Response to Stressful Experiences Scale (RSES), 290
reward system
altered responses, 8–9
motivation to adapt, 112–113
risk factors, 108–110
cumulative risk, 105
in development, 105–106
mediating effects, 110
PTSD, 221–222
following rape, 222–223
risk gradients, 105
risk prevention, 115
robustness, 163
Rochester Resilience Project, 266
rumination, 33–34, 36

Sago Mine disaster, 348–353
Haddon matrix application, 350
savoring, 283
scenario-based training, 297–298
schizophrenia, 276, *see also* serious mental illness
schools, 113
secondary appraisal, 46
selective attention, 35–36
training, 35–36
see also attention control (AC)
selective serotonin reuptake inhibitors

side-effects, 7
self-appraisal, 47
self-blame, following rape, 230
self-determination, 278
self-efficacy, 47–49
changes in, 51
demands and, 50–51
traumatic demands, 49–50
environmental context, 49–51
in children
promotion of, 314
stress relationships, 311–312
personality factors, 51–52
self-enhancement, 142
self-esteem, improvement with serious mental illness, 282
self-regulation, 46–47, 113
children living in poverty, 267
social cognitive theory, 47–49
see also emotion regulation
self-respect, 278
sense of community, 284
sense of humor, 284
September 11 terrorist attack, New York, 122, 141, 208
family meetings as community intervention, 158
Haddon matrix application, 343–347
Lower Manhattan Community Recovery Project, 158
serious mental illness, 276
objections to traditional hierarchical decision making, 277
recovery, 276
limitations of medical definitions, 276–277
themes, 278–279
resiliency in, 279
resiliency factors, 279–280
treatment, 280
broadening the focus, 277–278
novel strategies, 282–284
resilient strategies, 280–281
targeting deficits, 282
targeting the effects of stress, 281
serotonin (5-HT), 6–7
allostatic contribution, 6
allostatic load, 6–7
factors promoting resilience, 7
receptor dysfunction, 7
serotonin transporter gene (5-HTTLPR) polymorphism, 7
sexual assault, *see* rape
single nucleotide polymorphisms (SNPs), 3
social capital, 164–165
index of, 169
measurement, 169–170
poverty effects, 269

social closeness, 66
social cognitive theory, 7, 47–49
social competence, 17–18
Social Health Index, 169
social indicator research, 168–170
social integration, 77–78
  behavioral effects, 79
  physiological effects, 80
  psychological benefits, 78
  see also social ties
social isolation, 78
social networks, 164
social potency, 66
social support, 66, 67–68, 76–78
  behavioral effects, 79
  community resilience and, 164–165
  emotional support, 77
  following rape, 229
  informational support, 77
  instrumental support, 77
  interventions, 293–295
  matching hypothesis, 77
  older adults, 142–143
  physiological effects, 80, 81
    evidence for in chronic disease,
      82–83
    resilience promotion, 84–85
  psychological benefits, 78
    evidence for in chronic disease,
      81–82
    resilience promotion, 84
  serious mental illness and, 281
  see also social ties
social ties, 76, 85
  attachment relationships, 112
  behavioral effects, 79
  buffering effects, 77
  evidence for effects in chronic
    disease, 81–83
  main effects, 77
  physiological effects, 79–81, 82–83
    cardiovascular system, 79–80
    immune system, 80
    neuroendocrine system, 80–81
  psychological benefits, 78, 81–82
  resilience promotion, 83–85
    physiological adjustment, 84–85
    psychological adjustment, 84
    see also social integration; social
      support
Social Vulnerability Index (SOVI),
  168–170
spirituality, 141
  definition, 90–91
  interventions, 97–98
    group therapy module, 96–97
  spiritual development, 92
    model, 91
    see also religion/spirituality

state-space grids, 116
stress, 2
  cardiovascular response, 79–80
    social ties and, 79–80
  disaster-related, 204
  preparatory interventions, 297–298
  reactivity in children related to
    caregiving, 309–311
  self-efficacy relationships in
    children, 311–312
  transactional theory of, 46
  workplace stress, 50
  see also acute stress response; stress
    inoculation theory
stress inoculation theory, 137
stress inoculation training, 292–293
stress vulnerability model, 279
stressful life events, 30–31
Stroop measure, 34
Study of Adult Development, Harvard
  Medical School, 266
suppression, 195–196
survivorship, 298
sympathetic–adrenomedullary system,
  80–81

TAFES program, 157
Taoism, 180
team sports, 315–316
terrorist events, 202
  engagement versus distress
    trajectories, 259–260
  engagement/distress interactions,
    260–261
  resilience and, 202
    conservation of resources theory,
      254–257
    engagement theory, 257–258
    versus post-traumatic growth,
      258–259
    see also September 11 terrorist
      attack, New York
testosterone, 10–11
  stress response and, 11
threats, 105–106
tight coupling, 164
training
  hardiness training, 291–292
  learned optimism training,
    295–296
  mental health, 324, 326, 331
    implementation, 331–336
  moral courage, 317
  resilience enhancement, 290
  scenario-based training, 297–298
  stress inoculation training, 292–293
Training and Doctrine Command, 335
transactional theory of stress, 46
transformational coping, 291

trauma
  heterogeneous trajectories following
    exposure, 121–123
    chronic dysfunction, 122–123
    delayed reactions, 123
    resilience and recovery, 123
  historical conceptions of
    psychological trauma, 120–121
  recovery
    culture significance, 182–183
    in older adults, 136–138
  societal response to, 143
  trauma-specific variables, 142
  see also potentially traumatic
    events
Trauma and Spirituality Group
  Module, 96–97
trauma intensity, 68–69
traumatic demands, 49–50
Trier Social Stress Test, 4

US Marine Corps Combat and
  Operational Stress Control
  (COSC) program, 242–249
  core leader functions, 246–249
  goals, 242
  rationale, 242–243
  stress continuum model, 243–246
US Navy Operational Stress Control
  (OSC) program, 242–249
  core leader functions, 246–249
  goals, 242
  rationale, 242–243

vigor, 257
vulnerability theory, 137

Walsh Family Resilience Framework,
  153–155, 158, 302
  communication, 155
  family belief systems, 153–154
  family organization, 154–155
warfare, 323
  former combatants and prisoners of
    war, 140
  PTSD, 121
    hardiness relationship, 63–64,
    see also military personnel
well-being, 66
well-being therapy, 296–297
wellness, 163
widowhood, 139–140,
  see also bereavement
workplace stress, 50
World Trade Center terrorist attack.
  see September 11 terrorist
    attack, New York
worldview, 127
  resilience promotion, 127